SHOULD I CALL THE DOCTOR?

SHOULD I CALL THE DOCTOR?

A Comprehensive Guide to Understanding Your Child's Illnesses and Injuries

CHRISTINE A. NELSON, M.D. and SUSAN PESCAR

WARNER BOOKS

A Warner Communications Company

A Warner Communications Company

Printed in the United States of America
First Printing: July 1986
10 9 8 7 6 5 4 3 2 1

Designed by Giorgetta Bell McRee

Library of Congress Cataloging-in-Publication Data

Nelson, Christine A.
    Should I call the doctor?

    1. Sick children—Care and treatment.
2. Pediatric emergencies.   I. Pescar, Susan C.
II. Title.   [DNLM: 1. Child Care—popular works.
2. Emergencies—in infancy & childhood—popular
works.   3. Pediatrics—popular works.   WS200 N425s]
RJ61.N37   1986   618.92   85-43177
ISBN 0-446-51262-1

To my father, **PAUL R. NELSON**, who, no matter how hard or long he had to work and no matter how many sacrifices had to be made, did so willingly, unselfishly, and lovingly—so that his children would have a better life and more opportunities. Along with my mother, Jane Nelson, he taught each of us what the true meaning of being a loving, giving parent was all about.

Thank you, Dad, for always being there and always listening; for gently questioning us; for warmly, but firmly, directing us when it was necessary; and for always being supportive and loving. I hope you know how much I love you.

Christine A. Nelson

To my mother, **ARLENE ELLA WEST PESCAR**, whose lifetime commitment to the well-being of children—both as a teacher and as a mother—has always been deeply rooted in warmth, tenderness, understanding, encouragement, and love. In a sense, she has been the mother of a thousand children. I was lucky enough to have a special place among them!

Thank you, Mother, for all that you've done—but most of all, for just being you! I love you.

Susan Christine Pescar

A SPECIAL TRIBUTE

is given by both authors—to **JANE NELSON**—who died suddenly before this book was completed. She was a very rare, wonderfully unpretentious, joyful, loving, and gentle person who always cared about others and always gave of herself.

Should I Call the Doctor? was very special to her, and she enthusiastically awaited the day that, as she said, she "could proudly see it in the bookstore." We would like to believe she can see it now—and that she knows how greatly she is missed and how much she will always be loved.

ACKNOWLEDGMENTS

A very special acknowledgment is warmly and lovingly given to *Christopher Paul Nelson* (Dr. Nelson's son), *David Pescar Swigart* (Susan Pescar's nephew), and *Caitlin McBride* (Kathy McBride's daughter). Because of their enormous influence, the authors and editor of this book were constantly reminded of the importance of meeting the needs of parents and others, really answering the questions and concerns we all have when it comes to helping our children and those of others, and providing information in the most clear, helpful, and practical way. Their presence transformed our work on *Should I Call the Doctor?* into an expression of love—not only for them, but for all children.

Every now and then, doing a book (the entire process) becomes a truly unique human experience—a very special experience. In a way, the following people represent a handful of the more than a hundred co-authors of this book not listed on the cover. Each deserves our gratitude and special recognition:

- All the *parents* and *their children, grandparents* and *other relatives, baby-sitters, teachers* and *other professionals who work with children,* who taught us so much and helped make this a unique book. They were largely responsible for "what" would be included in the book, and "how" the "what" needed to be presented in order to be the most helpful and easy to read and use. We thank them for the countless hours they spent talking about what they needed and wanted in the book; for readily sharing their personal experiences, fears, frustrations, and hopes; and for reviewing the manuscript (over and over again) and making suggestions until we got it right! Their contributions and commitment were truly remarkable and greatly appreciated. We only wish there was enough room to list each person by name.

- *Kathy McBride*, executive managing editor, Warner Books, New York, for her enthusiasm and commitment to *Should I Call the Doctor?* and for ensuring that the book was done "right"; for always finding time in her already too busy schedule to listen to ideas and talk through concerns; for her excellent ideas and constant help and support; for being such a joy to work for and with (not to mention being a special person overall); for her talent, creativity, intelligence, and ability to always find a way to build a new or better path when we feared we had come to a dead end with an idea or a difficult concept; and for making *Should I Call the Doctor?* a better book than it would have been without her! The book is truly as much hers as ours.

- *Glenn Cowley*, Authors and Artists Group, New York, who not only played his usual role as a talented literary agent, but also jumped in from the very beginning with incredible enthusiasm and an inspiring commitment to the book. We thank him for going far beyond his professional responsibilities by giving countless hours of time and energy in helping develop concepts and ideas, as well as working out problems; for always being there when either one of us needed a pep talk throughout the four years of work on *Should I Call the Doctor?*; and most importantly, for being a special person and a special friend.

- *Valerie Pescar Swigart*, whose title, "research assistant," does not aptly represent all that she contributed to this book. We affectionately thank her for always being there whenever either one of us needed her help; for putting up with bad moods, exhausted authors, impossible requests, and continual pressure; for spending endless hours helping in any way she could —doing research, tirelessly making phone calls, collecting statistics, and reading the manuscript over and over and over again, then giving frank criticism, suggestions, and ideas from both a mother's and a professional's point of view—all of which surely made this a better book; and for providing constant moral support and encouragement. She is a very, very special person who should be quite proud of her work on *Should I Call the Doctor?* We couldn't have done it without her.

- *Mary Neiswender*, award-winning investigative reporter, two-time Pulitzer Prize nominee in journalism, and owner of KNWZ All News Radio, for her idea that we co-author a book for parents (and others who care for children of all ages) that would be helpful and easy to use and understand (a resource that she and her grown children could trust to help them care for her grandchildren); for being an extraordinary example of a "great" writer (her talent, skill, discipline, creativity, dedication, sensitivity, awareness, and love for her art and craft are virtually impossible to describe); for being an unselfish teacher over the years, explaining how to approach the work, research the subject, and include the audience for which a book was intended ("Who better knows what is needed and wanted?"); for being a kind and understanding friend who always had faith in us and in this book; and most of all, for being a wonderful, warm, and caring human being. We hope she finds *Should I Call the Doctor?* all that she thought it would be—and more. If it is, she played a major role in making it special.

- *Paula J. Nelson*, who could always be counted on whenever we needed help, ideas, or suggestions, for coming through time and time again, no matter how busy or tired she was; for her moral support and encouragement; and for being a very energetic and caring one-person cheering section when we needed it most. She should be very proud of what she did. We thank her for being such a special person.

Very special thanks is also warmly given to the following people, who have, over the years, devoted an enormous amount of time, skill, talent, and energy toward the betterment and well-being of children (and therefore had a significant impact on us and this book); and/or committed time and made personal sacrifices on behalf of the development and completion of *Should I Call the Doctor?*; and/or offered suggestions, ideas, or information; and/or provided continual moral support, encouragement, and enthusiasm. In alphabetical order: Ed Amend; David and Kathy Channell and their children, Kimberly and Sherry; Fay Hogan Conley and her children, Will and Meghan; Patricia Deatherage, R.N.; Kay Joncich Foubert; Michael and Donna Gilbert and their children, Lisa and Nikki; Ann Gronowski; Petty Officer Tom Heflick, U.S. Coast Guard, 11th Coast Guard District; Mrs. Eunice R. Hogan; Jim and Meg Hogan and their children, Brennan, Seamus, and Mark; Andy, Connie, Cathy, and Luke Joncich; Mrs. Katie Joncich; Edwin Kleinman, M.D.; Nord S. Nation, M.D.; Manuel Navarro, M.D.; Mercedes Navarro, M.D., child-adolescent psychiatrist and director of the Pediatric Therapy Center in Long Beach, California; Kate Neiswender and her daughter, Candace; Mark and Kristy Neiswender and their children, Loren, Luka, and Marissa; Jim Mand; Paul and Jane Nelson; John and Barb Nelson and their children, Eric and Saralyn; Jackie Nesthus; Harry W. Orme, M.D., medical director of Miller Children's Hospital in Long Beach, California, and clinical professor of pediatrics, University of California, Irvine; Arlene West Pescar; Mark D. Pescar; Val Pescar; Michele Predisik, illustrator of this book and others; John Samson, M.D., clinical professor of pediatrics, University of Southern California School of Medicine; Ann Schuler, R.N.; Robert L. Swigart; Susan B. Tully, M.D., director of the Pediatric Emergency Room and associate professor of clinical pediatrics and emergency medicine, University of Southern California School of Medicine; Earlene West Waddell; Ruby Langley West; and Brad and Mary Wing and their children, Amy and Michael. The efforts of each and every person were greatly appreciated.

CONTENTS

THE PUZZLE:

Putting the Pieces Together

It was cold, dark, and damp. The baby's cries and coughs could be heard over the pouring rain beating the ground outside the cave. "What is wrong?" the parents worried. "What should we do for our baby?"

They grew anxious and more and more concerned. The baby refused to breast-feed and seemed very weak. The father built a fire—a new and marvelous discovery that produced warmth and made food taste better when put over the flames. As the cave grew warmer, the baby settled down a little. The coughing, however, became more frequent and violent. "Now what?" they asked. The mother crushed eucalyptus leaves and made a paste with mud she had warmed by the fire. Together they packed the baby's chest and back with this paste. They did not know why, but it seemed to help for the moment.

Now there was nothing more they could do than keep the baby warm, breast-feed her when she would accept it, reapply the warm eucalyptus mud pack—and wait. Waiting is never easy, especially when there is little you can do and nowhere to turn for help.

Much has changed over the centuries! More is known today than ever before about illness, injury, home treatment, and taking on-the-spot action in true medical emergencies, as well as about diagnosis and treatment of mild to serious health-care problems.

Nonetheless, one very human feeling has not changed and seems to have transcended the ages. Parents (and others who care for children) worry! They worry about how best to care for their children when ill or injured—often feeling insecure, uncomfortable, or even helpless.

The fact is, whether you are a parent, grandparent, relative, friend, teacher, baby-sitter, or other professional who works with or cares for children, you want to do all you can to safeguard the health and well-being of children. You want to be knowledgeable and well informed, leaving little to chance. You want to make decisions that will be in the best interest of your children and/or the children of others. From the time a child is born until he or she reaches eighteen years of age (at least), *each of us is constantly faced with making important health-related decisions*. We don't want to overreact, nor do we want to underreact.

WHAT WE ALL NEED TO KNOW

When it became clear that illness and injury (and related areas) were the problems that concerned, worried, and often frightened parents (and others) the most, we asked them what they really wanted and needed to know in order to feel less frightened and more self-assured about their role. From their responses, we developed the following "we want to know" list to ensure that all they said they needed and wanted to know would be (and is) included in *Should I Call the Doctor? We want to know:*

- how to modify our children's environment as a means of better preventing accidents and injuries;

- how to prevent disease (when possible) and to control its spread;

- how to recognize symptoms that may point to serious illness or injury in contrast to those that signal a mild to moderate problem;

- what steps to take based on the symptoms we see;

- how to be prepared for (and what actions to take in) true medical emergencies;

- how to decide when and what kind of medical care is needed (call the paramedics or an ambulance; rush the child to the nearest emergency room; call the doctor immediately, within a few hours, or wait until regular office hours to make an appointment; treat the child at home);

- what to expect when we take our children to the doctor's office or emergency room or admit them to the hospital;

- the risks versus the benefits of prescribed and over-the-counter drugs and common diagnostic tests and procedures;

- how to help our children if they ever need to be hospitalized;

- all we can about home treatment and how to make our children more comfortable when ill or injured.

We want to know a lot—because there is a lot to know! All of the points on the "we want to know" list are simply pieces of the puzzle. The problem is that we often *think* that the puzzle is overwhelming and that putting the pieces together is too difficult—if not impossible. *Not true!* This puzzle is put together like *any other* puzzle.

IT'S LIKE ANY OTHER PUZZLE

In *Should I Call the Doctor?* we begin putting the pieces of the illness and injury puzzle together by first putting in place the largest and most recognizable pieces. These represent the vital foundation of the puzzle and include safety and prevention, how to be prepared and respond in a true life-threatening medical emergency, and what to do when specific life-threatening or potentially life-threatening medical emergencies occur. The next largest and most recognizable pieces of the puzzle are those that teach us how to recognize and evaluate symptoms (the body's special way of communicating with us) and those that help us learn how best to respond to certain symptoms or set of symptoms. With the large pieces in place, we are easily able to recognize, understand, and respond to them, even without the rest of the pieces in place.

Putting the remainder of the many smaller (but very important) pieces together requires a basic understanding of the symptoms and treatment of common illnesses and injuries, and the answers to all the other questions on the "we want to know" list (for example, home treatment, making a child more comfortable, prescribed and over-the-counter medications, and so on). The puzzle, however, is still not totally complete. In fact, it will fall apart unless we build (from the beginning) a strong and sturdy frame around it—one made of common sense, trust in our instincts, and an excellent relationship with our children's doctor.

Once all the pieces are in place and held together by a sturdy frame, we have mastered the puzzle. And this is what *Should I Call the Doctor?* is really all about.

BOTH AN IN-DEPTH GUIDE AND A QUICK REFERENCE RESOURCE

Why write a book about how to put the pieces of the illness and injury puzzle together? Simply, it became clear that parents (and others who care for children) wanted and needed a tool that would be *both* an in-depth guide *and* a quick reference resource to help answer the "we want to know"s. Also, practically speaking, as much as pediatricians and family physicians would like to provide everyone with all the in-depth information and education wanted and needed, they simply cannot do so. Unfortunately, there aren't enough hours in the day. Doctors must meet the immediate needs of all their patients, and this means busy office schedules, caring for children in the hospital, constant emergencies, and continual telephone calls (twenty-four hours a day).

Should I Call the Doctor? was developed and designed to complement the information given by your child's doctor and to assist the doctor by helping you (and others) become more knowledgeable, aware, better informed and prepared, and more active participants in your child's health care.

As one parent put it, "My mother once told me that when my brothers, sisters, and

I were children, the minute we coughed, sneezed, or had a fever—she reached for the telephone, day or night, and called the doctor. Our well-being, she said, was in his hands, not hers or my father's. Then parents knew very little about illness or injury and really weren't encouraged—and sometimes not even allowed—to play an important role in their children's medical care. My mother and father,'' she said, laughing, ''were really amazed that my husband and I wanted to know as much as we could and be so involved. But it's finally rubbed off on them. Now, we get quizzed about every little detail whenever one of their grandchildren has even the most minor problem. I think their interest and involvement is wonderful.''

Times have changed! As medicine and science have become increasingly sophisticated and complex, and more and more is known about illness, injury, diagnosis, and treatment, a slow but sure revolution (or evolution) has taken place in public and patient education. The ''we want to know''s had to be answered, and being involved in our children's (as well as our own) health care became an integral part of quality medical care.

IT'S A BOOK FOR EVERYONE!

We should also say that although *Should I Call the Doctor?* was written for parents —because they must make decisions, provide for their children's needs, and work hand-in-hand with their children's doctor—it was also written for others who care for children of all ages. Today, more than ever before, many others help care for our children. They must be well-informed and prepared to take action and assist parents when necessary.

Think about it! Do your parents, another relative, a friend, or a baby-sitter ever take care of your child? Does your child go to a child care center, nursery school, preschool, group care setting, or is he or she cared for by a nanny or housekeeper? Is your youngster in grammar school, junior high, or high school? Indeed, many others are often responsible for the care and well-being of our children. The more *they* know, the more confident they will be about caring for your children, particularly ill or injured children—and the more confident *you* will be in their ability to respond to a medical crisis, as well as to common problems.

Therefore, if you are a grandparent, other relative, friend, teacher, baby-sitter, or someone who cares for or works with children, then *Should I Call the Doctor?* is as much a resource for you as it is for parents. The fact is, if you are a ''significant other'' in a child's life and are reading this book and intend to use it as a continual resource, it means you care deeply and want to be well-informed, prepared, and involved. Hurray for you!!

WHY FOCUS ON ILLNESS AND INJURY?

It's important for anyone reading this book and using it as a continual resource to know the scope of the book. *Should I Call the Doctor?* does not (and was not meant to) provide either a very general view or an in-depth view of "total child care." It was specifically designed to give you very useful and detailed information on how to recognize, evaluate, and respond to medical emergencies, symptoms, illnesses, injuries, and common problems/conditions that children may experience (from birth through eighteen years of age).

There were several reasons the scope of the book was intentionally focused. For one, if we had covered all areas of child care, using the same format of providing both in-depth information as well as quick reference guides for each problem covered, this book would have been as large as the *Oxford English Dictionary* and you would have needed to use a magnifying glass. Furthermore, there are excellent "general child care" books already available that touch on a wide spectrum of information (for example, toilet training, diet when well, thumb-sucking, basic first aid, breast-feeding, some common illnesses, basic information on growth and development, the role of discipline, the do's and don'ts of raising children, bed-wetting, and the effects that violence has on children).

Also, when we talked to parents and others about what they needed and wanted, we heard the same responses over and over again. The "we want to know" list details their responses. Of all the points listed, most parents emphasized the need to learn how to recognize and evaluate symptoms, then be able to take action based on the symptoms they have identified; how to be prepared for true life-threatening medical emergencies; and when to treat the child at home (and how), call the doctor, take the youngster to the nearest emergency room, or call the paramedics or an ambulance. They also said they needed and wanted both an in-depth guide and a quick reference resource together in the same book: one that teaches and explains, so they would have an overall grasp of the information, *and* that can be used time and again as a quick reference resource to refresh their memory or when they needed information promptly.

Again, the point of *Should I Call the Doctor?* is to help you feel more confident and self-assured about the decisions you make and the actions you take. It is meant to be a special tool—a vital resource that's there when you need it.

YOU AND YOUR CHILD'S DOCTOR: A SPECIAL TEAM

Should I Call the Doctor? is not meant to replace your child's doctor but to assist him or her. Obviously, every attempt was made to ensure that this book be as complete and thorough as possible. Great care was taken to provide both in-depth information and step-by-step quick reference guides; to assist you in caring for your child when ill or injured; to help you make prompt and correct decisions about when to seek medical care and what level of care; to teach you how to become prepared for life-threatening medical emergencies and what actions to take when they occur; and to answer all of the "we want to know" questions. Nonetheless, this book was not meant to and should not replace your child's doctor. Certainly, you can refer back to the book for information or clarification, but if what you want isn't there (or you have other questions or concerns), do not hesitate to call the doctor.

You and the doctor should be true partners in assuring the health and well-being of your child. The doctor is a vital part of the frame that holds together the pieces of the illness and injury puzzle. He or she knows your family medical history and the present health status of your child, and has the education, training, knowledge, and skill to diagnose problems, make recommendations, provide appropriate treatment—and answer your questions and concerns.

Therefore, whenever you have questions about your child's health or well-being, call the doctor and get them answered. The doctor is an excellent resource and the person to turn to when your child needs evaluation and medical care.

YOU CAN MAKE A DIFFERENCE

You are the one who must manage your child's day-to-day activities and care for her when it comes to mild or moderate illnesses and injuries. You must decide what steps are necessary to make a child's environment as safe as possible in order to prevent accidents. You must direct the young person and teach him about safety and good health habits. You must continually make decisions regarding your child's health.

Only you can decide to follow a recommended schedule for well visits and determine whether or not your youngster will receive recommended immunizations. Only you can decide when it is necessary to call the doctor, go to the emergency room, or call the paramedics. And only you can respond—right on the spot and within seconds—if your child suddenly experiences a life-threatening medical emergency for which your preparation and ability to take action may make all the difference.

The fact is, the decisions you make and the actions you take can make a big difference. We hope you find *Should I Call the Doctor?* to be *the* in-depth guide and quick reference resource you've been looking for—the practical, easy-to-use-and-understand tool that puts the pieces of the illness and injury puzzle together and helps give you the confidence you need to make a difference.

True, the days of cave-dwelling parents struggling to help their child—not knowing what to do and frankly not having much they could do—are gone forever. But some things never change! How we feel about our children, how much we worry about their health and well-being, how we want to know all we can and do all we can to prevent illness and injury, and how much we want to help them in any way we can whenever they are ill or injured—all are things that will never change. Being a parent isn't easy—but even with all its hardships, worries, frustrations, and demands, it's still tremendously rewarding, and our children oh so wonderful.

HOW BEST TO USE THIS BOOK

Should I Call the Doctor? is broken down into six sections, each representing pieces of the illness and injury puzzle. The book was designed so that it could be used based on the needs, wants, and preferences of each reader. In other words, use it in the manner that is most helpful and comfortable to you!

You may find it most useful to read the book in its entirety. In this way, you will become familiar with the overall principles of caring for your child whenever he or she becomes ill or injured. This may also help you become more confident in your ability to handle what are sometimes very stressful situations. Once you've read the book, you may want to review the broad-based Emergency Quick Reference guides in Chapter 1, the Assessment Checklists and Emergency Quick Reference guides in Chapter 12, and the Emergency Quick Reference Guide on Assessing Injury in Chapter 15. By doing so, you will become quite comfortable and familiar with these if you ever have to immediately refer to them in more urgent situations.

You may, however, feel more comfortable mastering the most recognizable and largest pieces of the illness and injury puzzle. You can do this by reading Chapters 1 through 12 (which cover getting help, safety, preventing illness, being prepared for life-threatening emergencies, specific life-threatening emergencies, and recognizing and assessing symptoms of serious or potentially serious illness) and Chapter 15 (how to assess injury). To round off the information, it would also be useful to read Chapters 18 through 20 (which cover helping your child feel more comfortable, prescribed and over-the-counter medications, and preventing or controlling the spread of infection). You can then refer to specific illnesses and injuries (as well as to information about medical tests and procedures, hospitalization, and so on) when you need or want this information. Again, it is helpful to review the broad-based Emergency Quick Reference guides in the chapters you have read.

Depending on your knowledge and experience, you may want to read only the sections or chapters you feel you need more information about, or those you deem most important to you. Being familiar with the broad-based Emergency Quick Reference guides in Chapter 1 (as well as others in the book) is still a good idea.

In *Should I Call the Doctor?* an Emergency Quick Reference or Quick Reference guide precedes the in-depth information on each topic. Each guide is easy to find and to read. All are boxed on the page, with EMERGENCY QUICK REFERENCE or QUICK REFERENCE at the top, followed by the topic/problem it covers (all in very large, bold type). An arrow points to the main steps or information, and dots set off additional important information.

These guides are very easy to use—and to refer back to when you need them. You may find it most helpful to read the Emergency Quick Reference or Quick Reference guide, the in-depth information next, and then to review the guide so it is clear to you.

We should also point out that an enormous emphasis has been placed on the ease and speed of finding the Emergency Quick Reference and Quick Reference guides throughout the book, as well as the Assessment Checklists (in Chapter 12). You will notice that the Contents is quite extensive and designed so you can find what you want quickly. Every Emergency Quick Reference and Quick Reference guide in the book and all Assessment Checklists are listed by topic/problem and page number. Also, the first page of each chapter on specific illnesses and injuries has a ''minicontents'' that lists the topic/problem and the page number for each Emergency Quick Reference and

Quick Reference guide in that chapter. The first page of Chapter 12 (about recognizing and assessing symptoms of serious or potentially serious illness) also has a "mini-contents" that lists the topic/problem and page number for each Assessment Checklist and Emergency Quick Reference in that chapter. Furthermore, the Index lists all the above information and more.

Overall, *Should I Call the Doctor?* was designed to have many options (and/or backup systems), so you could use the book in the manner most useful and comfortable for you. When you need to review or refer back to information, you have many options. You can go directly to Chapter 1 and the broad-based Emergency Quick Reference guides; or you can turn to a specific Emergency Quick Reference or Quick Reference guide based on the problem you have recognized; or when you are not sure what the problem is, how serious it may be, and what action(s) you should take, you can turn to a specific Assessment Checklist (based on the child's most obvious major symptom) and its corresponding Emergency Quick Reference guide.

The bottom line is for you to approach the book in the manner most comfortable for you and to know how to find the quick reference information when you need it.

[*Please Note:* Where possible we have used the phrase "he or she" throughout the book. However, at times, this became very awkward and made sentences more difficult to understand. When this was the case, we used "he" only or "she" only. These two pronouns are used interchangeably throughout the book, but the information refers to both sexes. If something affects a male only or female only, we have been very clear in saying so.

Also, "child," "youngster," and "young person" are used interchangeably throughout the book and represent children of all ages (from birth through eighteen years of age). If something applies to a specific age group only, then it is specifically stated as such (infant or baby, toddler, young child, older child, or teenager).]

S E C T I O N 1

Getting Help, Safety, Preventing Illness, and Being Prepared for Life-Threatening Emergencies

In your lifetime, you may never experience a true medical emergency. But that would make you quite unique! The fact is, the number of medical emergencies that occur every year—not to mention every day—is staggering. Unless you live in a total vacuum—which is virtually impossible today—you will more than likely be faced with a serious situation at least once in your life and more likely a few times. There will be many other minor to moderately serious situations when your preparedness, knowledge, and ability to take action will be put to the test.

Each year approximately *24,000 deaths* result from *24 million injuries in the home*. In this overall group, children less than five years old are the second most commonly affected group. These rather grim statistics point to the need for more emphasis on prevention, safety, and preparedness.

Although it's a cliché, *prevention is always the best medicine*. Being prepared, knowing how to respond and how to evaluate a situation, taking a first aid course, and learning CPR (cardiopulmonary resuscitation) are really all special aspects of prevention. Another aspect of prevention involves making the environment (home, school, parks, playgrounds, streets, and so on) as safe as possible for our children. Chapters 1 through 4 give you vital information about how and when to get medical help and how you can better prevent accidents and illness; they also explain the tools and knowledge you need to respond calmly and efficiently if faced with a minor to major medical emergency.

True, you may never be faced with a life-threatening emergency. But is it really worth taking the chance? It's a lot easier to prevent accidents and illness where possible, by knowing all you can and being as prepared as you can to help your children and others—if they ever need you.

1

C H A P T E R 1
How and When to Get Help

IMPORTANT: In this chapter, you will find (in addition to other invaluable information) several *Emergency Quick Reference* lists that were designed to be useful guidelines as to *when to call the paramedics or ambulance, when to go to an emergency room, when to call the doctor immediately, when to call the doctor within an hour or two,* and *when to call the doctor for an appointment.*

While these guidelines may seem confusing to you right now, they will become clear as you read through the book—which covers this information in detail.

When this book was first being developed, a great deal of time was spent talking to parents, grandparents, relatives and friends of children, baby-sitters, and those who work with children. Therefore, much of what is covered in this book is based on what parents and others said they wanted and needed to know about caring for children when they are sick or injured.

One consistent concern was expressed by the vast majority of people. As one mother put it: "To be honest, I'm never sure whether I should call the doctor or handle the problem myself; and if the problem is serious enough to call the doctor, I can't tell whether I should call right this minute, in a few hours, or simply call for an appointment to have my son or daughter seen in a day or two. In fact, I'm not positive I'd know when to call the paramedics or take my child to the emergency room. My husband feels the same way. It's a frustrating feeling; at times, a helpless one. You just aren't sure what is best to do. So, you see, what I really need is a special list or some sort of guidelines that would help me make these often difficult decisions or at least reinforce my gut feeling."

Based on this need, expressed by so many people, special Emergency Quick Ref-

4

GETTING HELP,
SAFETY,
PREVENTING
ILLNESS, AND
BEING
PREPARED FOR
LIFE-
THREATENING
EMERGENCIES

erence guides on getting help were developed. These have been put in the front of the book so you can find them easily—anytime you need them.

It may be helpful to review them several times before and after you have read the entire book. In this way, you will become quite familiar with the guides and find them more useful to you.

EMERGENCY QUICK REFERENCE

When to Call the Paramedics or Ambulance

In all the following situations, have someone else call the *paramedics* or *ambulance* (if there are no paramedics in your area) while you treat the youngster. If no one is with you, continue treating the child while you periodically shout for help. When help arrives, have that person call the paramedics or ambulance.

▶ **BREATHING AND/OR PULSE HAVE STOPPED (FOR ANY REASON).** (If you are certified in CPR and are unable to remember the details of the procedure, turn to the Emergency Quick Reference on page 113, entitled "A Review of the Six Steps of CPR.")

▶ **SEVERE BREATHING DIFFICULTY (FOR ANY REASON).** This may be associated with:

 ● Complete airway obstruction. (If you are unable to remember the details of managing this problem, turn to the Emergency Quick Reference on page 127, entitled "Managing Airway Obstruction/Choking," for a review.)

 ● Extreme blueness or paleness of the skin.

 ● A chest injury, with the chest moving in an unusual way. (If you are unable to remember the details of managing this problem, turn to the Emergency Quick Reference on page 519, entitled "Chest (Thoracic) Injuries," for a review.)

 ● Hives and/or swelling of the tongue or lips. (If you are unable to remember the details of managing this problem, turn to the Emergency Quick Reference on page 324, entitled "Anaphylaxis," for a review.)

 ● A near-drowning episode, following which the youngster is not fully alert and/or is coughing and gagging. (If you are unable to remember the details of managing this problem, turn to the Emergency Quick Reference on page 191, entitled "Managing Drowning," for a review.)

▶ **CONVULSION/SEIZURE LASTING LONGER THAN FIVE MINUTES.** (If you are unable to remember the details of managing this problem, turn to the Emergency Quick Reference on page 337, entitled "Convulsions/ Seizures," for a review.)

▶ **UNCONSCIOUSNESS OR EXTREME DIFFICULTY IN AROUSING A YOUNGSTER (FOR ANY REASON).** (If you are unable to remember the details of managing this problem, turn to the Emergency Quick Reference on page 160, entitled "Managing Unconsciousness," for a review.)

▶ **SIGNS OF SHOCK (FOR ANY REASON).** (If you are unable to remember the details of managing this problem, turn to the Emergency Quick Reference on page 152, entitled "Managing Shock," for a review.) The signs to look for include:

- Skin color that is pale, pasty, or mottled.

- Cool and clammy skin.

- Severe weakness, dizziness, or light-headedness.

- Anxiety or extreme listlessness.

- Signs of agitation, irritability, irrationality, or fear.

- Nausea or vomiting.

- Weak, thready pulse with rapid heartbeat.

- Signs of dehydration.

▶ **SEVERE BLEEDING (OPEN WOUND).** (If you are unable to remember the details of managing this problem, turn to the Emergency Quick Reference on page 141, entitled "Managing Serious Bleeding," for a review.)

▶ **VOMITING LARGE AMOUNTS OF BLOOD OR PASSING LARGE AMOUNTS OF BLOOD IN THE STOOL (INTERNAL HEMORRHAGING).** (If you are unable to remember the details of managing this problem, turn to the Emergency Quick Reference on page 141, entitled "Managing Serious Bleeding," for a review.)

▶ **SUDDEN, SERIOUS ILLNESS WHERE YOU CANNOT SAFELY OR QUICKLY MOVE THE YOUNGSTER.**

GETTING HELP,
SAFETY,
PREVENTING
ILLNESS, AND
BEING
PREPARED FOR
LIFE-
THREATENING
EMERGENCIES

▶ **SEVERE HEAD, NECK, OR BACK INJURY OR THE POSSIBILITY OR SUSPICION OF THIS TYPE OF INJURY BECAUSE OF SOMETHING THAT OCCURRED,** for example, a fall from a high place. (If you are unable to remember the details of managing this problem, turn to the Emergency Quick Reference on page 573, entitled "Head, Neck, and Back Injuries," for a review.)

▶ **KNOWN OR POSSIBLE MULTIPLE INJURIES.** (If you are unable to remember the details of managing this problem, turn to the Emergency Quick Reference on page 503, entitled "Assessing Injury," for a review.)

▶ **SERIOUS FRACTURE (BROKEN BONE), DISLOCATION, OR OTHER SERIOUS INJURY.** (If you are unable to remember the details of managing this problem, turn to the Emergency Quick Reference on page 551, entitled "Fractures, Dislocations, and Growth-Plate Injuries," for a review.)

▶ **ANY SITUATION YOU PERCEIVE AS LIFE-THREATENING, CRITICAL, OR POTENTIALLY DISABLING.**

EMERGENCY QUICK REFERENCE

When to Go to an Emergency Room

Take your infant, child, or teenager to an *emergency room* in the following situations:

▶ YOU BELIEVE A PROBLEM NEEDS URGENT MEDICAL EVALUATION AND TREATMENT, BUT YOU HAVE NO PERSONAL PHYSICIAN.

▶ A POTENTIALLY SERIOUS PROBLEM ARISES WHILE YOU ARE TRAVELING.

▶ A SERIOUS OR POTENTIALLY SERIOUS PROBLEM OCCURS, AND YOU ARE UNABLE TO REACH YOUR DOCTOR.

▶ IT IS UNCLEAR TO YOU HOW SERIOUS AN INJURY OR ILLNESS IS.

▶ YOUR CHILD'S DOCTOR INSTRUCTS YOU TO GO TO THE EMERGENCY ROOM.

8

GETTING HELP,
SAFETY,
PREVENTING
ILLNESS, AND
BEING
PREPARED FOR
LIFE-
THREATENING
EMERGENCIES

EMERGENCY QUICK REFERENCE

When to Call the Doctor Immediately

The following symptoms and signs are serious enough that your infant, child, or teenager will usually need to be evaluated *within an hour or so*. Call your child's doctor for advice *immediately*. If you are unable to reach the doctor within fifteen to thirty minutes, take the youngster to an emergency room for evaluation.

▶ **MODERATE TO SEVERE BREATHING DIFFICULTY WITHOUT BLUE-NESS.** This can involve:

- Very rapid or very labored breathing.

- Grunting sound with breathing.

- Unusual chest motion or a sucking in of the spaces between the ribs or under the chest cage when the child breathes.

- Severe stridor (a crowing sound when the child breathes in) or severe wheezing (a whistling or musical sound when the child breathes out).

- Severe difficulty with breathing in, associated with anxiety, fever, refusal to swallow, or drooling.

▶ **TENSE OR BULGING FONTANEL (SOFT SPOT ON THE TOP OF THE HEAD) WHEN A SICK OR INJURED INFANT IS SITTING UPRIGHT AND QUIET.**

▶ **STIFF NECK IN A YOUNGSTER WHO SEEMS VERY ILL.**

▶ **RASH CAUSED BY BROKEN BLOOD VESSELS IN A YOUNGSTER WHO APPEARS ILL.** These broken blood vessels can look like tiny red dots that don't disappear when you press on the skin, or they may consist of larger blood spots that look like bruises.

▶ **SIGNS OF SEVERE DEHYDRATION,** including:

- Very dry mouth.

- Sunken eyeballs.

- Failure to urinate for more than eight hours for an infant or twelve hours for an older child when there are other signs of dehydration or when a youngster has had vomiting or diarrhea or refuses to drink.

- Very sunken fontanel (soft spot).

- Irritability and extreme listlessness.

- Doughy, wrinkled skin.

CONVULSION, WITH OR WITHOUT FEVER, IF A YOUNGSTER HAS NEVER HAD CONVULSIONS BEFORE—EVEN IF IT STOPPED ON ITS OWN.

SEVERE LETHARGY—SLEEPINESS OR LISTLESSNESS FAR OUT OF PROPORTION TO OTHER SYMPTOMS OF AN ILLNESS.

EXTREME IRRITABILITY THAT CANNOT BE EXPLAINED, ESPECIALLY IN A YOUNG INFANT.

UNUSUAL CRY.

- Weak or whimpering constant cry.

- High-pitched cry.

REFUSAL OF A YOUNG INFANT TO EAT (FAILURE TO TAKE TWO OR MORE REGULARLY SCHEDULED FEEDINGS).

FEVER OVER 105 DEGREES.

- Take steps to try to reduce the fever while you wait for the doctor to reach you or before you go to an emergency room.

FEVER OVER 101 DEGREES IN A SICK INFANT WHO IS UNDER TWO MONTHS OLD.

HEAD INJURY IN WHICH THE YOUNGSTER LOST CONSCIOUSNESS, EVEN BRIEFLY, *AND*

- Has not returned to his usual level of awareness.

- Has vomited more than twice after the injury.

- Has abnormal pupils.

- His condition has worsened in any way.

GETTING HELP,
SAFETY,
PREVENTING
ILLNESS, AND
BEING
PREPARED FOR
LIFE-
THREATENING
EMERGENCIES

▶ **THE YOUNGSTER HAS EXPERIENCED A NEAR-DROWNING EPISODE BUT IS AWAKE AND BREATHING WITH LITTLE OR NO DIFFICULTY.** Remember, a youngster should *always* be evaluated by a doctor after a near-drowning episode because of the possibility of later serious complications.

▶ **ABNORMAL BLEEDING (VOMITING BLOOD, BLOODY DIARRHEA, EXCESSIVE BRUISING) AND/OR AN OPEN WOUND THAT MAY REQUIRE STITCHES.**

▶ **YOU KNOW OR SUSPECT THAT THE CHILD HAS BEEN POISONED, AND THE CHILD IS CONSCIOUS AND NOT HAVING TROUBLE BREATHING.** In this case, call your local poison control center for advice *immediately*, and follow the instructions that the staff gives you.

EMERGENCY QUICK REFERENCE

When to Call the Doctor Within an Hour or Two

In the following situations, an infant, child, or teenager may require evaluation *within a few hours*. Call your doctor for advice or arrange for the youngster to be seen in an emergency room.

► **MODERATE BREATHING DIFFICULTY.**

- Wheezing (whistling noise when the child breathes out or, less commonly, when the child breathes in).

- Moderate or mild stridor (a crowing sound when the child breathes in) without color change or other signs of distress.

► **UNUSUAL OR WORRISOME BEHAVIOR,** such as:

- Lethargy or severe listlessness, but you are able to arouse the child for brief periods of time.

- Unusual or clumsy movements.

- Persistent refusal to eat or drink anything (in twelve to twenty-four hours).

- Unusual irritability.

- Persistent crying without apparent cause.

► **SEVERE OR PROLONGED VOMITING AND/OR DIARRHEA.**

► **SIGNS OF MILD DEHYDRATION,** including:

- Severe reduction in the amount of urine.

- Dry, sticky mouth and lips.

- Listlessness and irritability.

► **SEVERE OR PERSISTENT PAIN ANYWHERE IN THE BODY** (such as headache, abdominal pain, earache, sore throat, or bone pain).

GETTING HELP,
SAFETY,
PREVENTING
ILLNESS, AND
BEING
PREPARED FOR
LIFE-
THREATENING
EMERGENCIES

▶ **HEAD INJURY IN WHICH THE YOUNGSTER LOST CONSCIOUSNESS BUT NOW SEEMS NORMAL OR NEARLY NORMAL.**

▶ **SUSPECTED BROKEN BONE WHEN THE YOUNGSTER CAN BE EASILY MOVED.**

▶ **FEVER OVER 103 DEGREES WITH OTHER SYMPTOMS THAT SUGGEST A POTENTIALLY SERIOUS ILLNESS.**

- Some youngsters experience very high fevers without having a serious illness. Therefore, *fever alone* should not cause you undue concern.

- Try to reduce the fever to under 102 degrees if the youngster seems uncomfortable. Then reevaluate him. If he seems much better, you may be able to continue home observation and treatment.

▶ **THE YOUNGSTER HAS SIGNS AND SYMPTOMS OF A POSSIBLY SERIOUS INFECTION.**

▶ **THE YOUNGSTER HAS A SYMPTOM THAT REALLY CONCERNS YOU, SEEMS SICK OUT OF PROPORTION TO WHAT YOU'D EXPECT WITH A PARTICULAR ILLNESS, OR YOU ARE NOT SURE IF THE SYMPTOMS WARRANT EXTREME CONCERN.**

EMERGENCY QUICK REFERENCE

When to Call the Doctor for an Appointment

In the following situations, an infant, child, or teenager requires evaluation *within a day or two*. Call your doctor's office to arrange an appointment.

THE INFANT, CHILD, OR TEENAGER DOES NOT APPEAR TO BE RECOVERING FROM A USUALLY MINOR ILLNESS OR INJURY AFTER SEVERAL DAYS.

YOU ARE UNCOMFORTABLE WITH HOW A YOUNGSTER IS BEHAVING WITH AN ILLNESS OR SYMPTOM.

SEVERE CONGESTION IN A VERY YOUNG INFANT, ESPECIALLY IF IT INTERFERES WITH FEEDING OR SLEEPING.

FEVER THAT LASTS LONGER THAN THREE DAYS WITHOUT OTHER SYMPTOMS THAT EXPLAIN IT AS A MILD OR SPECIFIC ILLNESS.

PERSISTENT OR RECURRING PAIN, MILD TO MODERATE BREATHING DIFFICULTIES, PERSISTENT VOMITING OR DIARRHEA, OR ANY OTHER BOTHERSOME SYMPTOM.

SIGNIFICANT LOSS OF APPETITE FOR OVER ONE WEEK OR UNEXPLAINED WEIGHT LOSS IN AN OLDER CHILD OR TEENAGER.

YOU SEE ANY SIGNS OR SYMPTOMS THAT YOU FEEL UNSURE ABOUT, AND/OR YOU FEEL THE YOUNGSTER JUST ISN'T HIMSELF OR HERSELF LATELY.

YOU ARE WORRIED ABOUT THE YOUNGSTER OR JUST "FEEL" THAT SOMETHING IS WRONG. In this situation, you need medical advice (that is, you need to have the young person seen to find out if something is wrong or at least talk to the doctor to be reassured that the youngster is fine or is not seriously ill or injured).

GETTING HELP,
SAFETY,
PREVENTING
ILLNESS, AND
BEING
PREPARED FOR
LIFE-
THREATENING
EMERGENCIES

Making Important Judgments

One of the most vital aspects of being prepared for an emergency is knowing when to get professional help. Other important decisions you have to make are what kind of help you need and how quickly you must act. Being able to make these judgments—while staying calm and being confident about your ability to help your child—will do a great deal to ensure that your youngster gets appropriate and timely medical attention when necessary.

As you can imagine, staying calm in a crisis is sometimes difficult—especially when a loved one is involved. But it's important not to panic. You can only help if you are calm enough to assess the situation first—then take action. Also, your calmness and confidence will be felt by the sick or injured youngster. This, in turn, helps the young person feel more secure and safe and allows him or her to stay calm, too. If you panic, the youngster will also panic. The fact is, the more you know about potential emergencies and the better prepared you are, the more confidence you will feel in a crisis—and the more help you will be able to give.

You will find specific information about recognizing and handling life-threatening emergencies in Section 2, while Sections 3 and 4 detail information about recognizing potentially serious problems, as well as common illnesses and injuries.

It is important that you read these sections carefully, so you have an overall concept of the kind of things you could face—what they are and what to do. In this way you will be better able to use the Emergency Quick Reference guides at the beginning of this chapter. It may be helpful to refresh your memory from time to time by reviewing the various Emergency Quick Reference guides throughout the book, as well. In any case, they are readily accessible when you need them.

How Do I Decide?

In many situations, it is obvious that a child or youngster is very ill and must have immediate professional attention. In other cases, the problem is bothersome but obviously minor. The majority of problems, however, are somewhere in between—requiring a decision from you. In situations where you aren't quite sure, you may find the Emergency Quick Reference guides in this chapter, as well as the Assessment Checklists and Emergency Quick Reference guides in Chapter 12 (Recognizing and Assessing Serious or Potentially Serious Illness) and the Step-by-Step Injury Assessment in Chapter 15 (How to Evaluate Your Injured Child), helpful to you.

If you find yourself in a situation where you just can't decide what is best to do—don't hesitate to call the doctor for consultation. While doctors don't want you to overreact to minor problems, they don't want you to take any unnecessary risks either. When truly unsure about what to do, call your doctor and get his or her recommendations. If your child does not have a doctor (you're new to an area or are traveling), then call the nearest emergency room and explain the situation. The emergency room staff is usually able to tell you whether or not you should bring the child in for evaluation or can give you a list of names of pediatricians or family practice physicians in the area. (Usually they give the names of several physicians on their list to people who request physician referral. You may then choose one to contact.)

What You Should Know When Calling the Paramedics

The most important aspect of calling the paramedics is *always being prepared* to do so. This allows you to take action quickly and not panic—because you know *exactly* what you need to do. First, always have *all* emergency numbers next to your phone (and it's reasonable to have these in your wallet or pocketbook, as well). They should include: *the police, fire department, and paramedics; the nearest hospital emergency room; and the name and telephone number of each family member's doctor*. If the "911" number is in effect in your area, learn to use it correctly—for true emergencies only.

Leave nothing to chance or memory. In stressful situations, it's easy to forget simple things like your phone number and address. Baby-sitters or houseguests need quick accessibility to emergency information, so everything should be written down or typed on *one* sheet of paper. Don't forget to put *your address and telephone number* on the Emergency Sheet! There's an Emergency Sheet for your use at the end of this chapter.

Easily accessible, too, should be the *medical history of each family member*. This information can often be invaluable to doctors who must treat someone in a crisis. This information is particularly significant if the youngster has a chronic disease or disability, is taking certain medications, or has specific allergies. Baby-sitters and houseguests should always be told where the family medical-history information is located. (Try to keep each history in a large envelope or at least in a folder with each family member's name on his or her envelope or folder.) If you're going on a trip and leaving the children with relatives or friends, also leave the emergency information sheet and the children's medical histories with them. A Medical History sheet is included for your use at the end of this chapter.

Always leave a Consent to Treat form—completely filled out—with a baby-sitter or houseguest when you are away. The form must be filled out for *each* child (under the age of eighteen). If your child is visiting a friend or relative or takes a vacation with friends or relatives, make sure that they also have a completed Consent to Treat form in their possession. These forms can be obtained from your doctor, a hospital emergency room, or a hospital public relations or public information department. If you do not have a form to use, you may write your own consent statement. A sample form can be found at the end of this chapter.

16

GETTING HELP,
SAFETY,
PREVENTING
ILLNESS, AND
BEING
PREPARED FOR
LIFE-
THREATENING
EMERGENCIES

Don't forget to give the baby-sitter, houseguest, friend, or relative who is watching your child (or children) instructions as to what steps to take in the event of an emergency. These are best written down! Make sure you add the phone number where you can be reached, as well. A Baby-sitter's Checklist is included at the end of this chapter.

If you or anyone else needs to call the paramedics, fire department, or police, you must be able to give them

- Your name.

- The address and telephone number *where* the emergency is occurring (or you can say "across the street from such and such address" if you don't know the address).

- The major cross streets nearest the address.

- A description of the problem (to the best of your ability). For example: "A three-year-old child is choking"; "A ten-year-old has just been pulled out of the swimming pool, and he's not breathing"; "A sixteen-year-old was hit by a car."

If at all possible, someone should stay with an ill or injured person while the paramedics are being called. Try to keep the youngster calm and do not move the youngster unless his or her life is imminently threatened (by fire, smoke, traffic, and so on). If you are performing CPR (cardiopulmonary resuscitation), do not stop to call the paramedics. Instead, shout for help until someone comes to assist you, and have that person call the paramedics while you continue your rescue efforts.

When Calling an Ambulance

Have the same information at hand as previously discussed. State whether this is an emergency or whether (for example) the youngster has broken his leg, can't be moved, and needs to be transported as soon as possible. This makes a difference in how fast the ambulance responds. If there are paramedics in your area, always call them in a life-threatening or potentially serious situation. The paramedics should not be called for more minor problems or in situations where the youngster is basically fine other than that she requires transport on a stretcher (as explained later in the book). In this situation, calling for an ambulance is wise, but you need to let them know the urgency or lack of urgency of the situation.

THE DON'TS

Don't forget to have all emergency information at hand (near the telephone and in your possession).

Don't forget to prepare baby-sitters, houseguests, friends, and relatives for what steps to take in an emergency, and tell them where all emergency information is kept.

Don't forget to get a handful of Consent to Treat forms, keep them on hand, and fill them out completely for each baby-sitter, relative, or other person who will be responsible for your child.

What to Expect in an Emergency Room

If you need to take a child to a hospital emergency room (ER), try to call your personal physician first (if you have one and there's time) so he or she can call the ER doctors in advance and explain any particular medical problem or vital medical history to them.

For many people, emergency rooms are frustrating places. One woman put it this way: "I just sat there and sat there with my sick child in my arms. Other people who I know got there after us kept going into the treatment area before us. Then there seemed to be no one else but us waiting. Another hour went by, and I hadn't seen one person go in or out of the treatment area. Everyone must have been taking a break. Finally, after being there for two and a half hours, we were called in and put in a treatment room. A nurse checked my son's pulse, did a few other things, asked a couple of questions, then left. I could hear voices down the hall and some noise, but we didn't see a doctor for another half hour. I was furious and felt my son's health meant little to these people. The doctor spent all of ten minutes with us and prescribed an antibiotic, cough medicine, lots of liquids, and plenty of rest. He said I should call and make an appointment with my son's doctor so he could be rechecked in five to seven days. Tommy had bacterial pneumonia, he said; and off he went, never to be seen again! All in all, we were there for four full hours. It was an expensive ten minutes and a very unpleasant experience."

This woman does have a few legitimate gripes. She wouldn't have been so upset if someone had taken a moment to explain what was happening. Emergency medicine, on the whole, is greatly misunderstood. All ERs work on a "triage" basis. *Triage* means to "sort out." In emergency rooms, that means identifying those people who have the greatest emergency (life-threatening or serious) and seeing them first—since they require immediate medical intervention. Any hesitation in these cases may result in disability, loss of limb or organ, or even death.

Therefore—*no matter who arrives first*—those in life-threatening situations will be seen first. Those with serious problems will be seen next and those with potentially serious problems after them. Non–life-threatening and less serious problems will be treated last. Even if you happen to be in a treatment room already, if someone is brought into the ER with a more serious or life-threatening problem, he or she will be treated first.

GETTING HELP,
SAFETY,
PREVENTING
ILLNESS, AND
BEING
PREPARED FOR
LIFE-
THREATENING
EMERGENCIES

Often what many people don't see (depending on the layout of the ER) are the people brought in by the paramedics or ambulances. Many hospitals have designed the emergency room so that there is a special and separate entrance that goes straight into the treatment area (not through the waiting room area) for patients to be brought in by the paramedics, ambulances, or police. This is done partly to speed up the care for these people—but it's also intended to increase the comfort and lessen the stress level of those waiting to be seen in the ER waiting room. There's nothing quite as distressing as having people rushed by broken and bleeding or seeing the paramedics performing CPR on someone as they hurry past you.

Therefore, it is important to keep in mind that even if you *don't see* seriously ill or injured people coming into the ER, that doesn't mean that they are not there or that the ER doctors and staff are simply sitting around ignoring everyone in the waiting room. Remember, anyone whose life is imminently threatened requires more time and more professionals to help. All available personnel must assist in these situations unless they are already involved in another life-threatening crisis. So if one or two people brought to the ER before you arrived required aggressive or immediate medical help, that's where the doctors and nurses would be—and that's the reason you would not see anyone in the halls or other areas of the ER.

In some hospitals, it is the job of the receptionist or admitting clerk to explain the delays to those in the waiting room, while other hospitals ask the nurse who sees the patient (to take vital signs and so on) to apologize for any delay and explain that there have been many serious cases that had to be seen first. In other ERs, no one explains anything—and that is both frustrating and unkind.

Therefore, if you have to take your child to an emergency room for a nonemergency or a less urgent problem, you will probably be asked to sit down in the waiting area until the admitting clerk can see you. If the admitting clerk is free, you will be sent directly to her or him. There you are asked information about insurance, billing, name of personal physician, your name, the child's name, your address, phone number, and so forth. You will then be asked to go back to the waiting room until you are called. Once called, you and your child will be escorted to a treatment room. A nurse will usually take the youngster's vital signs, obtain a brief medical history, and (sometimes) perform a brief physical examination.

If there are obvious laboratory tests that need to be done, the nurse often orders them with the physician's approval. After any lab tests, your child is usually brought back to the treatment room. The physician may either wish to receive the lab reports before examining the child or may examine the youngster, then wait for the test results to verify or rule out a certain diagnosis. If your child's doctor has been called (either by you before going to the ER or by the ER staff), he or she may choose to come into the ER to evaluate your child or be waiting for the diagnosis and work with ER physician (over the phone) to determine the best treatment or decide if hospitalization is necessary.

If the youngster is to be admitted, then you will have to go through a hospital admissions procedure. If the youngster is to be discharged, you are most often given home-care instructions and any necessary prescription slips to be filled. If the youngster needs follow-up care, often those instructions as well as the diagnosis, any tests performed, and treatment administered are also given to you on an "after-care" or information sheet. This sheet is to be given to your child's doctor, either at the follow-up visit you arrange or at the child's next appointment (if follow-up care is not necessary).

However, if your child has a serious or potentially life-threatening illness or injury and is brought to the emergency room (or hospital trauma center) by the paramedics, ambulance, or you—then the youngster will have priority and be rushed into a treatment room. In this situation (if you are with the child when he or she arrives), you will see doctors, nurses, and other medical professionals moving around, doing things, and giving orders. There always seems to be a great deal of movement—professionals often moving, working, and talking fast. Some have described this intense experience as a fantasy or dream.

As one father vividly described it: "Our twelve-year-old son was hit by a car that went out of control and jumped the curb where Jimmy was playing catch with one of his friends. I just happened to be watering the lawn. It was a terrible feeling—it all seemed like slow motion—and I was helpless—frozen. I told Jimmy's friend to run into the house and have my wife call the paramedics while I tried to comfort and help Jimmy. It seemed as if hours had gone by before the paramedics arrived. Our neighbor said it was only four minutes. It's amazing how your mind just doesn't perceive time, place, or even reality when your whole world's been turned upside down.

"When we reached the emergency room, we seemed to be instantly surrounded by people in white coats—some working on Jimmy, other asking questions of the paramedics, someone shouting commands—all while Jimmy was raced down the hallway toward a treatment room.

"All of a sudden," the father said quietly, "it seemed like the treatment room door was slammed in our faces. In fact, a nurse had gently taken my wife and me by the arm and said we needed to wait outside—that we would only be in the way in there. It's odd, but I only remember the door to that room slamming. As we were led away, I kept trying to look back—to get a look at our son—as those in white coats moved in and out of the room.

"The nurse was very kind," he continued, "and sat us down. She said she was the liaison between us and the team working on Jimmy and that she would be back and forth trying to give us news as she could. Again, it seemed like an eternity before she came back. Jimmy was holding his own, she said, and left again. I looked at my watch. Only five minutes had gone by. I looked at my watch again. One minute had passed.

"Finally, the liaison nurse and a doctor appeared. The doctor explained that Jimmy needed immediate surgery for his internal injuries—and that the broken bones would be treated later—after he was out of danger. He assured us that Jimmy's vital signs were now stable and that they had been able to get the shock under control. From the time we pushed through the emergency room doors until Jimmy was in surgery—a

20

GETTING HELP,
SAFETY,
PREVENTING
ILLNESS, AND
BEING
PREPARED FOR
LIFE-
THREATENING
EMERGENCIES

mere forty-five minutes had passed. That's still difficult for me to believe. In my fear, confusion, and panic—it seemed like several hours.

"Jimmy, thank God, is fine today—out riding his bicycle as if nothing had ever happened. To all of us, it now seems like a dream. But at the time," the father said, "it was a terrible nightmare—the kind you simply want to wake up from and never, never remember."

This father's descriptions are quite vivid and express the feelings of helplessness, loneliness, emotional shock, grief, fear, confusion, and real pain that spell a true "emergency" for those who must wait and see if everything will be all right. It's important to remember that serious or life-threatening emergencies not only affect the young person who is actually ill or injured—but also his or her family and friends.

In the midst of all this fear and panic, the parent, legal guardian, or person watching the youngster must be able to answer questions about the youngster's name, age, medical history, address, doctor, insurance coverage, and so on. That may seem very cruel and insensitive, but unfortunately, the hospital must have a complete record. In addition, parents may find themselves answering more questions if the child requires admission to the hospital. They may also be asked to make very quick decisions about their child's care. In some situations, there is no decision to be made—in that a surgery or procedure must be done in order to save the child's life or to lessen the possibility of a lifelong disability.

Hopefully you will never find yourself in an emergency room or trauma center having to make decisions. However, if you do find yourself in the middle of a serious medical emergency—always ask questions and re-ask the questions if you don't understand or didn't hear the answers. If you find that the emergency room doesn't have a nurse or other professional to act as a liaison between you and the doctors, try to remember that the doctor will see you as soon as he or she can. The first priority, as we would all want it to be, is the care of the youngster.

A word about billing procedures. Depending on the hospital, you may receive one bill for the ER visit or many separate bills. It's best to ask so you won't be confused when billed. Some emergency medicine physicians are doctors under contract with the hospital to provide services, and their bill is sent separately from the hospital bill. You may also be billed separately for lab tests, X rays, and so on.

Many hospitals today expect full or partial payment upon receiving medical services. Others require you to pay the amount not covered by your insurance. For example, if you have insurance that covers 80 percent of usual, customary, and reasonable charges (as determined by your insurance company), then you will be expected to pay for 20 percent of the bill before leaving. You would then receive a bill for any other charges your insurance didn't cover. Other hospitals bill your insurance company first and then send you a bill for all charges not covered by your insurance. If you do not have insurance, always ask if arrangements can be made for you to pay for the services rendered (for example, so much money per month).

Remember, emergency room care is much more expensive than seeing your child's doctor at his or her office. Costs are greater because of the need for sophisticated equipment, tests, and treatment, as well as the staff, which must be available twenty-four hours a day.

THE DON'TS

Don't hesitate to take your child to an emergency room if you feel a problem requires evaluation immediately and you cannot reach your doctor, do not have a doctor, or are out of town.

Don't hesitate to ask questions when at the emergency room. Whether it be about how long (an estimate) it will be before the doctor sees the youngster or you need more of an explanation about what is wrong—make sure you ask until you are satisfied.

Don't forget that the most serious or life-threatening problems are always seen and treated first. Therefore, try to be patient, tolerant, and understanding if you must wait for long periods of time or if others are seen before your child.

Don't hesitate to insist that your child be reevaluated by a nurse or doctor if the child's condition worsens while you are waiting in the emergency room to see a doctor, or if you feel the youngster was not properly triaged and requires prompt or immediate medical attention. Remember that a youngster (or adult) is triaged based on the symptoms described and how he or she looks and acts. It is possible for a child's status to change or for the professional doing the initial triaging to misread the child's need for prompt or immediate medical attention.

What to Expect When Calling Your Doctor

Often people are confused by the procedures of a doctor's office and become uncomfortable about calling the office—particularly after hours or on weekends or holidays. Understanding the mechanisms of telephone communications in a doctor's office may put you more at ease and make you less frustrated.

OFFICE HOURS

First of all, office hours are those times when someone (or the entire staff) is in the office to receive calls, answer questions, make appointments, and see patients. Doctors have different office hours, based on the needs of their practice.

If the doctor routinely has a large number of patients in the hospital, then his or her office hours may start later than another doctor's. If, for example, the doctor also teaches at a nearby hospital or university, then his or her office hours may be a little different from the hours of a doctor who does not do this. Some doctors, then, start their office hours early in the morning, take a two-hour break (often from noon to 2:00

22

GETTING HELP,
SAFETY,
PREVENTING
ILLNESS, AND
BEING
PREPARED FOR
LIFE-
THREATENING
EMERGENCIES

P.M. to see patients in the hospital and/or to have lunch), and end their office hours at 5:00 P.M. or 6:00 P.M. Others may spend their mornings seeing hospital patients and begin their office hours at 11:00 A.M. or noon. Others have almost standard business hours—9:00 to 5:00 (office hours) without breaks. You might find some doctors with Saturday or evening hours and others who arrange for a time each day in which you may call to ask your questions without worrying about interrupting another person's office visit.

Find out what the doctor's office hours are and write them down (it's best to put them in the phone book next to the office phone number and address). In that way, when you need to make an appointment for a well-visit or a nonemergency illness, injury, or problem, then you would call *during office hours*. If you're waiting for test results or feel you need to talk to the doctor about a problem that is not an emergency, again you would call during office hours and explain what you need.

When you call and ask to speak to the doctor, the receptionist will ask you to explain the situation. If it is a nonurgent or nonemergency problem, one of several things usually happens. The receptionist may ask if you can bring the child into the office that same day or make an appointment for the following day. Or you may be asked to wait on the telephone in order to talk to the doctor's nurse/assistant. After you explain the situation and express your feeling about the urgency or nonurgency of the problem, the nurse/assistant may have you bring the child to the office or feel that you should talk to the doctor right away or indicate that the doctor will call you back later. If the doctor is going to return your call, make sure you leave the correct telephone number (have it repeated) and tell the receptionist or nurse/assistant how long you will be at that number. (Some receptionists are trained sufficiently to know whether the doctor should talk to you before anything else is done.)

Don't forget to ask approximately *when* the doctor will be calling you back. You have a right to know whether it will be in twenty minutes, the next three hours, or anytime all day until 6:00 P.M. There is nothing more frustrating than anxiously awaiting a call from the doctor when you have *no idea* when it might be.

On the other hand, when you know the doctor is supposed to be calling you back— *stay off the telephone*. If you are told your call will be returned within the next fifteen minutes to one hour, that means the doctor will probably try to call you between seeing patients. If you're on the telephone, he or she will not be able to get through to you. There's nothing more frustrating to a doctor than trying to return a patient's call (over and over again) and getting a busy signal.

If the doctor has not returned your call within a reasonable time *after* you were told he or she would phone, then call the office back. In very busy offices, messages can sometimes be misplaced, the importance of the message might not be relayed to the doctor, or the wrong telephone number could even be written down accidentally, so it's best to call back. Remember, too, if the situation suddenly changes and you feel the youngster is getting progressively worse, then call the doctor's office back, explain the situation, and let the receptionist or nurse/assistant know that you feel you need to talk to the doctor right away or bring the child in or whatever the case might be.

It is vitally important to have your child seen in the office whenever possible. This is *not* simply a matter of convenience! The young person's records are available at the doctor's office, as well as some diagnostic tools.

No one wants to perform "telephone diagnosis," and no one wants to see you at, or send you to, the nearest emergency room—unless there is no other, less expensive, choice. Therefore, if your child is ill or injured and you're not sure he or she needs to be seen, it is still a good idea (if at all possible) to call the doctor's office (as early as you can) during office hours to find out if the youngster should be evaluated or what further symptoms would warrant calling the doctor's office back—whether or not it is during office hours.

The reason this is important is because so many parents wait and wait and wait until the very last minute and then decide they'd better call the doctor. No one should worry all day long, wondering if his or her child should get medical attention. It's much better to know that, at this point, the child doesn't need to be seen, but here is what you can do at home and here are the symptoms to look for that would signal a need to call the office immediately, before the end of the day, the next day, or for an appointment to have the child seen within a few days.

THE ANSWERING SERVICE

Whenever the doctor's office is closed (whether that be on certain afternoons or mornings, lunchtime, evenings and overnight, weekends, or holidays), a telephone answering service receives the doctor's calls. It's important to remember that the operators of a doctor's answering service are there to take messages and to contact the doctor in the event of an urgent or emergency situation.

These operators cannot determine whether or not you *need* to talk to the doctor, whether your child should be seen by the doctor the next day or immediately, or whether he or she needs to be seen in an emergency room. They cannot give medical opinions or advice because they are not trained or authorized to do so. Essentially, the answering service is the liaison between you and the doctor when the office is closed.

Therefore, you must be specific in explaining your problem and needs. Remember, the answering service may be getting several to many calls an hour and must be able to tell the doctor which calls appear to be more urgent and must therefore be returned first. *You* must tell the answering service operator that this is an emergency and you must speak with the doctor right away. *You* must say that you feel this is an urgent situation and need to talk to the doctor within the hour. *You* should tell the operator that you're not sure what is going on but fear it may be serious and would feel better if you talked with the doctor in the next two or three hours.

The point is, you should not be afraid to call the answering service—but you should not mislead the operator, either. Don't say it is an emergency if it isn't. Don't say it's urgent if it can wait until regular office hours. But then again, don't hesitate to be *insistent* if you think the youngster is seriously ill or injured, or you're not sure if this

24

GETTING HELP,
SAFETY,
PREVENTING
ILLNESS, AND
BEING
PREPARED FOR
LIFE-
THREATENING
EMERGENCIES

is a potentially serious problem, and you really feel you need to speak to the doctor immediately or before the office opens again. Make sure you give the operator your name, your child's name, and your correct phone number. Ask when the doctor will be returning your call, so you won't be anxious or frustrated waiting. Again, if your call is not returned within a reasonable time *after* you were told the doctor would call you—then call back! If the situation worsens (at any point) and you feel you must talk to the doctor "right now," then call back and relay that message. If you feel the child is worsening rapidly and you have been unable to reach the doctor—go to the nearest emergency room. Make sure you tell the ER staff that you have been trying to reach your doctor. They will then try to contact your doctor to advise him or her of the situation.

If you are calling for an appointment and, to your surprise, the answering service picks up your call, still feel free to leave a message (for example, "When they get back into the office could they please call Mrs. Smith at such and such phone number. My son Mark is sick, and I think he needs to be seen today"). However, it is always best to call back yourself when the office opens to make the appointment. Sometimes the receptionist is so busy taking calls that she or he cannot get to making callbacks.

Many people panic and slam down the phone because they don't expect the answering service to pick up the call and are suddenly speechless or embarrassed. You are not imposing by calling and reaching the answering service. If it's a matter of not knowing the doctor's office hours, simply ask when you can call to talk to someone in the office.

WHEN ANOTHER DOCTOR IS "COVERING"

In group practices, most doctors take turns covering nights, weekends, and holidays. Your family doctor or child's doctor, even if in "solo" practice, does have a "coverage" system worked out whenever he or she is out of town or takes time off. Therefore, there may be times when you call the doctor about a problem that you feel cannot wait until the next morning or until office hours and ask to speak to him or her, only to be told that Dr. Johnson is covering for your doctor tonight (sometimes they just say Dr. Johnson is "covering" or available and ask whether you would like to speak to him or her).

Don't let coverage confuse you. The only thing you need to remember is that the doctor covering may only have seen your child once or twice or never before. Therefore, when you talk to the doctor, make sure you tell him or her about any chronic problems your child has, any medications currently being taken, any allergies or sensitivities to medications or other things, and the age and weight of the youngster. Remember, the doctor won't have the patient chart in front of him or her, so getting this information from you is very important. (Your own doctor might also ask you this information if the chart is not immediately available, just to ensure that he or she doesn't get your children mixed up.)

What Not to Do When Dealing with Your Doctor

There are a few things that you should avoid (if at all possible) when dealing with the doctor's office, the answering service, or the doctor.

If you know the youngster is sick and may need to be seen, don't wait until the office is about ready to close. Call and talk to the receptionist about the problem as early in the day as possible so an appointment can be arranged if the youngster does need to be evaluated.

Don't wait until late Friday afternoon or the weekend to call to have a prescription refilled. Check your supply ahead of time when a child has a chronic problem for which he or she is required to take medicine daily. In a situation where the doctor has instructed you to call if the child hasn't improved substantially, call early in the day so treatment can be changed or your child can be reevaluated. If you know you have no more refills at the pharmacy and the medication is starting to run out (or if for whatever reason you need to talk to the doctor about a refill or a prescription), call the doctor's office as soon as you recognize the need to do so.

All physicians prefer to look at a patient's chart before refilling or prescribing a medication. It's important, then, that your request be made during office hours (as previously noted)—when the patient chart is available. Obviously, if it's a sudden problem, then call the doctor! (For example, one father accidentally spilled his daughter's medication one Saturday morning and had little choice but to call. A mother once called the doctor hysterically because she and her husband had left their son's medicine in another city while visiting relatives and were now panicked.)

When making appointments for well-visits or minor illnesses, call as far in advance as possible, particularly if you know there are only certain times or days you can take the youngster to the doctor. This makes it more probable that the doctor will be able to see the child when you can most conveniently bring him or her in to the office.

When Talking to Your Child's Doctor

Under most circumstances, your child's doctor is the best resource for you. He or she knows your child's health history and can assess the seriousness of the situation. The doctor can help you decide if the youngster should be seen immediately or can wait until a later time. He or she may have suggestions for how you can try to make the young person more comfortable. The doctor can and will direct you to an appropriate emergency room or health care facility for urgent care if that is needed.

In order to best assess the problem, either by telephone or in person, the doctor needs important information from you. Sometimes only one or two questions will be asked, while at other times you might be asked many, many questions—depending on what the doctor is trying to determine (if the child needs to be seen immediately,

GETTING HELP,
SAFETY,
PREVENTING
ILLNESS, AND
BEING
PREPARED FOR
LIFE-
THREATENING
EMERGENCIES

what the extent of the problem is, and so on). You may find it helpful to look at the list of questions—found below under *What You Need to Tell the Doctor About the Problem*—before you call the doctor and write down your responses on a piece of paper. In this way, you have a moment to think carefully about each question and answer it as specifically as possible. When you call the doctor, you can have your responses right in front of you. (If the youngster has to be seen, take the list with you, as well.) The list is helpful, since many people panic a bit the minute the doctor gets on the telephone, or they go "blank."

Others say doctors tend to "fire questions" too fast, and this compounds the situation for them. And you may have had the experience of hanging up, then realizing there were some questions you had wanted to ask but simply forgot. It is best, then, to write down (on this same piece of paper) any specific questions you might have for your child's doctor. In this way, you will feel more comfortable when talking to him or her.

WHAT YOU NEED TO TELL THE DOCTOR ABOUT THE PROBLEM

- *When did the problem start?* Be as specific as possible—for example: "a week ago today," "two days ago," "last night," or "yesterday morning."

- *What exactly are the symptoms?* Give them in their order of occurrence. For example: "First I noticed that Tommy was quite inactive and irritable. Then he complained of a stomachache and wouldn't eat. He started vomiting yesterday and hasn't been able to keep anything down since. He seems very weak." Make sure you tell the doctor what bothers the child the most and what else you have noticed.

- *How severe are the symptoms?* For example: "His fever has been 104 degrees for three hours"; "She has vomited five times in the last twelve hours"; or "He just can't seem to stand on his leg, the pain is so severe."

- *Is the situation getting worse, staying the same, or seemingly getting better?* For example: "The fever hasn't gone down"; "The pain has lessened a little, but she still hurts"; or "I don't see any change one way or the other."

- *How quickly is it getting better or worse?* For example: "It seemed like nothing to worry about, but suddenly his fever shot up to 105 degrees this morning"; or "She seems to slowly be getting better over the last four hours but is still complaining of pain in her stomach."

- *Exactly what have you done for the young person?* For example: "I've used an ice pack and splinted her knee"; "We put pressure on the cut"; "We've been giving him half a teaspoon of children's Tylenol every six hours since eight o'clock last night."

- *What was the effect of your actions?* For example: "The pain in her knee seems to be better"; "The bleeding stopped"; or "The Tylenol has reduced the fever two degrees, but we can't get it down any further."

- *How does the child look right now?* For example: "He seems to be having some trouble breathing"; "Her color is normal," or "She is pale" (or bluish, flushed, or rashy); "There seems to be swelling in the abdomen" (or groin or some other place); "The abdomen is enlarged, hard, and tender"; "He doesn't seem to be responding normally"; or "His cry doesn't seem normal—he seems to be really hurting."

- *What is it about the child in this situation that worries you the most?* For example: "The fever doesn't bother me too much, but I can't get him to drink anything"; or "I can understand everything except that she seems so listless and lethargic."

- *Does the young person have any known medical problems or a chronic disease?* For example: "He has a tendency to get ear infections"; or "She's an asthmatic"; or "He has sickle-cell disease"; or "Often she has a urinary infection when she runs a fever."

- *Does he or she take any medication on a routine basis?* For example: "He takes medicine for asthma." (Be sure you know what kind, how much, and how often.)

- *Does the young person have any allergies?* For example: "She's allergic to penicillin"; or "He's allergic to milk products."

- *Do you have the telephone number of your nearest pharmacy in case the doctor wants to call in a prescription for the child?* Make sure you have this next to the phone and don't have to go get it after you've called the doctor. It is also helpful to know the pharmacy's hours if your call is late at night or on a weekend.

- *Do you know the present weight of your child?* The doctor needs this in order to prescribe the proper amount of medication if a prescription is necessary.

- *If this isn't a life-threatening emergency, have you written down any questions you might have for the doctor?*

THE DON'TS

Remember that your observations are very important and you need to be able to carefully assess the situation. Therefore, the following apply:

Don't panic. Stay calm at all costs. That's the only way you can act appropriately in order to help and comfort the child.

Don't forget to call the doctor's office during office hours if you are trying to

28

GETTING HELP,
SAFETY,
PREVENTING
ILLNESS, AND
BEING
PREPARED FOR
LIFE-
THREATENING
EMERGENCIES

make an appointment; find out test results; have a question that is not urgent; or have questions on billing, insurance, well-care information, and so on.

Don't hesitate to call the doctor after office hours, on weekends, or on holidays—if you really feel the youngster's condition warrants an immediate discussion with the doctor. In other words, call if you feel the problem is such that waiting until office hours the next day or until after the weekend might jeopardize the child's safety or well-being.

Don't overreact. Except for serious illness and injury (as discussed in the Emergency Quick Reference guide for When to Call the Paramedics or Ambulance or When to Go to an Emergency Room in this chapter and later in Section 2), taking immediate action may not be as important as staying calm and carefully determining the best action to take.

Don't underreact. Pay attention to the serious symptoms your child might have and act accordingly.

Don't hesitate to ask your doctor any questions you may have. No question is "silly" or "stupid" if you are worried and don't know the answer. You have a right to have your questions answered.

Don't underestimate your role in your child's health care. With knowledge and confidence, you can and will have good judgment about how serious a problem is and how to act in your youngster's best interests. You are quite important and serve as a special partner in your child's health care.

EMERGENCY SHEET

Emergency Numbers

ALL EMERGENCIES: *911* (Check to see if this applies in your area.)

Police: _____

Fire: _____

Paramedics: _____

Poison control center: _____

Nearest hospital: _____

   Phone: _____ Address: _____

_____

Ambulance: _____

Pharmacy: _____ Phone: _____

   Address: _____ Hours: _____

All-night pharmacy: _____ Phone: _____

   Address: _____

Home Information

Family name: _____

Telephone: _____

Address: _____

Nearest cross streets: _____

_____

_____

GETTING HELP,
SAFETY,
PREVENTING
ILLNESS, AND
BEING
PREPARED FOR
LIFE-
THREATENING
EMERGENCIES

Family Physicians

Family member(s): _____

_____

Dr. _____ Phone: _____

Family member(s): _____

_____

Dr._____ Phone: _____

Family member(s): _____

_____

Dr._____ Phone: _____

Relatives or Friends to Call for Assistance or Notify in an Emergency

Name: _____ Phone: _____

Address: _____

Relationship: _____

Name: _____ Phone: _____

Address: _____

Relationship: _____

Name: _____ Phone: _____

Address: _____

Relationship: _____

Other Information

Location of fire extinguishers: _____

_____

Fire evacuation plan: _____

_____

MEDICAL HISTORY

Name of child: _____

Date of birth: _____

Parents or legal guardian(s): _____

_____

Address: _____

Home phone: _____ Bus. phone: _____

Personal doctor: _____

  Phone: _____ Address: _____

General Information

Known allergies or sensitivities (list all medications, foods, plants, animals, and so on):

_____

_____

Medications taken on a regular basis (include dosage and how often taken):

_____

_____

Any chronic illnesses or problems (be specific) and date identified: _____

_____

Any surgeries (type and date): _____

_____

Any hospitalizations (give reason or problem and date): _____

_____

Any serious injuries (broken bones, dislocations, head injuries, and so forth, and dates):

_____

_____

Current weight (also include date weighed): _____

GETTING HELP,
SAFETY,
PREVENTING
ILLNESS, AND
BEING
PREPARED FOR
LIFE-
THREATENING
EMERGENCIES

Immunization Record

DTP (diphtheria, tetanus, pertussis) or DT (diphtheria, tetanus) (date)

Any reaction? If yes, what?

1st _____ no   yes _____

2d _____ no   yes _____

3d _____ no   yes _____

Booster _____ no   yes _____

Booster _____ no   yes _____

Booster _____ no   yes _____

Polio (date)

	Oral?	*Injected?*
1st _____	yes	yes
2d _____	yes	yes
3d _____	yes	yes
4th _____	yes	yes
5th _____	yes	yes

Others (dates)

Any reaction? If yes, what?

Measles _____ no   yes _____

Rubella _____ no   yes _____

Mumps _____ no   yes _____

MMR (measles, mumps, rubella) _____ no   yes _____

"Hib" (Hemophilus influenzae b) _____ no   yes _____

_____ no   yes _____

TB tests (dates)

Reaction?

_____ negative   positive

_____ negative   positive

_____ negative   positive

_____ negative   positive

_____ negative   positive

SAMPLE CONSENT TO TREAT FORM

I (we) authorize _____

name of person watching/caring for minor

to consent on my (our) behalf for any necessary medical evaluation and treatment and/
or surgical treatment for _____ in my (our) absence.

name of minor

_____

signature(s)

_____

printed name(s)
parent(s) or legal guardian(s)

_____

date

PLEASE NOTE: Some hospitals/doctors require that their particular Consent to Treat form be completed; others will accept a handwritten consent; while still others want more information included (such as from what date and time until what date and time the consent is authorized). Therefore, it is always best to check with your doctor and the hospital (emergency room) in the area where the child would be seen if a problem occurred. In this way, you can ensure that the young person will be treated by meeting both your doctor's requirements (if the child needs to see the doctor) and the requirements of the hospital. Find out also if the hospital will not treat a minor (anyone under age 18) even with a Consent to Treat form unless the problem is considered life-threatening or potentially life-threatening. In other words, they will not treat the child without the parents' (parent's) or legal guardians' (guardian's) knowledge of the problem and personal consent to provide treatment. Finally, it is always wise to *leave insurance information* with the Consent to Treat form.

34

GETTING HELP,
SAFETY,
PREVENTING
ILLNESS, AND
BEING
PREPARED FOR
LIFE-
THREATENING
EMERGENCIES

BABY-SITTER'S CHECKLIST

☐ HAVE YOU SHOWN THE BABY-SITTER WHERE ALL EMERGENCY IN-FORMATION IS LOCATED, INCLUDING THE EMERGENCY SHEET AND MEDICAL RECORDS?

☐ HAVE YOU LEFT THE TELEPHONE NUMBER WHERE YOU CAN BE REACHED IN CASE OF EMERGENCY?

☐ HAVE YOU GIVEN THE BABY-SITTER A COMPLETED *CONSENT TO TREAT* FORM FOR EACH OF THE CHILDREN HE OR SHE IS WATCHING?

☐ HAVE YOU CAREFULLY EXPLAINED HOW TO GIVE A CHILD HIS OR HER MEDICATION IF NEEDED?

☐ HAVE YOU SHOWN THE BABY-SITTER WHERE ALL WORKING FIRE EXTINGUISHERS ARE LOCATED IN THE HOUSE AND HOW TO OPERATE THEM?

☐ HAVE YOU SHOWN THE BABY-SITTER YOUR FIRE EVACUATION PLAN AND ROUTE?

☐ HAVE YOU EXPLAINED WHAT STEPS YOU WISH HER OR HIM TO TAKE IN CASE OF AN EMERGENCY (DEPENDING ON WHAT KIND OF EMER-GENCY)?

☐ HAVE YOU DETAILED THE DOS AND DON'TS FOR YOUR CHILDREN (IN TERMS OF USING APPLIANCES, PLAY BOUNDARIES, CURFEWS FOR PLAYING OUTSIDE THE YARD, TAKING BATHS AND SHOWERS, AND SO ON)?

CHAPTER 2

Safety: Preventing Accidents and Injuries

Accident is a word we misuse a great deal. We often call something an accident that in actuality could have been avoided with some careful planning and specific precautions. A true accident involves an incident that could not have been prevented, controlled, or avoided—*even when the most careful precautions had been taken.*

Is it truly an accident when a child is seriously hurt or killed in an automobile collision—if the child was not secured in an approved child restraint (car seat, infant seat, or seat belt if an older youngster)? Is it really an accident, in the true sense, if a young person meets a telephone pole head on—while traveling well over the speed limit on his or her motorcycle or minibike? What about the three-year-old who finds and swallows a bottle of prescription pills—pills left easily within the child's reach and not in a childproof container? How about the youngster who is pushed to play a sport while hurt? Is it an accident that he or she then sustains a more serious injury or even a lifelong disability? The list of examples goes on and on.

The point is, even though none of these incidents was intentional, each had a cause. Under a different set of circumstances, these "accidents" might have been prevented. The child might not have been killed or even seriously injured if properly secured in an approved child restraint. The young person might not have hit the telephone pole if he or she had not been speeding. The three-year-old could not have been poisoned if the pills had been locked in a cupboard and the container secured by a childproof cap. The youngster might not have experienced a serious injury or lifelong disability if he or she had not been forced to play the sport while hurting or already injured.

That is not to say "true" accidents do not occur—even when the best precautions and preventive measures have been taken. They do! However, we can greatly reduce the odds of certain accidents' occurring by taking some preventive steps.

GETTING HELP,
SAFETY,
PREVENTING
ILLNESS, AND
BEING
PREPARED FOR
LIFE-
THREATENING
EMERGENCIES

Babies, toddlers, small children, youngsters, and even teenagers are naturally curious and have little regard for danger. Because of their agility, energy, and healthfulness, teenagers have no sense of their mortality. They simply feel invincible and are risk-takers—even when they know danger lurks. Crawlers, toddlers, and small children, on the other hand, have absolutely no sense of danger. Therefore, they cannot be expected to perceive and sidestep threats to their safety. Only as they grow can they be taught what to fear or how to better protect themselves.

Of course, parents and others cannot be expected to watch a youngster every minute of the day and night. It would simply not be humanly possible to "never take your eyes off" a young person. It would also be impractical.

For the young ones, we can better protect them by taking specific steps to modify their environment. In other words, we must, when possible, try to entirely eliminate some potential hazards and reduce the likelihood of injury from others. For the older child and teenager, we must try to teach them good safety habits (the whys, wherefores, and possible consequences of their actions). Where necessary, we need to step in and use our better judgment on behalf of the young person. (For example, you do have control over whether or not your child will be allowed to purchase or ride on a minibike or motorcycle—both known to be extremely dangerous.)

One fact is clear—childhood injury is at an epidemic level. It *is* a serious problem and not simply a matter of minor bumps and bruises. The statistics are staggering and should serve as a warning to all of us. Preventing these incidents is a formidable challenge, but a task well worth the time and effort.

Another consideration: It is more reasonable to eliminate potential hazards than to cope with their often deadly and crippling results. The time, trouble, and expense involved in eliminating some hazards and modifying the risks of others are trivial compared to the physical and mental pain (not to mention the financial drain) that can be caused by a serious or disabling injury—or, even worse, the loss of a loved one.

You may have heard people say that preventive measures simply don't work and are therefore not worth the trouble. The truth is, they *do* make a significant difference. Here are a few examples.

Tennessee, which passed the first law requiring the use of federally approved safety seats for children under four years of age, saw a 55-percent reduction in automotive deaths in children under four years old and a 30-percent reduction in injuries. These impressive figures were based on only a 32-percent increase in the use of safety seats/ child restraints. Imagine the number of lives that would have been saved and the injuries avoided if there had been 100-percent compliance with the law.

New York City's Health Department began a special program in 1973 under which easy-to-install window safety-guards/locks were given free of charge to families with young children who were living on upper floors. In a two-year period, there was a 50-percent decline in reported falls and a 35-percent reduction in deaths due to falls.

As another example, in 1972, the childproof cap (safety cap) was introduced. These safety caps used on medication bottles significantly reduced the incidence of childhood poisoning. Deaths (due to the ingestion of analgesics and antipyretics) declined 41 percent for all age groups (between 1971 and 1977). The decline was even more impressive in aspirin poisonings, which were reduced 75 percent. The reduction would have been greater yet if everyone had used the safety caps and made sure the caps were returned to the container properly rather than being left half-on, half-off.

In Ontario, Canada, a study was done to determine the lifesaving potential of smoke detectors. Smoke detectors were installed in 97,000 homes. Eighty-five percent of the time, the initial warning that fire threatened came via the smoke detectors. The Missouri Division of Health developed a major prevention program to reduce the rate of burn injuries (from hot water, grease, hot liquid, stoves, irons, building fires, and so on). During the period the program was in effect, the annual death rate due to burns dropped 43 percent.

So you see, preventive measures do make a significant difference and are well worth pursuing. It is important to mention that taking preventive steps is important not merely for parents but for grandparents, relatives, friends—everyone, in fact, who has infants, toddlers, young children, or youngsters of all ages visiting their homes.

The remainder of this chapter contains a series of safety checklists for your use. You will notice that each preventive measure is preceded by a "yes" or "no" answer. The more "yes" answers you have, the safer the environment is for young people. The more "no" answers you have, the more substantial the risks that a serious problem may occur. If something does not apply to you or your family, do not answer it. For example, if you do not have an infant or toddler, the questions on nursery furniture do not apply to you, and you need not answer them. (However, it's a good idea to read all the questions.) You will also notice that after each question there is a short discussion about why anyone would want to spend the time, take the trouble, or go to the expense (in some situations) of taking these safety precautions.

We hope that, after completing all the questions, you will use these checklists as guidelines for better ensuring the safety of young people in the home, on the playground, and when away from home. If at all possible, try to change many of the "no" answers to "yes"—as you complete the checklists. It may be helpful to refer to these safety checklists periodically to make sure that all possible safety precautions have been taken. It's also an excellent way to refresh your memory, from time to time, about those measures that require continual or periodic examination. In this way, you can learn the odds of avoiding accidents and injuries in your favor and better protect the health and well-being of your children.

GETTING HELP,
SAFETY,
PREVENTING
ILLNESS, AND
BEING
PREPARED FOR
LIFE-
THREATENING
EMERGENCIES

MOTOR VEHICLE SAFETY CHECKLIST

yes no DO YOU SECURE YOUR INFANT OR YOUNG CHILD IN A CHILD
☐ ☐ SAFETY SEAT THAT MEETS OR EXCEEDS FEDERAL STANDARDS
FOR AUTOMOBILE SAFETY—EACH AND EVERY TIME HE OR SHE
RIDES IN YOUR CAR, TRUCK, OR OTHER MOTOR VEHICLE?

Very few parents take this simple step to ensure their children's safety. In
fact, most people place infants and small children on their laps and feel they
can protect the child in the event of a collision. Consider this: a child weighing
thirty pounds in a car going thirty miles per hour will actually weigh three-
quarters of a ton upon impact (due to the force). How many people can hold
on to a three-quarter-ton object that is thrusting forward? Most children in
such situations are crushed between the parent and the dashboard or thrown
through the windshield.

yes no IS IT AN ABSOLUTE RULE THAT YOUR INFANT OR YOUNG CHILD
☐ ☐ NOT BE ALLOWED IN ANYONE ELSE'S CAR OR OTHER MOTOR
VEHICLE UNLESS HE OR SHE IS SECURED IN AN AUTHORIZED
SAFETY SEAT?

Either grandparents, relatives, and friends must purchase their own safety seat
for the child or you must *always* leave your safety seat for their use when the
child is visiting. If they suddenly need to run an errand, the youngster will
not be properly restrained. Also, consider the fact that of children needing
emergency room treatment after motor vehicle incidents, almost 20 percent
experienced injuries from noncrash situations (for example, fast stops, swerves,
turns). All of these injuries more than likely could have been avoided if the
youngsters had been properly restrained.

yes no HAVE YOU CHECKED THE RECOMMENDED WEIGHT OR AGE LIM-
☐ ☐ ITS ON YOUR CHILD SAFETY SEAT, TAKING CARE TO USE A SEAT
ONLY IF IT FITS YOUR CHILD CORRECTLY?

Seats designed for young infants are safe only until a baby reaches seventeen
to twenty pounds, and are meant to face rearward in the car. Seats which can
be used for infants, then converted for later use with toddlers and young
children, as well as safety booster seats, carry weight limits and directions for
correct usage. Most seats for young children carry an upper weight limit of
forty pounds.

yes no DO YOU ALWAYS USE INFANT SAFETY SEATS, CHILD SAFETY
☐ ☐ SEATS, AND APPROVED BOOSTER SEATS CORRECTLY?

Studies have shown that as many as one-third of approved safety seats are
used incorrectly. Incorrect use of a seat (for example, facing an infant seat
forward, not using a tether strap on a seat requiring one, or not using a clip
to lock an interlocking car belt system) is sometimes no better than not using
a seat at all. Be sure to read the instructions carefully and follow them precisely
every time you install a safety seat in the car or place a child in an installed
seat.

yes no ARE ALL CHILDREN REQUIRED TO SIT IN THE BACK SEAT WHEN
☐ ☐ POSSIBLE AND USE SEAT BELTS OR SAFETY SEATS?

The safest passenger position is center rear, with seat belt attached or safety
seat in proper use. The least safe place for a child is in the front seat and
unrestrained. The highest injury and death rates occur there.

yes no DO YOU REQUIRE YOUR OLDER CHILDREN TO WEAR A LAP BELT
☐ ☐ (AND SHOULDER HARNESS IF OVER FIFTY-FIVE INCHES TALL)
WHEN THEY RIDE IN YOUR CAR OR ANYONE ELSE'S?

Each year, disabling injuries are experienced by 150,000 children (up to fourteen years of age) as a result of motor vehicle incidents. Studies have shown
that a substantial number of these injuries could be prevented or their severity
reduced if infants and children (under forty pounds) were restrained in approved
safety seats, children over forty pounds but shorter than fifty-five inches tall
wore lap belts, and all other children (over forty pounds and taller than fifty-
five inches) wore both seat belts and shoulder harnesses. Children shorter than
fifty-five inches tall can suffer neck injuries or suffocate if shoulder harnesses
are used, unless they are also sitting in an approved car booster seat designed
to be used with a shoulder harness.

yes no IF YOU ARE NOW EXPECTING A BABY, HAVE YOU PURCHASED A
☐ ☐ FEDERALLY APPROVED SAFETY SEAT, LEARNED HOW TO USE IT
PROPERLY, AND PLANNED TO TAKE YOUR NEWBORN INFANT HOME
FROM THE HOSPITAL IN IT?

Children less than six months of age have the highest death rate among American children, and many of these deaths are due to automobile accidents and
mishaps. The fact is, children under five years of age die more often in motor
vehicle incidents than they do from accidental poisonings (there are five motor
vehicle–related deaths to every one fatal poisoning). Using safety seats from

40

GETTING HELP,
SAFETY,
PREVENTING
ILLNESS, AND
BEING
PREPARED FOR
LIFE-
THREATENING
EMERGENCIES

the time a baby is born—each and every time he or she rides in a car or other type of motor vehicle—would decrease the likelihood of serious injury or death if an accident occurred.

yes no DO YOU INSIST THAT EVERYONE WHO RIDES IN YOUR CAR (FAMILY MEMBER OR NOT) WEAR A SEAT BELT (OR USE A SAFETY SEAT)?

☐ ☐

If all adolescents and adults wore seat belts (including the shoulder harnesses), it is estimated that there would be a 50-percent reduction in motor vehicle deaths and a 65-percent reduction in injuries. Infants and children restrained properly are 50 to 70 percent less likely to be injured or killed. It is a grim reality, though, that only 30 percent of American adults and adolescents, and only 13 percent of infants and children, actually use motor vehicle safety restraints. Imagine the number of lives that could be saved and injuries avoided if seat belts/shoulder harnesses and safety seats were actually used by everybody.

yes no DO *YOU* USE A SEAT BELT AND SHOULDER HARNESS EVERY TIME *YOU* GET INTO A CAR—WHETHER YOU ARE DRIVING OR NOT?

☐ ☐

It's important for you to realize that if something happens to you (lifelong disability or death), it dramatically affects the lives of your children. Abstractly speaking, then, safeguarding your own health and well-being is really safeguarding the health and well-being of your children, as well. Also, your chance of being thrown from the car and killed is 25 percent greater if you are not wearing a seat belt and shoulder harness, so there's every reason to wear them. Your good example dramatically influences your children's behavior, too.

yes no DO YOU ALWAYS CHECK TO SEE THAT EVERY PASSENGER IN YOUR CAR (INCLUDING YOU) IS PROPERLY BELTED IN, EVEN FOR VERY SHORT TRIPS (THOSE TO THE BANK, POST OFFICE, SHOPPING CENTER, A FRIEND'S HOUSE AROUND THE CORNER, AND SO ON)?

☐ ☐

Seventy-five percent of injuries and deaths take place within twenty-five miles of home, and 80 percent of serious injuries and deaths occur in cars traveling less than forty miles per hour. Remember, too, that children should never be allowed to ride in the back of trucks, station wagons, vans, flatbeds, and hatchbacks unless they are designed with proper seats and seat belts and are meant to carry passengers.

yes no ARE YOU CAREFUL TO COMPLY WITH THE FIFTY-FIVE-MILE-PER-HOUR SPEED LIMIT?

☐ ☐

This not only saves gas, but more important, it also significantly reduces the number of deaths and serious injuries due to traffic accidents. The fifty-five-mile-per-hour speed limit is an excellent means of safeguarding yourself and your children.

yes no HAVE YOU FRANKLY DISCUSSED WITH YOUR TEENAGER THE
☐ ☐ DANGERS OF DRIVING AFTER DRINKING ALCOHOL OR USING DRUGS, AS WELL AS THE DANGERS OF RIDING WITH HIS OR HER FRIENDS WHO HAVE BEEN DRINKING OR USING DRUGS?

One study noted that more than 40 percent of high school students drink alcohol at least once a month, and 5 percent are drunk at least once a week. Drinking and driving is a deadly combination that accounts for one-half of all motor vehicle deaths each year. Many of those killed or seriously injured are innocent victims—either people in the car with the driver who has been drinking, occupants of another car involved in the collision, or pedestrians.

yes no ARE YOU CAREFUL NEVER TO LEAVE YOUR KEYS IN THE CAR,
☐ ☐ TO USE SAFETY LOCKS ON REAR CAR DOORS, TO PUT SPECIAL LOCKS ON WINDOWS—AND TO ENFORCE REASONABLE RULES FOR BEHAVIOR WHEN CHILDREN ARE IN THE CAR?

Many children open car doors when the car is moving or roll down a window and fall out. When keys are left in the ignition, inquisitive youngsters start cars and play with the controls—resulting in injury and sometimes death. Also, children who are not restrained by seat belts or car seats and are allowed to play around in the car have actually caused accidents by interfering with or distracting the driver.

GETTING HELP,
SAFETY,
PREVENTING
ILLNESS, AND
BEING
PREPARED FOR
LIFE-
THREATENING
EMERGENCIES

PEDESTRIAN SAFETY CHECKLIST

yes no
☐ ☐ HAVE YOU TAUGHT YOUR CHILDREN TO STOP AT EVERY CURB AND CROSS THE STREET *ONLY AFTER* THEY HAVE LOOKED AND LISTENED FOR CARS?

Forty-five percent of pedestrian deaths involve youngsters one to fourteen years of age. Those children most vulnerable are five years old and under.

yes no
☐ ☐ HAVE YOU TAUGHT YOUR CHILDREN TO OBEY ALL SAFETY RULES? TO ALWAYS CROSS LARGE INTERSECTIONS IN THE CROSSWALK? TO CROSS ONLY AFTER THE LIGHT IS GREEN AND THEY HAVE LOOKED TO MAKE SURE ALL CARS HAVE STOPPED FOR THE RED LIGHT? TO WAIT UNTIL CARS AT A STOP SIGN HAVE PASSED OR GIVEN THEM THE RIGHT OF WAY?

Research has shown that anywhere from 50 to 75 percent of pedestrian deaths occur when rules are violated by the pedestrian.

yes no
☐ ☐ HAVE YOU MADE IT CLEAR THAT DAYLIGHT DOES NOT GUAR-ANTEE GREATER SAFETY AND THAT RULES SHOULD BE FOL-LOWED WHETHER IT IS DAYTIME OR NIGHTTIME?

It is always news to most people that a shocking 80 percent of pedestrian deaths take place during the day, not at night.

yes no
☐ ☐ HAVE YOU INSTRUCTED YOUR CHILDREN NEVER TO DART INTO THE ROAD AND EMPHASIZED THE DANGER OF THIS PRACTICE?

Young people should be taught that the street is "off limits" in terms of play and that it is not an extension of their yard, a park, or whatever. They should learn to respect the roadway and always cross with great care. The fact is, the majority of pedestrian deaths in children are due to their darting into the street or darting across the street.

yes no
☐ ☐ HAVE YOU PURCHASED REFLECTIVE ARMBANDS OR JACKETS WITH REFLECTIVE TAPE TO BE WORN BY YOUR CHILDREN AT NIGHT? OR HAVE YOU PUT REFLECTIVE TAPE ON YOUR CHILDREN'S COATS, JACKETS, HATS, OR OTHER ARTICLES OF CLOTHING TO BE WORN AT NIGHT?

Sweden initiated a program under which reflective tape was sewed on jackets and these were worn at night. The pedestrian death rate decreased 25 percent.

SAFETY IN THE HOME AND CHILDPROOFING THE HOME CHECKLIST

yes no HAVE YOU GOTTEN DOWN ON YOUR HANDS AND KNEES AND
☐ ☐ LOOKED FOR POTENTIAL HAZARDS (FROM A CHILD'S PERSPEC-
TIVE)?

Approximately 839,000 children were injured by home structural products in 1978. You'd be surprised how enlightening it is to get down on all fours and see things as toddlers and small children see them. It's easier to spot the hazards and the temptations children face.

yes no HAVE YOU REMOVED ALL POTENTIALLY HARMFUL OBJECTS—
☐ ☐ THOSE THAT ARE HEAVY OR SHARP—FROM COFFEE TABLES,
KITCHEN TABLES, END TABLES, ALL COUNTERS, BARS, DRESS-
ERS, DESKS, AND OTHER AREAS?

In 1978, 546,000 youngsters were treated in emergency rooms for head injuries. Some of these were the result of pulling things down on their heads.

yes no DO YOU BUY FURNITURE AND FIXTURES THAT DO NOT HAVE
☐ ☐ SHARP EDGES?

In 1978, there were 625,000 children injured by furniture and fixtures.

yes no HAVE YOU COVERED SHARP EDGES (ON EXISTING FURNITURE)
☐ ☐ WITH SPECIAL RUBBER GUARDS OR PADS?

Sharp-edged coffee tables alone caused injuries to 55,000 children in 1978.

yes no ARE ALL FREESTANDING BOOKCASES, BARS, WINE RACKS,
☐ ☐ SHOWCASES, AND SO ON BOLTED TO THE FLOOR AND/OR WALL
SO THAT THEY WILL WITHSTAND A YOUNGSTER'S CLIMBING,
FALLING AGAINST, OR PUSHING ON THEM?

A young child can easily be crushed by large, heavy objects such as these, so all possible care must be taken to secure such objects and avoid serious or even life-threatening injuries to children (as well as adults).

yes no ARE THERE SAFETY LOCKS ON ALL CUPBOARDS OR AT LEAST ON
☐ ☐ THOSE CONTAINING KNIVES, SILVERWARE, UTENSILS, AND OTHER
OBJECTS POTENTIALLY HARMFUL TO CHILDREN?

GETTING HELP,
SAFETY,
PREVENTING
ILLNESS, AND
BEING
PREPARED FOR
LIFE-
THREATENING
EMERGENCIES

Remember, children fear nothing. Utensils, knives, silverware, and other sharp objects are extremely dangerous in their hands. They can fall or impale themselves on these objects, causing serious injury (such as the loss of an eye or damage to the inside of the ear) or even death.

yes no HAVE YOU PUT SPECIAL LOCKS OR SAFETY DEVICES ON ALL WINDOWS TO PREVENT SMALL CHILDREN FROM FALLING OR CRAWLING OUT?

☐ ☐

Children are naturally curious and natural climbers. Windows provide a fascinating view of the outside world, and they love to "see out." For children, falling out of open windows is not a rare occurrence, and the only way to prevent this is to use safety locks that allow windows to open only a small amount.

yes no ARE ALL WINDOWS AND SLIDING GLASS DOORS IN YOUR HOME MADE OF SHATTERPROOF SAFETY GLASS?

☐ ☐

In 1984, approximately 40,000 children were injured by broken windows, sliding glass doors, shower doors, and so forth.

yes no ARE THERE COLORED DECALS ON ALL SLIDING GLASS DOORS, AND ARE THESE LOW ENOUGH FOR A YOUNG PERSON TO SEE?

☐ ☐

Often children do not see the glass, and significant injuries occur when they walk or run into or even through glass doors.

yes no HAVE YOU REMOVED OR SECURED FAR BEYOND THE REACH OR CLIMBING ABILITY OF INFANTS OR CHILDREN ALL DRAPERY AND WINDOW BLIND CORDS?

☐ ☐

Remember, cords like these that hang down are potentially very dangerous and can cause serious injury or even death if, for example, the young person climbs on a chair or tabletop, puts the cord(s) around his neck, and then falls—hanging himself.

yes no IF THERE ARE STAIRS IN YOUR HOME, ARE THEY CARPETED? IS THE CARPET SECURELY FASTENED TO THE STAIRS?

☐ ☐

If a child accidentally falls, carpet will at least partially cushion the fall. It may not prevent injury in all cases, but it may reduce the degree of injury.

yes no ARE THERE SAFETY GATES AT BOTH THE TOP AND BOTTOM OF ALL STAIRS, AT ANY DOORWAY THAT GOES TO STEPS, AND AT THE ENTRANCES TO ROOMS THAT SMALL CHILDREN SHOULD NOT ENTER?

☐ ☐

In 1978, approximately 147,000 children fell down stairs and were injured. Many children crawl up stairs, only to fall back down.

yes no ARE THE SAFETY GATES AT THE TOP AND BOTTOM OF THE STAIRS
☐ ☐ BOLTED TO THE WALL? DO THEY HAVE A CLOSURE OR LOCKING-TYPE DEVICE TO ENSURE THAT THE CHILD CANNOT OPEN THEM?

Permanently installed gates are, in general, more secure and safe than portable gates.

yes no HAVE YOU MEASURED THE SPACE BETWEEN ALL RAILS OR RAIL-
☐ ☐ INGS (SUCH AS ON STAIRWAYS) TO MAKE SURE A CHILD COULD NOT SQUEEZE BETWEEN THEM OR GET HIS OR HER HEAD STUCK?

Again, falls account for a great number of childhood injuries. If the child's head gets stuck and the rest of the body slips free, a serious head or neck injury resulting in lifelong disability or even death can occur.

yes no ARE YOU CAREFUL NOT TO LEAVE THE CHILD ON A CHANGING
☐ ☐ TABLE OR OTHER HIGH, FLAT SURFACE FOR EVEN ONE SECOND?

It is estimated that annually approximately 1,750,000 infants experience falls in the first year of their lives. These falls most often occur from adult beds, tabletops, changing tables, cribs, couches, high chairs, people's arms, and other elevated surfaces. Most falls are the result of human error, in which the infant was left alone for only a moment!

yes no ARE ALL STOOLS, STEPLADDERS, AND LADDERS KEPT IN THE
☐ ☐ GARAGE, AND IS THE GARAGE LOCKED AND OFF LIMITS TO YOUR CHILDREN AND ALL OTHER CHILDREN?

As noted above, falls are extremely dangerous for youngsters and occur all the time. Stools, stepladders, and ladders also allow youngsters to reach areas and objects potentially dangerous to them.

yes no ARE THERE SAFETY PLUGS IN ALL ELECTRICAL SOCKETS NOT IN
☐ ☐ USE?

Children are intrigued by electrical sockets and will put metal and other objects in them—only to electrocute themselves. Some children will even try to put their tongues in the sockets.

yes no ARE ALL APPLIANCES UNPLUGGED WHEN NOT IN USE? HAVE YOU
☐ ☐ MADE SURE APPLIANCE CORDS ARE NOT HANGING DOWN OR WITHIN THE REACH OF CHILDREN?

GETTING HELP,
SAFETY,
PREVENTING
ILLNESS, AND
BEING
PREPARED FOR
LIFE-
THREATENING
EMERGENCIES

Children can easily pull a cord and end up with an appliance and its contents on their heads and all over them. Serious head injuries and burns occur this way.

yes no ARE ALL ELECTRIC FRYING PANS, COFFEEPOTS, TOASTERS, CAN ☐ ☐ OPENERS, IRONS, CURLING IRONS, HAIR DRYERS, AND ELECTRIC TOOTHBRUSHES KEPT FAR BEYOND THE REACH AND CLIMBING RANGE OF CHILDREN?

Youngsters are quick to imitate the actions of adults and may plug in and try to use an appliance. To say nothing of the harm that can result from improper use of the appliance, this is critically dangerous if children drop the appliance in water when operating it, reach for it, and get electrocuted.

yes no ARE YOU CAREFUL NOT TO OVERLOAD EXTENSION CORDS AND ☐ ☐ ELECTRICAL OUTLETS?

Overloaded cords and outlets can result in electrical fires, which tend to break out and spread rapidly, giving no warning.

yes no HAVE YOU MADE SURE ALL LARGE APPLIANCES, SUCH AS ☐ ☐ REFRIGERATORS, FREEZERS, WASHERS, AND DRYERS, ARE GROUNDED?

This reduces the risk of electrical fires.

yes no HAVE YOU MADE SURE THERE ARE SAFETY FEATURES ON ALL ☐ ☐ OUTDOOR ELECTRICAL OUTLETS?

The moisture naturally present out of doors increases the risk of electric shock unless outlets are designed to prevent this.

yes no DO YOU PERIODICALLY CHECK FUSES? ARE YOU CAREFUL TO ☐ ☐ REPLACE BLOWN FUSES WITH FUSES OF THE CORRECT SIZE? DO YOU FOLLOW PROPER PROCEDURES WHEN WORKING WITH LIGHTING FIXTURES, ELECTRICAL SOCKETS, TELEVISIONS, AND ALL OTHER ELECTRICAL DEVICES?

We tend to forget that electricity can be dangerous. It can cause electrocution, and it can spark a fire. The greatest respect for its potential power is warranted when working with it. Many fires are the result of faulty electrical work or the use of incorrect fuses—most often done by the homeowner.

yes no DO YOU EXAMINE YOUR ELECTRIC BLANKETS TO MAKE SURE NO
☐ ☐ WEAR OR DAMAGE IS VISIBLE?

Approximately 2,200 fires are caused by electric blankets every year.

yes no DO YOU PERIODICALLY CHECK TO MAKE SURE VENTILATION IS
☐ ☐ ADEQUATE FOR FIREPLACES, WOOD AND COAL STOVES, SPACE
HEATERS, AND OTHER HEATERS?

Carbon monoxide is an odorless, colorless gas that can easily poison and kill.
Unfortunately, this is a situation where preventive action is the only answer,
since there is no warning that the level of carbon monoxide is high or going
up, and most people won't notice that there is a problem.

yes no ARE YOU CAREFUL NOT TO LEAVE SMALL OBJECTS AND FOOD
☐ ☐ THAT YOUNG CHILDREN CAN ASPIRATE (INHALE) LYING AROUND
THE HOUSE?

Aspiration of foreign objects resulting in suffocation is the greatest cause of
accidental death in the home for children less than six years old. Foreign
objects to beware of include coins; straight pins and safety pins; toy parts and
small toys; plastic bags; balloons; corn, popcorn, peanuts, other nuts, and hard
candies; marbles; small bottle caps; erasers; tape; matches; paper clips; small
scissors; letter openers; small batteries.

yes no DO YOU MAKE IT A RULE THAT CHILDREN MUST NOT TALK, WALK,
☐ ☐ OR RUN WHILE EATING?

The grinding motion of chewing is not mastered until age four or older.
Considering this and the ease with which a youngster can aspirate when not
concentrating on chewing and swallowing food, it becomes clear that many
children can aspirate and die while trying to talk, walk, or run and eat at the
same time.

GETTING HELP,
SAFETY,
PREVENTING
ILLNESS, AND
BEING
PREPARED FOR
LIFE-
THREATENING
EMERGENCIES

POISONPROOFING THE HOME CHECKLIST

yes **no** DO YOU KNOW HOW PREVALENT ACCIDENTAL INGESTION (POI-
☐ ☐ SONING) IS IN THE UNITED STATES?

More than 5 million children are victims of accidental ingestion each year,
and over 75 percent of these children are under five years old. Considering
these alarming statistics, it is vital that all possible measures be taken to protect
our children from the threat of death or disability as a result of accidental
poisoning.

yes **no** HAVE YOU ENSURED THAT YOUR CHILDREN CANNOT REACH THE
☐ ☐ PRODUCTS *MOST OFTEN* INVOLVED IN POISONING INCIDENTS?

Household cleaners, perfumes, cosmetics, plants, fertilizers, insecticides, paints,
and medicines are the usual culprits. Perfumes, cosmetics, and medicines are
all too often easily available in women's purses; men's slacks and jacket
pockets; and on top of dressers, cabinets, and bathroom sinks.

yes **no** IS THE NUMBER OF THE NEAREST POISON CONTROL CENTER
☐ ☐ POSTED AND EASILY WITHIN REACH?

If you need to use the poison control center number, you will not want to
spend time searching for it. In poisonings, time is vital and should not be
needlessly wasted.

yes **no** HAVE YOU REMOVED ALL POISONOUS OR POTENTIALLY HARM-
☐ ☐ FUL PRODUCTS FROM THE KITCHEN AND LOCKED THEM UP ELSE-
WHERE IN THE HOUSE OR IN THE GARAGE?

The kitchen represents good food to a young person, and he or she is likely
to believe that anything in the kitchen is tasty and OK to eat.

yes **no** HAVE YOU BEEN CAREFUL NOT TO STORE ANY POISONS, GASO-
☐ ☐ LINE, TURPENTINE, PAINT THINNER, OR OTHER HARMFUL PROD-
UCTS IN UNMARKED CONTAINERS OR FOOD CONTAINERS (SODA
BOTTLES, MILK CARTONS OR BOTTLES, JUICE CONTAINERS, AND
SO ON)?

Liquids stored in this manner are easy for anyone—even adults—to drink by
mistake.

yes **no** HAVE YOU BEEN CAREFUL NOT TO PUT ANY MEDICINE IN FOOD
☐ ☐ CONTAINERS?

This, too, is a very dangerous practice and can result in a serious tragedy. Keep all medications in their original containers.

yes no HAVE YOU BEEN CAREFUL NOT TO PUT ANY FOOD OR CANDY IN ☐ ☐ MEDICINE BOTTLES OR CONTAINERS?

This is another very dangerous practice. Some parents do this to deceive youngsters, so that when they have to take medicine, they will think it will taste good—like candy. But by confusing children, this practice could result in tragedy.

yes no ARE YOU CAUTIOUS ABOUT *NEVER* CALLING ANY KIND OF MED- ☐ ☐ ICINE (INCLUDING VITAMINS) CANDY?

Children need to understand that medicine is not candy but something given them by mother or father when they don't feel well. Never say "mmmm, candy." Not only is it deceptive, but worse, it gives children the wrong signals. This practice, too, could later result in tragedy.

yes no ARE YOU CAREFUL NEVER TO TAKE MEDICINE IN FRONT OF YOUR ☐ ☐ CHILDREN (UNTIL THEY ARE MUCH OLDER AND CAN UNDER- STAND WHAT "MEDICINE" REALLY IS AND THAT THEY SHOULD NEVER TAKE IT UNLESS YOU GIVE IT TO THEM)?

Ironically, the pills our children most often see us take are the same ones that are most often implicated in poisoning incidents. These include aspirin, acetaminophen (Tylenol, Datril, and other brands), vitamins, Dimetapp (and other cold and congestion products), diazepam (Valium), flurazepam (Dalmane), and Percodan (a narcotic pain reliever). Isopropyl alcohol (rubbing alcohol) is another major culprit in poisonings.

yes no DO YOU INSIST THAT ALL MEDICINES YOU PURCHASE (BOTH PRE- ☐ ☐ SCRIBED AND OVER-THE-COUNTER) HAVE SAFETY (CHILD-RE- SISTANT) CAPS? ARE YOU CAREFUL *ALWAYS* TO SECURE THE SAFETY CAP PROPERLY EACH AND EVERY TIME YOU CLOSE THE MEDI- CATION?

The safety cap has proved to be an excellent preventive measure. The use of safety caps on aspirin has, as noted earlier, reduced aspirin poisoning by 75 percent. And that figure would be even higher if everyone replaced the cap properly after every use.

yes no DO YOU MEASURE YOUR CHILDREN'S LIQUID MEDICATIONS WITH ☐ ☐ A DROPPER/SYRINGE OR THE MEASURING DEVICE THAT COMES WITH THE PRODUCT?

GETTING HELP,
SAFETY,
PREVENTING
ILLNESS, AND
BEING
PREPARED FOR
LIFE-
THREATENING
EMERGENCIES

If not, your child could be getting either too little or too much medication. Studies show that a household teaspoon does not provide an accurate dosage. The amount of medicine dispensed can vary from 40 percent too much to 40 percent too little. With some medicines, the "too much" can result in poisoning and/or complications. The "too little" will not provide the child with the proper effects of the drug. Therefore, accurate measuring is a must for both prescribed and over-the-counter medications. Safe and accurate measuring devices are very inexpensive and are available in many markets, most drugstores, and pharmacies.

yes no ARE ALL MEDICINES *LOCKED UP* FAR BEYOND THE REACH OR
☐ ☐ CLIMBING ABILITY OF YOUNG PEOPLE? DO YOU HAVE ALL OF THE FOLLOWING IN A SAFE AND LOCKED PLACE? (AS YOU GO THROUGH THIS LIST, CONSIDER THE FACT THAT MEDICINES ACCOUNT FOR MORE THAN 60 PERCENT OF DEATHS DUE TO ACCIDENTAL POISONING.)

yes no All prescribed medications?
☐ ☐

yes no Iron pills and supplements?
☐ ☐

yes no Aspirin or acetaminophen (as-
☐ ☐ pirin substitute)?

yes no Sleeping pills?
☐ ☐

yes no Cough medicines?
☐ ☐

yes no Laxatives?
☐ ☐

yes no Antacids?
☐ ☐

yes no Medicated creams and oint-
☐ ☐ ments?

yes no Diet pills?
☐ ☐

yes no Anesthetic creams?
☐ ☐

yes no Antihistamines?
☐ ☐

yes no Nose sprays and inhalers?
☐ ☐

yes no Cold medications?
☐ ☐

yes no All aerosols?
☐ ☐

yes no Vitamins, especially those with
☐ ☐ iron?

yes no HAVE YOU FLUSHED DOWN THE TOILET ALL OUTDATED MEDI-
☐ ☐ CINES OR UNUSED PRESCRIPTIONS IN YOUR HOME, CAR, AND
OFFICE? (WOMEN SHOULD CHECK THEIR PURSES, TOO.) DO YOU
PERIODICALLY RECHECK ALL THESE AREAS AND DESTROY OUT-
DATED MEDICINES OR UNUSED PRESCRIPTIONS?

It's a good idea to remind grandparents, relatives, and friends to do this as
well. Remember, the more medications you have around, the greater the risk
that a poisoning will occur.

yes no ARE ALL HOUSEHOLD CLEANERS, INSECTICIDES, AND OTHER PO-
☐ ☐ TENTIALLY DANGEROUS HOUSEHOLD, GARDEN, OR OTHER PROD-
UCTS *LOCKED UP* AND FAR BEYOND THE REACH OR CLIMBING
ABILITY OF YOUNG PEOPLE? DO YOU HAVE ALL OF THE FOLLOW-
ING IN A SAFE AND LOCKED PLACE?

yes no Rug cleaner?
☐ ☐

yes no Powder laundry detergent?
☐ ☐

yes no Oven cleaner?
☐ ☐

yes no Laundry spray aids?
☐ ☐

yes no Solvents?
☐ ☐

yes no Dry cleaning agents and spot re-
☐ ☐ movers?

yes no Acids and alkalis?
☐ ☐

yes no Floor polish and wax?
☐ ☐

yes no Drain cleaner?
☐ ☐

yes no Metal polish (silver, copper and
☐ ☐ the like)?

yes no Toilet bowl cleaner?
☐ ☐

yes no Dish soap and detergent?
☐ ☐

yes no Lye?
☐ ☐

yes no Automatic dishwasher deter-
☐ ☐ gent?

yes no All bleaches?
☐ ☐

yes no Scouring powder and liquid?
☐ ☐

yes no Liquid laundry detergent?
☐ ☐

yes no Ammonia?
☐ ☐

GETTING HELP,
SAFETY,
PREVENTING
ILLNESS, AND
BEING
PREPARED FOR
LIFE-
THREATENING
EMERGENCIES

yes no Shoe polish?
☐ ☐

yes no Rubbing alcohol?
☐ ☐

yes no Furniture polish and wax?
☐ ☐

yes no Aerosol and pump-type contain-
☐ ☐ ers?

yes no Cleaning agents?
☐ ☐

yes no Perfume/cologne?
☐ ☐

yes no Rust remover?
☐ ☐

yes no Hair shampoo?
☐ ☐

yes no Mothballs?
☐ ☐

yes no Toothpaste?
☐ ☐

yes no Fingernail polish remover and
☐ ☐ cuticle remover?

yes no Mouthwash?
☐ ☐

yes no Hair spray?
☐ ☐

yes no Rough-skin remover?
☐ ☐

yes no Suntan lotion/oils?
☐ ☐

yes no Talc powder?
☐ ☐

yes no Instant-bonding glue, plastic
☐ ☐ glue?

yes no Air freshener?
☐ ☐

yes no Facial scrubs?
☐ ☐

yes no Lighter fluid?
☐ ☐

yes no Cosmetics/makeup?
☐ ☐

yes no Batteries—especially small, but-
☐ ☐ tonlike batteries?

yes no Deodorant?
☐ ☐

yes no Diaper pail deodorant?
☐ ☐

yes no ARE THE FOLLOWING PRODUCTS FAR BEYOND THE REACH OF
☐ ☐ CHILDREN AND PREFERABLY LOCKED UP IN THE GARAGE OR
OTHER STORAGE AREA AWAY FROM THE HOUSE?

yes no Industrial cleaners? ☐ ☐

yes no Fertilizer? ☐ ☐

yes no Pesticides? ☐ ☐

yes no Boric acid? ☐ ☐

yes no Weed killer? ☐ ☐

yes no Charcoal starter? ☐ ☐

yes no Kerosene? ☐ ☐

yes no Gasoline? ☐ ☐

yes no Turpentine? ☐ ☐

yes no Paint, stain, varnish, and so forth? ☐ ☐

yes no Paint thinner? ☐ ☐

yes no Varnish, paint, and stain removers? ☐ ☐

yes no Plant food? ☐ ☐

yes no DO YOU PURCHASE HOUSEHOLD PRODUCTS THAT HAVE SAFETY ☐ ☐ CAPS OR CLOSURES ON THEM?

Like the safety (child-resistant) caps used on medications, safety caps or closures on household products have greatly reduced the incidence of poisoning with those products that have them. Again, it is vital that care be taken to replace the cap or closure properly each time the product is used.

yes no DO YOU KNOW WHAT KIND OF HOUSEHOLD, GARDEN, AND LAWN ☐ ☐ PLANTS, SHRUBS, AND BUSHES YOU HAVE? HAVE YOU CHECKED TO MAKE SURE THAT NONE IS POISONOUS?

Some very common ornamental and flowering plants are quite poisonous. Many poison control centers have lists of poisonous and nonpoisonous plants. Call the center to see if it has such a list or book or can tell you where to get one.

yes no DO YOU KNOW THE BOTANICAL NAMES OF THE PLANTS IN YOUR ☐ ☐ HOUSE AND YARD, AS WELL AS THE TREES IN YOUR YARD?

If a child eats a plant or part of a plant or nibbles at it, the poison control center would need to know *what plant* (botanical name) was involved if you're

54

GETTING HELP,
SAFETY,
PREVENTING
ILLNESS, AND
BEING
PREPARED FOR
LIFE-
THREATENING
EMERGENCIES

not sure whether it is poisonous. An easy way to remember the plants is to tape the botanical name *to the bottom* of the plant container. It's always best, though, to simply eliminate all known poisonous plants from the *house and yard*. Take a list of poisonous and nonpoisonous plants with you to the nursery, so you can be sure of what you are buying. If a certain plant or flower is not on your list—don't buy it until you find out *for sure* that it is not poisonous. Ask at a reputable nursery, or call the poison control center, giving the botanical name. The staff will usually be happy to tell you whether or not the plant is poisonous (if they are not involved in an emergency or urgent situation).

yes no ARE YOU CAREFUL *NOT* TO SHAKE BABY POWDER OR TALC PROD-
☐   ☐   UCTS NEAR A BABY'S FACE OR ALLOW THE BABY TO SHAKE THE POWDER NEAR HIS OR HER FACE?

Baby powder and talc products can cause severe respiratory distress if inhaled.

yes no DO YOU AVOID USING TOILET-TANK CLEANERS?
☐   ☐
Many toddlers (and pets) find drinking or playing in this water inviting.

yes no DO YOU PURCHASE ONLY THOSE ART SUPPLIES WITH AN AP OR
☐   ☐   CP SEAL OF APPROVAL ON THE PACKAGING BOX OR BOTTLE?

These seals tell you that the Crayon, Water Color, and Craft Institute, Inc., has tested the product and has found it not to be acutely toxic. Products with the approval seals do not contain any *known* carcinogen (cancer-causing agent) or mutagen (agent know to cause mutations). To obtain a complete list of art supplies with the AP or CP seal of approval, write: Crayon, Water Color, and Craft Institute, Inc., 715 Boylston Street, Boston, Massachusetts 02116.

yes no DO YOU KNOW WHICH ART SUPPLIES WOULD BE DANGEROUS FOR
☐   ☐   CHILDREN?

The best rule of thumb is, if the product is safe to eat or smell, then children can use it. Some dangerous art materials include rubber cement; oil paints; india inks; epoxy and polyurethane adhesives; permanent (indelible) felt-type markers; aerosol fixatives and aerosol paints (in fact, any aerosol); most dyes used for batik or tie dye; airplane glue; and anything containing lead, mercury, uranium, manganese, chromium, and countless other chemicals; and all cleaning and thinning solvents. For more-detailed information, the handbook *Artist Beware*, by Dr. Michael McCann, has an excellent chapter on art materials and children.

yes no IF YOU DO ART OR PHOTOGRAPHIC WORK AT HOME, ARE *ALL* ART
☐ ☐ SUPPLIES AND PROCESSING CHEMICALS LOCKED UP WHEN NOT
IN USE?

Since many art supplies are dangerous if ingested or inhaled, they should
always be under lock and key. It's best to have one room set aside for working
on art or other projects, so it can be locked at all times. Set up a system so
that you always know where your child is whenever art supplies or photographic
chemicals are in use.

BURN-PREVENTION CHECKLIST

yes no ARE THERE PROPERLY WORKING SMOKE DETECTORS IN YOUR
☐ ☐ HOME?

In a fire, inhalation of smoke or toxic gases is the cause of death more often
(74 percent of the time) than the fire itself. Smoke detectors give an early
warning signal, long before smoke might be seen or smelled or heat from the
fire might be felt—particularly if you are in another part of the house or
everyone is asleep. Considering the fact that 1,500 children die and another
48,000 are injured by fire each year in the United States, it's important to do
everything possible to prevent fires and to provide early warning when fires
do break out.

yes no DO YOU HAVE FIRE EXTINGUISHERS WITHIN REACH IN YOUR
☐ ☐ HOME?

It's important to remember that 75 percent of all fires occur in the home
(residential fires).

yes no DO YOU HAVE A FIRE ESCAPE (EVACUATION) PLAN THAT EVERY-
☐ ☐ ONE UNDERSTANDS?

It is estimated that 90 percent of deaths due to fire could be prevented if all
fire safety measures were diligently followed.

yes no DO YOU AND ALL FAMILY MEMBERS PERIODICALLY PRACTICE
☐ ☐ HOME FIRE DRILLS SO ESCAPE WOULD BE AUTOMATIC IF A FIRE
BROKE OUT?

Research and experience show that there is a critical four-minute time period
in which to get out. Remember, too, that any child under the age of five is

GETTING HELP,
SAFETY,
PREVENTING
ILLNESS, AND
BEING
PREPARED FOR
LIFE-
THREATENING
EMERGENCIES

four times more likely to die in a fire than his or her parents. It's vital to plan in advance who will get a young child out of the house. Older children and teenagers must know where to go (the escape route), so they do not panic.

yes no HAVE YOU TAUGHT YOUR CHILDREN SAFETY RULES AROUND
☐ ☐ THE STOVE, OVEN, OTHER COOKING APPLIANCES, THE WASHER, DRYER, AND ALL OTHER APPLIANCES?

For very young children, safety rules should mean they are not allowed even to be near these appliances. This is particularly true of the stove, where the vast majority of scald burns are the result of hot foods or liquids spilling on youngsters. Children most vulnerable are between nine and nineteen months of age. Older children and young people should be taught how to cook and use appliances safely but should *not* be allowed to do so without your presence and supervision. Teenagers should be taught to cook and use these appliances and should understand safety precautions so they do not injure themselves or others (particularly little ones) who are nearby.

yes no DO YOU ALWAYS USE THE BACK BURNERS OF THE STOVE AND
☐ ☐ TURN ALL POT AND PAN HANDLES TO THE REAR?

A frightening number of children experience serious head injuries every year because objects fall on them or are pulled down on top of them. When cooking is involved, potential injuries become even more serious and would include severe burns.

yes no HAVE YOU TURNED DOWN YOUR HOT WATER HEATER TO 120
☐ ☐ DEGREES FAHRENHEIT?

Did you know that it takes only two seconds of contact with water 150 degrees Fahrenheit to cause deep second- and third-degree burns in an adult? Imagine the severe damage an infant or young person could experience!

yes no IN YOUR HOME, DO YOU USE ONLY COOL-MIST HUMIDIFIERS
☐ ☐ (RATHER THAN STEAM VAPORIZERS) FOR YOUR CHILDREN?

They are effective in adding moisture to the air while eliminating burn hazard.

yes no DO YOU TEST THE TEMPERATURE OF CAR SEATS AND CHILD-
☐ ☐ RESTRAINT SEATS BEFORE PLACING A CHILD IN OR ON THE SEAT?

Many burns result from contact with hot car seats, with children under one year old experiencing the highest rate of this kind of burn. Some child-restraint seats are available in corduroy, which tends to stay cool. You can also simply cover the child-restraint or car seat with a towel or blanket, to protect the seat from overheating, or use a commercial cloth seat cover.

yes no ARE ALL MATCHES, LIGHTERS, CIGARETTES, CIGARS, AND PIPE
☐ ☐ TOBACCO KEPT IN A CUPBOARD FAR BEYOND THE REACH OR
CLIMBING ABILITY OF YOUNG CHILDREN? IS THERE A SAFETY
LOCK OR LATCH ON THE CUPBOARD?

Matches and lighters are serious fire hazards. You should also realize that tobacco products are poisonous. If a young person ingests enough tobacco, it can make him or her quite ill.

yes no IF YOU OR OTHERS IN YOUR HOME (OR VISITORS) SMOKE, ARE
☐ ☐ YOU ALWAYS CAREFUL TO THOROUGHLY SOAK CIGARETTE BUTTS
BEFORE EMPTYING THEM INTO THE TRASH OR SEAL THEM IN
ALUMINUM FOIL? DO YOU CHECK AROUND AND DOWN THE SIDES
OF FURNITURE CUSHIONS FOR SMOLDERING CIGARETTES AFTER
PARTIES OR WHEN YOU'VE HAD GUESTS WHO SMOKE? IS IT A
RULE IN YOUR HOUSE THAT *NO ONE* SMOKES IN BED—EVEN
GUESTS?

Improper handling of cigarettes and matches is the cause of almost half of all home (residential) fires.

yes no DO YOU PERIODICALLY CHECK ALL GAS APPLIANCES (SUCH AS
☐ ☐ STOVES, HEATERS, AND BARBECUES) FOR DEFECTS, POOR PIPING,
LEAKS, AND IMPROPER VENTILATION?

Leaks into closed rooms present hazards for explosions and fires. Natural gas can also cause brain damage and death due to lack of oxygen.

yes no DO YOU PERIODICALLY CHECK ALL ELECTRICAL CORDS AND RE-
☐ ☐ PLACE THEM IMMEDIATELY IF DAMAGED, FRAYED, OR TORN IN
ANY WAY? DO YOU PROPERLY TAPE OR REPLACE CORDS WITH
EXPOSED WIRES? PERIODICALLY CHECK THE WIRING AND CORDS
OF ELECTRIC HEATERS AND REPLACE DAMAGED ONES?

All of these measures decrease the risk of electrical fires, electric shock, and severe burns. In particular, youngsters who chew on damaged electrical cords can get serious mouth burns, which usually require extensive plastic surgery to repair.

yes no IF YOU HAVE A WOOD OR COAL STOVE, DO YOU EXERCISE EX-
☐ ☐ TRAORDINARY CAUTION IN ITS USE?

Each year, 14,000 fires are caused by wood or coal stoves.

GETTING HELP,
SAFETY,
PREVENTING
ILLNESS, AND
BEING
PREPARED FOR
LIFE-
THREATENING
EMERGENCIES

yes no IS THERE A STURDY METAL SCREEN ON YOUR FIREPLACE?

Crawlers and toddlers are especially at risk for crawling or falling into un-protected fireplaces.

yes no IS GASOLINE FOR LAWN MOWERS AND OTHER EQUIPMENT KEPT IN SAFETY CANS (WITH FLAME ARRESTERS AND PRESSURE-RE-LEASE VALVES) AND LOCKED IN THE GARAGE? DO YOU DRAIN THE GASOLINE FROM ALL EQUIPMENT AFTER EACH USE AND START MOTORS ONLY OUTDOORS?

One gallon of gasoline exploding has the same force as twenty sticks of dynamite. Gasoline builds up pressure inside containers not meant for storing it. This includes gasoline-operated equipment, which is not designed for storing the fuel. Gasoline is much more sensitive than we tend to think, and accidents take place all the time. Never allow your children to be near when you start gas-operated equipment.

yes no WHENEVER POSSIBLE, DO YOU PURCHASE FLAME-RETARDANT SLEEPWEAR AND CLOTHING FOR YOUR CHILDREN?

Make sure to tell children that if their clothes ever catch on fire, they should never run but should immediately shout for help as they drop to the ground and roll until the fire is out. It is prudent to have them periodically demonstrate this technique for you.

yes no DO YOU FORBID YOUR CHILDREN TO PLAY WITH FIRECRACKERS AND FIREWORKS OR AT LEAST HANDLE SUCH ITEMS YOURSELF AND LET THE CHILDREN ENJOY JUST WATCHING THEM?

Thousands of children lost fingers, hands, and eyes and experienced severe burns from playing with fireworks each year—until many states restricted their use. In states without restrictions, the injuries continue. From smoke bombs to roman candles to sparklers—every kind of fireworks has been directly associated with serious injuries. It is ''safe and sane'' to go to a public fireworks display rather than to let a child or young person risk serious injury or even lifelong disability.

INFANT AND CHILD FURNITURE, EQUIPMENT, AND SUPPLIES SAFETY CHECKLIST

yes no DO YOU KNOW HOW PREVALENT INJURIES ARE THAT ARE DI-
☐ ☐ RECTLY RELATED TO NURSERY FURNITURE, EQUIPMENT, AND
SUPPLIES?

More than forty thousand infants and young children were treated in emergency
rooms in 1982 for injuries sustained from nursery furniture, equipment, and
supplies. In fact, 87 percent of recorded injuries and deaths could probably
have been avoided if equipment, furniture, and supplies had been properly
selected and safety precautions followed. Information about the safety of nursery furniture or toys can be requested from the U.S. Consumer Product Safety
Commission. It has a toll-free "Hot Line" number (1–800–638-CPSC) and
its staff will be happy to answer any question(s) you may have.

yes no DOES YOUR CHILD'S CRIB HAVE A LABEL SAYING THAT IT MEETS
☐ ☐ THE "FEDERAL CRIB STANDARD"?

Cribs with this label meet basic safety requirements and should be the cribs
of choice.

yes no ARE THE SLATS OF THE CRIB NO MORE THAN 2 ⅜ INCHES APART?
☐ ☐
This distance prevents infants from slipping through the slats and strangling
or getting their heads stuck.

yes no WHEN THE SIDES OF THE CRIB ARE LOWERED, ARE THEY FOUR
☐ ☐ INCHES ABOVE THE MATTRESS?

This ensures that there is at least a low barrier to prevent rolling.

yes no ARE YOU VERY CAREFUL NOT TO LEAVE THE BABY IN THE CRIB
☐ ☐ WITH THE RAIL(S) DOWN—EVEN WHEN YOU ARE "JUST ACROSS
THE ROOM," "A FEW STEPS AWAY," OR "GONE FOR A SECOND"?

The first time a baby rolls over is always a "surprise," and many infants are
very fast about rolling right onto the floor.

yes no HAVE YOU CHECKED TO SEE THAT THERE ARE NO GAPS BETWEEN
☐ ☐ THE MATTRESS AND THE SIDES OF THE CRIB?

Infants have slipped down into such gaps and suffocated or been trapped.

GETTING HELP,
SAFETY,
PREVENTING
ILLNESS, AND
BEING
PREPARED FOR
LIFE-
THREATENING
EMERGENCIES

yes no DO YOU PERIODICALLY CHECK TO SEE THAT THERE ARE NO LOOSE
☐ ☐ SPRINGS IN THE CRIB?

This makes the mattress surface unstable, increasing the possibility of falls if
an infant can stand or walk around the crib.

yes no HAVE YOU CAREFULLY CHECKED THE CRIB FOR SPLINTERS,
☐ ☐ CRACKS IN THE PAINT, OR PEELING PAINT?

Each of these can cause a serious injury, and if lead-based paint is swallowed,
poisoning and even death can result. If it is an older crib, it is best to remove
all old paint and repaint the entire crib with lead-free paint.

yes no IS THERE A LOCKING, HAND-OPERATED LATCH ON THE CRIB THAT
☐ ☐ CANNOT BE RELEASED ACCIDENTALLY?

Serious injury can occur if the child leans on the rail and it releases. The child
tumbles to the floor, and in most cases, a head injury results.

yes no ARE ALL MOBILES FAR OUT OF REACH, AND ARE LARGE TOYS
☐ ☐ AND STUFFED ANIMALS REMOVED FROM THE CRIB WHEN THE
BABY IS ASLEEP?

Aspiration of parts is always possible, as is suffocation from large stuffed
animals. To prevent hanging injuries, remove mobiles when the infant can
pull himself or herself up and stand.

yes no HAVE YOU BEEN LOWERING THE CRIB MATTRESS AS THE BABY
☐ ☐ GROWS?

When the child reaches thirty-five inches tall, the crib should no longer be
used, since he or she can crawl and then fall out of the crib.

yes no DOES THE HIGH CHAIR HAVE A LABEL ON IT THAT STATES THAT
☐ ☐ THE CHAIR MEETS THE SAFETY REQUIREMENTS OF THE "VOL-
UNTARY STANDARD"?

Unfortunately, head injuries occur in 75 percent of high chair–related accidents, so care should be taken to purchase a safe high chair.

yes no IS THERE A WIDE BASE ON THE HIGH CHAIR?
☐ ☐ Active youngsters can tip narrow-based chairs, and these falls can result in
serious head and other injuries.

yes no DOES THE HIGH CHAIR HAVE A SECURE WAIST STRAP AND A
☐ ☐ CROTCH STRAP THAT RUNS BETWEEN THE CHILD'S LEGS? DO YOU
SECURELY FASTEN THE CHILD IN WITH *ALL* SAFETY STRAPS EVERY
TIME HE OR SHE IS PUT IN THE HIGH CHAIR?

Falls from high chairs are a serious problem, and care must be taken to prevent
such falls by carefully securing the child so he or she doesn't slip out of the
chair and tumble to the floor.

yes no IF YOU HAVE ONE OF THE OLDER CHAIRS (ONE THAT DOES NOT
☐ ☐ MEET VOLUNTARY SAFETY REQUIREMENTS), HAVE YOU PUR-
CHASED A SAFETY HARNESS FOR YOUR CHILD?

These older high chairs do not comply with present safety standards. A child
can more easily slip under the tray; the crotch strap that attaches to the tray
may not hold well; or the child can more easily climb out of the chair. It is
best to buy a safety harness to attach to these older high chairs.

yes no DO YOU PERIODICALLY CHECK ALL HIGH-CHAIR SAFETY DEVICES
☐ ☐ (THE STRAPS, THE ATTACHMENT POINTS, THE CONDITION OF THE
TRAY) TO ENSURE THAT THEY ARE STURDY AND SECURE AND
THAT THEY WORK PROPERLY?

Many accidents are due to frayed straps, deteriorating attachment points, and
a broken or warped tray.

yes no DO YOU TEST THE TRAY TO MAKE SURE IT LOCKS SECURELY AND
☐ ☐ PROPERLY—*EVERY TIME* YOU PUT THE CHILD IN THE HIGH CHAIR?

If the tray is not securely latched, the child can easily fall out.

yes no IF YOU HAVE A FOLDING HIGH CHAIR, DO YOU CHECK TO MAKE
☐ ☐ SURE THE LOCKING DEVICE IS SECURE EACH TIME YOU SET UP
THE CHAIR?

If the locking device fails, the chair will collapse, and the potential injuries
to the child could be serious.

yes no DO YOU PUT THE HIGH CHAIR (FOLDING OR NOT) IN A CORNER
☐ ☐ OUT OF THE WAY WHEN IT IS NOT IN USE?

Other children (and even adults) have been seriously injured by an unoccupied
high chair that fell on them.

GETTING HELP,
SAFETY,
PREVENTING
ILLNESS, AND
BEING
PREPARED FOR
LIFE-
THREATENING
EMERGENCIES

yes no HAVE YOU MADE IT A RULE THAT YOUR OTHER CHILDREN NOT
☐ ☐ BE ALLOWED TO RUN OR PLAY NEAR, CLIMB ON, HANG ON TO,
OR LEAN AGAINST THE HIGH CHAIR?

In these situations, injuries can be sustained not only by the young child in
the chair but also by others if the chair and child fall on them.

yes no IS IT A POLICY IN YOUR HOME THAT *NO ONE* CLIMB INTO THE
☐ ☐ HIGH CHAIR WITHOUT ASSISTANCE?

Children should never be allowed to climb into the high chair by themselves.
It can easily tip while the young person is in it or getting into it.

yes no DO YOU ALWAYS CHECK TO SEE WHERE THE CHILD'S HANDS AND
☐ ☐ FEET ARE WHEN ATTACHING AND DETACHING THE HIGH CHAIR'S
TRAY?

Many injuries occur when fingers and toes are caught or skin is trapped.

yes no IF YOUR CHILD SEEMS TO SLIP AROUND ON THE SEAT OF THE
☐ ☐ HIGH CHAIR, HAVE YOU PUT ROUGH-SURFACED ADHESIVE STRIPS
OR ANTISLIP RUBBER SPOTS (LIKE THOSE USED FOR SHOWERS
AND BATHTUBS) ON THE HIGH CHAIR SEAT?

Doing this makes the chair seat more slip-resistant and reduces the likelihood
of the child's sliding out of the chair and experiencing a serious head, neck,
back, or other injury.

yes no ARE YOU CAREFUL *NEVER* TO PLACE AN INFANT SEAT ON AN
☐ ☐ ELEVATED SURFACE (TABLE, CHAIR, BED, SINK, AND SO ON)?

Even a very young infant can move the seat on a slippery surface, and other
people can bump into the infant, knocking the seat off the surface.

yes no ARE YOU CAREFUL NOT TO PLACE AN INFANT SEAT ACROSS THE
☐ ☐ TOP OF A SHOPPING CART?

The seat can easily be jarred by a passing shopper or a child, throwing the
baby out of the cart.

yes no IF YOU HAVE OR ARE GOING TO PURCHASE A BABY WALKER
☐ ☐ (BABY BOUNCER, WALKER-JUMPER, OR SIMILAR PRODUCT), HAVE
YOU CHECKED THAT IT DOES NOT HAVE ANY OF THE FOLLOWING
POTENTIALLY DANGEROUS FEATURES: SCISSOR-ACTION BRACES
(WHICH CAN PINCH, SHEAR, OR—EVEN WORSE—AMPUTATE FIN-
GERS, TOES, AND OTHER AREAS WHEN CLOSING), EXPOSED
SPRINGS, BREAKABLE PLASTIC SEATS, IMPROPER WHEEL ALIGN-
MENT, LOOSE OR MISSING SCREWS, AND THE POTENTIAL TO COL-
LAPSE WHILE IN USE?

Avoiding these dangerous features could prevent needless injury to your infant.

yes no ARE YOU CAREFUL TO SUPERVISE THE BABY AT ALL TIMES WHILE
☐ ☐ HE OR SHE IS IN THE WALKER?

Many serious injuries related to walkers occur when unsupervised infants go
outdoors and fall down steps, tip over, and so on. Approximately 15,000
infants and young children required emergency room care for walker and
jumper injuries in 1984.

yes no ARE YOU CAUTIOUS ABOUT NEVER LEAVING A CHILD ALONE
☐ ☐ WHILE HE OR SHE IS IN A STROLLER?

The vast majority of injuries occur when the child attempts to climb out and
falls (often on his or her head).

yes no DO YOU CHECK THE RESTRAINING STRAPS TO MAKE SURE THEY
☐ ☐ ARE IN GOOD CONDITION AND STAY SECURE WHEN THE CHILD
IS IN THE STROLLER?

Remember also to check for sharp edges and corners and possible pinch points
when purchasing a new stroller.

yes no IS THE CHILD'S PLAYPEN *FREE OF* PINCH POINTS, BREAKABLE
☐ ☐ PLASTIC DECORATIONS OR DECORATIONS THAT CAN BE PULLED
OFF, SHARP CORNERS, SPLINTERS, TOXIC PAINT, OR SLATS THAT
ARE MORE THAN 2 ½ TO 3 INCHES APART?

Such concerns are very real, and you should make sure the playpen presents
none of these hazards. Playpens with mesh sides and padded floors, rails, and
supports are the safest choice.

64

GETTING HELP,
SAFETY,
PREVENTING
ILLNESS, AND
BEING
PREPARED FOR
LIFE-
THREATENING
EMERGENCIES

yes no IF YOU HAVE A PLAYPEN WITH MESH SIDES, DO YOU ALWAYS
☐ ☐ MAKE SURE THE SIDES ARE SECURELY LOCKED IN THE "UP"
POSITION WHEN A LITTLE ONE IS INSIDE?

Suffocation has occurred when young infants were left with the mesh side
down. Their heads were caught between the soft mattress and the mesh side.

yes no IS THE TOY CHEST *FREE OF* A LID, SHARP CORNERS AND EDGES,
☐ ☐ AND HINGES WITH SCISSORLIKE ACTION?

Open containers (without lids) with rounded edges and corners or padding are
much safer and usually do not cause injury. Lids, hinges, and sharp corners
present rather serious hazards. An estimated 4,800 injuries related to toy chests
were serious enough to require emergency care in 1984. Sixty-seven percent
involved children less than four years of age.

yes no IF YOUR INFANT OR CHILD HAS A PACIFIER, IS IT A SINGLE-PIECE
☐ ☐ PACIFIER THAT DOES NOT COME APART WHEN YOU PULL HARD
ON IT? HAVE YOU REMOVED ANY CHAINS OR CORDS FROM THE
PACIFIER? (THESE ARE OFTEN PUT AROUND THE LITTLE ONE'S
NECK SO THE PACIFIER WON'T BE LOST.)

Aspiration (inhalation of an object) can occur if the pacifier can be pulled
apart, and having a chain or cord around the neck of an active child puts him
at risk for strangulation. Pin or tie the string to the child's clothing if you feel
you must attach the pacifier to him. (Better yet, restrict pacifier use to "quiet
time" or bedtime.)

yes no ARE YOU USING PLASTIC RATHER THAN GLASS BOTTLES IF YOUR
☐ ☐ CHILD HOLDS HER OWN BOTTLE? DO YOU PERIODICALLY CHECK
THE CONDITION OF THE NIPPLES AND THROW OUT THE ONES
THAT ARE BEGINNING TO TEAR OR BECOMING SOFT ENOUGH TO
BITE OFF?

Glass bottles can cause serious injury if children throw them or even hit them
on the floor while sucking on them, because they might break and the glass
might shatter if they are not shatterproof. Nipples that tear or are too soft or
worn can easily be bitten off and aspirated or choked on.

yes no ARE ALL SAFETY PINS AND OTHER SMALL OR POTENTIALLY DAN-
☐ ☐ GEROUS ITEMS AND SUBSTANCES (INCLUDING LOTIONS, COTTON
BALLS, COTTON SWABS, ROOM DEODORANTS, AND SO ON) KEPT
FAR BEYOND THE REACH AND CLIMBING RANGE OF YOUNG-
STERS?

Serious injury, poisoning, and aspiration (inhaling an object) can result from many infant supplies. These need to be kept away from cribs, dressing tables, and so forth and preferably secured in a high cupboard or locked in a dresser drawer in the child's room. Watch the child carefully when these supplies are out and being used. Be especially careful with toddlers and preschoolers, who can get into the supplies meant for a smaller infant.

BICYCLES, ROLLER SKATES, AND OTHER "WHEELS" SAFETY CHECKLIST

yes no HAVE YOU MADE IT CLEAR THAT A BICYCLE IS NOT A TOY BUT
☐ ☐ A VEHICLE? DO YOUR CHILDREN UNDERSTAND ALL RULES OF THE ROAD AND SAFETY PRECAUTIONS?

Ninety percent of bicycle-related deaths are the result of accidents where the young person was at fault. Most often the rider does not stop at a stop sign or red light, darts out of a driveway or alley or into the middle of an intersection, or suddenly pulls in front of a car without looking.

yes no WERE YOU CAREFUL TO BUY A BICYCLE THE CORRECT SIZE FOR
☐ ☐ YOUR YOUNGSTER, NOT ONE HE OR SHE CAN "GROW INTO"?

Many accidents are the result of a bicycle's being too big for the rider. He or she cannot control the bike well and cannot stop fast enough because the brakes are too far away. The youngster should be able to place his or her feet flat on the ground (without stretching) when comfortably seated on the bicycle seat. There should be at least a one-inch clearance between the center bar and the youngster's crotch. And handlebars and hand brakes should be easy to reach.

yes no DO YOU INSTRUCT YOUR CHILDREN NOT TO RIDE DOUBLE, SHOW
☐ ☐ OFF, OR DART ACROSS STREETS BUT RATHER TO WALK THE BIKE AT MARKED INTERSECTIONS AND FOLLOW ALL SAFETY RULES AND TRAFFIC LAWS?

It is estimated that in 1982 approximately 447,000 people experienced bicycle-related injuries serious enough to be treated in an emergency room.

GETTING HELP,
SAFETY,
PREVENTING
ILLNESS, AND
BEING
PREPARED FOR
LIFE-
THREATENING
EMERGENCIES

yes no ARE YOU CAREFUL TO PROVIDE PERIODIC MAINTENANCE OF YOUR
☐ ☐ YOUNGSTER'S BICYCLE TO ENSURE PROPER MECHANICAL FUNC-
TIONING? DO YOU MAKE SURE THAT ALL FENDERS ARE RE-
PAIRED; BOLTS ARE TIGHT; THE TENSION ON THE CHAIN IS
CORRECT AND THE CHAIN IS OILED ROUTINELY; THE BRAKES
WORK PROPERLY AND ARE NOT TOO WORN (THEY ALLOW THE
BICYCLE TO STOP EASILY AND SAFELY); THE HANDLEBARS ARE
SECURED (NOT LOOSE) AND AT THE PROPER HEIGHT; THE SEAT
IS NOT LOOSE AND IS AT ITS PROPER HEIGHT; THE TIRES ARE
INFLATED TO THE CORRECT PRESSURE AT ALL TIMES; THE WHEELS
ARE NOT UNSTABLE (WIGGLY AND WOBBLY); AND THERE IS A
CHAIN GUARD ON THE BICYCLE?

Countless bike injuries occur as a result of mechanical failures. Bicycles have
been ranked number one or two on the U.S. Consumer Product Safety Commission's Hazard Index for the past five years. Proper maintenance, then, is
vital for the protection of our children, considering the fact that bicycles have
a significant risk factor for injury anyway.

yes no DOES YOUR YOUNGSTER'S BIKE HAVE LIGHTS AND REFLECTORS,
☐ ☐ AND DO YOU INSIST THAT REFLECTIVE CLOTHING BE WORN WHEN
THE BICYCLE IS RIDDEN AT NIGHT?

In many car–bike accidents that occur at night, the driver of the car was really
not at fault because he or she couldn't see the youngster on the bicycle in
time. Considering this, no youngster should be allowed to ride a bicycle at
night unless it is properly equipped with lights and reflectors. The youngster
should have a reflective armband or reflective tape on his or her jacket (both
front and back), as well.

yes no IS IT A RULE IN YOUR HOME THAT NO INFANT UNDER SIX MONTHS
☐ ☐ OLD BE CARRIED ON A BICYCLE?

These infants are much too small to be safely carried on a bicycle. Also, any
fall might prove to be life-threatening.

yes no IF YOUR CHILD IS SIX MONTHS TO ONE YEAR OLD AND YOU CARRY
☐ ☐ HIM OR HER ON A BICYCLE, DO YOU USE A BACKPACK-TYPE
CARRIER?

This is the safest way to carry a child in this age group. It is important, too,
that you be an excellent bicycle rider and that you have the strength to carry
the child safely.

yes no IF YOU HAVE A CHILD BETWEEN ONE YEAR AND FOUR YEARS
☐ ☐ OLD (UP TO FORTY POUNDS) AND YOU CARRY HIM OR HER ON
YOUR BICYCLE, DO YOU PUT THE CHILD IN A SEAT DESIGNED
AND MANUFACTURED FOR THAT PURPOSE?

There are special bicycle carriers for children on the market. Care should be
taken to purchase one that is sturdy, protects the child's hands and feet from
the wheels and spokes, and is built to be stable. Some have protective guards
for knees also. The seat should have a strong seat belt, which should always
be secured when the child is in the seat. Some experts also recommend that
a helmet and knee and elbow pads be worn by the child whenever riding on
the bicycle.

yes no WHEN YOUR CHILD IS A PASSENGER ON YOUR BICYCLE, DO YOU
☐ ☐ RIDE SLOWLY AND CAREFULLY AND BEGIN BRAKING LONG BE-
FORE YOU NEED TO STOP?

Whenever there is a passenger on a bicycle, it takes longer to stop, and speeds
can easily increase rapidly. Care should be taken to go *slowly* around corners.

yes no DOES YOUR CHILD'S TRICYCLE FIT HIS OR HER BODY SIZE AND
☐ ☐ HAVE WIDELY SPACED WHEELS, A SEAT THAT IS CLOSE TO THE
GROUND, HANDGRIPS AND PEDALS WITH NONSLIP (ROUGH) SUR-
FACES, AND NO SHARP EDGES ANYWHERE ON THE TRICYCLE?

These safety measures help prevent injuries. Remember, a tricycle can easily
tip over if the child cannot control it or the tricycle is unstable.

yes no HAVE YOU ESTABLISHED VERY SPECIFIC SAFETY RULES FOR RID-
☐ ☐ ING THE TRICYCLE?

Experts estimate that twelve thousand youngsters required emergency room
treatment in 1984 as a result of injuries due to tricycles. Most occurred because
the child was going too fast, couldn't stop, hit an obstacle or collided with
another tricycle or bicycle, or tipped over while going around a corner or turn.

yes no IF YOUR YOUNGSTER RIDES A SKATEBOARD, IS IT A RULE THAT
☐ ☐ HE OR SHE USE PROTECTIVE EQUIPMENT (HELMET, ELBOW AND
KNEE PADS, GLOVES)? CLOTHING SUCH AS LONG PANTS AND LONG-
SLEEVED SHIRTS, AS WELL AS PROPERLY FITTED SNEAKERS, ADD
MORE PROTECTION.

There are more than 100,000 skateboard injuries each year that are serious
enough to require emergency room treatment. The vast majority are fractures
of the leg or forearm, head and abdominal injuries, and serious cuts and bruises.
Protective equipment is vital to reducing these injuries.

GETTING HELP,
SAFETY,
PREVENTING
ILLNESS, AND
BEING
PREPARED FOR
LIFE-
THREATENING
EMERGENCIES

yes no **IF YOUR YOUNGSTER HAS A SKATEBOARD, DO YOU INSIST THAT**
☐ ☐ **IT BE WELL MAINTAINED MECHANICALLY AND BE THE CORRECT SIZE FOR THE YOUNGSTER?**

A great many skateboard injuries occur as a result of mechanical failure. Also, youngsters should not ride their skateboards on wet, rough, rocky, or sandy surfaces with holes or cracks. Night skateboard riding should be prohibited unless lighting is exceptional.

yes no **IF YOUR YOUNGSTER HAS ROLLER SKATES, ARE THEY SHOE**
☐ ☐ **SKATES THAT FIT HIS OR HER FOOT SIZE (NOT TOO BIG OR TOO SMALL)? HAVE YOU EXAMINED THE SKATES FOR SHARP EDGES? DO YOU ROUTINELY CHECK THE SKATES TO MAKE SURE THEY ARE MECHANICALLY IN GOOD WORKING ORDER?**

Often accidents and injuries occur because the skates are the wrong size or are tie-on or clip-on skates that slip off the youngster's feet, or because they are not in good working order and cause a fall.

yes no **DO YOU REQUIRE YOUR YOUNGSTER TO USE PROTECTIVE EQUIP-**
☐ ☐ **MENT WHENEVER HE OR SHE GOES ROLLER-SKATING? THIS WOULD INCLUDE A HELMET AND KNEE AND ELBOW PADS (AND SOME WOULD RECOMMEND MOUTH GUARDS TO PROTECT TEETH, AS WELL AS WRIST BRACES).**

Alarmingly, experts estimate that 93,000 people (children and adults) were seen in emergency rooms last year with injuries sustained from roller-skating.

yes no **DO YOU KNOW HOW DANGEROUS MINIBIKES ARE AND THAT**
☐ ☐ **CHILDREN UNDER FOURTEEN YEARS OF AGE SHOULD NOT BE ALLOWED TO RIDE THEM (FOR THEIR OWN SAFETY)?**

The Consumer Product Safety Commission noted that 31,000 people are treated in emergency rooms each year for minibike-related injuries. Sixty-five percent of those injuries were experienced by children less than fifteen years of age. The American Academy of Pediatrics, the National Highway Traffic Safety Agency, the American Motorcycle Association, and the Insurance Institute for Highway Safety supported a proposal to the effect that minibikes be designed so that no one under fourteen years old could operate them; that horsepower be limited; that steps be taken to make minibikes safer and more stable; and that minibikes have warning labels detailing the risks related to their use.

yes no **DO YOU REQUIRE THAT YOUR TEENAGERS WEAR HELMETS AND**
☐ ☐ **PRACTICE GOOD SAFETY HABITS IF THEY INSIST ON RIDING MOPEDS OR MINIBIKES (WHETHER ON THE STREETS OR OFF THE ROAD)?**

Many serious injuries, including permanently disabling head injuries, occur when these precautions are not taken.

yes no DO YOU KNOW THAT MOTORCYCLES HAVE STARTLING INJURY
☐ ☐ AND DEATH RATES?

Personal injury or death occurs in 90 percent of *all motorcycle accidents*, compared to the 9 percent injury/death rate in *all other motor vehicle accidents*. That makes motorcycles very dangerous. The highest death rate occurs in fifteen- to twenty-four-year-old males.

yes no DO YOU INSIST THAT YOUR CHILDREN NOT BE ALLOWED TO DRIVE
☐ ☐ A MOTORCYCLE (IF OLD ENOUGH) OR RIDE ON ONE (IF YOUNGER)?

The risk of injury or death is so high that it is prudent not to allow youngsters to own, operate, or be a passenger on a motorcycle. If you have no other choice, however, make sure the youngster (whether a passenger or a driver) wears a helmet and is taught all safety precautions for the motorcycle's operation and maintenance.

TOY SAFETY CHECKLIST

yes no BEFORE YOU BUY YOUR CHILD (OR ANOTHER CHILD) A TOY, DO
☐ ☐ YOU CONSIDER THE SAFETY OF THE TOY, THE YOUNGSTER'S AGE AND MATURITY, AND WHETHER OR NOT OTHER CHILDREN WHO ARE TOO YOUNG FOR IT MIGHT BE PLAYING WITH IT, AS WELL?

The U.S. Public Health Service estimates that 7 million injuries occur each year from toys. Be sure to carefully examine toys you might purchase in another country, since they may not have standards for toy safety to protect the consumer.

yes no ARE YOU CAREFUL TO PURCHASE TOYS THAT *DO NOT* HAVE SMALL
☐ ☐ PARTS, AREAS OR PARTS THAT CAN BREAK OFF, OR SHARP EDGES?

Although toys that can fit into a 1.25-inch (inside diameter) cylinder are banned from sale (because they could be aspirated or ingested by small children), you should also watch for toys whose parts can be broken off or stuffed animals whose eyes, nose, and so on can detach or be broken off—all presenting a serious hazard.

70

GETTING HELP,
SAFETY,
PREVENTING
ILLNESS, AND
BEING
PREPARED FOR
LIFE-
THREATENING
EMERGENCIES

yes no ARE YOU CAREFUL TO CHECK THE SAFETY OF OLDER TOYS THAT
☐ ☐ HAVE BEEN SAVED FOR YEARS OR HANDED DOWN OVER THE
YEARS?

Literally thousands of unsafe toys have been banned from sale in the United
States since the Child Protection and Toy Safety Act went into effect. You
should, however, be careful not to purchase a banned toy that is sold illegally.
Also, check older toys carefully before allowing a child or youngster to play
with them (since you have no way of knowing if they are safe or not unless
you examine them). The U.S. Consumer Product Safety Commission has a
free publication available on banned toys. (The commission also has free
information on child furniture, poisons, playground equipment, and child safety.)
Write the U.S. Consumer Product Safety Commission, Washington, D.C.
20207.

yes no ARE YOU CAREFUL TO BUY TOYS MADE OF NONTOXIC MATE-
☐ ☐ RIALS AND PAINTED WITH LEAD-FREE PAINT? DO YOU THROW
AWAY TOYS THAT ARE DAMAGED OR BROKEN (OR AT LEAST
REPAIR THEM PROPERLY)?

Since young children suck on or chew on toys, it's important to make sure
the material cannot poison the child. It is also vital for the safety of our children
that damaged or broken toys be repaired or thrown away—before they cause
injuries. Again, be particularly wary of toys that are purchased in other countries and that might have toxic components.

yes no HAVE YOU TAKEN THE TIME TO TEACH YOUR CHILDREN TO PLAY
☐ ☐ WITH AND PUT AWAY TOYS SAFELY? DO YOU SUPERVISE THEIR
PLAY OFTEN TO ENSURE THAT THEY ARE FOLLOWING THESE RULES
AND THEREFORE LEARNING HOW TO PLAY SAFELY WITH TOYS?

If not instructed in the safe use of toys, children will throw them, beat on
things with them, hit other children with them, and leave them lying around,
creating the danger that other children and/or adults may slip on them and
fall.

PLAYGROUND AND BACKYARD SAFETY CHECKLIST

yes no IF YOU HAVE A SWING SET IN YOUR BACKYARD, HAVE YOU MADE
☐ ☐ SURE THAT IT IS AT LEAST SIX FEET AWAY FROM WALLS, WALK-
WAYS, FENCES, OTHER PLAYGROUND EQUIPMENT, AND SO ON?
ARE THE SEATS MADE OF A SOFT MATERIAL? ARE ALL S HOOKS
PINCHED SHUT AT EACH END? IS THERE A SOFT SURFACE (SAND
OR GRASS) UNDER THE SWING SET?

In 1982 there were 196,000 youngsters who required emergency room treatment as a result of injuries from playground equipment. Another study showed
that 43 percent of injuries due to playground equipment occurred on swing
sets. The biggest culprit appears to be falls.

yes no ARE YOU CAREFUL TO PROPERLY ASSEMBLE AND MAINTAIN ALL
☐ ☐ PLAYGROUND EQUIPMENT? DO YOU ROUTINELY CHECK TO SEE
THAT ALL SCREWS, BOLTS, AND NUTS ARE PROPERLY TIGHT-
ENED? HAVE YOU MADE SURE ALL EQUIPMENT IS SECURELY AN-
CHORED?

Proper installation and maintenance are vital preventive measures and should
not be overlooked. With more than $200 million spent on medical costs each
year as a result of injuries from playground equipment, not to mention the
pain and trauma to the youngsters who sustain these injuries, all possible
preventive measures are worth our time and efforts.

yes no HAVE YOU INSTRUCTED YOUR CHILDREN HOW TO PROPERLY PLAY
☐ ☐ ON PLAYGROUND EQUIPMENT (SUCH AS SWINGS, CLIMBING
EQUIPMENT, SLIDES, SEESAWS, AND MONKEY BARS), WHETHER
THE EQUIPMENT IS IN YOUR BACKYARD OR ON A PUBLIC PLAY-
GROUND?

You should know that one-half of playground injuries take place on home
equipment and the other half on public equipment. Much of the time the
youngster is using the equipment improperly—showing off, taking risks,
roughhousing with friends, taking dares, and generally breaking all the safety
rules. Therefore, your ability to teach your children safety habits and impress
on them the need to practice these habits may someday make the difference
between safe and fun play and a potentially serious injury.

72

GETTING HELP,
SAFETY,
PREVENTING
ILLNESS, AND
BEING
PREPARED FOR
LIFE-
THREATENING
EMERGENCIES

DROWNING-PREVENTION CHECKLIST

yes no HAVE YOU OR A CERTIFIED INSTRUCTOR TAUGHT YOUR CHIL-
☐ ☐ DREN (INCLUDING THE LITTLE ONES ONE YEAR OF AGE OR OLDER)
HOW TO FLOAT ON THEIR BACKS? DO THEY KNOW TO DO THIS
IMMEDIATELY IF THEY FALL INTO WATER OR GET INTO TROUBLE
SWIMMING? DO YOU PERIODICALLY TEST THEIR ABILITY TO DO
THIS ON COMMAND?

If children could learn this technique and it became second nature to them,
many drownings and near-drownings could be prevented. Even if children
know this skill, however, they *should not* be trusted around water. It is only
a help, not a guarantee of water safety.

yes no ARE YOU AND YOUR CHILDREN WELL INSTRUCTED IN SWIMMING,
☐ ☐ WATER SAFETY AND RESCUE, AND LIFESAVING TECHNIQUES?

All children should be given swimming lessons and should, when old enough,
learn water safety and lifesaving techniques. This is particularly true if you
own a pool; if there are pools in your neighborhood; or if you spend time at
an ocean, river, lake, or other body of water.

yes no ARE YOU CERTIFIED TO PERFORM CPR (CARDIOPULMONARY RE-
☐ ☐ SUSCITATION)?

CPR (which involves rescue breathing and chest compressions) is not difficult
to learn, although you must be taught the technique in a training course. It
can make the difference between life and death in many situations. Drowning
is only one example. Everyone over the age of eleven should be trained in
CPR.

yes no HAVE YOU MADE IT A RULE, AND DO YOUR CHILDREN UNDER-
☐ ☐ STAND, THAT THEY *ARE NOT ALLOWED* TO SWIM IN OR PLAY NEAR
WATER (SUCH AS IN A SWIMMING POOL, SPA, OCEAN, RIVER,
LAKE, OR ICE POND) UNLESS AN ADULT IS PRESENT WHO IS A
PROFICIENT SWIMMER, KNOWS WATER RESCUE TECHNIQUES AND
FIRST AID, AND IS CERTIFIED IN CPR?

This rule protects your children and would prevent many drownings. Remember, just because someone is an adult doesn't mean that person is capable of
saving a drowning child or youngster—unless he or she is trained to do so.

yes no HAVE YOU MADE IT CLEAR THAT *NO ONE* IS TO SWIM ALONE—
☐ ☐ NO MATTER HOW SKILLED A SWIMMER HE OR SHE HAPPENS TO
BE?

Supervision is the key to preventing unnecessary death or disability when it comes to swimming and water sports, regardless of the age of the swimmer. Often it is the excellent, strong swimmer who gets into trouble (hits his or her head on something, gets a severe cramp from very cold water, or simply tires). With no one there to help, the young person can quickly drown.

yes no IF YOU OWN A POOL OR SPA, IS IT FENCED IN ON ALL SIDES? IS
☐ ☐ THE FENCE HIGH ENOUGH AND CONSTRUCTED SO IT CANNOT BE
CLIMBED? DOES THE GATE TO THE FENCE HAVE AN AUTOMATIC
SELF-LATCHING MECHANISM (OUT OF THE REACH OF CHILDREN),
AND IS THE GATE LOCKED WHEN THE POOL IS NOT IN USE?

Most people make the error of using one side of their house as part of the fence that encloses the swimming pool. This makes it easy for a youngster to go out back or side doors, sliding glass doors, windows, and even "pet" doors (if a toddler). The vast majority of home drowning incidents could have been prevented with proper fencing of the pool, along with proper supervision of children.

yes no HAVE YOU PROHIBITED DIVING INTO YOUR SWIMMING POOL?
☐ ☐

Most home pools (both built-in and above-ground) were not designed for diving and do not have deep enough water in a long enough area to make diving safe. It is estimated that at least 800 people break their necks diving into pools each year. Permanent paralysis or drowning can result. The groups most commonly involved are older children and teenagers.

yes no IF YOU HAVE AN INFLATABLE KIDDY POOL, DO YOU EMPTY IT
☐ ☐ WHEN IT IS NOT BEING USED AND TURN IT UPSIDE DOWN OR
DEFLATE IT? DO YOU OR ANOTHER ADULT *ALWAYS* SUPERVISE
THE CHILD WHEN HE OR SHE IS PLAYING IN OR AROUND THE
POOL?

It's important to remember that it only takes one inch of water for a child (or an adult) to drown.

yes no DO YOU *ALWAYS* WATCH AND SUPERVISE YOUR CHILDREN WHEN
☐ ☐ THEY ARE IN OR NEAR ANY BODY OF WATER?

Ninety-five percent of *all* reported drownings (or near-drownings) take place in swimming pools or bathtubs or at beaches or swimming holes.

74

GETTING HELP,
SAFETY,
PREVENTING
ILLNESS, AND
BEING
PREPARED FOR
LIFE-
THREATENING
EMERGENCIES

yes no ARE YOU CAREFUL NEVER TO LEAVE THE ROOM AND TO WATCH
☐ ☐ A CHILD CLOSELY WHEN HE OR SHE IS TAKING A BATH?

Infants and toddlers—in particular, children under three years old—account
for the majority of bathtub drownings. However, no child under six years old
should be left unsupervised while taking a bath. Often, too, the person supervising is a sibling too young to respond properly if a problem occurs. An
older teenager or adult should always supervise a child closely and know what
to do if a problem arises.

yes no HAVE YOU TALKED TO YOUR OLDER CHILDREN AND TEENAGERS
☐ ☐ ABOUT THE OFTEN DEADLY OR CRIPPLING RESULTS OF DRINKING
ALCOHOL AND SWIMMING OR DIVING?

Older children and teenagers are the second largest age group involved in
swimming accidents—but alarmingly, they have the *highest death rate*. Most
often they swim unsupervised, in more dangerous areas, are risk-takers, and
are often drinking alcohol—a deadly combination.

yes no DO YOU HAVE A RULE THAT ALL NONSWIMMERS AND YOUNG
☐ ☐ CHILDREN MUST WEAR APPROVED LIFE JACKETS IN AND AROUND
THE SWIMMING POOL AND THAT *ALL* PEOPLE ON A BOAT MUST
WEAR APPROVED LIFE JACKETS?

This rule would prevent a substantial number of drownings each year.

yes no DO YOU HAVE A HEAVY COVER OVER YOUR HOT TUB, SPA, OR
☐ ☐ JACUZZI WHEN IT IS NOT IN USE?

Young children have drowned in these when parents weren't even aware that
the youngsters were in or near them. A heavy cover that cannot be moved by
anyone but an adult is an excellent preventive measure.

yes no DO YOU KNOW THAT CHILDREN HAVE DROWNED IN HOT TUBS
☐ ☐ AND OTHER SIMILAR DEVICES BY BEING SUCKED TO THE BOTTOM
OF THE TUB?

In tubs with a large single outlet and strong suction, a vacuum can form against
the skin and hold a youngster underwater or entrap the hair so he or she cannot
get free. Therefore, great care should be taken whenever you allow children
to use the hot tub or spa, and they should be told *not* to submerge themselves
or try to find the center of the tub underwater (which is a game they often
play).

yes no HAVE YOU MADE IT A RULE THAT YOUR TEENAGERS AND THEIR
☐ ☐ FRIENDS NOT BE ALLOWED IN THE HOT TUB OR SPA IF THEY HAVE
BEEN DRINKING ALCOHOL AND THAT THEY *NOT BE ALLOWED TO
DRINK* WHILE IN THE HOT TUB OR SPA?

The combination of hot water and alcohol can be deadly—producing unconsciousness, then death from drowning.

yes no ARE YOU CAREFUL TO KEEP TOILET LIDS DOWN AND EMPTY
☐ ☐ BUCKETS OF WATER IMMEDIATELY AFTER USE?

Each year a small number of toddlers are victims of drowning or near-drowning
because they fall into toilets or buckets and cannot get out.

GUNS (FIREARMS) SAFETY CHECKLIST

yes no IF YOU OWN A GUN, DO YOU KEEP IT UNLOADED AND LOCKED
☐ ☐ UP? IS THE AMMUNITION STORED SEPARATELY FROM THE GUN?

Consider the fact that 30 percent of all firearm-related deaths that occur in the
home involve youngsters under fifteen years of age. Most often the gun and
ammunition are easily accessible.

yes no DO YOU ALLOW YOUR CHILDREN TO FIRE THEIR BB GUNS, PELLET
☐ ☐ GUNS, AIR RIFLES, AND SO ON ONLY WHEN YOU ARE PRESENT
AND ONLY UNDER YOUR SUPERVISION?

In 1980, there were 23,000 injuries serious enough to require emergency room
treatment because of BB guns, pellet guns, air rifles, and so on, and two-
thirds of those injuries were in young people under sixteen years of age. Many
of these incidents involved significant or quite serious eye injuries.

yes no HAVE YOU TAUGHT YOUR CHILDREN AND TEENAGERS THAT A
☐ ☐ GUN (ANY KIND OF GUN OR RIFLE) IS NOT A TOY BUT A DAN-
GEROUS WEAPON THAT CAN KILL OR MAIM? DO THEY UNDER-
STAND THAT THE POWER OF A GUN OR RIFLE MUST BE RESPECTED
AT ALL TIMES AND THAT THEY SHOULD NEVER POINT A GUN OR
RIFLE (LOADED OR PRESUMABLY UNLOADED) AT OTHERS OR
THEMSELVES?

In the United States, in 1975, there were 2,500 accidental deaths involving
firearms. Of those, more than half occurred in or around the home. Most often
the people were playing with or cleaning the gun.

76

GETTING HELP,
SAFETY,
PREVENTING
ILLNESS, AND
BEING
PREPARED FOR
LIFE-
THREATENING
EMERGENCIES

yes no IF YOU HAVE DECIDED TO ALLOW YOUR CHILD TO HAVE A GUN,
☐ ☐ HAVE YOU TAUGHT HIM OR HER ALL FIREARM SAFETY PROCE-
DURES AND PRACTICES AND MADE IT QUITE CLEAR THAT THESE
WILL BE FOLLOWED *AT ALL TIMES?*

The National Rifle Association has teaching manuals available on firearm safety
in the home and outdoors. You can request these by writing the National Rifle
Association, 1600 Rhode Island Avenue, Washington, D.C. 20036.

EQUIPMENT AND TOOLS SAFETY CHECKLIST

yes no DO YOU KEEP ALL CHILDREN AWAY FROM POWER LAWN MOW-
☐ ☐ ERS AND TAKE THE STRICTEST SAFETY PRECAUTIONS AROUND
THEM?

There are 77,000 injuries (in all age groups) from power lawn mowers each
year. In 1976, 2,400 children under five years old and 10,447 youngsters five
to fourteen years old sustained injuries from power lawn mowers. Objects
(such as rocks and glass) can be propelled by the blades, or part of a blade
itself can rip off and shoot out with the speed of a bullet. Young people can
sustain chain injuries, wounds, and even burns. New safety measures on the
machines, which will be instituted soon, as well as greater caution when
running the mowers or when children are in the area, are expected to reduce
injuries by 75 percent.

yes no IS IT A RULE IN YOUR HOME THAT NO YOUNGSTER BE ALLOWED
☐ ☐ TO OPERATE THE POWER MOWER?

The vast majority of injuries are the result of operator carelessness. Only 30
percent (a significant proportion, but still a minority) are due to projectiles.

yes no ARE ALL TOOLS FOR THE YARD, HOUSE, OR GARDEN LOCKED IN
☐ ☐ THE GARAGE? IS THE GASOLINE DRAINED FROM ALL GAS-OP-
ERATED EQUIPMENT EACH TIME THE EQUIPMENT IS PUT AWAY?
ARE ALL ELECTRICAL CORDS KEPT IN A LOCKED CABINET AND
STORED SEPARATELY FROM THE ELECTRICAL TOOLS?

Children love to imitate their parents, so if they have seen mother or father
sawing, trimming, sanding, drilling, and so on, it is a normal desire to want
to do these things, as well. Injuries occur when children can get to this

equipment and simply plug it in or attempt to start the gas-operated tools. They have no idea that these tools can easily "get away" from them—and cause injury.

yes no ARE YOU CAREFUL NEVER TO ALLOW A SMALL CHILD AROUND POWER TOOLS (SUCH AS SAWS AND DRILLS)?

Although very young children are somewhat frightened by power tools, they always seem to want to watch. Watching is fine if it's from a great and safe distance where you are sure they cannot be injured by flying debris or a malfunction in the equipment. It is better to keep them away from all power tools until they are *much older* and can be taught how to use them safely and protect themselves when around them.

PREVENTING SPORTS INJURIES CHECKLIST

yes no DO YOU INSIST THAT YOUR YOUNGSTER WEAR ALL PROTECTIVE EQUIPMENT FOR THE SPORT HE OR SHE IS PLAYING? DO YOU CHECK TO ENSURE THAT THE EQUIPMENT IS IN EXCELLENT CONDITION, GETS REPAIRED WHEN NEEDED, AND IS USED PROPERLY?

Protective equipment developed over the years has made a substantial contribution to preventing and lessening injuries. It's a must for any sport that requires it.

yes no HAVE YOU MADE IT VERY CLEAR TO YOUR YOUNGSTER (AS WELL AS TO COACHES) THAT HE OR SHE NOT BE TAUGHT OR ENCOURAGED TO PLAY ANY SPORT WHILE IN PAIN?

Remember, pain is our body's way of warning us that something is wrong. Continued participation when a youngster is injured or in pain is foolish and may result in further injury—or even permanent disability.

yes no DO YOU CHECK TO SEE WHETHER THERE IS PROPER SUPERVISION WHENEVER YOUR CHILD OR TEENAGER IS PARTICIPATING IN A SPORT? IF THERE IS A LOCAL PARK, HAVE YOU CHECKED THE VARIOUS PLAYING FIELDS FOR REAL AND POTENTIAL HAZARDS AND REQUESTED THAT THESE BE REMOVED?

Proper supervision lessens the number of injuries because rules are followed and care is taken to respect the other players. You should also know that

GETTING HELP,
SAFETY,
PREVENTING
ILLNESS, AND
BEING
PREPARED FOR
LIFE-
THREATENING
EMERGENCIES

young people often get injured when playing in poorly kept-up areas—where there are rocks, holes, ditches, torn fences, trees too close to playing fields, and other hazards.

yes no HAVE YOU TAUGHT YOUR CHILDREN HOW TO WARM UP PROP-
☐ ☐ ERLY BEFORE BEGINNING PLAY?

Many injuries occur because muscles, tendons, and ligaments are not properly stretched and warmed up *before* a youngster starts to play or race. Children learn by example, and you can make a big difference by playing games with your children and stretching and warming up before you begin.

yes no DO YOU ENCOURAGE YOUR YOUNGSTER TO PLAY SPORTS FOR
☐ ☐ THE JOY OF FEELING HIS OR HER BODY MOVE, THE OPPORTUNITY OF SHARING WITH OTHERS, AND THE BENEFITS OF FITNESS? HAVE YOU BEEN CAREFUL NOT TO MAKE "WINNING" THE ONLY THING?

Physical fitness and sports should be fun for young people. The more they are pressed to win, win, win—at all costs—the more likely it is that they will get hurt. We have a responsibility to protect our children from lifelong disabilities that would permanently prevent them from enjoying and participating in sports.

WINTER SPORTS SAFETY CHECKLIST

yes no ARE YOU CAREFUL TO CLOTHE YOUR CHILDREN PROPERLY TO
☐ ☐ PROTECT THEM FROM COLD INJURIES WHEN THEY ARE INVOLVED IN WINTER SPORTS OR ACTIVITIES OR ANYTIME THEY ARE OUT IN VERY COLD WEATHER AND/OR SNOW?

Most people do not realize that infants, children, and even teenagers are more prone to cold injuries (frostbite and hypothermia) than adults. Frostbite can result in loss of fingers, hands, arms, toes, feet, or legs (as well as nerve damage in other areas of the body), and hypothermia, at worst, can result in death.

yes no DO YOU INSIST THAT YOUR CHILDREN OR TEENAGERS TAKE TIME
☐ ☐ OUT TO REST WHEN THEY ARE INVOLVED IN WINTER SPORTS OR PLAY?

Young people are more likely to ignore being cold and/or wet and will push themselves to the point of exhaustion without ever recognizing it. Both these problems—being cold and/or wet and tired/exhausted—greatly increase the possibility of hypothermia.

yes no HAVE YOU TAUGHT YOUR CHILDREN THE SIGNS AND SYMPTOMS
☐ ☐ OF FROSTBITE AND HYPOTHERMIA?

No matter what age a child is, he or she can be taught what danger signs to be aware of when playing in the snow, in very cold weather, and when the windchill factor drops the temperature to life-threatening levels. It's important for children to know when it's time to come in and (if they are older) what to do if a friend experiences a problem.

yes no IF YOUR CHILDREN GO TOBOGGANING, SLEDDING, ICE SKATING,
☐ ☐ SKIING, AND/OR SNOWMOBILING, DO YOU INSPECT ALL EQUIP-
MENT BEFORE THE WINTER SEASON BEGINS TO MAKE SURE IT IS
SAFE AND IS THE PROPER EQUIPMENT FOR THE YOUNG PERSON,
BASED ON HIS OR HER SIZE AND AGE?

Equipment should not be too big or too small for the young person; it should not be falling apart or too worn out; there should be no loose or protruding parts; and great care should be taken to repair equipment properly (if possible) and replace it when it cannot be properly repaired or the youngster has outgrown it.

yes no HAVE YOU TAUGHT YOUR CHILDREN HOW TO USE WINTER SPORTS
☐ ☐ EQUIPMENT CORRECTLY AND EMPHASIZED THE IMPORTANCE OF
STOPPING THEIR ACTIVITIES IF SOMETHING GOES WRONG WITH
THE EQUIPMENT?

Each year, countless minor and a number of major injuries, and even deaths, are due to faulty equipment or the incorrect use of equipment. Many such incidents could be avoided if children were instructed in the proper use of equipment and taught to recognize when something is wrong with the equipment, so they stop their activities *before* somebody gets hurt.

yes no HAVE YOU TAUGHT YOUR CHILDREN SAFETY RULES FOR EACH
☐ ☐ ACTIVITY THEY ARE INVOLVED IN AND EMPHASIZED THE IM-
PORTANCE OF FOLLOWING THESE RULES?

Serious injury often occurs when a child, youngster, or teenager breaks a safety rule or challenges himself or is "dared" to do something by a friend: tobogganing or sledding through a heavily forested area; skiing down a mountain when her level of skill and experience doesn't match the mountain's challenge; ice skating on a pond with areas of thin ice; attempting jumps in

80

GETTING HELP,
SAFETY,
PREVENTING
ILLNESS, AND
BEING
PREPARED FOR
LIFE-
THREATENING
EMERGENCIES

snowmobiles; taking an unknown trail when cross-country skiing; or climbing a snow-covered mountain without the skill to do so.

yes no DO YOU (OR ANOTHER QUALIFIED ADULT) ALWAYS SUPERVISE
☐ ☐ CHILDREN WHEN THEY ARE INVOLVED IN WINTER SPORTS OR ACTIVITIES?

Many problems can be avoided when an adult is present and is involved in the activity or carefully watches the young people—making it clear that safety rules will be observed. There have been children, for example, who have drowned or died from hypothermia because they fell through thin ice while ice skating—and no one could help them (or another child tried to help and was injured or died, as well). The adult needs to be "qualified"—meaning he or she must know the sport and be trained in rescue techniques, first aid, and hopefully CPR (cardiopulmonary resuscitation).

yes no HAVE YOU TAUGHT YOUR CHILDREN WHAT TO DO IF THEY EVER
☐ ☐ FIND THEMSELVES IN A DANGEROUS OR LIFE-THREATENING SITUATION WHILE INVOLVED IN A WINTER SPORT OR ACTIVITY?

It's vital that children know what to do if they fall through thin ice while ice skating (or a friend does); if fog or a blizzard suddenly strands them on a mountain while skiing or they are caught in an avalanche; if they become lost on a cross-country trail or separated from the group; if they become cold or begin to have symptoms of hypothermia while mountain climbing, hiking, or playing in the snow or cold weather; and if they or a friend are injured while tobogganing, sledding, and so on.

yes no IF YOU ALLOW OLDER CHILDREN OR TEENAGERS TO DRIVE OR
☐ ☐ RIDE ON A SNOWMOBILE, HAVE YOU MADE IT CLEAR THAT A SNOWMOBILE IS *NOT* A TOY, BUT A POWERFUL VEHICLE—AND THEREFORE, GREAT CARE SHOULD BE TAKEN IN OPERATING IT?

Snowmobiles can cause very serious injury or even death if they hit someone, flip, or meet a tree head on. Anyone who drives or rides on a snowmobile should wear protective equipment and be taught how to handle this machine safely. Often youngsters are hurt when they try to race each other (and lose control or crash into each other) or when they try dangerous maneuvers or stunts.

WILDERNESS SAFETY CHECKLIST

yes no DO YOU ALWAYS TAKE A WELL-STOCKED FIRST AID KIT WITH
☐ ☐ YOU WHENEVER YOU GO TO THE MOUNTAINS, DESERTS, OR OTHER
WILDERNESS AREAS?

Particularly if you will be far from medical help, you must be able to provide
basic first aid until you can get a child or adult to medical care.

yes no WHEN PREPARING FOR A TRIP, DO YOU LOOK UP INFORMATION
☐ ☐ ON THE AREA TO WHICH YOU ARE GOING; DETERMINE WHAT (IF
ANY) KINDS OF POISONOUS SNAKES, SPIDERS, REPTILES, IN-
SECTS, OR OTHER ANIMALS ARE KNOWN TO BE IN THE AREA;
AND FIND OUT WHAT TYPE OF FIRST AID SUPPLIES YOU WOULD
NEED AND WHAT TREATMENT PROCEDURES YOU WOULD HAVE
TO KNOW IN ORDER TO HELP A YOUNGSTER UNTIL PROFESSIONAL
ASSISTANCE COULD BE FOUND?

Being prepared may spare a youngster (or adult) serious complications and
prevent unnecessary pain.

yes no ARE YOU CAREFUL TO ENSURE THAT PROPER PROTECTIVE
☐ ☐ CLOTHING FOR BOTH WARM AND COLD WEATHER IS AVAILABLE
TO ALL CHILDREN WHEN THEY ARE CAMPING, BACKPACKING,
OR ENGAGING IN OTHER WILDERNESS ACTIVITIES?

Often children *and* adults get into trouble because they are ill prepared for the
weather conditions, and cold or heat injuries occur. These can be dangerous
and even life-threatening.

yes no ARE YOU CAUTIOUS ABOUT PURCHASING OR RENTING PROPER
☐ ☐ AND SAFE EQUIPMENT FOR CAMPING, BACKPACKING, AND SO ON
(SUCH AS TENTS, SLEEPING BAGS, STOVES, AND LANTERNS)?

Small children should never be allowed to carry a lantern or be near the camp
stove. All campfires and lanterns should be kept away from tents, sleeping
bags, and other flammable materials, since injuries and deaths occur each year
when fires break out in such situations.

yes no HAVE YOU TAUGHT YOUR CHILDREN SAFETY RULES FOR CAMP-
☐ ☐ ING, BACKPACKING, OR AN OUTING IN THE WILDERNESS? ARE
THEY TRAINED IN FIRST AID AND RESCUE TECHNIQUES?

The more children know about how to protect themselves and what to do when
an injury occurs, the safer they will be.

GETTING HELP,
SAFETY,
PREVENTING
ILLNESS, AND
BEING
PREPARED FOR
LIFE-
THREATENING
EMERGENCIES

ANIMAL SAFETY CHECKLIST

yes no DO YOU MAKE SURE YOUR PETS RECEIVE ALL NECESSARY IM-
☐   ☐ MUNIZATIONS (SHOTS) AT THE PROPER RECOMMENDED INTER-
VALS?

Vaccinating our animals protects not only them but also our children and
ourselves. It is therefore vital that we be diligent about having our pets vaccinated and given their booster shots as recommended by a veterinarian.

yes no DO YOU TAKE ANIMALS TO THE VETERINARIAN WHENEVER THEY
☐   ☐ ARE ILL OR HAVE A HEALTH PROBLEM?

Having pets checked and treated when they are ill or have a health problem
not only is humane but also in some cases prevents certain problems from
spreading to children. Diseases and problems that can be transmitted from pets
to children and adults include ringworm (a fungus infection of the skin);
roundworm (a parasite that can cause serious problems in children from one
to four years old if not treated); sarcoptic mange (a form of scabies, a skin
infestation); Cheyletiella mites (called ''walking dandruff'' in the animal, they
cause skin bumps in youngsters); psittacosis (a relatively rare disease of birds
that causes flulike symptoms in humans); toxoplasmosis (a parasitic disease
that affects the unborn human fetus if the mother is infected and is not immune);
and rabies (a viral encephalitis that is often deadly and is a rightfully feared
disease).

yes no DO YOU KNOW WHAT MEASURES YOU CAN TAKE TO BETTER
☐   ☐ ENSURE THAT YOUR PETS DON'T GET THESE DISEASES OR TRANS-
MIT THEM TO CHILDREN AND OTHERS?

All of the previously mentioned problems (ringworm, roundworm, rabies, and
so on) are preventable and/or treatable with proper pet hygiene, routine veterinary visits, and vaccinations. Specifically, you can reduce your child's
chances of catching a pet's disease if you routinely vacuum the house and
dispose of the vacuum bags appropriately; are careful about handling and
disposing of animal feces; keep your animals away from other animals that
are ill or have a health problem; make sure your children don't eat or play in
dirt contaminated by dog or cat feces (or eat the feces either); do not feed
your animals raw or undercooked meat; purchase your animals from reputable
pet shops or breeders; keep your animals clean; keep your children away from
wild animals (such as skunks, foxes, raccoons, coyotes, cats, dogs, and bats);
and discourage them from petting or approaching dogs, cats, and other animals
that are strangers to them.

yes no HAVE YOU TAUGHT YOUR CHILDREN WHAT TO DO IF THREAT-
☐ ☐ ENED BY A DOG?

It is estimated that approximately 500,000 to 1 million dog bites occur in the United States each year. However, the exact number is unknown and is thought to be substantially higher. Children should learn not to run but rather to hold still, face the dog, stay calm, and start talking gently to the dog. They should never move toward the dog, even if it appears to be calmed down. If attacked, children should cross their arms in front of their face and neck. They should also be told never to put their faces down close to an animal's face, since the animal might be frightened or might panic and bite, snap, or claw.

THE DON'TS

Don't forget to review the Safety Checklists periodically, paying particular attention to any steps you haven't yet taken (those you did not check off). Determine whether you can now take these steps to better ensure your youngster's safety. Be sure to check off each item as you complete it.

Don't forget to refer back from time to time to the Safety Checklists to refresh your memory about those measures that require continual or periodic examination or diligence.

Don't neglect to review the Safety Checklists as your child reaches new milestones in his or her life. For example, your child may now be ready for a bicycle, roller skates, or other "wheels" or have reached the age where he or she is getting involved in sports, but those were Safety Checklists you previously skipped because they did not apply to your child.

Don't hesitate to suggest to anyone who cares for or works with children (such as grandparents, other relatives, friends, teachers, and baby-sitters) that they read the Safety Checklists and, where necessary, institute the suggested safety measures.

C H A P T E R 3
Preventing Illness

QUICK REFERENCE

Recommended Schedule for Immunizations*

2 months of age	DTP (diphtheria, tetanus, pertussis)
	Oral polio (OPV)
4 months of age	DTP
	Oral polio
6 months of age	DTP
12 months of age	Test for TB (tuberculosis)†
15 months of age	MMR (measles, mumps, rubella)
18 months of age	DTP
	Oral polio

*Recommendations of the American Academy of Pediatrics, 1985.

†A TB test is recommended every one to two years.

2 years of age	"Hib" (Hemophilus influen-zae b)
4 to 6 years of age	DTP Oral polio
14 to 16 years of age	Td (so-called adult DT—tet-anus and diphtheria)
Every 10 years thereafter	Td

Since dates are difficult to remember as time passes, it is a good idea that as your child receives the necessary immunizations, you record them on the Immunization Record section of the Medical History form found at the end of Chapter 1. Remember, you need a Medical History/Immunization Record for *each* of your children.

Immunization Against Preventable Diseases

In the past, many serious diseases were simply a "normal" part of childhood. Parents hoped their children wouldn't get these often deadly diseases and could only pray that they would not be killed or crippled if they did. There was simply nothing parents could do to prevent them, and little could be done to treat them. Because many of these "childhood diseases" can now be effectively prevented, we tend to forget how frightening and devastating these illnesses were and *can still be* without immunization against them.

Many people have forgotten or don't know that measles is a very serious disease—with complications found in as many as one in every ten children who get it. Measles carries with it a risk for convulsions, permanent hearing loss, and other serious problems for children. It's easy to forget that there once was a polio epidemic that killed literally thousands of children each year and crippled countless others. The word *croup* no longer rings of terror as it did fifty years ago. Then it usually meant diphtheria—and diphtheria meant death. The list goes on and on, but the fact remains that countless lives were lost, while those who survived had to learn to live with serious, lifelong, crippling problems—all because of a handful of devastating childhood diseases.

Today the problem is a little different. Parents who did not live through the grim epidemics and know very little about them often become complacent about having their children immunized. This is not to say that some parents don't have very legitimate concerns and questions about immunizations. They do! However, there are those who simply don't believe immunizations are necessary or don't realize how important they are to them and to their children.

86

GETTING HELP,
SAFETY,
PREVENTING
ILLNESS, AND
BEING
PREPARED FOR
LIFE-
THREATENING
EMERGENCIES

A great deal of misunderstanding is also to blame. We hear things like: "Aren't those diseases wiped out now?"; "Baby shots aren't necessary anymore. They had more germs back then"; "The risk of getting polio is greater with the immunization than without it"; "I haven't heard of anyone getting diphtheria in years"; "Oh, they make a big deal out of nothing"; "The risks of pertussis vaccine are too high"; or "Those diseases weren't so bad!"

True, it's hard to remember how really terrible these diseases once were and easy to relax our vigilance to the point where we don't complete our children's "baby shots." The less we hear about these deadly and crippling diseases, the more likely it is that we will put off having our children immunized. It's easy to feel "too safe." It's also easy to forget that the reason we don't hear very much about these problems is because our parents were diligent about having *us* immunized—as soon as the immunizations were available.

Ask your parents or grandparents about what the polio, measles, diphtheria, or whooping cough epidemics were like. Ask them about how the public responded to the development of immunizations. They will probably tell you what a medical miracle immunizations were and how relieved people were that something could finally be done. These diseases were as feared as cancer and heart disease are today. And before the development of immunizations, they were the number-one killer of children and took the lives of many adults, as well. Parents and grandparents may also tell you that the only way we can avoid having these epidemics again is to diligently continue immunizing our children.

Where Do We Stand Today?

Smallpox—a frightening killer of young and old—is now considered completely eradicated worldwide because of successful immunizations. Other devastating childhood diseases are not yet eradicated, but polio, measles, and diphtheria can be effectively prevented with immunizations. Tetanus is unheard of in people effectively immunized against it. Rubella (German measles)—which can cause serious and often deadly problems for the fetus—can be completely prevented if the mother is immune, either because she was immunized long before she became pregnant or because she has had proven rubella in the past. Mumps is presently under control, and pertussis (whooping cough) can be prevented in the majority of susceptible youngsters by immunizing them. Other new vaccines are in the testing stages, and there is hope for controlling or preventing other common childhood diseases in the future.

The problem is, many people are not having their children immunized today. Even though most states have laws that require youngsters to be completely immunized when they enter school for the first time, somehow a number of children have slipped by without being immunized, or the parents have refused to have their children immunized for religious or other reasons. (Day-care centers, nursery schools, and preschools are also bound by this same law, which helps stress immunizations at an earlier age.) Now the laws are being more stringently enforced each year, and those who do not want their children protected because of religious or other convictions must sign a document specifying that they understand the risks of not having their children vaccinated.

The reason it is so important that children be immunized *before* they enter school or preschool is that any large group of children presents a perfect place for infectious diseases to spread and epidemics to start. Unimmunized schoolchildren can easily bring home these serious diseases and give them to other family members—in particular, to young infants, who are highly susceptible to them. Just think about how you most often get a cold or the flu. Children have a way of being very generous about sharing their colds, flu, and other illnesses! Imagine how easy it would be to spread a serious, devastating disease such as polio, measles, whooping cough, or diphtheria if there were no immunizations against them.

It's also important to remember that certain childhood diseases present greater risks to young infants and become less serious problems if contracted later in life. Pertussis is one of these that has a high potential for causing serious, life-threatening illness in very young infants. Therefore, immunization against this disease is most crucial for young infants. Continuing protection until school age reduces the risk of exposure to infant siblings or to the infants of friends and relatives.

Other diseases are less threatening to young infants because of natural immunity (acquired through the placenta and reinforced by breast feeding), which is passed on from an immune mother to her infant. This temporary immunity disappears by the end of the first year, and vaccines must take over. For example, immunization against measles becomes important in the second year of life, when this temporary immunity from the mother has disappeared. Principles like this determine when each particular immunization is recommended.

How Immunizations Work

When an infection (bacteria or virus) invades the body, our "immune system" gears up and attacks. In order to do this, the body must first *recognize* the invaders as *foreign*. Once this has occurred, the body can circulate more blood to the area so the white blood cells can join defenses and "swallow up" and destroy the invading germs. While this happens, special cells begin to make substances called *antibodies*—unique compounds that instantly recognize the germ and destroy it. Antibody formation is gradual and takes several days to weeks. However, once it has occurred, it is usually very long-lasting, often permanent. Once the process is completed, the body is able to recognize that particular germ and destroy it. In other words, the body becomes immune to that germ.

Immunizations use this same principle and are designed to force the body to actively make antibodies against a disease. When a person is exposed to a mild or harmless

GETTING HELP,
SAFETY,
PREVENTING
ILLNESS, AND
BEING
PREPARED FOR
LIFE-
THREATENING
EMERGENCIES

form of the illness-producing germ, the body is able to make antibodies. If the person is exposed to the actual disease later, his or her immune system immediately attacks and destroys the germs—because it recognizes them. Some immunizations must be given in small, repeated doses to build immunity, while others are effective and safe when given only once.

This theory was proved by Edward Jenner, who developed the earliest immunization against smallpox. Jenner discovered that milkmaids were strangely resistant to smallpox. He found that exposure to cowpox—a mild disease similar to smallpox—produced resistance to the more serious disease, smallpox. To test his theory, he first inoculated himself, then others, with the fluid from cowpox sores. None developed smallpox. This was a major medical breakthrough. While smallpox vaccination is no longer recommended (because the disease is considered totally eradicated, and the vaccination now poses a greater risk than the disease), the principles confirmed by Jenner's experience still apply and are the basis for immunization against other diseases.

How Vaccines Are Made

Some vaccines are made by using the killed bacteria or viruses (or their by-products) to stimulate immunity. These vaccines usually require several doses at specific intervals in order to result in initial, reliable antibody formation. Some require ''booster'' doses to keep the level of immunity high enough to protect a person against a disease. DTP (diphtheria, tetanus, and pertussis) vaccines and inactivated polio (Salk) vaccine are examples of this kind of vaccine.

However, most vaccines against viral diseases now rely on live, modified viruses to stimulate immunity. Live-virus vaccines actually cause a very mild, usually harmless, case of the disease. The vaccine viruses are weakened (called ''attenuated'') to a safe level in the production process. Current evidence suggests that the immunity that results from these vaccines is more permanent than that from killed-virus vaccines (that is, the immunity appears to be lifelong). Vaccines against measles, mumps, and rubella (German measles) and the oral polio vaccine (Sabin) are live, attenuated viral vaccines. As noted previously, smallpox vaccine was also a live-virus vaccine.

Another kind of protection is also available for certain diseases for which so-called active immunization is not possible or is simply too risky. This ''passive immunization'' is temporary but can at times prevent a disease or lessen its seriousness when given to an exposed person. Injections of gamma globulin provide this kind of protection. This form of immunization is most often used for those exposed to hepatitis and is helpful for youngsters and adults whose immune systems do not work properly.

It is given to them when they have been exposed to a potentially life-threatening disease (such as chickenpox or measles). The gamma globulin used for these purposes is very special and high in antibodies against the specific disease. The reason that the protection provided by passive immunization is only temporary is because the "artificial" antibodies disappear in time, and the body cannot make more of its own.

The Risks of Immunizations

Are the risks associated with the immunizations much less than the possible harmful effects of the various diseases? This is a very important question that each and every parent needs to ask and to have answered. While each immunization indeed carries risks (some minor, others more worrisome) that cannot be overlooked, current recommendations to immunize children are based on statistics and experience that show the risks associated with the immunizations to be much less than those of the diseases in question.

The *most common problems* children experience with immunizations are "side effects"—rather unpleasant (mild to moderate) problems that don't have any long-term consequences. These include aches and pains; mild fever; rashes; pain, swelling, or discomfort around the injection; or just not feeling well. These side effects are probably due to specific features of the vaccines and are relatively predictable.

"Adverse reactions," on the other hand, are much more rare. When they occur, they are usually more serious and can leave permanent damage. While no one is sure why some youngsters have adverse reactions, the cause is probably an idiosyncrasy— an unusual combination of the vaccine itself and the child receiving it. Unfortunately, adverse reactions are not usually predictable and are therefore the target of concern for both professionals and parents. Most of these reactions must run their course and have no specific treatment other than to make the youngster more comfortable.

An "allergic reaction" is another type of problem that can occur in some children. In these cases, the child is usually allergic to some ingredient in the vaccine and can respond adversely immediately after the immunization is given, or the response may be delayed. Allergic reactions can be prevented by not giving the vaccine to a youngster known to be allergic to one of its components. Allergic reactions can also be treated if promptly recognized. True allergic reactions to vaccines are rare.

The DTP Vaccine

The *DTP vaccine* combines components to protect an infant or young child against diphtheria, tetanus, and pertussis (whooping cough). The immunization is given by injection into the muscle (usually in the thigh of young children or the arm of older ones). Children need a "basic series," then boosters to keep up their immunity.

The vaccine uses modified toxins to trigger immunity to diphtheria and tetanus.

90

GETTING HELP,
SAFETY,
PREVENTING
ILLNESS, AND
BEING
PREPARED FOR
LIFE-
THREATENING
EMERGENCIES

These two parts of the vaccine are considered safe and cause few side effects (other than soreness at the spot where the injection was given, as well as a slight fever and achiness). Some people who have had an excessive number of tetanus boosters, however, experience a severe reaction at the injection site. This is thought to be an allergic or hypersensitivity reaction. Both diphtheria and tetanus are very easy to prevent with the immunizations, and immunity lasts for a long time. After a basic series of immunizations, a booster every ten years throughout life is quite effective.

To set the record straight, you need not have your child get a tetanus booster every time he or she sustains a wound—unless it has been ten years since the last immunization *or* the injury carries a particularly high risk for tetanus and five years have passed since the last booster. Particularly high-risk injuries include such mishaps as a cut while working or playing on a farm, or when working with fertilizer, or a puncture wound from a rusty metal object. Information now available makes it clear that there is no need to get a tetanus booster more often than this. When a booster dose is given to a youngster as a result of injury (before the scheduled immunization time), then the next booster is scheduled from that date.

Try not to panic about the tetanus shot if your youngster gets a cut or puncture wound. First check his or her immunization schedule, and if you're still not sure about what to do—call your doctor and ask. One note regarding timing: you do have some leeway in which to get a booster if it's needed, so it doesn't require an emergency room visit unless the injury itself needs emergency medical attention. It's always worthwhile to get a booster of diphtheria at the same time (or diphtheria and pertussis for young children).

Pertussis (whooping cough) *vaccine* is made with products of the killed pertussis bacteria and, as noted, is part of the DTP immunizations. Currently, pertussis vaccine is the focus of a great deal of controversy—as to both its effectiveness and its risks. In fact, when an infant or child has an adverse reaction to the DTP immunization, the "P" (pertussis) portion is usually to blame. While not as effective as many other vaccines, it is a good vaccine, which can be given in early infancy. Recent controversy has stimulated a new look at this vaccine, and steps are being taken to study it again and hopefully to improve it.

It is not given after the age of seven years, except in very unusual circumstances. In this case, the risk that an older youngster will have serious complications from pertussis is low, and the risk of bothersome to more serious reactions to the vaccine is higher. It is also not given to infants who have had a previous *serious* reaction to it, nor is it given to youngsters with certain central nervous system problems. These youngsters should all receive immunization against diphtheria and tetanus *without* pertussis vaccine.

Mild to moderate side effects of the pertussis vaccine are common and should not worry you or make you concerned about your child's receiving the vaccine in the future. The usual side effects of pain at the shot site, fever over 100 degrees, and fussiness for several hours are seen in about half of the youngsters who receive pertussis vaccine. About one-third of infants become very drowsy during the first day after the shot, and about one in five loses his or her appetite. Acetaminophen (Tylenol, Panadol, and other brands), in the proper dosage for the child's weight, can be administered every four to six hours for one to two days from the time the immunization was given. This can be of great help in making a youngster who is experiencing the usual side effects of DTP vaccine more comfortable.

Serious reactions to pertussis—high fever (over 103 degrees); convulsions; collapse; high-pitched, unusual cry; excessive sleepiness; or persistent screaming (over three hours)—are rarely seen. *If your child experiences ANY of these serious adverse reactions, then call the doctor (for advice) immediately.*

About one in seven thousand youngsters has these kinds of serious reactions. Permanent brain damage occurs once for every 310,000 doses of vaccine given. These reactions, while serious, occur less often than the serious complications seen with pertussis itself, and brain damage or death is much more likely with the disease itself. However, the serious reactions to pertussis vaccine, while rare, are still real. But so is the disease! For many, this presents a terrible dilemma.

In countries where pertussis vaccine has been eliminated from the routine immunizations, the disease is on the rise. For example, British authorities who stopped giving the vaccine routinely are now recommending that it be reinstituted, since so many pertussis cases have been seen and serious complications have followed.

It is prudent, though, to avoid giving pertussis vaccine to youngsters who are at a higher than usual risk for problems from the vaccine. Currently, *no* further pertussis vaccine is recommended for infants who have had any of the following reactions to DTP vaccine: (1) convulsions, (2) encephalitis (brain inflammation), (3) certain nervous system signs, and (4) collapse. In addition, most doctors would also avoid further pertussis vaccine if there had been fever over 103 degrees, excessive sleepiness, or a screaming or crying episode lasting longer than three hours. These infants should receive combined tetanus and diphtheria vaccines, which are available in two forms, depending on the youngsters' age.

It is best to be alert for any new information about the pertussis vaccine, as well as any updated recommendations. Be sure that you are careful to weigh the risks and benefits of this immunization for your child and discuss your concerns with your doctor.

The Polio Vaccines

LIVE POLIO VACCINE

Oral polio vaccine (OPV) contains three types of live polioviruses that have been "weakened" to generally safe levels. The vaccine is given by mouth as liquid drops and causes the body to make antibodies against the polioviruses—just as if there had been exposure to the "real" poliovirus. One dose usually is effective in causing immunity to all three poliovirus types, but more doses ensure that the immunity is

92

GETTING HELP,
SAFETY,
PREVENTING
ILLNESS, AND
BEING
PREPARED FOR
LIFE-
THREATENING
EMERGENCIES

complete. OPV protects against polio in two ways: it causes resistance to infection in the nose and intestine and also allows the body to make antibodies if the virus somehow gets past these barriers. It is easy to give and provides long immunity—perhaps for a lifetime.

However, there are several risks associated with this vaccine. Although quite rare, there is a risk for getting paralytic polio from this vaccine. One case of paralytic polio is seen for about each four million doses of vaccine given. This "vaccine-associated polio" affects nonimmune household members and other close contacts somewhat more often than the youngster who actually got the vaccine. This occurs because the vaccine virus is excreted into the bowel movement of the immunized youngster and is therefore passed to the household contacts. Therefore, nonimmune adults caring for youngsters who have been immunized—particularly those in diapers—are at risk for this vaccine-associated polio.

Another problem seen with oral polio vaccine (and other live-virus vaccines) is that certain individuals whose immune systems are faulty cannot make antibodies against this virus and are therefore at greater risk for vaccine-associated paralytic polio. Therefore, oral polio vaccine is not recommended for the following groups of people without first checking with the doctor:

- Those with cancer, leukemia, or lymphoma.

- Those with diseases where the body's resistance to infection is lowered.

- Those taking medications that lower the body's resistance to infection (such as cortisone or prednisone).

- Children who live in the same house with people who have the problems mentioned above.

- Pregnant women.

- Those who are sick with any kind of infection (more serious than an uncomplicated cold) at the time the vaccine is to be given.

- Most people over eighteen years old, because of the increased risk for paralytic polio related to the vaccine. (However, there are times when this caution might not apply.)

For those adults who have never been immunized against polio, and for people listed previously, inactivated polio vaccine (IPV) is available and can be used. Check with your doctor if you need further information.

INACTIVATED POLIO VACCINE (SALK)

Salk vaccine—*inactivated polio vaccine (IPV)*—is effective in producing protection against paralytic polio. Given by injection, it causes the body to make antibodies against polio. To be effective, it requires a series of three injections two months apart (and all can be given with DTP), followed by a booster a year later and then scattered throughout life. While it is effective in stimulating the body's production of antibodies, it does not lead to protection against poliovirus invasion in the nose or intestine (which can lead to acute gastroenteritis—vomiting and diarrhea).

The major advantage of IPV is that it presents no risk of producing paralytic polio. It can therefore be safely used in all people, both youngsters and adults, including those who cannot receive live-virus vaccines. This safety, along with its good effectiveness, has led to many people's strongly recommending that IPV replace live oral polio vaccine in routine immunization programs. While IPV was not available in the United States for several years, it is now available again. It is recommended when polio vaccination is needed but oral vaccine is not to be used.

CURRENT RECOMMENDATIONS ABOUT POLIO IMMUNIZATION

While IPV is safe and quite effective, oral polio vaccine is still preferred and recommended for routine use in infants and children in the United States. Inactivated polio vaccine should be used in adults who are unimmunized (and can be given to unprotected parents of infants who are to receive OPV) and in those youngsters with the risks mentioned earlier. It can and should also be used in youngsters whose parents choose not to use the OPV because of the risk of possible paralysis. The progress in controlling polio has been very impressive and must continue. Regardless of which vaccine is used, we cannot afford to relax our guard against this potentially deadly disease.

MMR (Measles, Mumps, Rubella)

The development of the *MMR vaccine*—a combined vaccine of live modified viruses of measles, mumps, and rubella (German measles)—followed the development of individual vaccines against these diseases in the 1960s. Because infants can have some protection against these diseases from their immune mothers, these vaccines are given after the first birthday (if given singly) or at fifteen months of age as combined MMR.

Rubella vaccine deserves some special attention. It is particularly important that all women who can and may someday wish to have children be immune to rubella. In this way, they cannot contract rubella during pregnancy nor put the fetus at risk for serious problems. Preteenagers who have not had this vaccine should receive it, and adult women whose blood shows no immunity should talk to their doctor about getting the immunization at a time when they are not pregnant and will diligently prevent pregnancy for at least three months. (Longer is even better, since a live virus is involved.) Adult men who are not immune should also be vaccinated. A simple blood test (called a rubella titer) can determine if a person has immunity to rubella.

GETTING HELP,
SAFETY,
PREVENTING
ILLNESS, AND
BEING
PREPARED FOR
LIFE-
THREATENING
EMERGENCIES

The side effects of MMR vaccine are mild and are related to the measles vaccine, the rubella virus, or both. The common reactions are mild fever and rash a week or two after the shot—in about one in every five to seven children. Rubella vaccine can cause mild neck gland swelling, as well. A few children (and about one in four adults) experience mild joint swelling and pain after rubella vaccination. Mumps vaccine very rarely leads to mild swelling of the cheeks and salivary glands.

Youngsters who have diseases that interfere with their immunity may face potentially serious risks with these vaccines. There is a *very* rare association between measles vaccine and a form of encephalitis (brain inflammation), convulsions, and nerve deafness. Allergic reactions to these vaccines are rare but possible. Ask your doctor about allergies to the vaccine if your youngster has serious, life-threatening (anaphylactic) reactions to eggs. Other persons who should not receive these vaccines without a doctor's recommendation include:

- Anyone who is sick with something more serious than a simple cold at the time the vaccine is to be given.

- Those with cancer, leukemia, or lymphoma.

- People taking medications that lower immunity to infections (such as cortisone and prednisone).

- People with diseases that cause lowered resistance to infection.

- People with allergy to neomycin (an antibiotic).

- People who have received a gamma globulin injection within the past three months.

All live-virus vaccines should be avoided during pregnancy. However, it is not dangerous to give an MMR vaccination to a *child* whose mother is pregnant, since these vaccines do not result in the production of harmful organisms that can be transmitted to others.

Hemophilus Influenzae Type b Vaccine

Hemophilus influenzae b polysaccharide vaccine is the newest vaccine recommended for routine use in children. Licensed in 1985, "Hib" vaccine will protect young children against serious and often life-threatening infections due to the bacteria Hemophilus influenzae, type b. (This bacteria is different from the so-called flu or influenza viruses—even though the names sound similar.)

Hib vaccine (given as an injection [shot]) is currently recommended for all children at two years of age. It is expected to be effective for 1½ years to 3½ years—during the time when young children are very susceptible to infections due to the so-called H. flu bacteria.

This new vaccine is somewhat effective when given to toddlers at eighteen months of age, but children who receive the vaccine at eighteen months of age may need a second dose of the vaccine six months to eighteen months later to ensure good protection throughout the preschool years. Because of this partial protection, the vaccine is recommended at eighteen months of age only for toddlers who are at greater than usual risk of H. flu disease. This includes little ones in day-care centers (nursery schools, preschools, or any type of group care), those who do not have functioning spleens (because of sickle-cell anemia or the removal of their spleens, for example), and those with certain cancers.

The advantages of Hib vaccine for children between two and five years old decrease with each year—that is, if youngsters are immunized at three or four years of age, their benefits are less than if they had received the vaccine at two years of age. However, it will still be of benefit if given until the age of five, especially for youngsters in day care or group care. Talk to your doctor about the possible benefits of this vaccine if your child is between two and five years old and has not received it.

The risks of the Hib vaccine are very small. Most children who receive it have no reaction at all, with some having a low fever (less than 101.5 degrees) and a sore injection site for twenty-four hours or so. No long-term side effects of this vaccine are known at this time.

One of the major disadvantages of Hib vaccine is that it is not effective in infants and toddlers younger than eighteen months—a time when H. flu infections are particularly common—and is not recommended before eighteen months of age. New vaccines to protect younger infants are being developed, but for the present time, protection can only be offered to older toddlers and preschoolers. However, this protection should be helpful, because younger infants are often infected by older brothers or sisters (or their school or neighborhood friends) who bring home the bacteria from other children.

There is some controversy about this new vaccine, mainly because it offers so little protection for young infants, who have approximately 75 percent of the serious H. flu infections. However, it seems to be a very good idea to protect toddlers and preschoolers, especially those who are in any type of day-care center or group care, against potentially serious or life-threatening H. flu infections. However, be sure to watch for changing recommendations about this important vaccine and for a new vaccine that will be helpful for young infants. Your child's doctor is an excellent resource for updating you on this type of information.

Other Vaccines

You may have heard about certain vaccines that are being used or tested against diseases other than those mentioned. New vaccines are constantly being developed and tested and will hopefully prove effective against many diseases. Some vaccines are currently available and useful in certain situations. A few of them are listed here.

96

GETTING HELP,
SAFETY,
PREVENTING
ILLNESS, AND
BEING
PREPARED FOR
LIFE-
THREATENING
EMERGENCIES

Influenza vaccine (to protect against influenza viruses) is recommended only for infants and children with certain chronic health problems that make it likely they would have serious complications from influenza. Included are those with serious heart disease, serious chronic lung disease, some kidney disease, certain cancers and immune problems, diabetes, and some serious forms of anemia.

Pneumococcal vaccine is designed to protect certain children against overwhelming infection with fourteen types of the pneumococcus bacteria. Children over two years old who have no spleen, those with sickle-cell anemia, nephrotic syndrome (a kidney problem), and immune problems might benefit from this vaccine. It is not very effective in infants under two years of age.

Smallpox vaccine, once used routinely, no longer has any recommended role in childhood immunization. It should not be given.

If you have any questions about these or any of the immunizations recommended now or in the future, contact your child's doctor.

About the Diseases Themselves

Diphtheria is a serious bacterial infection of the respiratory system and involves the nose, throat, and windpipe. The infection can make a thick membrane of pus that obstructs breathing. In addition, the diphtheria bacteria produce a toxin (poison) that causes serious problems with the heart (inflammation of the heart muscle—called myocarditis) and the nervous system (possible paralysis of various areas of the body).

Before the discovery of antibiotics and antitoxins and other kinds of treatment, death from diphtheria was quite common. It is still fatal for those who experience serious heart or nervous system complications. Unfortunately, there are people who can get this disease and yet not be protected from getting it a second time. For both children and adults, the diphtheria immunization is a successful preventive measure against this serious disease.

Tetanus (also called "lockjaw") is a disease caused by a toxin (poison) made by the tetanus bacteria. This toxin damages the nervous system and causes severe muscle spasms. Tetanus bacteria are found everywhere. They become a serious threat when they enter wounds that have not been carefully cleaned and that do not allow air inside (for example, puncture wounds), because the germs grow best where there is no oxygen. Therefore, careful washing of all wounds helps to prevent this disease, but the immunization is the most effective means of protection. Tetanus, like diphtheria, can affect a person more than once (if the person has not been immunized against it).

Pertussis (whooping cough) is a serious respiratory disease that is most dangerous for young infants but can be serious in children and even adults. Of greatest concern are infants under one year old, since they are more likely to have serious, life-threatening problems with the disease. Pertussis starts much like a cold (with runny nose and congestion, then a cough). This coldlike illness usually gets worse over a two-week period (unlike a normal cold, which generally improves in the second week). The second stage of the disease usually lasts another two weeks.

It is this second stage that gave whooping cough its name. Coughing becomes very severe and occurs in spells. The youngster coughs so hard and so constantly that he or she can't catch a breath until the end of the spell and turns very blue. At the end of the spell, the child takes a sharp breath, making a loud "whooping" sound. There may be many spells in a day during the worst part of the illness. Many children vomit after the coughing spells. Young infants under six months old may not make the "whooping" noise but still have very serious coughing spells and experience lack of oxygenation.

In the third stage of the disease (which also lasts about two weeks), the coughing spells become less frequent.

The complications of the disease include pneumonia; ear infection; slowing of the heart during the coughing spells; and a very serious brain disorder (called pertussis encephalopathy), which results in seizures and mental retardation. The most serious problems with pertussis result from lack of oxygen during the coughing spells, which leads to the heart's slowing and possible brain damage. Sometimes, too, the force of the coughing is associated with small hemorrhages (bleeding) in the eyes, on the face, and probably in the brain as well. If the lack of oxygen is severe, death can occur, or there can be such extensive brain damage that the child will be left in a coma.

Poliomyelitis is a potentially serious disease that killed or crippled thousands of children and young adults each year until an effective vaccine was developed to prevent it. Now the number of cases reported annually in the United States is about twenty-five—but the disease is still a serious problem in many parts of the world. In the United States, the risk of getting the disease is low, but this will continue only if we keep our children protected.

Polio is caused by one of three related viruses, which are spread by contact with either nose and mouth secretions or bowel movements of people with the virus. While most cases are actually mild and go unrecognized, some youngsters who get the disease suffer brain inflammation (meningoencephalitis), and about one in ten dies from it. Polio produces permanent paralysis and crippling in many who are not immunized against it.

Measles is a serious viral disease that was quite common before the vaccine was available. It starts like a very bad cold with high fever, red eyes, very runny nose, and severe cough. About four days later, a rash develops—both on the skin and on the linings of the mouth, respiratory tract, eyes, intestines, and urinary tract. The youngster is usually *very* sick for ten to fourteen days. Complications are serious, with one of every ten children getting ear infections and others getting pneumonia. About one in one thousand youngsters develops brain inflammation and has lasting damage. One in ten thousand who get the disease dies from it. Unfortunately, there is no cure and no effective treatment. Therefore, prevention is the best medicine.

Mumps is a relatively mild viral disease that usually infects the salivary (saliva-producing) glands of the mouth and leads to slight fever and pain and swelling of the

GETTING HELP,
SAFETY,
PREVENTING
ILLNESS, AND
BEING
PREPARED FOR
LIFE-
THREATENING
EMERGENCIES

cheeks in front of the ears. Some youngsters get more serious problems, such as inflammation of the pancreas (which is an organ in the abdomen that produces enzymes for digestion as well as the hormone insulin). About one in ten youngsters gets a mild inflammation of the brain and spinal cord. About one-fourth of teenage and adult men who get mumps get inflammation of the testicles, and a few older girls and women get a similar inflammation of the ovaries. These problems are painful but rarely if ever cause total sterility, as was believed earlier. One of the most common and serious aftereffects of mumps is deafness (usually partial, not total).

One attack of mumps causes permanent immunity, and many adults have immunity without ever knowing they had the disease. Contrary to popular belief, having gland swelling on only one side of the face does not mean you will have to get the disease again (with swelling on the other side) to be completely immune. A condition often confused with mumps is neck swelling caused by inflammation of the lymph nodes of the neck.

Rubella (so-called German measles or three-day measles) is a mild disease for children and most adults. They have a low fever; swelling of the lymph nodes (so-called glands) at the back of the neck; and a mild rash, which lasts about three days. A few people—most often adults—also have a mild arthritis with joint pain and swelling for several weeks.

At highest risk for serious problems from this disease is the fetus whose mother gets rubella during pregnancy—particularly early pregnancy. Miscarriage may result, or the fetus can suffer serious, permanent damage. Congenital rubella causes such conditions as blindness, deafness, mental retardation, heart defects, and other serious deformities. So, you see, it is vital that females be immunized before childbearing age (preferably during childhood) to avoid exposing their unborn children to potentially serious problems, if not death in some cases.

Hemophilus influenzae type b (*"H. flu"*) is a very strong, resilient bacteria that can cause serious, life-threatening infections in infants, toddlers, and older children. The risk for infection with this devastating germ is especially great early in life but continues throughout childhood and even into adulthood (although it is rarely seen in adults). About one in one thousand children suffers a serious H. flu infection each year, and even effective antibiotic therapy cannot always prevent death or permanent damage for certain of these children.

Meningitis (infection of the covering of the brain and spinal cord), epiglottitis (infection of the epiglottis, which is located at the base of the tongue), and sepsis (overwhelming general body infection—so-called blood poisoning) are the most serious of the diseases that can be caused by the H. flu bacteria. However, this dangerous bacteria can also cause infections of the soft tissues around the eye, cheek, and face (called cellulitis); pneumonia; pericarditis (infection in the sac that surrounds the heart); bone infections (osteomyelitis); and joint infections (septic arthritis).

H. flu bacterial infections are spread by contact with nose and mouth secretions. We now know that some children can carry this bacteria without actually getting the infection or any of the diseases it causes. The problem is that those who carry the bacteria do present a risk to other young children with whom they come into contact. Unfortunately, H. flu infections spread quite easily in groups of children, such as those in day care or preschool, and even in families. The vaccine, then, is a major break-through in helping to prevent infection by H. flu bacteria, as well as the spread of its potentially deadly and/or disabling diseases.

The Bottom Line on Immunizations

The availability and widespread use of immunizations have been responsible for a significant decline in death and disability due to "childhood diseases." It's important that infants and children continue to be protected with vaccines if that trend is to be maintained. If we relax our stand, the diseases will return. This is well documented in the case of pertussis vaccine (in Great Britain).

On the other hand, while vaccines have many benefits, they also have risks. For the average youngster, the benefits of routine immunization far outweigh the potential risks. However, there may be situations in which the risks are significant and warrant careful decision making and, at times, avoidance of the immunization.

As parents, you have an important role in deciding whether your youngsters will be immunized or not. You also have the responsibility to be well informed and to weigh the evidence as it is now known. Armed with the facts—from reading, as well as from asking questions of your doctor—you can make an informed decision on behalf of your children.

The Importance of Teaching Our Children Good Health Habits

Now, more than at any other time in history, we have become keenly aware that *prevention* of illness and injury *is always the best and most practical medicine!* It has, over the years, become even more clear that certain life-styles and daily habits have a great deal more to do with our health and well-being (or lack of it) than we ever before imagined.

Good health habits are learned. How we treat our bodies early in life determines a great deal about how healthy we will be later in life. Starting from the moment of conception, the human body is dependent on good nutrition (from the mother) to develop and grow. Even then, the little being can be affected by an adverse environment—cigarette smoking, alcohol, drugs, and other chemicals can cause damage to the fetus.

Once the baby is born, the learning process begins. At this point, infants and children have very little to say about what they eat and drink or even what they are allowed to

GETTING HELP,
SAFETY,
PREVENTING
ILLNESS, AND
BEING
PREPARED FOR
LIFE-
THREATENING
EMERGENCIES

do. They are totally dependent on our best judgments and are essentially at our mercy until they are old enough to make their own choices. If we encourage proper nutrition, exercise, and other good health habits, these become routine (a type of life-style) for the young person.

If, on the other hand, a child is not encouraged to eat properly, exercise, and follow sound health principles, he or she will more than likely not follow these later in life. We now know that the diet of infants and children not only determines their nutritional habits but also has a lot to do with the size and number of fat cells they will have in their bodies. Roly-poly babies—those truly fat—are more likely to be overweight teenagers and adults. If children are allowed to continually indulge in ''junk food'' or even too much ''good'' food, then they will more than likely eat the same way all their lives.

This principle is true in most other areas as well. Good examples from parents are important. If parents exercise daily and include their children in these activities (at the level of their physical and mental maturity), then the children will enjoy exercise and make it part of their lives. If children see that their parents do not smoke or drink alcohol excessively and that they do not use drugs, at least they will have a solid foundation of good health habits on which to base personal decisions.

Establishing good health habits requires time, patience, and a commitment to do so. It requires active participation from us—not just a ''Do as I say, not as I do'' philosophy. We all know children are too smart for that and will only throw it back at us someday. Therefore, we must make a decision early on, when our children are born. It is then that we establish our priorities and help form our children's daily habits. If we are physically inactive, careless about what kinds of food we eat and when we eat, and don't follow reasonable guidelines for good health, chances are we will teach our children to live their lives the same way.

Therefore, it is vital that we actively participate in our children's daily lives and encourage them to practice good health habits. If we can be good examples and ensure that they learn to enjoy healthy food, exercise, and respect safety rules, then we have given them a giant head start toward good health—and the prospects for a longer, healthier life.

An example: One father mentioned that he couldn't understand why his son and daughter were content to sit around the house on weekends—watching television, downing one soda after another, and eating junk food. When asked if he would describe what he and his wife thought was an enjoyable time, he said they like sitting around the house watching television on the weekends. When asked if meals were served on weekends, he replied that there were plenty of snacks available and they sometimes ran out to a local hamburger stand and brought back dinner. The point here is not to criticize but rather to point out that children do follow our examples, even when we aren't aware that we are sending certain signals.

Another example: One couple expressed concern that their children were never home and were too active in a variety of after-school activities. They felt they rarely got to spend time with them. After talking about this for a while, it became clear to both parents that they had set the example for this. Both were committed to their work. Each belonged to social groups and fitness centers and was also involved in a variety of other activities. The children had learned that it was important to be involved, active, and busy. After thinking it over, both parents decided that the children had simply followed their example, and they were glad to see that they were active in sports and involved in school activities and social organizations. They only regretted one thing: they hadn't set aside activities and times for the family to be together. They hadn't made relaxation a part of their life-style and feared that the children would be too goal oriented and enormously stressed later in life by the need to continually achieve.

Therefore, we must take care to send the signals we wish to send—whether they are about the kind of food to eat, the best ways to relax, the importance of physical activity and fitness, or the amount of work that is healthy but not overly stressful. We can have a major impact on how our children see themselves and how they choose to live their lives. These concepts are learned quite early in life and form a solid resource upon which the youngsters can draw as they grow older.

THE DON'TS

Don't neglect your infant's or child's immunizations. If you have serious concerns, talk to your doctor. No one wants to put his or her children at needless risk for serious diseases.

Don't hesitate to get all the facts about immunizations—both their risks and their benefits. Ask your child's doctor to clarify any points you don't understand and help guide your decisions.

Don't forget to establish the framework for your child's good health habits. Children learn by example, and the process starts early in infancy.

PLEASE NOTE: Now that you have a grasp of what immunizations are all about it would be extremely helpful for you to go back to the Quick Reference and review it carefully. Reviewing the Recommended Schedule for Immunizations will help you determine if your child has received immunizations on schedule and/or allow you to discuss with your doctor certain immunizations your child may require.

C H A P T E R 4

Being Prepared for Emergencies

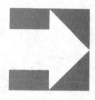

QUICK REFERENCE

Being Prepared

▶ **SERIOUSLY CONSIDER THE IMPORTANCE OF BECOMING CERTI-FIED IN CPR (CARDIOPULMONARY RESUSCITATION).** Find out where and when there is a convenient training course available for you and other members of your family and friends.

▶ **THINK ABOUT TAKING A FIRST AID TRAINING COURSE.** This is particularly important for anyone who feels insecure or is fearful he or she might panic in a medical emergency. Hands-on training is very helpful in alleviating these fears!

▶ **CHECK YOUR HOME FIRST-AID SUPPLIES (AT LEAST ONCE A YEAR) TO MAKE SURE ALL THE BASIC SUPPLIES YOU NEED ARE READ-ILY AVAILABLE.** Also, consider putting together a first aid kit for your car and/or for trips/vacations where you might need one.

▶ **HAVE CONFIDENCE IN YOUR ABILITY TO STAY CALM AND HANDLE ANY MEDICAL EMERGENCY.** Remember, the more you know, the better you will be able to respond calmly and remain in control—no matter how difficult the situation.

Learning to Save a Life

Taking the time to learn how to perform CPR (cardiopulmonary resuscitation) is one of the very important ways you can really make a difference—between life and death (in many situations). CPR is essentially a technique whereby you breathe for the person who is not breathing and physically pump his or her heart when the heart has stopped. It requires learning how to perform mouth-to-mouth resuscitation (now called rescue breathing) and external cardiac compression. These techniques are also known as providing "basic life support"—a good definition for them.

Mouth-to-mouth resuscitation is a way of forcing needed oxygen into another person's lungs. External cardiac compression is a technique involving compression of the outside of the chest (at a very specific point) for a certain number of times each minute. When the outside of the chest is compressed properly, the heart is squeezed between the rib cage and the backbone. When the heart is squeezed, it pushes the oxygen-enriched blood throughout the body. These two techniques together form the basis for CPR—*c*ardio (heart), *p*ulmonary (lungs), *r*esuscitation (revival).

The development of this lifesaving technique was a major medical breakthrough. It gave medical professionals a means of keeping someone in what is called the gray area—between life and death—until further steps could be taken to treat him or her and restart the heart. Brilliantly, someone thought to take this idea one step further—by having nonmedical people taught how to perform CPR. Some said this could not be done, but others were determined that the public could easily learn CPR and that the result of this training would be the saving of a significant number of lives each year.

The testing ground was Seattle, Washington, where approximately 125,000 people went through a citizens' CPR training course. It was found that 20 percent of resuscitations from cardiac arrest (outside of the hospital) were being initiated by someone other than the paramedics. Time is a critical factor when the heart and lungs stop working. The study showed that when CPR was started one to two minutes after the cardiac arrest occurred, 40 percent of those resuscitated walked out of the hospital after treatment. When the delay was greater (until the paramedics arrived—even considering how fast they respond), only 18 percent of those resuscitated later walked out of the hospital.

104

GETTING HELP,
SAFETY,
PREVENTING
ILLNESS, AND
BEING
PREPARED FOR
LIFE-
THREATENING
EMERGENCIES

Why the difference? Simply, when cardiac arrest occurs, it takes only four to six minutes for death or severe, permanent brain damage to follow. The longer the brain and other organs are without oxygen, the greater the risk for serious damage or death. If every person eleven years of age and older knew how to perform CPR, many, many more lives could be saved each and every day.

Despite this enormous lifesaving potential, CPR is surprisingly easy to learn. It doesn't take any athletic ability or great strength. It doesn't require unusually skillful coordination. You don't need to know much about human physiology to perform it. What it does require, however, is formal training! Training takes only four to eight hours and is well worth the time and trouble.

There is no way CPR can be taught in this or any other book alone. All we can do is explain what CPR is in general terms and how vital it is for you to be trained. It requires learning and practicing the correct techniques through hands-on experience with specially designed mannequins that stimulate the actual "feeling" of compressing the chest properly (without causing injury) and breathing for someone. It takes, most of all, learning the correct mechanical techniques and practicing them—until they become second nature to you.

Knowing how to perform CPR doesn't just help your children if they experience a crisis. In fact, becoming certified in CPR is probably one of the single most important public services you could perform. The chances are actually pretty good that you will be faced sometime in your life with a situation where a loved one, a friend, or even a stranger needs your help. Whether or not you are certified in CPR may make the difference between that person's living to talk about what happened to him or her that day—or death. Whether it's a heart attack suffered by an adult or those mishaps anyone at any age can experience (like drowning, electrocution, shock, airway obstruction/choking, drug overdose, or poisoning) where the heart and lungs stop working—you *can* make the difference.

In many situations, you may be the only hope someone has for survival. *If you are certified in CPR,* then that person—youngster or adult—has the best chance to survive. *If you are not certified in CPR,* the person's chance for survival is drastically reduced, and in some situations, there would be little or *no* hope if you could not immediately perform CPR.

Remember, you have only a matter of moments to really help someone in this type of situation. If you decide not to take a CPR course, there's really no going back. If something happens, it's simply too late then. It won't do any good to say, "I should have taken that course." In reality, it's a decision either to be able to do something or to stand by and do nothing. It's a terribly helpless feeling when you are not able to assist someone in this kind of critical situation. For the sake of our children, other loved ones, and friends, each of us should take the time to make a difference.

CPR courses are frequently offered by the American Heart Association, the National Red Cross and its local or regional chapters, area medical centers or hospitals, colleges, civic groups, and even some gyms and fitness centers. Just call one of these places in your area, and the staff can tell you when the next course begins.

First Aid Training

First aid training is excellent for everyone—because it gives hands-on experience. Most classes don't just involve lectures; more often, they emphasize how to do things—such as how to apply a compression wrap, a splint, and a tourniquet; how to manage shock, stop bleeding, treat a snakebite; how to transport someone who is injured or ill; and how to check vital signs (heart rate and breathing), make someone more comfortable, and keep the victim as calm as possible. Some first aid classes also teach CPR (cardiopulmonary resuscitation). If you're looking for a first aid class that includes CPR, make sure you ask whether CPR certification training is part of the course.

Because most junior (city) colleges (and sometimes four-year colleges and universities) offer "emergency medical technician" training (called EMT training), they often provide quite excellent first aid courses. Other places to consider are community organizations, such as the Red Cross, local medical associations, your community hospital, the parks and recreation department, and even some fitness centers and gyms. If a place you contact does not provide first aid training, ask who does in the local area.

The real importance of first aid classes and CPR training is that both prepare you for medical emergencies. You no longer feel helpless when something occurs—but take proper action without hesitation. These classes and CPR training are quite helpful for new or expectant parents who feel anxious about meeting the health care needs of their family. Most people say they feel a great deal more secure after first aid and CPR training and feel confident that they are well prepared to do what is necessary if a crisis occurs. Baby-sitters really should have both first aid and CPR training, as should all coaches (whether or not they are coaching an organized sport) and all others who work with children.

The real answer to this problem would be to require first aid and CPR training in junior high school and high school, as well as at the college level. Businesses could provide training for their employees, as could all government agencies for their employees. Requiring training would be a giant step toward preventing unnecessary death and, in some cases, unnecessary lifelong disability or chronic conditions. Until then, each of us should take the first step by completing the courses ourselves, so we can be prepared for medical emergencies.

Your Mini–Medicine Centers

Many people feel that "having first aid supplies available" means keeping a small box of Band-Aids somewhere around the house. The problem is that most injuries and illnesses give little or no warning. Then, just when you need something most—it simply isn't there. That problem can easily be alleviated with some advance planning

106

GETTING HELP,
SAFETY,
PREVENTING
ILLNESS, AND
BEING
PREPARED FOR
LIFE-
THREATENING
EMERGENCIES

and attention. Your medicine cabinet and first aid kit should really be ''mini–medicine centers.'' Both should be well stocked with proper supplies, which must be updated and maintained carefully.

THE MEDICINE CABINET

First, start with your medicine cabinet. Most often a medicine cabinet becomes a potpourri of pills, ointments, creams, and out-of-date prescriptions—instead of a resource center. Clean it out carefully, discarding *all old or unused* prescriptions, over-the-counter drugs, ointments, and medicated creams. If there is no expiration date, take a look at the condition of the container. If it's old or damaged—discard it. (Some people mark the date of purchase on all these items themselves and throw out everything more than a year old.) Check all labels on over-the-counter medications, ointments, and creams to determine their expiration dates. It's important for you to realize that the chemical contents of drugs *do* age and can act differently if they are past their expiration date. You really wouldn't want to take them or give them to your children. It is best to clean out the medicine cabinet at least once a year and replace items as needed.

Whether your medicine cabinet is in the bathroom or elsewhere in the house—make sure it is always locked. The key should be kept far from the reach, climbing ability and ingenuity of toddlers and young children. All medicines should be kept in one place—the locked medicine cabinet. This is not only a safety precaution but makes it quite easy to find something when you need it.

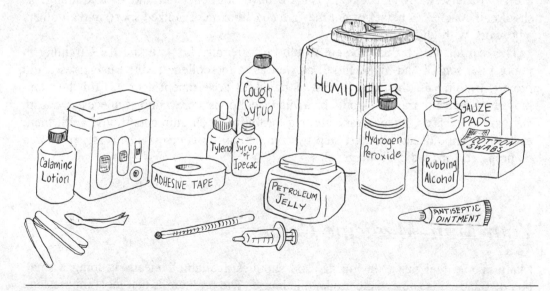

Stock and maintain your mini–medicine centers so you are always prepared to deal with an illness or injury.

THE FIRST AID KIT

Your next step should be to put together a first aid kit. Although prepackaged first aid kits are available for purchase, most do not have all the needed supplies in them, and some can be quite expensive. Plastic (fishing) tackle boxes are inexpensive, and the many compartments in them make it quite easy to organize supplies accessibly. You can use the First Aid Supplies Shopping List in this chapter as a guide for buying supplies.

All first aid supplies should be stored in the case you buy for that purpose, not scattered all over the house, making it difficult to find them. And since these supplies and medicines can be dangerous in the hands of children, you must observe the same precautions that you do with the medicine cabinet. Namely, once you have the kit together, make sure you put a lock on it; make sure the lock is always used; and make sure both the kit and the key are in a safe place (keeping in mind the young person's reach, climbing ability, and often creative thinking when his or her curiosity is aroused).

As with your medicine cabinet, check your first aid kit at least once a year, discarding damaged or old supplies and all out-of-date medications. Restock supplies that are low or missing. You may want to check the kit before going on vacation or long trips — to make sure all needed supplies are there. It is also a good idea to go through the first aid kit after returning from a vacation and replace anything you had to use while gone. You may wish to review the First Aid Supplies Shopping List at your yearly supply check, since it would help to refresh your memory about what items should be included.

You may want to consider having two first aid kits—one for the home and one for the car. If this would be financially impossible, then it would be best for you to take the first aid kit with you on all trips or vacations and put it back in the house when you return.

One note about the keys to the medicine cabinet and the first aid kit: Some people have extra keys made so they can have a key for their key chains, as well as keys for in the house. Usually they place one key for the medicine cabinet and another for the first aid kit on a hook or nail inside a high cupboard or cabinet. It's best to tape a piece of paper identifying the keys above the hook or nail as well as mark the keys themselves with fingernail polish (*M* for medicine cabinet and *1st* or *A* for the first aid kit).

First Aid Supplies Shopping List

Your first aid kit should include the items listed below. (Those items in boldface are the bare minimum supplies you should have in your first aid kit.)

- **One or two rolls of adhesive tape.**

- One roll of gauze.

GETTING HELP,
SAFETY,
PREVENTING
ILLNESS, AND
BEING
PREPARED FOR
LIFE-
THREATENING
EMERGENCIES

- **A package of sterile gauze pads (separately wrapped).**

- **A box of small adhesive strip bandages (like Band-Aids).**

- One or two elastic wraps (like an Ace bandage).

- Cotton balls.

- Cotton swabs (like Q-Tips).

- **A bar of plain soap (unperfumed).**

- **A bottle of antiseptic cleaner** (like hydrogen peroxide or Betadine).

- An antiseptic cream (for minor cuts and burns).

- A jar of petroleum jelly (for chapping, chafing, or blisters).

- Calamine lotion.

- **A bottle of liquid acetaminophen** (like children's Tylenol, Panadol, Tempra, Liquiprin, or the store brand available) **for the infant or young child.**

- **A bottle of chewable children's acetaminophen for older children.**

- **A bottle of regular aspirin or acetaminophen for teenagers and adults.**

- **A one-ounce bottle of syrup of ipecac** (to induce vomiting).

- Sunscreen.

- Lip balm (like Chap Stick).

- **A rectal thermometer.**

- Safety pins.

- Tweezers.

- **Scissors.**

- Snakebite kit.

- A man's tie, cheesecloth, or a long piece of a sheet (useful as a tourniquet).

- Tongue depressors (useful as splints for injured fingers and toes).

- **A good flashlight (with extra, sealed batteries for backup).**

- **A chemical "ice bag" if the kit will be used outside the house where ice is not available.**

- An anaphylaxis kit (if prescribed by your doctor for a family member who is very allergic to bee stings and so on).

- A backup supply of a prescription drug if someone in the family has a chronic condition that requires daily medication. (Mark this *carefully* as to what it is and its date of expiration. Dispose of this when the expiration date passes, and replace the supply with new medication.)

Handling an Emergency

Many people think they simply cannot "handle" a medical emergency. You may feel that you would go blank, panic, just stand there, get sick, faint, do the wrong thing, or even run! The truth is, none of these things happens when you're *prepared* and *know that you can help.* The best way to be prepared and feel confident about your ability to respond promptly and correctly is to be certified in CPR and take first aid training, as well as learn all you can about taking care of a child when he or she is sick or injured. The more you know, the better equipped you are to respond and to stay calm and alert.

It's when people feel helpless that they go blank, panic, get sick, just stand there, faint, do the wrong thing, or run. Since they don't know how to help, they respond in the only way they know—by fleeing from the trauma (in their own way). You've probably heard people say, "I just can't handle it." The irony of that statement is that if they were trained and knowledgeable, they *would* handle it.

This gets more complicated when you realize that some people, believing they can't handle an emergency, don't take CPR and first aid training or even read about how to respond. It becomes a vicious cycle. Because they *feel* they can't handle such a situation, they don't take the training courses or read about what to do—so then they *really* can't handle it. It becomes a self-fulfilling prophecy. The way to break the vicious cycle is to become as prepared as possible—by taking the training and learning all you can about emergency care. These steps really do make you feel much more confident, and you find that the principles and techniques become second nature to you.

It's important to remember that when they are in training, even medical professionals have moments when they wonder if they could "handle" some things. They find they are so well trained and prepared, though, that they respond well and do what they were trained or prepared to do. You may also be surprised to know that it is perfectly normal to feel shaky, nauseated, sick, dizzy, faint, or panic-stricken *after* the emergency is over. Some people can be totally calm, totally efficient throughout a medical emergency—then faint or vomit once the crisis is past. Others simply become weak in the knees or get the shivers.

The bottom line, however, is that those who are well trained and knowledgeable— prepared for the unexpected—do stay calm, alert, and responsive during a medical emergency. The only way you can help someone—particularly a child whom you love—is to stay calm no matter how difficult it is to do so. Your first priority must be the safety and well-being of the injured or ill person. You *must* be able to control

110

GETTING HELP,
SAFETY,
PREVENTING
ILLNESS, AND
BEING
PREPARED FOR
LIFE-
THREATENING
EMERGENCIES

the situation so you can help the young person—above all else. If you panic or don't think clearly, you won't be able to do anything useful.

THE DON'TS

Don't let the fear that you might not be able to handle emergencies stop you from learning how you actually can handle them.

Don't let anxiety stop you from taking CPR training and a first aid course. The hours you set aside may someday prove to be the most worthwhile time you'll ever spend.

Don't forget that everybody worries about how they will react and whether they will do what is necessary to help in a medical emergency. The fact is, each of us can learn how to handle an emergency—and feel really good about ourselves for doing so.

PLEASE NOTE: Now that you have a better grasp of being prepared for emergencies, it would be extremely helpful for you to go back to the Quick Reference and review the points that are important reminders.

SECTION 2

Life-Threatening Emergencies:
Only a Matter of Moments

Seconds and minutes tick off quickly. We don't think much about this precious time or how important it can be—until we face a serious medical emergency. There is a handful of medical emergencies where seconds and minutes can make the difference between life and death—or between full recovery and a serious, lifelong disability or even irreversible brain damage.

Your ability to respond effectively to these life-threatening emergencies is essential. Cardiopulmonary arrest due to many causes—airway obstruction/choking, serious bleeding, shock, unconsciousness, poisoning, and drowning—all require immediate action by someone who is knowledgeable and trained in basic life-support procedures.

As you read Chapters 5 through 11, imagine yourself facing these kinds of situations, and in your mind, put yourself through the rescue steps. This is often a helpful way to remember what steps you would need to take if actually confronted with these crises. It is best to review the information until you feel comfortable and confident that you could do what needs to be done. The greater your ability to imagine yourself in a similar situation, the easier it is to "see" the rescue steps (visualize yourself performing them), which makes it far easier to remember them. You really have only a matter of moments in some situations—moments that can save a life.

C H A P T E R 5

Cardiopulmonary Arrest

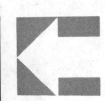

EMERGENCY QUICK REFERENCE

With the Steps in Detail

A Review of the Six Steps of CPR (Cardiopulmonary Resuscitation)

The following discussion will not teach you how to perform CPR but will review the six basic steps for those already trained in CPR. It will also familiarize you with the procedure if you have not as yet taken the CPR training course. In this way, you will be more comfortable in the CPR course, and the language won't be as foreign to you. By the way, the *ABC*'s of CPR are *airway*, *breathing*, and *circulation*—an easy way to remember the basic components of this lifesaving technique!

114

LIFE-
THREATENING
EMERGENCIES:
ONLY A
MATTER OF
MOMENTS

Step One of CPR

▶ **DETERMINE IF THE YOUNGSTER IS UNRESPONSIVE.**

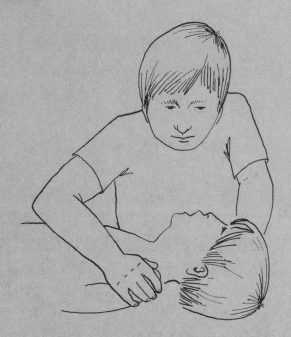

Shout the youngster's name and gently shake his shoulder to determine if he is unresponsive.

- Kneel next to the young person and shout his or her name a few times. For example, "Johnny, Johnny! Are you OK, Johnny?"

- At the same time you are trying to arouse the youngster by shouting, gently shake or tap on her shoulder (as you would do when trying to awaken someone) or pinch the foot or skin under the arm. *Do not shake an infant or a young child*, since this can result in serious injury. You are only trying to see if the youngster is unresponsive or unconscious— *not* to "shake her into consciousness" (which won't work anyway).

- If the young person is unconscious, you will also notice that his legs and arms are limp and that he will not move, moan, or cry when you touch or shout at him.

Step Two of CPR

▶ **SHOUT FOR HELP.**

- If someone else is with you, have that person call the paramedics while you treat the child.

- If no one is with you, continue treating the child while you periodically shout for help. When help arrives, have that person call the paramedics.

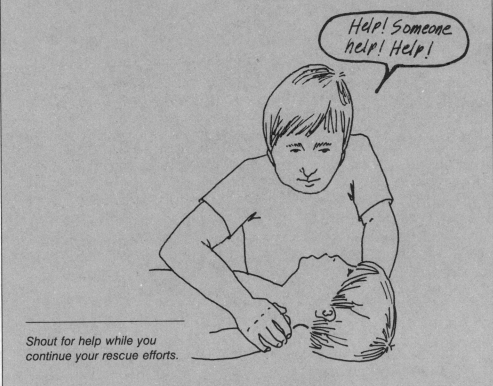

Help! Someone help! Help!

Shout for help while you continue your rescue efforts.

Step Three of CPR

▶ **POSITION THE YOUNGSTER.**

- If there is a potential head, neck, or spine injury, then the youngster should not be moved—*unless* she is not breathing or is having serious difficulty breathing (and the airway must be opened to alleviate this).

116

LIFE-
THREATENING
EMERGENCIES:
ONLY A
MATTER OF
MOMENTS

- The youngster needs to be placed on his back. It's important that the surface on which the child is placed be hard and flat.

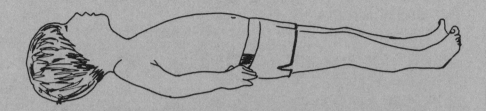

Position the youngster on his back on a hard, flat surface. Use extreme caution if you have any reason to believe he may have a head, neck, or back injury.

- Take care in moving the youngster. If he is lying facedown or on his side, you must *move him as a unit*—while supporting the head and neck. You can do this by placing one hand under the neck and head. Hold this area securely so it does not twist, roll, or move as you roll the youngster onto his back.

Step Four of CPR

▶ **OPEN THE AIRWAY AND DETERMINE WHETHER OR NOT THE YOUNGSTER IS BREATHING.**

- Open the airway (as you were taught in CPR training).

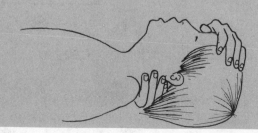

To open the airway: Lift the neck gently with one hand while you tip the head back with your other hand.

- Remember that you must use a different technique based on whether or not there is or may be a head, neck, or serious back injury.

- In most situations (where there is no head, neck, or serious back injury), you open the airway by putting one hand under the youngster's neck and the other hand on his or her forehead. Then, gently and carefully lift the neck while your other hand pushes back on the forehead. Do not tip the child's head too far back, since this can actually block the airway.

- If, however, this technique for opening the airway is not successful, you'll have to attempt the other techniques you learned in CPR training.

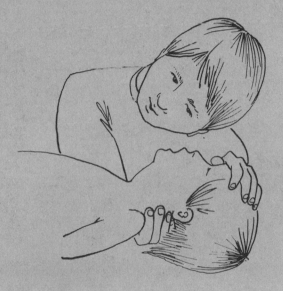

Checking for breathing: Look to see if the chest is rising. Listen and feel for air movement through the youngster's nose and mouth.

- Now see whether the chest rises and falls. Put your ear and cheek near the young person's mouth and nose and see if you can feel or hear air moving in or out.

Step Five of CPR

▶ **RESCUE BREATHING (MOUTH-TO-MOUTH RESUSCITATION).**

- If the youngster *is not breathing*, then deliver four rapid rescue breaths.

118

LIFE-
THREATENING
EMERGENCIES:
ONLY A
MATTER OF
MOMENTS

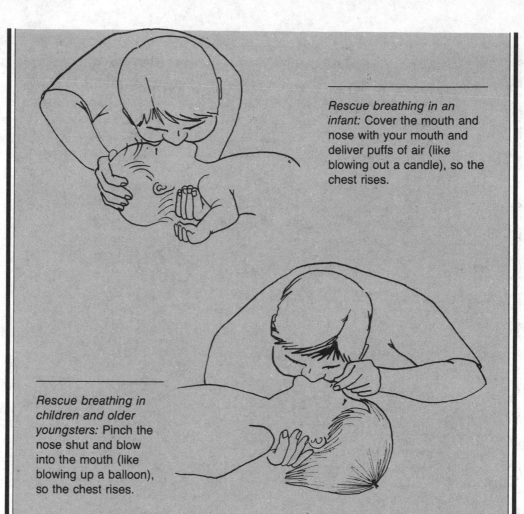

Rescue breathing in an infant: Cover the mouth and nose with your mouth and deliver puffs of air (like blowing out a candle), so the chest rises.

Rescue breathing in children and older youngsters: Pinch the nose shut and blow into the mouth (like blowing up a balloon), so the chest rises.

- If the *delivered air doesn't go in*, then there are two possibilities: (1) the airway is not properly open; (2) there is an airway obstruction (foreign body in the airway). Readjust the airway and try to deliver four more rescue breaths. If there appears to be an airway obstruction, relieve the obstruction immediately (as you were taught in CPR training) and deliver another four rescue breaths. Before you can go any further, *you must have an open airway and be able to perform rescue breathing.* Continue to repeat the steps to open the airway and relieve an obstruction (if present) until you have established an open airway. (If you are unable to remember the details of managing this problem, turn to the Emergency Quick Reference on page 127, entitled "Managing Airway Obstruction/Choking," for a review.)

- If the youngster *is breathing*, then maintain an open airway and watch for changes in her status (until the paramedics or ambulance arrive).

Step Six of CPR

▶ **CHECK FOR A PULSE.**

- Use the carotid artery (found in the neck) for children, adolescents, and adult-sized young people. Use the brachial artery (found in the upper arm) for infants.

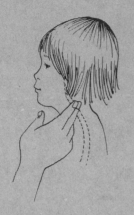 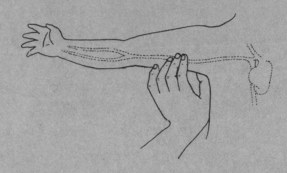

In children and older youngsters: Feel for the carotid pulse—found in front of the large muscle on either side of the neck.

In infants: Feel for a pulse on the inside of the upper arm.

- You can take up to ten seconds to determine if there is a pulse (see if the heart is working or not).

▶ **BEGIN CHEST COMPRESSIONS.**

- If cardiac arrest has occurred (there is no pulse), begin chest compressions in combination with rescue breathing (as you were taught in CPR certification training).

▶ **AS A REMINDER, THE RATIOS OF RESCUE BREATHS TO CHEST COMPRESSIONS ARE AS FOLLOWS:**

Infants (Under One Year of Age)

- Chest compression rate is one hundred compressions per minute.

- Compression-ventilation (rescue breathing) ratio is 5:1 (five compressions to one rescue breath).

120

LIFE-
THREATENING
EMERGENCIES:
ONLY A
MATTER OF
MOMENTS

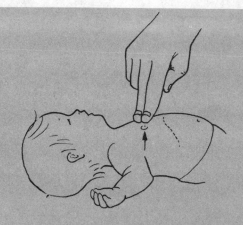

In infants: Compress the chest with your index and middle fingers. Position them on the middle of the breastbone between the nipples, as you were taught in your CPR course.

- Cadence used: "one, two, three, four, five, breathe, one, two, three, four, five, breathe," and so on.

- Depth of compressions: one-half inch to one inch.

- *The above are for both one- and two-rescuer CPR.*

Children (One to Eight Years of Age)

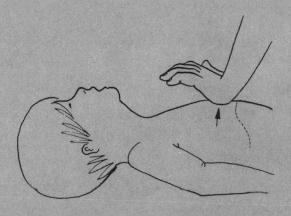

In children: Place the heel of one hand on the lower part of the breastbone, two finger widths above the notch of the ribcage, as you were taught in your CPR course.

- Chest compression rate is eighty compressions per minute.

- Compression-ventilation (rescue breathing) ratio is 5:1 (five compressions to one rescue breath).

- Cadence used: "one and two and three and four and five and breathe and one and two and three and four and five and breathe," and so on.

- Depth of compressions: 1 inch to 1½ inches.

- *The above are for both one- and two-rescuer CPR.*

Older Child, Adolescent, Adult-Sized Young Person (and Adult) (Anyone over Eight Years Old)

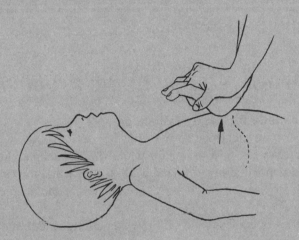

Older children and adolescents: Compress the chest with heels of both hands. Position your hands on the lower part of the breastbone, two finger widths above the notch of the ribcage, as you were taught in your CPR course.

One-Rescuer

- Chest compression rate is eighty compressions per minute.

- Compression-ventilation (rescue breathing) ratio is 15:2 (fifteen compressions to two rescue breaths).

- Cadence used: "one and two and three and four and five and six and seven and eight and nine and ten and eleven and twelve and thirteen and fourteen and fifteen and breathe and breathe," and so on.

- Depth of compressions: 1½ to 2 inches.

Two-Rescuer

- Chest compression rate is sixty compressions per minute.

122

LIFE-
THREATENING
EMERGENCIES:
ONLY A
MATTER OF
MOMENTS

- Compression-ventilation (rescue breathing) ratio is 5:1 (five compressions to one rescue breath).

- Cadence used: "one–one thousand, two–one thousand, three–one thousand, four–one thousand, five–breathe, one–one thousand, two–one thousand, three–one thousand, four–one thousand, five–breathe," and so on.

- The rescue breath is delivered on the upbeat of "five." Therefore, one rescuer compresses the chest on "five," and as he or she releases that compression on "breathe," the rescue breath is given by the second rescuer.

Cardiopulmonary Arrest: A Look at the Problem

A four-year-old peddles her tricycle into the family swimming pool. A six-year-old chokes on a piece of meat. A live wire electrocutes a young boy as he plays with daddy's tools. A teenager falls partway down a mountain while she is backpacking. A curious toddler walks out the patio door and falls into the wading pool while mommy is on the phone and daddy is rushing to answer the door. A seventeen-year-old staggers from a car crash, then collapses.

The list of possible serious injuries is endless, and all have something in common. Because of the seriousness of the injuries, each young person may be facing sudden death or serious, lifelong disability. Your ability to immediately initiate basic life-support procedures—CPR (cardiopulmonary resuscitation)—may be the youngster's only hope for survival.

As we discussed in Chapter 4, when a young person or adult stops breathing—it's only a matter of moments before his or her heart stops, too. The reverse is also true—once the heart stops, breathing will cease rather rapidly. When the heart and lungs cease to function, it's called "cardiopulmonary arrest." (*Cardio* means heart, *pulmonary* means lungs, and *arrest* means *both* stop!) Even if the young person is later revived, permanent brain damage could already have occurred because of lack of adequate oxygen to the brain for a period of time. Other organs can suffer irreparable damage because of lack of oxygen, as well.

Four to six minutes! That's all it takes for someone to die or experience profound and irreversible brain damage (and other serious physical problems) as a result of cardiopulmonary arrest. Fortunately, youngsters *may* tolerate oxygen deprivation longer than adults (usually death occurs six to fifteen minutes after the oxygen supply is lost). However, the sooner you start your rescue efforts, the better!

If a youngster chokes on a piece of meat, obstructing the airway—he will stop breathing. After breathing has ceased, the heart will arrest rather quickly. If you are able to remove the obstruction (see Chapter 6 for details), you may be faced with one of two serious problems. If his heart hasn't stopped as yet but the child isn't breathing, you must be able to breathe for him. If both lung and heart function have ceased, then you must not only be able to breathe for him but circulate the delivered oxygen through the body by physically pumping the heart. You must be able to do this until the paramedics or other help arrives and takes over your life-support efforts.

If neither you nor anyone else there is able to perform CPR, the youngster's chance for survival is rather slim. With each minute that passes, the possibility of survival becomes even less. As seconds tick away, the risk for very serious and permanent brain damage becomes greater—even if emergency medical personnel are able to restart heart and lung function when they arrive at the scene or later at the hospital.

Most often, infants, children, and teenagers experience cardiac arrest as a result of hypoxia (lack of adequate oxygen intake). In other words, their lung function stops, and heart failure follows. The lungs can cease to function for many reasons. The major events that cause pulmonary arrest are: *airway obstruction* due to a foreign body, such as large chunks of food (in particular, peanuts, popcorn, hot dogs, and other large pieces of meat), coins, buttons, plastic covers, balloons, beads, rubber bands, paper clips, Band-Aids, and small toys or toy parts; *drowning* or *near-drowning; poisoning; drug overdose; smoke inhalation; automobile accidents; other accidents, especially those involving serious head injuries; infection* that blocks the airway; *allergic reaction* to a substance; or *sudden infant death syndrome* (SIDS). *Electrocution* can essentially stop heart function directly.

Cardiopulmonary Arrest: Signs and Symptoms

It's an experience almost every parent has had: quietly entering the baby's room to make sure he or she is breathing. Parents talk about how they simply stand there for a few minutes and stare at the baby's tiny body. When they see the chest and abdomen rise and fall a few times, they smile with relief and quietly leave. Parents also talk about doing the same thing when their children are sick, injured, or just not feeling well (no matter what the young person's age).

The point is, the most obvious way to tell whether someone is breathing or not is to *see if his or her chest and abdomen rise and fall.*

Another way to tell whether someone is breathing or not is to put your ear and cheek close to his or her mouth and nose—to see if you can *feel* or *hear air being exhaled.* Also, if the young person's lips, fingernails, toenails, and skin are blue—he or she either is not receiving enough oxygen or is not breathing at all.

Determining if the heart is functioning or not is a little more difficult. Trying to ''hear'' the heartbeat with your ear against the young person's chest is not a very

124

LIFE-
THREATENING
EMERGENCIES:
ONLY A
MATTER OF
MOMENTS

effective way to determine whether the heart is functioning. Someone's heart can be working—although in a weakened state—but you still won't be able to "hear" a heartbeat. The only way you can really determine if the heart is functioning is to *feel for a pulse*. Every time the heart contracts (squeezes down), it pushes blood through the arteries (large blood vessels), which transport the oxygenated blood to all organs and tissues. If slight pressure is put on one of the major arteries just below the skin, you can feel the pulse.

What you are really feeling is an increase in pressure at that spot as the blood is pushed by. For example, if you put your hand on or around a garden hose, then turned the water off and on in a rhythmic manner (let's say, one second on, then one second off), you would feel the "pulse" of the water going through the garden hose. This same basic principle applies to the heart and the arteries. Each time the heart pushes blood into the arteries, there is a rise in pressure in the arteries (a throb is felt), and anytime the heart is filling up with newly oxygenated blood from the lungs, there is a release in pressure (a pause is felt). People call this "feeling the heartbeat." Feeling for a pulse, then, is the best way (without special instruments) to tell if someone's heart is functioning.

One important aspect of CPR (cardiopulmonary resuscitation) training is to show you the easiest and most efficient way to find and feel the pulse. The way to do this differs, based on a person's size. A different artery is used to detect the pulse in an infant or child as compared to the older child, adolescent, or adult-sized young person.

Why CPR Requires Hands-on Training

Again, it is very important for you (and everyone over eleven years old) to be certified in CPR—because it *does* save lives. Although we have described the six steps of the CPR procedure, this was done as a resource to refresh the memory of those who have already been trained and certified in CPR, *not as an attempt to actually teach this lifesaving procedure*. It does take hands-on training, and it would be very deceptive if we in any way implied that you could learn to perform CPR simply by reading about it. Reading this information, however, will give you an idea about how it is performed so you will be more familiar with the procedures when you take your CPR certification training. After CPR training, you can use this information as a review.

People often ask why CPR can't be taught by reading alone and really don't understand why everyone is hesitant to do this. Here are some of the reasons. First, if the wrong part of the sternum (breastbone) is compressed, it is possible to puncture or lacerate (cut) the liver or other internal organs, causing severe and often deadly internal bleeding. Second, if your hands are positioned incorrectly on the chest, it is possible to fracture ribs and damage other areas of the chest, as well as puncture the lungs or even the heart if a fractured rib is thrust into one of these organs. Third, if chest compressions are performed in a jerky fashion (like quick jabs) instead of smoothly and rhythmically, the possibility of injury increases, and the blood from the heart is not effectively moved throughout the body.

Fourth, if you do not know how to properly position yourself and perform both chest compressions and rescue breathing (previously known as mouth-to-mouth resuscitation), you will quickly become fatigued and may in fact cause unnecessary and serious damage. Fifth, the timing of rescue breathing interspersed between a specific number of chest compressions is vital in order for this lifesaving procedure to be effective. Sixth, if you perform chest compressions on a weak but beating heart, you're actually working *against* the heart and may force the heart to stop altogether.

Properly performed CPR poses less risk for causing damage but does require careful attention to the details of the procedure. These details *are not difficult* to learn or remember when you are actually shown how to do CPR and can practice it on specially designed mannequins, which simulates the actual "feel" of performing CPR on a human. (*Never* "practice" CPR on a well person—this is extremely dangerous.)

Besides all these reasons—there's one more potential problem to consider. The real purpose of CPR is to keep oxygenated blood circulating through the body until advanced medical care can be provided. If this is done, then the person has a good chance of not experiencing brain damage or other serious central nervous system damage if he or she is revived. The point is to be *effective*. If CPR is improperly performed or the initiation of the procedure is delayed, it is very likely that severe brain damage (or other serious central nervous system damage) will occur. If brain damage is severe enough, the person's heart and lung function may subsequently be reestablished with medical treatment, but he or she may never regain consciousness and may stay in a coma until death occurs (possibly) years later. Of course, there are varying degrees of brain damage, and sometimes—even with the best efforts of a person certified in CPR—brain damage or death can still occur. But at least in this case, the rescuer did everything possible—giving the victim every ounce of his or her knowledge, training, and involvement.

More than anything else, we owe it to ourselves, our families, and our friends to learn the procedures correctly, so we can do all we can if a life-threatening situation occurs. But remember, it does take hands-on experience, so that all steps in the CPR procedure are second nature to you and you are able to perform them efficiently and rapidly.

THE DON'TS

Don't forget to take a CPR training course without delay if you are not already certified in CPR. It is recommended that everyone already certified in CPR take a refresher course for recertification.

Don't forget that you must initiate CPR rapidly. Severe, irreversible brain damage or death can occur within four to six minutes after cardiopulmonary arrest.

126

LIFE-
THREATENING
EMERGENCIES:
ONLY A
MATTER OF
MOMENTS

Don't stop your CPR efforts unless the paramedics or someone else certified in CPR takes over for you. Once CPR is started, it must be continued—unless you become so exhausted that you simply cannot keep it up.

Don't forget that you cannot learn and perform CPR without taking the training course. Learning the proper techniques is not difficult, but it does require hands-on instruction, and nothing can take the place of that four to eight hours of training.

PLEASE NOTE: Now that you have a better grasp of how to recognize and manage cardiopulmonary arrest, it would be extremely helpful for you to go back to the Emergency Quick Reference With the Steps in Detail and review it. The more familiar you are with that material (even if you are certified in CPR or simply want to become more familiar with the information before you take the CPR training course), the more useful it will be to you when you need it.

CHAPTER 6

Airway Obstruction/Choking

EMERGENCY QUICK REFERENCE

With the Steps in Detail

Managing Airway Obstruction/Choking

When airway obstruction occurs, your first step is to determine whether there is *complete obstruction* or *partial obstruction* (page 128). Then take appropriate action based on the following categories in this Emergency Quick Reference:

Complete Obstruction in the Infant/Baby (Birth to One Year of Age) (page 128)

Complete Obstruction in the Child (over One Year Old), Adolescent, or Adult-Sized Young Person—The Heimlich Maneuver (page 131)

Partial Obstruction—And the *Youngster Is Blue* (page 134)

Partial Obstruction—And the *Youngster Is Not Blue* (page 135)

128

LIFE-
THREATENING
EMERGENCIES:
ONLY A
MATTER OF
MOMENTS

Determine Whether There Is Partial or Complete Airway Blockage

▶ IN COMPLETE AIRWAY BLOCKAGE, THE YOUNGSTER MAY STRUGGLE AT FIRST, BUT NO AIR MOVES IN AND OUT OF THE LUNGS, AND HE MAKES NO NOISE. THE CHILD'S COLOR IS BLUE, AND HE RAPIDLY BECOMES UNRESPONSIVE AND UNCONSCIOUS.

▶ IN PARTIAL AIRWAY BLOCKAGE, THE YOUNGSTER COUGHS AND GAGS, MAKING NOISE, AND OFTEN CRIES. AT LEAST SOME AIR MOVES IN AND OUT OF THE LUNGS. MOST OFTEN, THE CHILD IS REDDISH OR PURPLE, ALTHOUGH WITH SEVERE DEGREES OF PARTIAL OBSTRUCTION, SHE MIGHT BE PALE OR BLUE. THE YOUNGSTER IS USUALLY VERY UPSET AND EXCITED, AS WELL.

Complete Obstruction in the Infant/Baby (Birth to One Year of Age)

▶ HAVE SOMEONE ELSE CALL THE PARAMEDICS WHILE YOU TREAT THE INFANT. IF NO ONE IS WITH YOU, CONTINUE TREATING THE BABY WHILE YOU PERIODICALLY SHOUT FOR HELP. WHEN HELP ARRIVES, HAVE THAT PERSON CALL THE PARAMEDICS.

▶ TURN THE INFANT OR BABY FACEDOWN OVER YOUR KNEES OR LAP, WITH HIS HEAD SLIGHTLY LOWER THAN HIS CHEST. (YOU MAY TURN A SMALL INFANT FACEDOWN OVER YOUR ARM AND SUPPORT HIS CHEST IN YOUR HAND.)

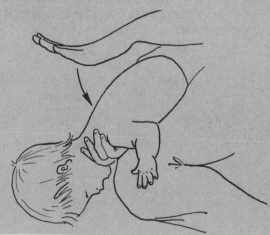

To relieve complete airway obstruction in an infant, turn him face down over your knees and with the heel of your hand, give four sharp blows to the back between the shoulder blades.

▶ **GIVE FOUR SHARP BLOWS TO THE BACK BETWEEN THE SHOUL-DER BLADES.** USE THE HEEL OF YOUR HAND AND HIT AS IF YOU WERE CLAPPING YOUR HANDS LOUDLY.

▶ **IMMEDIATELY TURN THE INFANT ONTO HER BACK AND GIVE FOUR QUICK CHEST THRUSTS.** USE THE HEEL OF YOUR HAND OVER THE LOWER PART OF THE BREASTBONE, AS IS DONE IN CPR.

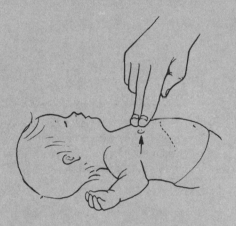

Use your index and middle fingers to give four quick chest thrusts.

▶ **OPEN THE BABY'S MOUTH TO LOOK FOR ANY FOREIGN MATE-RIAL.** WITH ONE HAND, GRASP THE LOWER JAW BETWEEN YOUR THUMB AND FINGERS AND LIFT IT UP AND FORWARD.

▶ **IF YOU SEE FOREIGN MATERIAL, USE ONE OR TWO FINGERS OF THE OTHER HAND TO SCOOP OR SWEEP IT FORWARD AND OUT OF THE MOUTH.** *DO NOT* REACH INTO THE MOUTH TO DO THIS *UNLESS YOU CAN SEE MATERIAL* THAT IS OR MAY BE BLOCKING THE AIRWAY. BE CAREFUL NOT TO PUSH THE MATERIAL FARTHER INTO THE THROAT.

To sweep the mouth: Use one or two fingers to remove any foreign material that you can see.

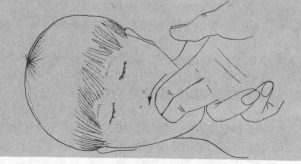

130

LIFE-
THREATENING
EMERGENCIES:
ONLY A
MATTER OF
MOMENTS

▶ **IF THE INFANT HAS NOT STARTED GASPING OR BREATHING ON HIS OR HER OWN, OPEN THE AIRWAY.** KEEPING THE JAW FORWARD, TILT THE HEAD BACK SLIGHTLY. YOU CAN DO THIS BY GENTLY LIFTING THE NECK WITH ONE HAND WHILE GENTLY PUSHING BACK ON THE FOREHEAD WITH YOUR OTHER HAND. YOU CAN GET THE SAME EFFECT BY PLACING A FOLDED (LENGTHWISE) TOWEL UNDER THE SHOULDERS. (This is sometimes called the "sniffing position.")

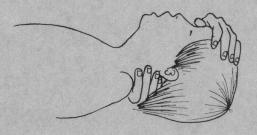

To open the airway: Lift the neck gently with one hand while you tip the head back with your other hand.

▶ **BEGIN RESCUE BREATHING BY MAKING A SEAL OVER THE BABY'S MOUTH (EITHER BY PINCHING THE NOSE WITH YOUR FINGERS OR BY COVERING THE NOSE AND MOUTH TOTALLY WITH YOUR MOUTH) AND DELIVERING FOUR RESCUE BREATHS IN RAPID SUCCESSION.** (THE RESCUE BREATHS SHOULD FEEL LIKE BLOWING OUT A CANDLE IN AN INFANT.) TRY TO MAKE THE CHEST RISE WITH EACH BREATH YOU DELIVER. (If you are unable to remember the details of rescue breathing, turn to the Emergency Quick Reference on page 113, entitled "A Review of the Six Steps of CPR.") IF YOU FEEL RESISTANCE TO BLOWING INTO THE MOUTH (THE AIR IS NOT GOING ANYWHERE) OR THE CHEST DOESN'T RISE, THE AIRWAY IS STILL BLOCKED.

▶ **REPEAT THE SAME SEQUENCE—FOUR SHARP BACK BLOWS, FOUR QUICK CHEST THRUSTS, AND FOUR RESCUE BREATHS IN RAPID SUCCESSION—UNTIL YOU SUCCESSFULLY PERFORM RESCUE BREATHING (MOVE AIR IN AND OUT OF THE LUNGS), THE INFANT GASPS AND BREATHES ON HIS OR HER OWN, OR THE PARAMEDICS OR AMBULANCE ARRIVES.**

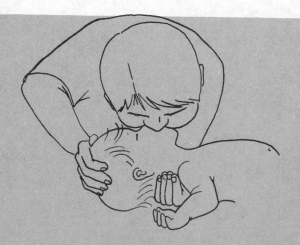

Rescue breathing in an infant: Cover the mouth and nose with your mouth and deliver puffs of air (like blowing out a candle), so the chest rises.

▶ **IF THE BABY'S HEART HAS ALSO STOPPED (THERE IS NO PULSE), BEGIN CHEST COMPRESSIONS WITH RESCUE BREATHING (FULL CPR) AS SOON AS YOU CLEAR THE AIRWAY OBSTRUCTION.** (If you are certified in CPR and are unable to remember the details of the procedure, turn to the Emergency Quick Reference on page 113, entitled "A Review of the Six Steps of CPR.")

Complete Obstruction in the Child (over One Year Old), Adolescent, or Adult-Sized Young Person— The Heimlich Maneuver

▶ **HAVE SOMEONE ELSE CALL THE PARAMEDICS WHILE YOU TREAT THE CHILD. IF NO ONE IS WITH YOU, CONTINUE TREATING THE CHILD WHILE YOU PERIODICALLY SHOUT FOR HELP. WHEN HELP ARRIVES, HAVE THAT PERSON CALL THE PARAMEDICS.**

▶ **PERFORM FOUR QUICK ABDOMINAL COMPRESSIONS.** THESE CAN BE DONE FROM ANY POSITION. MAKE YOUR COMPRESSIONS FORCEFUL ENOUGH TO PUSH AIR SUDDENLY OUT OF THE LUNGS.

- If the youngster is standing or sitting, stand behind him and put your arm around his midsection. Make a fist with one hand and put it over the youngster's upper abdomen between the navel and the ribs, with the thumb side inward. Cover your fist with your other hand, and in a sudden motion, pull upward and inward—pulling toward his shoulders. Be careful not to squeeze in on his sides with your arms!

132

LIFE-
THREATENING
EMERGENCIES:
ONLY A
MATTER OF
MOMENTS

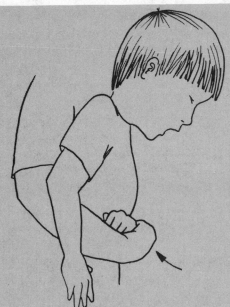

Hug the youngster from behind and place your fisted hands on the upper abdomen. A swift, sharp upward and inward thrust forces air out of the lungs to dislodge a foreign object.

- If the young person is lying down, turn her face up, if necessary. Put one hand on top of the other, then place the heels of your hands on her upper abdomen. Now, in a rapid motion, push upward and inward—as if to knock the wind out of her.

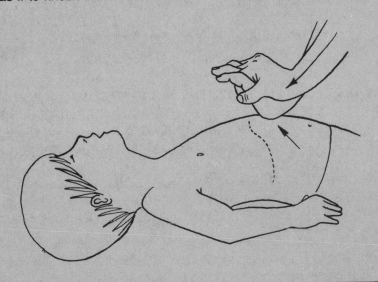

Place the heels of your hands one on top of the other, on the upper abdomen. In a swift, sharp motion push upward and inward—as if to knock the wind out of the youngster.

- **Adjust the force of the abdominal compressions based on the youngster's size.** Your goal is to compress the upper abdomen enough to forcefully push air out of the lungs and up the airway—thus pushing out the foreign object. The concept is the same as "knocking the wind out of someone." In very young infants and children, use only a small amount of force. Compress harder for larger children and teenagers.

▶ **OPEN THE YOUNG PERSON'S MOUTH AND LOOK FOR FOREIGN MATERIAL.** WITH ONE HAND, GRASP THE LOWER JAW BETWEEN YOUR THUMB AND FINGERS, THEN LIFT THE JAW UP AND FORWARD. IF YOU SEE FOREIGN MATERIAL, USE ONE OR TWO FINGERS OF YOUR OTHER HAND TO SCOOP OR SWEEP IT FORWARD AND OUT OF THE MOUTH. *DO NOT* REACH INTO THE MOUTH *UNLESS YOU CAN SEE MATERIAL* THAT IS OR MAY BE BLOCKING THE AIRWAY. BE CAREFUL NOT TO PUSH THE OBJECT FARTHER INTO THE THROAT.

▶ **IF THE YOUNGSTER HAS NOT STARTED GASPING OR BREATHING ON HIS OR HER OWN, OPEN THE AIRWAY.** KEEPING THE JAW FORWARD, TILT THE HEAD BACK SLIGHTLY. YOU CAN DO THIS BY GENTLY LIFTING THE NECK WITH ONE HAND WHILE GENTLY PUSHING BACK ON THE FOREHEAD WITH YOUR OTHER HAND.

▶ **BEGIN RESCUE BREATHING BY MAKING A SEAL OVER THE YOUNG PERSON'S MOUTH (PINCH THE NOSE WITH YOUR FINGERS AND COVER THE YOUNG PERSON'S MOUTH WITH YOUR MOUTH) AND DELIVERING FOUR RESCUE BREATHS IN RAPID SUCCESSION.** THE RESCUE BREATHS SHOLD FEEL LIKE INFLATING A BALLOON IN A CHILD, WITH A LITTLE MORE FORCE NECESSARY IN THE ADOLESCENT OR ADULT-SIZED PERSON. TRY TO MAKE THE CHEST RISE WITH EACH BREATH YOU DELIVER. (If you are unable to remember the details of rescue breathing, turn to the Emergency Quick Reference on page 113, entitled "A Review of the Six Steps of CPR.") IF YOU FEEL RESISTANCE TO BLOWING INTO THE YOUNGSTER'S MOUTH (THE AIR IS NOT GOING ANYWHERE) OR THE CHEST DOESN'T RISE, THEN THE AIRWAY IS STILL BLOCKED.

134

LIFE-
THREATENING
EMERGENCIES:
ONLY A
MATTER OF
MOMENTS

Rescue breathing in children and older youngsters: Pinch the nose shut and blow into the mouth (like blowing up a balloon), so the chest rises.

▶ **REPEAT THE FOUR ABDOMINAL COMPRESSIONS AND FOUR RES-CUE BREATHS IN RAPID SUCCESSION—UNTIL YOU SUCCESS-FULLY PERFORM RESCUE BREATHING (MOVE AIR IN AND OUT OF THE LUNGS), THE YOUNGSTER GASPS AND BREATHES ON HIS OR HER OWN, OR THE PARAMEDICS OR AMBULANCE ARRIVES.**

▶ **IF THE YOUNGSTER'S HEART HAS ALSO STOPPED (THERE IS NO PULSE), BEGIN CHEST COMPRESSIONS WITH RESCUE BREATH-ING (FULL CPR) AS SOON AS YOU CLEAR THE AIRWAY OBSTRUC-TION.** (If you are certified in CPR and are unable to remember the details of the procedure, turn to the Emergency Quick Reference on page 113, entitled "A Review of the Six Steps of CPR.")

Partial Obstruction—And the Youngster Is Blue

▶ **PROCEED AS IF THERE WERE COMPLETE BLOCKAGE.**

- **In infants and babies (birth to one year of age): Perform four sharp back blows, then four quick chest thrusts, then four rescue breaths in rapid succession. Repeat this sequence if obstruction contin-ues. Once the obstruction is relieved, perform rescue breathing (or full CPR if the heart has also stopped [there is no pulse]) until the infant gasps and breathes on his or her own or the paramedics or ambulance arrives.** (If you are certified in CPR and are unable to remember the details of the procedure, turn to the Emergency Quick Reference on page 113, entitled "A Review of the Six Steps of CPR.")

- **In children (over one year of age), teenagers, and adult-sized youngsters: Perform four quick abdominal compressions, then four rescue breaths in rapid succession. Repeat this sequence if obstruction continues. Once the obstruction is relieved, perform rescue breathing (or full CPR if the heart has also stopped [there is no pulse]) until the child gasps and breathes on his or her own or the paramedics or ambulance arrives.** (If you are certified in CPR and are unable to remember the details of the procedure, turn to the Emergency Quick Reference on page 113, entitled "A Review of the Six Steps of CPR.")

Partial Obstruction—And the Youngster Is Not Blue (All Ages)

▶ **KEEP CALM AND TRY TO REASSURE AND CALM THE YOUNG-STER.** TELL THE YOUNGSTER THAT SHE WILL BE ALL RIGHT AND THAT THINGS ARE UNDER CONTROL.

▶ **ASK THE YOUNGSTER TO OPEN HIS MOUTH AND LET YOU LOOK.** IF THE YOUNGSTER COOPERATES, LOOK FOR THE BLOCKING OBJECT OR MATERIAL AND SWEEP THE MOUTH TO REMOVE IT—BUT *ONLY* IF YOU SEE IT.

▶ **HAVE THE YOUNGSTER SIT OR STAND AND LEAN FORWARD SLIGHTLY IF THAT IS COMFORTABLE.** AS SHE CONTINUES TO COUGH AND GAG, WATCH CAREFULLY FOR SIGNS OF COMPLETE OBSTRUCTION (THE YOUNGSTER TURNS BLUE, CAN NO LONGER MAKE NOISE OR TALK, OR LOSES CONSCIOUSNESS).

▶ **IF THE AIRWAY BECOMES COMPLETELY BLOCKED, TAKE IMME-DIATE ACTION TO RELIEVE IT,** as indicated on page 128 (Complete Obstruction in the Infant/Baby [Birth to One Year of Age]), or page 131 (Complete Obstruction in the Child [over One Year Old], Adolescent, or Adult-Sized Young Person).

▶ **EVEN WITHOUT COMPLETE OBSTRUCTION, IF THE YOUNGSTER IS CONSIDERABLY UNCOMFORTABLE OR HAVING TROUBLE BREATHING, CALL THE PARAMEDICS OR AN AMBULANCE.**

▶ **IF COUGHING, CHOKING, NOISY BREATHING, OR WHEEZING PER-SISTS, EVEN WITHOUT COMPLETE BLOCKAGE, TAKE THE YOUNGSTER TO THE NEAREST EMERGENCY ROOM.**

136

LIFE-
THREATENING
EMERGENCIES:
ONLY A
MATTER OF
MOMENTS

➡ **IF THERE IS LESS DIFFICULTY BUT THE PROBLEM HAS NOT COMPLETELY CLEARED UP, CALL THE YOUNGSTER'S DOCTOR (OR GO TO AN EMERGENCY ROOM IF YOU DO NOT HAVE A DOCTOR OR CANNOT REACH YOUR DOCTOR).**

Please Note:

➡ **IF SIGNS OF AIRWAY OBSTRUCTION ARE SEEN IN AN INFANT OR CHILD WHO IS SICK (HAS A COLD, CONGESTION, AND FEVER OR HAS A SORE THROAT, DROOLING, AND FEVER), CALL YOUR DOCTOR FOR INSTRUCTIONS OR GO TO AN EMERGENCY ROOM.** (If you are unable to remember the details of managing this problem, turn to the Emergency Quick Reference on page 344, entitled "Croup," for a review.)

- *However*, if you know or suspect that the child has put something in his or her mouth that is or may be obstructing the airway, proceed as if there were an airway obstruction (based on whether obstruction is partial or complete).

- If breathing and/or heart function stops (there is no pulse), have someone else call the paramedics while you treat the infant or child. (Attempt to open the airway and perform rescue breathing or full CPR, as necessary, until the child gasps and breathes on his or her own or the paramedics arrive to take over for you.) (If you are certified in CPR and are unable to remember the details of the procedure, turn to the Emergency Quick Reference on page 113, entitled "A Review of the Six Steps of CPR.")

➡ **IF SIGNS OF AIRWAY OBSTRUCTION ARE SEEN IN *ANY YOUNGSTER* WHO HAS HAD CONTACT WITH SOMETHING TO WHICH HE OR SHE IS KNOWN TO BE SERIOUSLY ALLERGIC, OR IF SIGNS OF AIRWAY OBSTRUCTION ACCOMPANY FACE AND TONGUE SWELLING, ITCHING, OR HIVES, CALL FOR PARAMEDIC ASSISTANCE.** (If you are unable to remember the details of managing this problem, turn to the Emergency Quick Reference on page 324, entitled "Anaphylaxis," for a review.)

- *However*, if you know or suspect that the youngster has put something in his or her mouth that is or may be obstructing the airway, proceed as if there were an airway obstruction (based on whether obstruction is partial or complete).

- If breathing and/or heart function stops (there is no pulse), have someone else call the paramedics while you treat the youngster. (Attempt to open the airway and perform rescue breathing or full CPR, as necessary, until the child gasps and breathes on his or her own or the paramedics arrive to take over for you.) (If you are certified in CPR and are unable to remember the details of the procedure, turn to the Emergency Quick Reference on page 113, entitled "A Review of the Six Steps of CPR.")

The Facts About Airway Obstruction

Airway obstruction (blockage of the windpipe) is a very common life-threatening emergency in people of all ages—and is the second greatest cause of accidental death in the home for children under five years of age. In infants and children, airway obstruction most often results from aspirating (inhaling) an object (such as a toy, food, a bone, a nut, or a button) that was in the mouth. Older children often aspirate if they laugh or "horse around" while eating or sucking on something. Adults usually aspirate large chunks of food. Some adults have swallowing problems, while others have been drinking alcohol, which slows reflexes (such as swallowing).

A foreign body can become lodged anywhere in the airway—from in the throat just above the vocal cords all the way to one of the smaller bronchi (breathing tubes) in one part of one of the lungs. The larger the object, the more likely it is to lodge high in the airway and completely block the passage of oxygen to the lungs.

When a person chokes on something, his or her body responds automatically by trying to clear away the foreign object—through coughing and gagging. The force of the coughing pushes the foreign object out of the airway into the throat, where it can be spit out or swallowed. The cough reflex is usually very efficient, and most objects (food, mucus, and so on) are pushed up and don't cause further difficulty. If, however, the foreign object becomes tightly lodged in the windpipe—totally blocking it—the situation is much more critical. In this case, oxygen cannot enter the lungs and therefore cannot reach the vital organs of the body.

Here's what usually happens. Within minutes, the young person's skin turns blue. Because the brain is without oxygen, he or she collapses and becomes unconscious. The heart slows down and stops.

The first few seconds and minutes after complete airway obstruction are vital if brain damage or death are to be avoided. Permanent brain damage can occur in as short a time as four minutes, although fortunately, youngsters may tolerate oxygen deprivation somewhat longer than adults. Death can take place in six to fifteen minutes after the

138

LIFE-
THREATENING
EMERGENCIES:
ONLY A
MATTER OF
MOMENTS

oxygen supply is lost. As you can imagine, immediate, effective action is critical in preventing this kind of needless death or brain damage.

However, you should know that until recently there had been a great controversy among doctors about what is the best, safest way to handle complete airway obstruction due to aspiration *in infants and children.* The latest official recommendation of the Committee on Accident and Poison Prevention of the American Academy of Pediatrics, the national committees that set the standards for cardiopulmonary resuscitation (CPR), the American Heart Association, and the American Red Cross is: *In infants* under one, complete airway blockage should be relieved by using a series of back blows and chest thrusts (as detailed earlier). They recommend abdominal compressions (better known as the Heimlich maneuver) in all other cases.

The techniques to relieve airway blockage, like those used in cardiopulmonary resuscitation, are not easily learned by reading alone. They must be learned through hands-on instruction. With practice, they become second nature to you. Techniques to relieve airway obstruction are taught as part of all CPR certification classes. If you have not done so already, take a CPR course. Also, ask your child's doctor to review the steps in relieving airway obstruction with you at your next visit. (*Do not* "practice" abdominal thrusts or chest thrusts on another person. They should only be practiced in a formal training course on special mannequins to get the "feel" of the methods.)

Airway Obstruction: Signs and Symptoms

As previously noted, when an object is accidently inhaled, it triggers a cough reflex and often gagging, as well. We commonly call this choking. Other symptoms depend on how large the inhaled object is and where in the airway it gets stuck.

Large objects that lodge high in the airway—in the throat, near the vocal cords, or high in the trachea (windpipe)—often completely block the passage of air to the lungs. The youngster will struggle to breathe or cough, but no sound will be heard, and you won't be able to feel or hear air rushing through the mouth or nose. The youngster soon turns blue and loses consciousness. If the airway is not cleared quickly, death or permanent brain damage is imminent.

Smaller objects or those that are irregularly shaped may only partially obstruct the air passage. If this occurs, the youngster is able to cough, cry, or speak, even though he is quite uncomfortable. His breathing is often noisy. There might be a loud, harsh, "crowing" noise when the child breathes in (called stridor) or a whistling or harsh noise when he breathes out (wheezing). The cough may sound like barking, or it may sound "metallic." The child is usually excited and upset, and bright red or purple— but can be pale or blue if there is serious lack of oxygen. In this situation, it is important to try to keep the young person calm.

Small objects (beads, peanuts, and the like) may travel down into the smaller airways of one of the lungs. When this happens, the youngster may seem fine for some time after the choking or coughing spell. Later, however, a "foreign body" should be suspected because of persistent cough, wheezing, or pneumonia. By this time, the choking spell is often long past and forgotten! It's important to evaluate the child off and on after a choking incident and call your doctor if other symptoms (as mentioned) occur.

You should also suspect aspiration of an object if you find your child blue and unconscious for no other apparent reason. If there are small toys or objects around, this is very likely the case. Be especially watchful when infants and toddlers are in the "mouthing" or "tasting" stage. At this point, *all objects* are likely to be tested by placing them in their mouths. These little ones—from 6 months to 2½ years of age—are especially vulnerable to upper airway blockage from aspiration, so be very careful about what is given them, and be diligent about watching for an aspiration incident.

Airway blockage in infants and children can also occur as a result of an infection or an allergic reaction. Infections such as croup and epiglottitis usually start gradually and often have fever and other signs of illness associated with them. When the problem is due to a serious allergic reaction to something, face and tongue swelling are usually found along with signs of airway obstruction. These problems are discussed in detail in Section 3, Chapter 13. It is best to review these problems carefully, so you feel comfortable about recognizing the difference between these problems and obstructions caused by choking and aspiration. In this way, you will be prepared to take appropriate action should airway obstruction occur and know what to do if the problem is related to an illness or allergy.

THE DON'TS

Don't panic. Your calmness helps the choking youngster stay calm and allows you to assess the situation and act accordingly.

Don't reach into a child's mouth blindly to remove an object. Look for an object, and go after it only if you can see it. Otherwise, you may push it farther into the airway and worsen the blockage.

Don't stop trying to dislodge an inhaled object if there are signs of complete airway blockage. The person has no chance to survive unless you keep trying. Remember, each second and minute without oxygen are critical.

Don't use back blows in a infant/baby unless there is complete blockage. Hitting the infant/baby on the back in this situation may make the object go farther down into the airway.

Don't neglect to have a child evaluated by his or her doctor or in an emergency room if noisy breathing or wheezing continues after a choking episode. A small foreign object may be stuck in one of the small airways in one of the lungs.

140

LIFE-
THREATENING
EMERGENCIES:
ONLY A
MATTER OF
MOMENTS

Don't forget to ask your doctor to review the technique for relieving airway obstruction.

PLEASE NOTE: Now that you have a grasp of how to recognize and manage airway obstruction/choking, it would be extremely helpful for you to go back to the Emergency Quick Reference With the Steps in Detail and review it carefully. The more familiar you are with that material, the more useful it will be to you when you need it.

C H A P T E R 7

Serious Bleeding

EMERGENCY QUICK REFERENCE

With the Steps in Detail

Managing Serious Bleeding

Treating Open Wounds

▶ IF BLEEDING IS OBVIOUSLY SEVERE OR LIFE-THREATENING, HAVE SOMEONE ELSE CALL THE PARAMEDICS WHILE YOU TREAT THE YOUNGSTER. IF NO ONE IS WITH YOU, CONTINUE TREATING THE CHILD WHILE YOU PERIODICALLY SHOUT FOR HELP. WHEN HELP ARRIVES, HAVE THAT PERSON CALL THE PARAMEDICS.

142

LIFE-
THREATENING
EMERGENCIES:
ONLY A
MATTER OF
MOMENTS

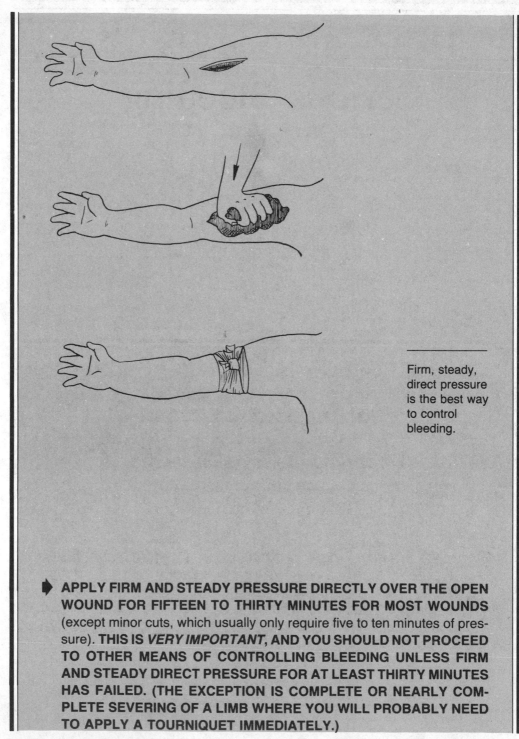

Firm, steady,
direct pressure
is the best way
to control
bleeding.

▶ **APPLY FIRM AND STEADY PRESSURE DIRECTLY OVER THE OPEN WOUND FOR FIFTEEN TO THIRTY MINUTES FOR MOST WOUNDS** (except minor cuts, which usually only require five to ten minutes of pressure). **THIS IS *VERY IMPORTANT*, AND YOU SHOULD NOT PROCEED TO OTHER MEANS OF CONTROLLING BLEEDING UNLESS FIRM AND STEADY DIRECT PRESSURE FOR AT LEAST THIRTY MINUTES HAS FAILED. (THE EXCEPTION IS COMPLETE OR NEARLY COMPLETE SEVERING OF A LIMB WHERE YOU WILL PROBABLY NEED TO APPLY A TOURNIQUET IMMEDIATELY.)**

- Use the heel of your hand (if possible) and gauze, strips of sheet, a towel, or even a piece of clothing to hold against the wound.

- If the blood soaks through the gauze or cloth, do not remove it, but add more gauze or cloth on top of the first layer and continue firm pressure.

- Elevate the wounded area above the level of the heart—*unless* there is also a fracture, dislocation, or other serious injury in the same area.

- Once bleeding has stopped or is under control, wrap the wound with gauze or strips of cloth—or tape down the existing cloth or gauze. Do *not* remove this dressing until medical personnel can care for the wound (if it is serious or may need stitches) *or* until you can carefully and thoroughly clean and re-dress the wound (if it is more minor).

▶ **IF AT ANY POINT IT BECOMES OBVIOUS THAT THE WOUND IS VERY SERIOUS OR THE YOUNGSTER CANNOT SAFELY AND EASILY BE MOVED—CALL THE PARAMEDICS OR AN AMBULANCE.**
IF THE WOUND IS MODERATELY SERIOUS OR IS ONE THAT MAY NEED STITCHES (BUT IS NOT LIFE-THREATENING) AND THE YOUNGSTER CAN EASILY AND SAFELY BE MOVED—CALL YOUR DOCTOR FOR INSTRUCTIONS OR GO TO THE NEAREST EMERGENCY ROOM (IF YOU HAVE NO DOCTOR OR CANNOT REACH YOUR DOCTOR).

▶ **IF BLEEDING IS LIFE-THREATENING AND CANNOT BE CONTROLLED EVEN WITH STEADY, DIRECT PRESSURE (YOU STILL HAVE GUSHING AND SPURTING OF BLOOD), THEN FIND THE NEAREST "PRESSURE POINT" AND APPLY PRESSURE.**

- *Never* use "pressure points" unless the bleeding is quite serious and direct pressure as well as elevation have *not* controlled it.

- **You need to find the "pressure point" closest to the wound but between the wound and the heart.** For example, if the wound were in the forearm, you would use the "pressure point" in the upper arm—not in the wrist, since pressure there would control blood flow to the hand only.

- "Pressure points" are found throughout the body (see diagram). Simply apply steady pressure over the "pressure point" with your fingers—until bleeding is controlled.

144

LIFE-
THREATENING
EMERGENCIES:
ONLY A
MATTER OF
MOMENTS

Arteries close to the surface, such as those in the upper arm or groin, can be used as "pressure points" when bleeding cannot be controlled by direct pressure on a wound.

Use your fingers or the heel of your hand to compress the pressure point on the inside of the upper arm.

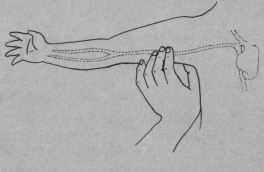

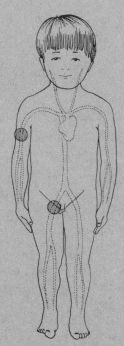

Use the heel of your hand or your fingers to apply firm, steady pressure to the "pressure point" in the groin.

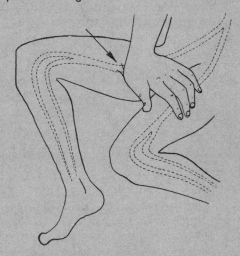

▶ **CONTINUE TO APPLY PRESSURE TO THE "PRESSURE POINT" UNTIL BLEEDING IS UNDER CONTROL. THEN RELEASE THE "PRESSURE POINT" SLOWLY, SO OXYGENATED BLOOD CAN REACH THE TISSUES IN THAT AREA. DON'T FORGET TO RELEASE THE "PRESSURE POINT" AT LEAST EVERY TEN TO FIFTEEN MINUTES.** Since "pressure points" are really areas where major arteries are near the surface of the skin, you are in essence "stopping" or "slowing down" blood flow to the area beyond the point where pressure is applied. Therefore, you should *not* apply continuous pressure over a "pressure point" but should instead release the pressure periodically.

▶ **CONTINUE TO APPLY DIRECT PRESSURE TO THE WOUND ITSELF AFTER YOU HAVE RELEASED THE "PRESSURE POINT." IF BLEEDING GOES OUT OF CONTROL AGAIN, ONLY THEN SHOULD YOU REAPPLY PRESSURE TO THE "PRESSURE POINT."** IF BLEEDING CAN ONLY BE CONTROLLED WITH PRESSURE ON THE "PRESSURE POINT," THEN REPEAT THIS PROCEDURE (PRESSURE ON "PRESSURE POINT" UNTIL BLEEDING IS CONTROLLED, THEN RELEASE OF "PRESSURE POINT") OVER AND OVER AGAIN.

▶ **APPLY A TOURNIQUET. (THIS IS A LAST RESORT—UNLESS THE LIMB IS OBVIOUSLY SEVERED OR NEARLY SEVERED.)**

- **Remember, a tourniquet can only be used on an arm or a leg.**

- **Apply a tourniquet *only* if you've tried everything else (direct pressure, elevation, and "pressure point")—*unless* the limb is obviously severed or nearly severed, in which case apply a tourniquet immediately.** If nothing has controlled the bleeding and the young person's life is seriously jeopardized—then you have no other choice but to apply a tourniquet. (Inappropriate use of a tourniquet—too tight a tourniquet or one left on too long—can lead to serious tissue damage or even loss of a limb because the blood supply is completely cut off.)

- You need a very *long* strip of cloth, man's tie, belt, scarf, or something similar. It should be at least two inches wide. Just above the wound, wrap the tourniquet around the arm or leg twice, and tie the ends into a half-knot (*not* a full knot).

- Place a stick or other straight and strong object on top of the half-knot and tie a full knot over the stick (or other straight object) to secure it. If the full knot doesn't hold, tie a double knot.

- Now, carefully and slowly twist the stick (or other straight object) *until* the bleeding slows to a trickle or stops. Do *not* tighten the tourniquet more than you need to—tighten it just enough to stop the life-threatening bleeding.

- Once you have found the position that will control the bleeding—tie the two ends of the tourniquet around the arm or leg (placing the knot on the side opposite the stick or straight object) to hold the tourniquet in place.

▶ **DO NOT REMOVE THE TOURNIQUET ONCE YOU HAVE APPLIED IT. LOOSEN IT FOR THIRTY TO SIXTY SECONDS EVERY TWENTY TO THIRTY MINUTES—IF YOU HAVE NOT BEEN ABLE TO GET MEDICAL ASSISTANCE BEFORE THEN.**

146

LIFE-
THREATENING
EMERGENCIES:
ONLY A
MATTER OF
MOMENTS

▶ **IF ICE IS AVAILABLE OR COLD, WET TOWELS, THEN APPLY ICE BAGS OR THE TOWELS TO THE AREA BELOW THE TOURNIQUET AND WOUND. (THIS HELPS PRESERVE THE LIMB.)**

▶ **WRITE THE TIME THE TOURNIQUET WAS APPLIED ON A PIECE OF PAPER OR CLOTH OR A PIECE OF CLOTHING—AND PIN IT IN PLAIN SIGHT ON THE YOUNGSTER.** You can also write "tourniquet" and the time on the young person's forehead (using a pen, lipstick, charcoal, or whatever is available).

Managing Internal Bleeding (Hemorrhaging)

▶ **INTERNAL BLEEDING REQUIRES IMMEDIATE MEDICAL INTERVENTION. SEEK MEDICAL ASSISTANCE PROMPTLY.**

▶ **IF YOU SUSPECT INTERNAL BLEEDING AND THE YOUNG PERSON IS BREATHING, CONSCIOUS, AND MOBILE, CALL YOUR DOCTOR FOR IMMEDIATE INSTRUCTIONS OR GO TO THE NEAREST EMERGENCY ROOM (IF YOU HAVE NO DOCTOR OR ARE UNABLE TO REACH YOUR DOCTOR).**

▶ **CALL THE PARAMEDICS WITHOUT DELAY IF THE YOUNGSTER CANNOT BE MOVED OR IS EXPERIENCING ANY LABORED BREATHING.**

Managing All Cases of Serious Bleeding

▶ **TREAT FOR SHOCK.** (If you are unable to remember the details of managing this problem, turn to the Emergency Quick Reference on page 152, entitled "Managing Shock," for a review.)

- Shock usually occurs with any severe bleeding problem, so expect and watch for it.

- The blood loss (as well as other possible serious injuries) is usually the major cause of the shock; therefore, the bleeding must be controlled *before* the shock can be treated.

▶ **IF AT ANY POINT THE YOUNGSTER STOPS BREATHING AND/OR THE HEART STOPS—BEGIN CPR IMMEDIATELY.** (If you are certified in CPR and are unable to remember the details of this procedure, turn to the Emergency Quick Reference on page 113, entitled "A Review of the Six Steps of CPR.")

Managing Cuts, Scrapes, and Abrasions

▶ **FOR INFORMATION ON MANAGING CUTS, SCRAPES, AND ABRASIONS, AS WELL AS OTHER MINOR WOUNDS, SEE THE QUICK REFERENCES IN CHAPTER 17.**

Serious Bleeding: A Frightening Experience

You've heard about people fainting or even vomiting at the sight of blood. You may even have done this yourself or know someone quite well who has done this. Although these people are relentlessly teased because they respond this way, in reality, it's nothing to laugh about. What most people don't realize is that panicking at the sight of blood is a perfectly natural response. Think about it: from the time we were very little children, we were taught that bleeding (any bleeding) was *a very serious thing*. "Blood," we learned early on, was synonymous with "life," and "losing blood" meant you could "lose your life."

With this kind of training, it can only be expected that most people will react with utter horror at the sight of blood—particularly when it involves their children. It can also be expected that many of us will panic—thinking that more minor bleeding is potentially serious or life-threatening. The truth is, when we see someone (or ourselves) bleeding, it frightens us. What makes matters worse is that, at times, it's very difficult to determine the degree of blood loss or the severity of a wound. This in part is due to the fact that "a little blood" often looks like "a lot of blood." This, of course, confuses and frightens people even more.

A notable example of the kind of fear and confusion that can occur involved a husband, his wife, and their five-year-old son. One Saturday afternoon, while the woman was working in the house, her husband calmly came through the back door holding a rag over a fairly serious wound on his upper arm. Apparently, he had slipped while trimming the backyard trees—bouncing off a few branches, with one cutting deeply into his arm. At the same time, the couple's five-year-old son ran through the front doorway yelling and holding his bloody nose. He had run into a friend's elbow while playing on the front lawn.

Obviously, neither of these situations is humorous or pleasant. What made both parents laugh later, though, was that in their panic they ignored the husband's potentially

148

LIFE-
THREATENING
EMERGENCIES:
ONLY A
MATTER OF
MOMENTS

serious wound and rushed their son to the nearest emergency room! Why? They said that blood was "all over" the child—all over his face, head, hands, arms, and shirt. The youngster had smeared the blood all over while trying to wipe it off. The problem was that neither parent stopped, cleaned the area, and evaluated the extent of the problem. They did not realize it was a nosebleed—because blood was everywhere.

The emergency room doctor was quite concerned, however, when he noticed the blood-soaked rag the father appeared to be holding. (The father had crossed his arms to maintain pressure on his own wound, but at a glance, it seemed as if he were simply holding a bloody piece of cloth.) "Was that cloth used to control the nosebleed?" the doctor asked. "Because that would be an extraordinary amount of blood for your son to lose, and that really does concern me." When the father lifted the blood-soaked cloth, the doctor was startled. The wound ultimately required twenty-two stitches! The father later admitted that he had felt weak and nauseated but hadn't really *looked* at the wound and was more concerned about his son.

The point is, in both cases, *not looking* was the basis for the error in judgment. When it comes to bleeding, then, it is vital that you calmly, carefully, and as rapidly as possible *evaluate* the extent of damage and the severity of blood loss. It's also important to remember that not all blood loss is serious or life-threatening. Although all of us were taught to associate the sight of blood with imminent danger to physical well-being, we have to look at the problem more logically and really assess the extent of the wound and the amount of blood loss.

The more you can learn about recognizing the difference between potentially serious and life-threatening bleeding as compared with less worrisome bleeding, the better equipped you will be to correctly assess a bleeding problem. Also, the more you know about managing and treating wounds and cuts, the more comfortable and confident you will feel when faced with even more serious situations.

As we discussed earlier, people get sick, go blank, freeze, or panic when they feel helpless—*not* when they feel able to help and *not* when they know what to do. Moreover, if you stay calm and in control, the injured young person will not panic, or if he does, you will be able to calm and reassure him by your actions and your tone of voice. You will also be sending an important message to your child: bleeding is *not* something to panic about, but to respond to—by looking at the problem and then doing something about it!

Serious Bleeding: Signs and Symptoms

The signs and symptoms of an open wound are obvious—because you can see the blood loss and the wound. The key to this, then, is to evaluate the *amount of blood loss* and the *extent of the wound*—in a rapid and efficient manner. Some serious and life-threatening wounds are quite apparent and can easily be identified.

A gaping wound on the trunk or limbs where there is profuse and often uncontrollable bleeding, as well as a severed or near-severed limb, is always clearly life-threatening. Gunshot, knife, and other wounds due to an object's being propelled or thrust into the body must always be considered potentially life-threatening. Multiple wounds due to a car accident, a fall from a high place, or other accidents where some sort of force to the body was involved should always be considered potentially serious or life-threatening, since internal bleeding (hemorrhaging) may also have occurred.

Usually, the problem does not lie in identifying the truly serious or life-threatening wounds. The problem lies instead in evaluating the vast spectrum of wounds found in between the minor cut and clearly life-threatening bleeding. These are the "iffy" situations that haunt parents and others. Your ability to assess these situations is vital. Here are some helpful guidelines to consider in evaluating the amount of bleeding and the extent of the open wound—when you're not sure about the severity of the problem:

- Assess the extent of the wound by quickly trying to wipe away some of the blood (if you cannot see the wound).

- If assessing the wound is impossible because bleeding is too great, immediately apply firm and steady pressure directly over the wound. *This is the cornerstone to treating almost all wounds and is the most important step you can take.*

- If you are able to see the wound, or if bleeding stops or comes under control, carefully look at the wound. Is it gaping, or does it have uneven edges? If so, it will more than likely require medical attention.

- If the bleeding has not stopped or is not under control (blood flow has not markedly decreased) after fifteen to thirty minutes of firm, steady, and direct pressure—then medical evaluation and care are usually necessary. In the vast majority of wounds—even those that are fairly severe—firm, steady, and direct pressure will control the bleeding. The key is in maintaining the firm and steady direct pressure *long enough*—which means *not releasing* direct pressure every few minutes to see if the bleeding is under control or has stopped. You'll know if the bleeding is under control—so don't look unless you are fairly confident that it is.

- "Pressure points" should only be used when firm, steady, and direct pressure for fifteen to thirty minutes has *not* controlled the bleeding and medical help has not arrived. Remember that when you use "pressure points," you are actually stopping blood—and hence oxygen—from going to the area. It is therefore imperative to use a "pressure point" only after you are *absolutely sure* that firm, steady, and direct pressure is not working and, consequently, you have no other alternative.

- If there is a serious wound to an arm or leg, apply a tourniquet only if you've tried everything else—direct pressure, elevation, and "pressure point." However, if the limb is obviously severed or nearly severed, then you will have to apply a tourniquet immediately.

150

LIFE-
THREATENING
EMERGENCIES:
ONLY A
MATTER OF
MOMENTS

- Remember to consider the size of the young person when evaluating the amount of blood loss. The smaller the youngster, the smaller the total blood volume she has—and therefore, the smaller the blood loss she can tolerate. Conversely, the larger the young person, the greater the blood loss she can tolerate—because the youngster has a greater total blood volume.

Severe blood loss is most often accompanied by other signs that point to a more serious problem. For example, the youngster may show one or more signs of shock: clammy, moist, or cold skin, which may be pasty or pale looking; nausea, dizziness, or even vomiting; general overall weakness; panic, anxiety, or fear; and he or she may complain about being thirsty or repeatedly ask for something to drink.

The paramedics or an ambulance should be called immediately when life-threatening bleeding occurs. Also, if serious bleeding occurs and the youngster cannot easily or safely be moved, or if he or she goes into shock—call the paramedics or an ambulance immediately. If bleeding is potentially serious, call the youngster's doctor for his or her recommendation or go to the nearest emergency room (if you do not have a doctor or are out of town).

If you are able to control or stop the bleeding but the wound is still gaping or its edges are ragged or uneven, call the doctor for instructions. In situations where the wound is *not* life-threatening, the doctor may want to see the youngster at the doctor's office or meet you at the emergency room. Or the doctor may want you to take the youngster to the emergency room and have the physician on duty there evaluate and treat the wound. If ever in doubt about the need for medical attention—call your doctor for advice without delay.

Internal bleeding (hemorrhaging) is much more difficult to identify, since you cannot see it—and assessing it therefore requires some attention to detail. Internal bleeding should be of concern if you notice: any very red or frothy blood being coughed up; bright red or black stools; dark, coffee ground–looking vomit; bloated-looking (distended) abdomen; tenderness in the abdomen or chest; weak but rapid pulse (heartbeat); signs of shock, such as clammy, cold, or pale skin, as well as anxiety, confusion, restlessness, and overall weakness; and breathing difficulty.

You should watch for signs of internal bleeding anytime a young person experiences a fall from an elevated surface (such as a tree, window, fence, or even a table, high chair, or dressing table if an infant or small child) or a moving object (such as a bicycle, minibike, skateboard, or roller skates). You should also watch for signs of internal bleeding if the youngster was involved in a car accident or other event that resulted in a collision with something or someone. If a young person falls on an object—such as a fence, handlebars, large rock, post, bench, or playground equipment—he or she should be watched for signs of internal bleeding.

Sometimes a young person seems perfectly fine right after an accident, then suddenly shows signs of internal bleeding, or even collapses, later. At the first indication of internal bleeding—call your doctor promptly for instructions. If the youngster suddenly has problems breathing, call the paramedics or an ambulance immediately. If cardiopulmonary arrest occurs (heart and lung function stop), perform CPR and have someone else call for the paramedics or an ambulance.

THE DON'TS

Don't forget to immediately apply steady and firm pressure directly on an open wound before you do anything else. Most often this will stop or control the bleeding, so it should be done promptly.

Don't hesitate to call the doctor if you're not sure whether a wound could be serious. Your doctor is the best resource when you are concerned and are not sure what steps to take.

Don't panic, or you will not be able to help the young person. Remember, your actions can make a major difference. The youngster needs your help and is relying on you. Remember also to evaluate the amount of blood loss and the extent of the wound.

Don't forget about the possibility of internal bleeding (hemorrhaging) with any significant blow to the body. Take care to watch for signs of this.

PLEASE NOTE: Now that you have a grasp of how to recognize and manage serious bleeding, it would be extremely helpful for you to go back to the Emergency Quick Reference With the Steps in Detail and review it carefully. The more familiar you are with this material, the more useful it will be to you when you need it.

CHAPTER 8

Shock

With the Steps in Detail

Managing Shock

Treatment of shock always depends on your ability to *recognize the cause(s) of the shock and control that problem (or those problems) first.* It's a matter of cause and effect. Shock is not the cause of the young person's condition (although it will worsen the situation). Shock is the effect that results from the problem(s). For example, if the young person is not breathing, or both pulmonary and cardiac (lung and heart) function have ceased, or there is massive bleeding—these must be treated *before* treating the shock. Therefore, you must treat the most life-threatening problem(s) first. By doing so, shock can more easily be managed or controlled.

▶ IF YOU SUSPECT SHOCK, HAVE SOMEONE ELSE CALL THE PARA-MEDICS WHILE YOU TREAT THE CHILD. IF NO ONE IS WITH YOU, CONTINUE TREATING THE CHILD WHILE YOU PERIODICALLY SHOUT FOR HELP. WHEN HELP ARRIVES, HAVE THAT PERSON CALL THE PARAMEDICS.

▶ **SUSPECT SHOCK WHEN THE SICK OR INJURED YOUNGSTER HAS:**

- Pale, clammy, cold, or mottled skin.

- Signs of agitation, irritability, and/or irrationality.

- Severe weakness, listlessness, and/or light-headedness.

- Signs of dehydration.

- Severe thirst.

- Nausea and vomiting.

- Weak, rapid pulse—with or without labored or rapid breathing (breathing difficulty).

▶ **HAVE THE YOUNGSTER LIE DOWN IF HE OR SHE IS NOT ALREADY DOING SO.**

▶ **ASSESS THE YOUNGSTER FOR PROBLEMS YOU *MUST* TREAT IMMEDIATELY:**

- **Make sure the youngster's airway is open and he or she is breathing. If not, open the airway and begin rescue breathing.** (If you are unable to remember the details of managing these problems, turn to the Emergency Quick References on page 113 [entitled "A Review of the Six Steps of CPR"] and page 127 [entitled "Managing Airway Obstruction/Choking"].)

- **Check his or her pulse. If there is no heartbeat, begin full CPR (both rescue breathing and chest compressions).** (If you are certified in CPR and cannot remember the details of the procedure, turn to the Emergency Quick Reference on page 113, entitled "A Review of the Six Steps of CPR.")

- **Look for signs of severe bleeding. Take appropriate measures to control the bleeding if found.** (If you are unable to remember the details of managing this problem, turn to the Emergency Quick Reference on page 141, entitled "Managing Serious Bleeding," for a review.)

- **Look for signs of serious injury—involving the head, neck, back, chest, or abdomen.** (If you are unable to remember the details of managing this problem, turn to the Emergency Quick Reference on page 503, entitled "Assessing Injury," as well as page 573, entitled "Head, Neck and Back, Injuries," page 519, entitled "Chest (Thoracic) Injuries," and page 513, entitled "Abdominal Injuries," for a review.)

154

LIFE-
THREATENING
EMERGENCIES:
ONLY A
MATTER OF
MOMENTS

➤ **IF THERE IS NO EVIDENCE OF HEAD, NECK, OR BACK INJURY, ELEVATE THE YOUNGSTER'S FEET ABOUT TEN TO TWELVE INCHES TO ALLOW SOME BLOOD TO RETURN TO THE HEART AND HEAD.** CRADLE A YOUNG INFANT IN YOUR ARMS—NOT OVER YOUR SHOULDER.

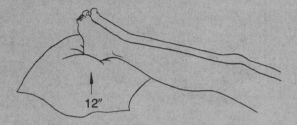

Elevate the youngster's feet 12 inches to help control shock.

➤ **IF THERE IS BREATHING DIFFICULTY, YOU MAY NEED TO ELEVATE THE YOUNGSTER'S SHOULDERS SLIGHTLY.** ROLL A TOWEL LENGTHWISE AND PLACE IT UNDER THE SHOULDERS.

➤ **IF POSSIBLE, KEEP THE YOUNGSTER WARM.** PUT A BLANKET UNDER AS WELL AS OVER HIM (IF YOU CAN). YOUR GOAL IS NOT TO OVERHEAT THE YOUNG PERSON BUT RATHER TO KEEP HIM FROM LOSING BODY HEAT UNNECESSARILY. (THIS WOULD ONLY MAKE THE SITUATION WORSE.)

➤ **CONTINUE TO WATCH THE CHILD CLOSELY FOR NEW AND PO-TENTIALLY SERIOUS PROBLEMS.**

- If she vomits, turn her head to the side, or roll her onto her side so she doesn't choke or aspirate (inhale) the vomitus (vomited matter).

- If breathing and/or heart function stop, begin rescue breathing and/or full CPR.

➤ **DO NOT GIVE THE YOUNGSTER ANYTHING TO EAT OR DRINK,** EVEN IF HE OR SHE REPEATEDLY ASKS FOR SOME-THING.

➤ **KEEP CALM AND BE REASSURING, BUT ALSO BE ATTENTIVE AND WATCHFUL.**

➤ **IF ONE OR MORE PEOPLE CAN ASSIST YOU, THEN PROCEED AS FOLLOWS:**

- If you must start CPR and there is also obvious bleeding or other serious injury, then have someone work on these other major problems—while you initiate and continue CPR. If there are no life-threatening injuries, have someone help you with CPR if he or she is trained to do so.

- If more than one person is going to be helping the youngster, then it is imperative that *only one person* be in charge. This person should direct all rescue activities, to ensure that no one gets in the way and that efforts are not duplicated. Usually the person to direct rescue activities is someone trained in CPR.

Understanding Shock

Shock is a very serious, potentially life-threatening medical emergency that requires a prompt response. It results when the blood supply—and therefore the oxygen supply—to various organs of the body has been reduced. Essentially, there is not enough blood circulating to keep the organs functioning properly. Because of this, anyone (regardless of age) who appears to be in shock must receive immediate medical evaluation and treatment.

Normally, blood circulation to the various organs of the body is quite steady, with only minor variations. Body chemicals and reflexes keep everything on an even, constant, uniquely balanced course. But when some form of stress is experienced, a special protective mechanism of the body is automatically triggered. Blood is shifted from the less vital organs and tissues to the more vital organs.

One of the more important regulators of the blood supply is the chemical epinephrine (also called adrenaline). We secrete it, along with related chemicals, in response to various kinds of stress—for example, fear, panic, injury, or illness. This has been called the "fight or flight" reaction. This chemical, produced by the adrenal gland, causes a complicated series of reactions in the blood vessels.

Similar kinds of "automatic" reflexes come into play when there is a disturbance in blood flow—for example, loss of blood. The body "knows" that remaining blood must be diverted from its less vital areas to the more critical areas. Blood vessels to the skin and intestines narrow and limit the amount of blood that goes there. (That's why a person's skin looks pale, pasty, or mottled and feels cool and clammy when he or she is in shock.) Arteries that lead to the more vital and sensitive organs—the brain, kidneys, liver, and heart—stay wide open to maintain a good oxygen supply to these organs for as long as possible.

As this occurs, fluid is released from the cells and the tissues and moves into the bloodstream. The kidneys reduce the amount of urine they are producing. The heart beats faster in order to circulate what blood is left, and the tissues attempt to extract

156

LIFE-
THREATENING
EMERGENCIES:
ONLY A
MATTER OF
MOMENTS

all the available oxygen from the blood. Various glands in the body produce hormones in an attempt to keep up the body's protective response.

The problem is, this response is just not efficient enough when shock is severe— and the vital organs may not receive enough blood and therefore not enough oxygen. Or instead of being shunted to vital organs, the blood may be trapped or pooled in the small blood vessels. If the shock is not quickly controlled, temporary or permanent damage to vital organs can occur. Also, when cells do not receive enough oxygen, they function poorly and produce excess acids, which cannot be effectively eliminated from the body. This condition, called "acidosis," further poisons the cells.

Certain organs and tissues are more susceptible to the harmful effects of shock than others. While loss of blood flow to the skin or intestines certainly can cause damage, these tissues are usually capable of rejuvenation and repair when circulation is restored. The kidneys, on the other hand, are particularly vulnerable to the effects of shock and can easily sustain damage. The brain is also quite sensitive, and brain damage can be very severe if the situation is not corrected quickly. The heart, however (especially in infants and children), is usually quite resilient.

The Causes of Shock

There are many possible causes of shock, some more common in infants and children than others. These causes can be grouped into three categories: (1) actual lack of blood volume, (2) faulty blood vessel function, and (3) heart failure (that is, the pump doesn't work). In youngsters, lack of blood volume and/or poor blood vessel function are most often the cause of shock, while heart failure is rarely the culprit. In older adults, on the other hand, heart disease is one of the leading causes of shock. It is often quite apparent *what* caused the shock to occur.

Shock due to low blood volume is usually caused either by rapid, *excessive blood loss* or by *serious dehydration*. With either of these situations, the youngster's body tries to compensate for the sudden loss of circulating blood by narrowing the blood vessels, increasing the heartbeat, reducing the urine production, and moving tissue fluid into the bloodstream. Since youngsters have such healthy bodies, they are, in fact, usually able to tolerate rather low blood volumes for a longer period of time than adults.

However, when a young person's body is no longer able to cope and compensate, his or her blood pressure drops, and deterioration takes place very suddenly (rather than gradually), and usually without warning. Because the effects of low blood volume can appear suddenly, it is important to quickly recognize the signs and symptoms of shock—which signal danger to a young person's well-being.

One of the most important things to remember when youngsters experience blood loss is that, because of their size, they have proportionately less blood circulating, and the loss of a rather small amount of blood can therefore get them into serious trouble— fast! For example, an adult who loses a quart of blood might be dizzy and weak—

and would certainly require treatment—but he or she would probably not go into deep shock. On the other hand, if the average one-year-old (who has less than a quart of blood) suddenly loses only eight ounces or so of blood, low blood pressure may well result, and shock might follow rather rapidly. It is therefore important to consider the size of the young person (and hence, his or her blood volume) when assessing the significance of the amount of blood lost.

Don't forget that blood loss can be the reason behind shock even when you can't see the blood. For example, a youngster who is hit by a car or falls over bicycle handlebars might experience serious internal bleeding in the abdomen, chest, or elsewhere. This can occur without there being one drop of blood visible. Remember, too, that while almost all internal bleeding in children results from injury, a few infants and children may hemorrhage (bleed internally) for other reasons, such as an ulcer, bowel disease, liver disease, or serious bleeding disorders.

Dehydration usually develops over several hours to days, but if shock follows, it most often occurs quite rapidly. The infant and/or young child is better able to compensate for lack of adequate fluid intake for a longer period of time than older youngsters and adults (although this is obviously not healthy and is potentially dangerous). However, when the little one's reserves run out, shock, low blood pressure, and collapse follow rather rapidly. He may not seem particularly sick over a period of time—but will then suddenly and dramatically crash. The older youngster or adult, in contrast, may slowly grow weaker and sicker—and go downhill more gradually. This is because the infant has such a healthy vascular system that he can hang on longer—on the brink of shock. The problem is, when shock finally occurs, it can be devastating.

Profound dehydration is usually seen in infants and young children who experience prolonged vomiting (with or without diarrhea), inadequate and inappropriate feeding, or serious burns. When infants become dehydrated, imbalances in body salts can also be a contributing factor to shock.

When *faulty blood vessel function* is the cause of shock, there is actually enough blood in the body, but it is inappropriately trapped or pooled in the small blood vessels away from the vital organs. This usually occurs when the muscles of the small arteries relax and dilate—allowing blood to pour out to nonessential areas of the body. This relaxation of the arteries results in low blood pressure (sluggish blood flow) and therefore inadequate oxygenation of tissues and organs.

In infants and young children, among the most common causes of shock due to faulty blood vessel function are *sepsis* (overwhelming infection)—also known as "blood poisoning"—and/or *meningitis* (inflammation and infection of the coverings of the brain and spinal cord).

The bacteria (or their by-products) that cause sepsis and meningitis seem to produce toxins (poisons) that cause the blood vessels to malfunction. Infants and children with this kind of shock often have had fever or other signs of illness before the shock occurred. Shock due to faulty blood vessel function can also result from metabolic disturbances, such as excessive acid production, abnormal salt levels, or unusual hereditary diseases.

158

LIFE-
THREATENING
EMERGENCIES:
ONLY A
MATTER OF
MOMENTS

In older youngsters and adults, *anaphylaxis* (overwhelming allergic reaction) can lead to severe shock due to blood vessel malfunction. In this kind of situation, you may know that the youngster is allergic to particular things (foods, medicines, or certain animals, plants, or insects). You may also have seen the youngster come in contact with or suspect that he or she has been in contact with the offending substance. Other symptoms—such as swelling of the face and tongue, difficulty breathing, hives, or itching—are also tip-offs that anaphylaxis caused the shock.

So-called *neurogenic shock*—simple fainting, or syncope—is a special kind of shock. It results from an abnormal drop in blood pressure due to poor blood vessel function (because of an abnormal reflex). This is one form of shock from which the body is usually able to recover quickly when simple measures (such as having the youngster lie down and calming him or her) are instituted. For further information on fainting, turn to page 164.

So-called *cardiogenic shock*—"pump failure"—is occasionally seen in youngsters with serious heart defects or in those with inflammation of the heart (myocarditis, endocarditis). However, in otherwise healthy youngsters, the heart is in fact more likely to withstand serious insults until their reserves are depleted—which is long beyond the period of time an adult could withstand the same kind and level of stress. When the youngster's reserves become depleted, the heart may suddenly slow down or beat irregularly, then fail to work as a *result* of the problem, not as its cause. True "pump failure" does, however, occur in adults.

Shock is a medical emergency and requires prompt intervention by skilled medical personnel. Your job is to do everything possible to halt the progression of the shock by initiating first aid measures and performing CPR if necessary. The cornerstone of medical treatment for shock is to stabilize the young person by giving large amounts of fluids intravenously (through the vein). These might include salt solutions, blood plasma, and protein solution (called albumin). These not only provide the body with needed blood and fluids but also rebalance the body chemistry and metabolism. Obviously, this kind of treatment must be given by medical personnel, the paramedics, or the emergency room staff. It is therefore imperative that the paramedics (preferably) or an ambulance be called immediately if a youngster goes into shock.

Shock: Signs and Symptoms

Your first indication that shock has occurred is usually the presence of very pale, cold, clammy skin—especially of the hands and feet. A youngster may have a gray or bluish look, as well. If you press your fingers against his or her skin (push the "color" out), you may find that the color returns very slowly. (Normally, after you push on the skin, the color returns instantly. When a person is in shock, it does not.) All these signs are indicators that the blood is being diverted away from the skin and other less vital tissues—and directed to the internal organs.

Changes in behavior and mood are other signs of shock. Youngsters who can talk may tell you that they feel weak and light-headed or are seeing spots. They may collapse and become unconscious if standing or sitting. Anxiety, fear, agitation, irritability, and irrationality may also be a part of shock. Young infants are likely to be very quiet and listless or lethargic, but irritable when disturbed. You may notice that an infant has a weak, irritable cry. These small ones often have a "worried" look, as well. When shock is severe, young infants do not arouse or respond to stimulation.

Because of the body's signals to conserve fluid, the youngster who is in shock does not urinate much—if at all. This is especially true if dehydration is the cause of the shock. He or she is also *very* thirsty and may ask for something to drink—only to become nauseated and vomit.

You may also notice that the heartbeat is very fast (even for a youngster, whose pulse is normally faster than an adult's). This is the body's means of responding to the shock by trying to pump blood to the vital organs faster. The pulse is usually weak and thready instead of strong and forceful, and breathing may be fast or labored. As shock progresses, breathing becomes more and more difficult and irregular. The heartbeat may become weaker and more irregular, as well. Unconsciousness follows rather rapidly because of lack of oxygen to the brain. Death is imminent if breathing stops or the heart becomes weak from lack of oxygen and/or from working too fast and too hard.

THE DON'TS

Don't panic. It's important that you remain calm and transfer the message of "calmness" to the youngster. This keeps him or her calm and allows you to assess the situation with a cool head. Also, if the youngster panics, the situation can worsen, since becoming excited further stresses the body's protective mechanisms.

Don't give the child any food or liquids—not even water. While the youngster may be thirsty, he will also have a tendency to vomit and aspirate (inhale) the vomited matter into his lungs. Serious aspiration can cause death or lung damage.

Don't allow the youngster to get up or move around. This "robs" the heart and vital organs of blood they need to get oxygen to the tissues. In addition, the child is likely to be dizzy and fall (further hurting herself) or lose consciousness (worsening the situation).

Don't give the youngster any medication, especially strong pain medication or sedatives. These can make the youngster sleepy, slow his or her breathing, and create confusion about how serious the situation is.

PLEASE NOTE: Now that you have a grasp of how to recognize and manage shock, it would be extremely helpful for you to go back to the Emergency Quick Reference With the Steps in Detail and review it carefully. The more familiar you are with that material, the more useful it will be to you when you need it.

C H A P T E R 9

Unconsciousness

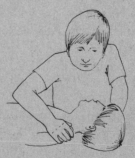

EMERGENCY QUICK REFERENCE

With the Steps in Detail

Managing Unconsciousness

When it comes to situations of unconsciousness, your ability to quickly and effectively evaluate the youngster's condition and initiate lifesaving procedures can mean the difference between life and death—particularly when the young person has stopped breathing and his or her heart function has ceased. Again, it is vital that you take a CPR course.

▶ **DETERMINE WHETHER OR NOT THE YOUNGSTER IS UNCONSCIOUS.**

- Shout the child's name and gently shake her shoulder. (If an infant or a very small child—*do not* shake her but pinch the bottom of the foot or squeeze the muscle on the shoulder near the neck.)

Be sure the youngster is really unconscious and not just sleeping.

- The child's response may vary from arousable but drowsy to totally unresponsive.

▶ **IF THE YOUNG PERSON IS UNCONSCIOUS, CHECK TO SEE WHETHER HE OR SHE IS BREATHING.** THIS DETERMINES HOW YOU SHOULD PROCEED FROM HERE.

If the Youngster Is Not Breathing

▶ **HAVE SOMEONE ELSE CALL THE PARAMEDICS WHILE YOU TREAT THE CHILD. IF NO ONE IS WITH YOU, CONTINUE TREATING THE CHILD WHILE YOU PERIODICALLY SHOUT FOR HELP. WHEN HELP ARRIVES, HAVE THAT PERSON CALL THE PARAMEDICS.**

▶ **LAY THE YOUNGSTER ON A FLAT, FIRM SURFACE (USUALLY THE FLOOR OR GROUND). TAKE GREAT CARE IN MOVING THE YOUNGSTER IF THERE IS ANY POSSIBILITY OF A HEAD, NECK, OR BACK INJURY.**

▶ **OPEN THE AIRWAY.**

- Either tilt the head back gently or place a folded (lengthwise) towel under the youngster's shoulders, so his or her head is in the "sniffing position" (chin jutted forward and head tilted slightly back, as people do when trying to smell something).

- Clear the mouth of any vomited material or secretions.

▶ **BEGIN RESCUE BREATHING.** (If you are unable to remember the details of managing this problem, turn to the Emergency Quick Reference on page 113, entitled "A Review of the Six Steps of CPR.")

- Deliver four quick rescue breaths.

- If air doesn't move down the youngster's throat or the abdominal area doesn't rise, readjust the airway and deliver four more rescue breaths. If there still seems to be resistance (air doesn't move down the youngster's throat and so on), then assume there is an airway obstruction.

- Relieve the obstruction and deliver four more quick rescue breaths. (If you are unable to remember the details of managing this problem, turn to the Emergency Quick Reference on page 127, entitled "Managing Airway Obstruction/Choking," for a review.)

LIFE-
THREATENING
EMERGENCIES:
ONLY A
MATTER OF
MOMENTS

▶ **CHECK FOR A PULSE.**

- If there *is no pulse*, begin full CPR (chest compressions with rescue breathing), as you learned in your CPR training course. (If you are certified in CPR and are unable to remember the details of the procedure, turn to the Emergency Quick Reference on page 113, entitled "A Review of the Six Steps of CPR.")

- Do not stop CPR until the paramedics or ambulance personnel or someone else certified in CPR takes over for you. You may also stop CPR if the young person begins breathing on his or her own (and has a pulse) or if you are so totally exhausted that you cannot continue.

- If there *is a pulse* but the youngster is not breathing, then continue rescue breathing until the paramedics or ambulance personnel or someone else certified in CPR takes over for you or the youngster begins breathing on his or her own.

- When treating the youngster, be sure to check frequently for a pulse, to make sure heart function has not suddenly stopped.

If the Youngster Is Breathing

▶ **HAVE SOMEONE ELSE CALL THE PARAMEDICS WHILE YOU TREAT THE CHILD. IF NO ONE IS WITH YOU, CONTINUE TREATING THE CHILD WHILE YOU PERIODICALLY SHOUT FOR HELP. WHEN HELP ARRIVES, HAVE THAT PERSON CALL THE PARAMEDICS.**

▶ **KEEP THE YOUNGSTER IN THE SAME POSITION IN WHICH YOU FOUND HIM OR HER UNTIL YOU CHECK FOR SERIOUS INJURIES.**

- Check the head for swelling, bumps, and bruises. Is there fluid or blood seeping from an ear or the nose?

- Is a neck injury possible? What about a back injury?

- If it is at all possible that the child was hurt, do not move him or her, since this could worsen a head, neck, or serious back injury. (If you are unable to remember the details of managing this problem, turn to the Emergency Quick Reference on page 573, entitled "Head, Neck, and Back Injuries," for a review.)

▶ **LAY THE YOUNGSTER DOWN (ON HIS OR HER BACK) IF THERE ARE NO HEAD, NECK, OR BACK INJURIES.**

▶ **CHECK FOR SIGNS OF SEVERE BLEEDING (BOTH OPEN WOUNDS AND INTERNAL HEMORRHAGING), AND TAKE STEPS TO TREAT IT.** (If you are unable to remember the details of managing this problem, turn to the Emergency Quick Reference on page 141, entitled "Managing Serious Bleeding," for a review.)

▶ **CHECK FOR SIGNS OF SHOCK**—PALE OR PASTY SKIN COLOR; COOL, CLAMMY SKIN; WEAK, THREADY PULSE; RESTLESSNESS; VOMITING; AND SO ON—**AND TAKE STEPS TO TREAT IT.** (If you are unable to remember the details of managing this problem, turn to the Emergency Quick Reference on page 152, entitled "Managing Shock," for a review.)

• If shock has occurred, elevate the youngster's feet slightly, only if there are no head, neck, or back injuries.

• Keep the young person warm by placing a blanket over her. (Place one under her, too, if possible.) Do not try to overheat the youngster, but attempt to retain her own body temperature.

▶ **WATCH CAREFULLY TO SEE THAT THE AIRWAY STAYS OPEN AND CHECK FOR A PULSE PERIODICALLY.**

▶ **IF VOMITING OCCURS, TURN THE YOUNGSTER ON HIS SIDE, SO THE VOMITED MATTER (AND FLUIDS) CAN DRAIN OUT OF HIS MOUTH AND NOT BE ASPIRATED (INHALED).**

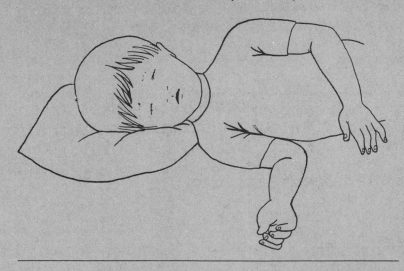

Turn the youngster on his side so he doesn't inhale (aspirate) vomited material. Use extreme caution in moving the youngster if you have any reason to believe he may have a head, neck, or back injury.

LIFE-
THREATENING
EMERGENCIES:
ONLY A
MATTER OF
MOMENTS

If the Youngster Wakes Up While You're Waiting for Help

▶ **KEEP THE CHILD CALM AND DO NOT ALLOW HIM OR HER TO MOVE OR GET UP. WATCH CAREFULLY FOR SIGNS OF BREATHING PROBLEMS.**

▶ **TRY TO DETERMINE WHY THE YOUNG PERSON WAS UNCON-SCIOUS.** IF HE IS OLD ENOUGH AND ABLE TO TALK, ASK HIM WHAT HAPPENED. IF THE CHILD IS TOO YOUNG OR UNABLE TO TALK, THEN BE A DETECTIVE.

- Are there signs of poisoning, serious infection, convulsions, electric shock, allergic reactions, injury, or chronic disease?

- If the youngster is your child, did you notice any events or problems in the few minutes, hours, and days before the incident that might be related to it?

▶ **IF YOU THINK THE YOUNGSTER EXPERIENCED ACCIDENTAL POI-SONING, GIVE ANY POISON, PILLS, OR VOMITUS (VOMITED MA-TERIAL) YOU FOUND TO THE PARAMEDICS OR AMBULANCE CREW. (IF YOU MUST TAKE THE YOUNGSTER TO THE EMERGENCY ROOM YOURSELF, TAKE ANY OF THESE WITH YOU.)** (If you are unable to remember the details of managing this problem, turn to the Emergency Quick Reference on page 172, entitled "Managing Poisoning," for a review.)

If the Youngster Was Unconscious Just Momentarily and It Appears that He or She Only Fainted

▶ **HAVE THE YOUNGSTER LIE DOWN.**

CHECK TO MAKE SURE THERE ARE NO INJURIES.

▶ **TRY TO DETERMINE *FOR SURE* WHETHER THIS WAS A CASE OF SIMPLE FAINTING.** IF THE CHILD IS OLD ENOUGH TO TALK, ASK HER WHAT HAPPENED. IF THE CHILD IS TOO YOUNG, THEN BE A DETECTIVE.

> ◗ HAVE HIM GET UP VERY SLOWLY IF YOU FEEL EVERYTHING IS
>   NOW OK.
>
> ◗ MAKE SURE YOU CALL THE DOCTOR IMMEDIATELY FOR ADVICE.
>   PARTICULARLY IF THIS IS THE FIRST FAINTING EPISODE, THE
>   DOCTOR MAY WANT TO EVALUATE AND EXAMINE THE YOUNG-
>   STER.

Unconsciousness: What Is It?

Finding a young person (or anyone) unconscious can be a very scary experience. What makes it even more difficult is that many times there are no obvious clues as to the cause of the problem. In this situation, you need to remember some basic life-support techniques and stay calm enough to play detective at the same time. It's also extremely helpful to better understand what unconsciousness means so you can be alert to any signs of potential problems.

Essentially, unconsciousness occurs when the brain stops functioning normally. For our brains to work properly (physiologically), we must have a normal flow of blood to all areas of the brain. This continual and adequate blood flow brings with it oxygen and nutrients that the cells of the brain need in order to perform their job. Any disturbance in this blood flow (or oxygenation of the cells) will cause faulty functioning of the brain cells.

This faulty functioning can either be temporary or permanent, depending on the degree of damage to the brain cells. Brain cells, unlike most other cells in the body, do not reproduce themselves. If a sufficient number of cells die in a certain area of the brain, then permanent damage is likely, and the function(s) affected will depend on the area of the brain damaged. On the other hand, if cells are damaged and they eventually revive, then the resultant problems may be temporary, or there may be degrees of permanent damage.

The scenario goes something like this. If a youngster falls off a bicycle and hits his or her head solidly on the concrete, two injuries to the head can actually occur (the old saying "adding insult to injury" appropriately applies here). The impact of the skull hitting the hard cement results in the first injury—that is, the injury to the skull and scalp itself. This is the injury we can often see and feel. The "insult" (or second injury) comes when the brain bounces against the inside of the skull. It is this blow that causes unconsciousness or stuns the youngster for a period of time. It is also this second injury that causes most of the problems.

If the force of the brain hitting the skull is great, then the youngster may remain

166

LIFE-
THREATENING
EMERGENCIES:
ONLY A
MATTER OF
MOMENTS

unconscious for minutes or even longer. The problem is, when the brain hits the skull, it may sustain a bruise (meaning it swells and may bleed), usually in the area where it hit the skull. The degree of swelling and the extent of the bruise (bleeding) depend on the severity of the blow to the head. But the problem doesn't end here. Brain swelling can increase pressure inside the head, which results in decreased blood flow to that area of the brain. Because these cells are then getting less oxygen, the problem is compounded.

A similar sequence of events can also occur whenever *lack of oxygen* (due to any number of reasons) is the basic cause of unconsciousness. It's a vicious cycle. Because the cells aren't getting enough oxygen, they swell. Swelling causes increased pressure, which results in decreased blood flow to the area and therefore decreased oxygenation. Hence, even if the initial reason for the lack of oxygenation is resolved (the airway obstruction is relieved, the near-drowning victim is revived, the youngster regains consciousness after the fall from the bicycle, or whatever), a problem may still be seen for a period of time or even permanently because of this second insult to the brain and the cycle of problems it can create.

Unconsciousness can result from anything that causes brain swelling or lack of adequate oxygenation to the brain, as well as "poisoning" or destruction of brain cells—for example: head injury; poisoning; severe shock; a disturbance in the body's metabolism (such as diabetic shock, hepatic coma, uremia, insulin shock, hypoglycemia, electrolyte imbalance); illness or injury; airway obstruction; hypothermia; serious bleeding; electric shock; intoxication; severe generalized infection; fever; drugs; carbon monoxide poisoning; anaphylactic shock; heatstroke; reaction to bites and stings; brain tumor; convulsive disorders (seizures); degenerative diseases; and cerebrovascular accidents.

Accidental poisoning with sedatives or barbiturates is particularly problematic, not only because this same process occurs but because those types of medications have the added effect of directly attacking the brain cells that control breathing. So you have not only lack of oxygenation due to the poisoning but also a diminished breathing pattern because of the type of medication (poison) taken. Again, this essentially starts a "domino effect"—one problem causing another and that problem another, and so forth. Brain injury, then, is frightening because it can snowball into a vicious cycle of problems.

Fainting: A Special Consideration

Fainting is a very momentary loss of consciousness. It is caused by faulty reflex actions in the blood vessels, leading to a temporary lack of an adequate blood supply (and thereby inadequate oxygenation) to the brain. Since the brain has not directly been injured (as occurs in many head injuries or cases of more severe oxygen deprivation), the situation can easily be resolved if you lay the youngster down and elevate his feet or if you place his head lower than his heart. (Both increase blood flow to the brain.)

Fainting has many causes, including fear, panic, hyperventilation (overbreathing), heat exhaustion, lack of adequate food intake (near-starvation), exhaustion, pain, or even illness. While it is most common in teenagers and adults, neurogenic shock can occur in younger children, as well. Certain individuals have a greater tendency to faint under any kind of pressure. While fainting is common, and the youngster usually wakes up right after lying down and calming down, it's important to have the young person evaluated by the doctor or in an emergency room (after the first episode) to make sure that there are no underlying physiological reasons for the problem. Also, certain people who faint easily can be taught how to recognize the signs of fainting and lie down soon enough to prevent the loss of consciousness.

Unconsciousness: Signs and Symptoms

Essentially, there are varying levels of loss of consciousness. In one level, known as lethargy, the youngster is slightly arousable but does not act like himself when awake. He quickly falls back to sleep and appears rather peaceful if not disturbed. In another level of loss of consciousness, the young person can be stimulated when pain is inflicted but only moves around without purpose, doesn't open her eyes, and doesn't seem to be aware of what is going on.

In yet another level of loss of consciousness, the young person will fight you or withdraw if pain is inflicted but do little else. Again, he doesn't open his eyes and doesn't seem to be aware of anything around him. In this situation, he only responds to painful stimuli. In the deepest level of unconsciousness, there is total unresponsiveness. The youngster does not respond to anything, including pain, although he may or may not have some unusual reflexes.

A word about coma. The term *coma* is usually used to refer to a rather prolonged loss of consciousness (hours, days, weeks, or even years). Most people think of coma as meaning *complete* lack of responsiveness. They are often correct, although a person who is in a coma can show some response to his or her surroundings or to stimulation and still have very severe brain malfunction. For example, some reflexes may be present, or the youngster may kick or move in response to pain or have body spasms or make chewing motions. Depending on other factors, all of these reflexes may be seen both in certain forms of coma and in certain stages of recovery from very deep unconsciousness. However, having these reflexes *does not* mean the young person will come out of the coma. This depends on many factors.

If you find a youngster who appears to be unconscious, the first thing you need to do is determine whether or not she is *really* unconscious—not just sleeping. If the young person does not respond to the shouting of her name or "hey you," gentle

168

LIFE-
THREATENING
EMERGENCIES:
ONLY A
MATTER OF
MOMENTS

shaking of the shoulder, pinching the skin of the foot, or squeezing the shoulder muscle near the neck—then she is unconscious. The legs and arms will also usually be limp. If you lift one slightly and let it go, the arm or leg will simply flop back down.

One mistake commonly made is a desperate attempt by the adult to "shake the young person into consciousness." This not only will fail but can actually hurt the youngster or cause further injury. In a panic, people have been known to "slap around," roll or push, violently shake, or sit up an unconscious youngster, then allow him or her to drop back down—all in an attempt to "awaken" the child. Infants and very small children are particularly vulnerable to serious and sometimes fatal injury if they are picked up and shaken. This shaking actually "bounces" the brain against the skull, causing bleeding and severe swelling.

So it is important not to panic but rather to make sure that the young person is unconscious and begin rescue steps. If he begins to revive or is moaning and moving when you find him, keep him lying down and watch how he acts while reviving. It is at this point that you need to look for neurologic or central nervous system problems.

It's important to look for the following: twitching or jerking of an arm, a leg, or the entire body; stiffness of an arm, a leg, or some other area of the body; weakness in an arm, a leg, or another area; failure to move an arm, a leg, or an area of the body or one entire side of the body; lack of sensation in arm(s), leg(s), or other areas of the body; a sensation of "tingling" or "pinpricks" in any area of the body; total disorientation (inability to remember where he is or what is going on); loss of memory (inability to remember her name, where she lives, phone number, or date and day); slurred, jumbled, or nonsensical speech; or the youngster starts fighting you or panics and shows signs of paranoia or distrust. It is also important to watch for convulsions or seizures (see Chapter 12 for details).

If your child experiences a head injury or an incident where lack of oxygenation to the brain occurred for any reason, it is vital that you continue to be a *good observer* for twenty-four to forty-eight hours after the incident (even if the youngster has been evaluated by your doctor or has been treated in an emergency room and released). Look for the problems previously mentioned and note any changes in behavior. If any occur, it is best to call your doctor immediately. Your observations are particularly valuable because you know how your youngster usually behaves and what is truly abnormal *for him or her*.

If the young person is sent home from the doctor's office or emergency room, you will probably be told to watch him closely and to awaken him every hour or two for the first twelve to twenty-four hours. This is done to make sure the young person can easily be awakened. When awakening him, it is also important to determine whether or not the young person is alert, makes sense when he responds to questions, and shows little or no sign of residual problems as a result of the incident. Do not try to keep the child awake—it is all right for him to doze or sleep. It is *how he wakes up* that tells about brain injury. Compare his response this time to his usual response to being awakened. Keep in mind, though, that a youngster who is normally hard to wake up will be hard to wake up whether or not he has experienced a brain injury.

For this particular child, then, grogginess *does not mean* a brain abnormality. On the other hand, a youngster who is usually easy to awaken probably has a problem if she is slow to wake up or fights and doesn't make sense when you talk to her.

Another way to identify a potential problem is by periodic evaluation of *pupil response*. The pupils are the black spots found in the center of the eyes. Normally, the pupils respond to changes in light intensity. They get smaller (constrict) when light

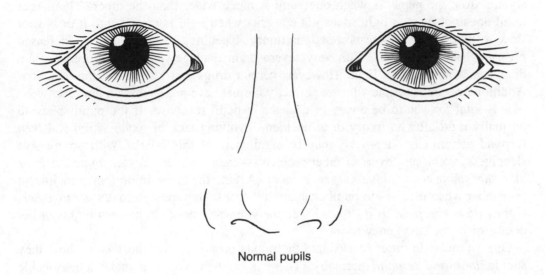

Normal pupils

Pupils that are equal and both react together are normal. If one pupil does not get smaller (constrict) when light is shined into the eyes, seek medical help immediately.

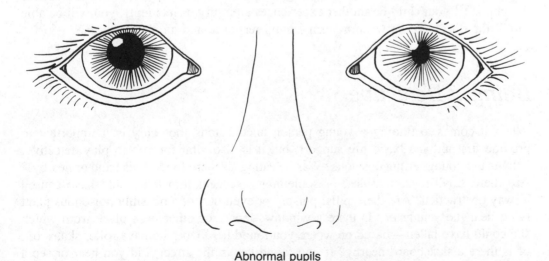

Abnormal pupils

170

LIFE-
THREATENING
EMERGENCIES:
ONLY A
MATTER OF
MOMENTS

gets brighter or a light is shined in the eye, and they get larger (dilate) when light is dimmed or the light is turned away from the eye. Brain injury (swelling and/or bleeding) can cause the pupil reflex to disappear or be abnormal.

Usually, both pupils work together and respond immediately to changes in light intensity. That means if you shine a flashlight into one eye—*both pupils* should quickly tighten down in response. When you remove the light from one eye—*both pupils* should promptly widen (dilate). One of the most worrisome and potentially serious signals from the pupils is when one pupil is much wider than the other. This larger pupil does not react to light (does not constrict when light is shined into it or is very slow to react). This suggests a serious injury, bleeding, swelling, and/or increased pressure inside the skull. With very severe brain damage, *both pupils* may remain dilated and not react to light. However, certain drugs can also cause this reaction. Additionally, some people who are perfectly normal have pupils that do not react well.

It is vital for you to be aware of changes in pupil response. If the pupils respond normally right after an injury or an incident involving lack of oxygenation and *then* respond abnormally later—this may be significant. If this is seen with progressive sleepiness, vomiting, fever, or other problems—then *call your doctor immediately or take the youngster to the emergency room*. Again, the most important principle to remember when it comes to pupil evaluation is that both pupils normally *act together*. If they *do not respond as a "unit,"* then the youngster needs to be seen by his or her doctor or in the emergency room.

One warning: In order to evaluate the pupils properly, you must know how they should *look and respond* normally. There is no way you can make a reasonable comparison or a correct judgment *unless* you have previously tested someone's pupils. The best way to do this is simply to evaluate your own child's pupils. Take a flashlight or penlight and shine it in one eye. Watch both pupils respond together. Turn the light away from the one eye (don't accidently shine it in the other eye!) and watch both pupils widen together. Do this in soft light. In this way, if you ever have to evaluate the pupils (if your child or another experiences an injury or incident), you will be able to tell the difference between a normal pupil response and an abnormal one.

Being a Detective

When it comes to finding a young person unconscious, not only is it important to provide first aid and basic life support, but it is also vital for you to play detective. Why is the youngster unconscious? Was he eating (is there food in his hand or nearby)? Are there small toys, marbles, or something else near him that could have caused airway obstruction? Are there pills, poison, or even part of a possibly poisonous plant lying near the youngster? Is there a window, fence, or other high place from which she could have fallen—based on where you found her? Does he have roller skates on, or is there a skateboard nearby? If you found her in the street, did you hear or see a car, or are there skid marks? Was he on playground equipment? Has she had any symptoms to suggest that she might have been sick? Has he lost consciousness before?

The point is to find out (as far as is humanly possible) what caused the unconsciousness. This helps the doctor treat the problem more specifically. It also gives you direction in terms of your rescue efforts. For example, if you think the youngster may have experienced airway obstruction, then you will need to relieve the obstruction before your other rescue efforts can be successful.

THE DON'TS

Don't panic. Your observations, as well as the actions you take, are very important. Make sure an unconscious infant or child is breathing. If not, it's vital that you start basic life-support procedures immediately.

Don't try to give an unconscious or semiconscious youngster anything to drink or eat. There is a serious risk of choking or aspirating (inhaling) the food or liquid or of causing vomiting.

Don't move an unconscious youngster without assistance unless you have no other alternative. Especially avoid the temptation to scoop up an infant or small child (who might have a serious neck, head, or back injury) and rush to an emergency room.

Don't hesitate to call the paramedics or an ambulance if you're unsure about the youngster's condition.

Don't fail to have a youngster who has lost consciousness evaluated by a doctor, even if he or she seems to have recovered completely. While a short lapse of consciousness may result from simple fainting or hyperventilation, it can also signal a more serious problem. If you have questions about this kind of episode, call your doctor.

PLEASE NOTE: Now that you have a grasp of how to recognize and manage unconsciousness, it would be extremely helpful for you to go back to the Emergency Quick Reference With the Steps in Detail and review it carefully. The more familiar you are with that material, the more useful it will be to you when you need it.

Poisoning

EMERGENCY QUICK REFERENCE

With the Steps in Detail

Managing Poisoning

▶ **WHEN FACTORS POINT TO POISONING AS A POSSIBILITY, ASSUME THAT IT *DID* HAPPEN RATHER THAN THAT IT DID NOT. TAKE APPROPRIATE ACTION.**

▶ **SUSPECT POISONING IN THE FOLLOWING SITUATIONS:**

- If a youngster is found with or near an open container of a drug or other poisonous substance.

- If a youngster is acting in an unusual way (for example, behavior changes, diarrhea, or breathing trouble) that is not explainable by a common illness (such as the flu or a cold). Even then, it is wise to look around to make sure a poison could not be involved.

▶ IF THE YOUNGSTER IS FOUND *UNCONSCIOUS, DELIRIOUS, HAVING CONVULSIONS, OR WITH ANOTHER SERIOUS PROBLEM*, CHECK TO SEE WHETHER HE OR SHE IS BREATHING AND HAS A PULSE (AS YOU WERE TAUGHT IN CPR TRAINING).

▶ IF THE *YOUNGSTER IS UNCONSCIOUS AND NOT BREATHING*, BEGIN RESCUE BREATHING IMMEDIATELY AND

- Have someone else call the paramedics while you treat the child. If no one is with you, continue treating the child while you periodically shout for help. When help arrives, have that person call the paramedics.

- If the youngster's heart has stopped as well (there is no pulse), initiate full CPR (rescue breathing with chest compressions). (If you are certified in CPR and are unable to remember the details of the procedure, turn to the Emergency Quick Reference on page 113, entitled "A Review of the Six Steps of CPR.")

- Continue CPR until the paramedics or someone else certified in CPR arrives and takes over for you (or assists you in two-rescuer CPR), or until the youngster gasps and breathes on his or her own.

▶ IF THE *YOUNG PERSON IS UNCONSCIOUS BUT IS BREATHING AND HAS A PULSE*, PROCEED AS FOLLOWS:

- Immediately have someone else call the paramedics while you treat the child. If no one is with you, continue treating the child while you periodically shout for help. When help arrives, have that person call the paramedics.

- Continue to check to see whether the youngster is breathing and has a pulse.

- If the youngster is vomiting and unconscious, turn him or her on one side to better prevent aspiration (inhalation) of the vomited matter or choking.

- If someone else is with you, have him or her search the house for a possible poison. If something is found, save the poison and the container. Give these to the paramedics or ambulance crew, together with any vomited matter you may have found.

- Never induce vomiting if the youngster is unconscious or is not fully alert. He or she may aspirate (inhale) what has been vomited.

174

LIFE-
THREATENING
EMERGENCIES:
ONLY A
MATTER OF
MOMENTS

Poisons Swallowed, Inhaled, or on the Skin:

▶ **IF THE YOUNGSTER** *MAY HAVE EATEN OR DRUNK A POISON AND IS CONSCIOUS AND NOT VOMITING*, **GIVE HIM OR HER FOUR TO EIGHT OUNCES OF WATER OR MILK.** THIS HELPS DILUTE THE POISON IF IT WAS INGESTED (EATEN OR DRUNK).

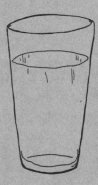

Dilute a poison by giving the youngster water or milk to drink.

- Do not attempt to "neutralize" a poison such as an acid or alkali. Just dilute it.

- Don't attempt to induce vomiting at this point. You will need to determine whether or not causing vomiting is necessary for this particular poison.

▶ **IF THE CHILD HAD A** *POISON IN HIS MOUTH BUT SPIT IT OUT:*

- Have him repeatedly rinse his mouth with water or milk. (Make sure he rinses, then spits out the water or milk.)

- After repeated rinsing, have him drink four to eight ounces of water or milk in case some of the poison was swallowed.

▶ **IF THE** *POISON IS ON THE SKIN*, **YOU NEED TO RINSE IT OFF IMMEDIATELY.**

- If the poison is on a large area of the body, then rapidly put the youngster (clothes and all) in the shower—under a steady stream of lukewarm water.

- While the child is under the stream of water, remove all clothing (as quickly as possible) and allow the water to run over the youngster for ten to fifteen minutes.

- Now call the poison control center for further instructions.

Try to Identify the Poison

▶ **DETERMINE WHAT WAS INGESTED (EATEN OR DRUNK), INHALED, OR GOTTEN ON THE SKIN OR IN THE EYES.**

- If the youngster is old enough to answer you, ask whether she ate, drank, or inhaled something, and ask her where it is.

- Look for the poison. Carefully check all rooms and areas of the house, including cupboards, cabinets, on top of sinks, tabletops, under beds, sofas, chairs, and on the floors.

- Check all plants to see if bites have been taken out or pieces of the plants have been pulled off.

- Don't forget to check usually locked areas of the house, as well. You never know when someone will have forgotten to lock a door or cabinet, or you might be surprised to find the youngster has learned how to open a lock.

- If you find no evidence during your search, try to determine whether the youngster could have been poisoned elsewhere. Where has he been in the last few hours? Was he visiting a neighbor, friend, or relative? Has he been playing in the yard or garage? Has he been at the grocery store with you or someone else? Any other place where he could have gotten into a poisonous substance in the last few hours?

If You Find the Poisonous Substance (Usually It Is Found Opened or Spilled)

▶ **READ THE "CAUTION" STATEMENT ON THE LABEL (IF IT IS A PRODUCT OTHER THAN A MEDICATION), WHICH USUALLY GIVES AN INDICATION OF HOW POISONOUS THE MATERIAL IS AND INSTRUCTIONS ABOUT WHAT TO DO IN CASE OF POISONING. *DO NOT* FOLLOW THESE INSTRUCTIONS AT THIS TIME.**

▶ **SAVE THE CONTAINER AND THE REMAINING POISONOUS SUBSTANCE.**

▶ **ESTIMATE (AS BEST YOU CAN) THE AMOUNT OF POISON TAKEN.**

176

LIFE-
THREATENING
EMERGENCIES:
ONLY A
MATTER OF
MOMENTS

▶ **CALL THE POISON CONTROL CENTER IN YOUR AREA.** (THE NUMBER SHOULD ALWAYS BE ON OR AT YOUR PHONE.) **IF THERE IS NO POISON CONTROL CENTER NEAR YOU, CALL THE NEAREST HOSPITAL EMERGENCY ROOM OR YOUR FAMILY DOCTOR FOR INSTRUCTIONS. YOU WILL NEED TO TELL THE PROFESSIONALS THE FOLLOWING INFORMATION:**

- **What type of poison was involved.**

- **How much was eaten, inhaled, or made contact with the skin.**

- **When the youngster was poisoned** (for example, twenty minutes ago, probably one hour ago).

- **Whether the young person is showing any signs or symptoms.** You'll need to describe these (if any have occurred) in as much detail as possible.

- **What steps you have taken so far to aid the youngster** (given milk or water, flushed water on the skin, and so on).

- **The age and weight of the young person.**

- **Whether or not you have syrup of ipecac** (a medicine used to cause vomiting) available in case you are instructed to give it to the youngster.

- **Your address and phone number, if requested.** (You should always know the major cross streets nearest your home.)

▶ **CAREFULLY FOLLOW THE INSTRUCTIONS GIVEN YOU BY THESE PROFESSIONALS.**

- Remember, they are highly trained and have all necessary information at hand.

- **Never hang up the phone unless instructed to do so.** Often the medical personnel will want to stay in contact with you—until they can establish that the child is out of danger, that it was a false alarm, or that other medical professionals (usually the paramedics) are on the scene and have taken over for them.

- **If you are given any instructions** (from the poison control center, the hospital emergency room personnel or the family doctor) **to follow in case a problem occurs later,** *write them down* **so you don't forget them.**

If the Youngster Has Ingested (Eaten or Drunk) a Poison and You Are in a Situation Where You Cannot Reach Medical Professionals for Advice and Must Act on Your Own (You Are Camping, Backpacking, Snowed In and the Phones Are Out of Order, or Whatever)

▶ **FIRST, GIVE THE YOUNG PERSON FOUR TO EIGHT OUNCES OF WATER OR MILK IF HE OR SHE IS FULLY CONSCIOUS AND NOT VOMITING.**

▶ **READ THE "CAUTION" STATEMENT ON THE PRODUCT TO DETERMINE WHETHER VOMITING *IS OR IS NOT* TO BE INDUCED.   READ ALL OTHER INSTRUCTIONS.**

▶ **IF VOMITING IS RECOMMENDED ON THE PRODUCT LABEL OR IF THE POISON IS A MEDICATION, INDUCE VOMITING IMMEDIATELY.**

▶ **USE SYRUP OF IPECAC IF YOU HAVE IT WITH YOU.** (This should be in your first aid kit.) **READ THE INSTRUCTIONS ON THE LABEL. HAVE THE YOUNGSTER DRINK MORE WATER OR MILK AFTER TAKING THE SYRUP OF IPECAC—UNTIL HE OR SHE BEGINS TO VOMIT.**   SYRUP OF IPECAC TAKES BETWEEN FIFTEEN AND THIRTY MINUTES TO INDUCE VOMITING. IF VOMITING DOES NOT OCCUR, THEN ADMINISTER ANOTHER DOSE OF SYRUP OF IPECAC. IF VOMITING STILL DOES NOT OCCUR, INDUCE VOMITING BY TICKLING THE THROAT (EXPLAINED BELOW), SINCE *IPECAC IS ALSO A POISON* IF IT STAYS IN THE SYSTEM.

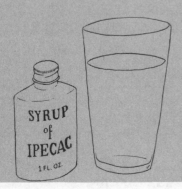

Syrup of ipecac is used to induce vomiting to remove poison from the stomach. Use it only as directed.

178

LIFE-
THREATENING
EMERGENCIES:
ONLY A
MATTER OF
MOMENTS

▶ IF YOU DO NOT HAVE SYRUP OF IPECAC, TICKLE THE BACK OF THE THROAT TO INDUCE VOMITING.   YOU CAN USE THE *HANDLE SIDE* OF A SPOON, FORK, KNIFE, OR OTHER UTENSIL (BUT DON'T USE THE OTHER SIDE OF ANY UTENSIL, SINCE THIS COULD CAUSE SERIOUS INJURY). TRY NOT TO USE YOUR FINGER UNLESS YOU HAVE NO OTHER CHOICE, SINCE YOU MAY BE SERIOUSLY BITTEN.

▶ GET THE YOUNGSTER MEDICAL HELP AS RAPIDLY AS POSSIBLE (HOPEFULLY AT THE NEAREST HOSPITAL EMERGENCY ROOM). MAKE SURE YOU TAKE THE POISON AND ITS CONTAINER WITH YOU.

You Should Not Induce Vomiting in the Following Situations

▶ IF YOU HAVE NOT YET CALLED THE POISON CONTROL CENTER, EMERGENCY ROOM, OR DOCTOR (ASSUMING THIS CHOICE IS OPEN TO YOU). IT IS IMPERATIVE THAT YOU SEEK THEIR ADVICE BEFORE YOU PROCEED IF AT ALL POSSIBLE.

▶ IF THE "CAUTION" STATEMENT ON THE CONTAINER SAYS NOT TO INDUCE VOMITING AND YOU CAN'T CALL THE POISON CONTROL CENTER. (THE SUBSTANCES INVOLVED IN SUCH CASES ARE USUALLY PETROLEUM PRODUCTS, HYDROCARBONS, CAUSTICS, ACID, OR OIL.) THESE SUBSTANCES ARE POTENTIALLY HARMFUL IF THEY ARE VOMITED WITHOUT MEDICAL SUPERVISION.

▶ IF THE YOUNGSTER IS UNCONSCIOUS OR SO SLEEPY THAT HE COULD ASPIRATE (INHALE) THE VOMITED MATTER OR CHOKE IF VOMITING WERE INDUCED.

▶ IF THE YOUNG PERSON IS ALREADY VOMITING, IS VOMITING BLOOD, OR HAS BLOODY DIARRHEA.

▶ WHEN VOMITING SHOULD NOT BE INDUCED, ALL YOU CAN DO IS HAVE THE YOUNG PERSON IMMEDIATELY DRINK AS MUCH MILK OR WATER AS POSSIBLE (IF SHE IS FULLY CONSCIOUS) AND GET HER MEDICAL ATTENTION AS QUICKLY AS YOU CAN.

- Keep watching for signs of shock, breathing trouble, or other serious symptoms.

- If the youngster stops breathing at any point, start rescue breathing. If both lung and heart function cease, initiate full CPR (rescue breathing with chest compressions). (If you are certified in CPR and are unable to remember the details of the procedure, turn to the Emergency Quick Reference on page 113, entitled "A Review of the Six Steps of CPR.")

Solvents, Poisons, and Chemicals in the Eye(s)

▶ **IMMEDIATELY FLUSH THE CHEMICAL FROM THE EYE(S).**

- If *both eyes* have been contaminated (assume they have if you find the young person rubbing his eyes), then run a steady stream of cool water through both eyes. (You can have the youngster put his head under the faucet or use a pitcher, glass, or cup.) Flush the eyes for at least ten minutes (make sure you time it by the clock, so you flush the eyes long enough).

- If *only one eye* is contaminated, care should be taken not to contaminate the unaffected eye. Again, flush the eye with a steady stream of cool water. Position the youngster's head so the affected eye is down. Aim the stream of water at the inside corner of the affected eye (next to the nose)—flushing toward the outside of the eye. This protects the unaffected eye. Make sure you flush the eye for at least ten minutes by the clock.

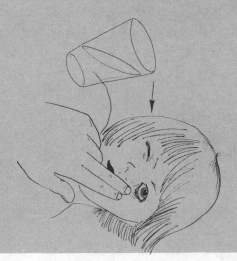

Flush the eye with water to remove a poison or chemical.

180

LIFE-
THREATENING
EMERGENCIES:
ONLY A
MATTER OF
MOMENTS

➡ **AFTER FLUSHING THE EYE(S) FOR A FULL TEN MINUTES, CALL THE POISON CONTROL CENTER OR YOUR DOCTOR FOR INSTRUCTIONS. MAKE SURE YOU TELL WHOMEVER YOU SPEAK TO WHAT THE YOUNG PERSON GOT IN HER EYE(S) AND WHAT STEPS YOU HAVE TAKEN (FLUSHED THE EYE[S] FOR TEN MINUTES).**

- Do not allow the youngster to rub or touch her eyes.

- Cover *both* eyes with a gauze wrap, scarf, strip of clean cloth, or other similar material to protect them.

➡ **IF INSTRUCTED TO DO SO, TAKE THE YOUNGSTER TO THE NEAREST EMERGENCY ROOM FOR EVALUATION AND TREATMENT.**

- Take the chemical, solvent, or poison bottle with you.

- Do not allow the youngster to rub or touch his or her eyes.

- Cover *both* eyes with a scarf, gauze wrap, strip of clean cloth, or other similar material to protect them.

Instant-Bonding Glue (Cyanoacrylate) in or near the Eye(s): A Special Case

➡ **INSTANT-BONDING ADHESIVES (THE SO-CALLED SUPER-GLUE PRODUCTS) CAN POTENTIALLY GLUE THE EYELIDS TOGETHER AND DAMAGE THE CORNEA ITSELF. UNFORTUNATELY, THEY FORM A SOLID BOND ALMOST INSTANTLY, STICKING THE TWO SURFACES THEY TOUCH FIRMLY TOGETHER.**

- Do not try to pry the stuck tissue apart, because you will only damage it.

- Do not panic, and keep the youngster calm.

➡ **TRY FLUSHING THE EYE(S) WITH WATER, BUT DON'T PRY THE LIDS APART.**

➡ **CALL YOUR OPHTHALMOLOGIST FOR AN OPINION, OR IF YOU DON'T HAVE AN OPHTHALMOLOGIST, TAKE THE YOUNGSTER TO AN EMERGENCY ROOM FOR EVALUATION AND TREATMENT.**

- Take the glue container with you.

- Cover both eyes with a cold, wet cloth or patch after you rinse with cold water.

What You Should Know About Poisoning

While having his diaper changed, Jimmy reached over, grasped an open tube of zinc oxide ointment, and sucked on it. As her mother picked out apples, Kate suddenly reached into the purse that was sitting next to her in the shopping cart, pulled out her mother's Valium bottle, and swallowed a few pills. Michael opened a kitchen cabinet and drank some drain cleaner while his daddy cooked dinner. As grandma answered the door, Michelle gulped down the glass of wine on the table. While the baby-sitter tried to soothe his upset infant sister, Eric grabbed the aspirin out of the medicine cabinet and started eating them.

These are not uncommon occurrences. It is estimated that 2 million childhood poisonings take place each year in the United States alone! In fact, poison-related incidents send approximately 600,000 children (under five years old) to hospital emergency rooms every year. The problem among teenagers (in the last few years) has dramatically increased—most often due to drug overdoses or abuse or as a means of suicide. So it's not simply a problem for the little ones.

Poison. The word itself has extraordinary power and conjures up our deepest fears. P-O-I-S-O-N—six little letters that can spell death. The fact of the matter is, we do have good reason to fear poisoning. However, if we are aware of how poisoning occurs, how best to prevent it, when to suspect it, and what to do when it does happen, then we can very often halt the disastrous effects of most poisons. By our quick and efficient actions, we can also help the young person avoid many of the lifelong disabilities or chronic conditions that can result from a serious poisoning incident.

There are a few noteworthy features of poisoning that we need to keep in mind. We are better armed to prevent a poisoning by being more aware of these special factors. It is important to realize that any one of these factors increases the likelihood that a poisoning incident will occur. If two or more of these factors are present at any one time—you can imagine how much the risk for poisoning increases.

First, children are much more vulnerable to accidental poisoning at certain ages than at other times. If your child is *between nine months and three years old* (crawler stage through curious toddler stage), then he is at the *highest risk* ever for poisoning. During this time span, the youngster is so curious that he puts *everything* directly into his mouth as a way of exploring his environment.

182

LIFE-
THREATENING
EMERGENCIES:
ONLY A
MATTER OF
MOMENTS

Intense curiosity overwhelms any common sense; it even overwhelms the normal reaction to bad taste! Most often these little ones don't stop long enough to even "taste" or "test" a substance or thing. Anything available is fair game. If a poison is involved, they simply get a mouthful and swallow *before* they realize it either tastes bad, hurts to swallow, or makes them cough, gag, or choke. With pills, they energetically and systematically shovel little handfuls into their mouths—then either chew and swallow or suck on them until they dissolve.

Older youngsters are at risk for slightly different reasons. Children *from three to six years old may imitate adult behavior* by taking "medicine" or giving it to their younger brothers or sisters. They—and older children—tend to do less tasting out of curiosity *unless* the poison is colorful, in an incorrect container, or offered by a friend. They might also be coerced into trying street drugs by older youngsters or adults. *Older children and teenagers* are usually subject to alcohol or drug overdose or abuse, sometimes accidentally, but often as a means of suicide or homicide.

The child's personality and temperament play important roles in increasing his or her risk for accidental poisoning. Children who are especially *curious, outgoing, active, inquisitive, aggressive, and seem to get into everything* tend to be involved in more accidental poisonings than less active, less curious, and more passive children. Therefore, if your child (or one of your children) has the personality and temperament that put him or her at greater risk for poisoning, you will need to be even more diligent than usual in your preventive measures and more watchful of the youngster.

It is important to know that poisonings most often occur *when things are in some sort of turmoil or when a change from the norm has taken place*. Even in the very best, most stable home environment, a set of circumstances can occur that easily sets the stage for accidental poisoning.

Think about it. How many times have you painted the house, a fence, or even furniture in the house? Things needed to be moved out of place, cans of paint or stain and solvents were sitting around, and the house or yard was understandably in a turmoil. How many times were those poisonous substances left unattended or not locked up? Did the phone ring, or did someone come to the door? Did you or another person drop everything (just for a moment) to answer the phone or door? Did you or someone else run to the bathroom (for only a second) or to the kitchen for a cup of coffee or a soda—and leave the poisonous substances with an unsupervised child loose in the house or yard? These are all easy things to do and seem quite harmless. It's easy for us to forget that poisoning can occur literally in the seconds it takes us just to turn our backs!

Ever performed the drudgery of spring cleaning? Ever decided to clean and straighten the kitchen cupboards or bathroom shelves or medicine cabinet? How about cleaning out the garage? Not only are the contents of these cupboards, shelves, and storage areas scattered everywhere, but cleaners and solvents are available, open, and in use. This spells "prime time" for a poisoning incident!

How many times have you had guests staying in your home for a few days—and it was necessary to move things around to meet their needs? Were poisonous items inadvertently left on shelves, the bathroom sink, the nightstand, or in an unlocked cupboard? Things *can* become a little confusing. Items that are normally locked up are suddenly left out, or your guests unthinkingly leave pills, toilet articles, or other poisonous substances within the reach or climbing ability of children.

What about grandpa's high blood pressure pills or other medication(s) on the night-stand or bathroom sink? Where are grandma's tranquilizers, sedatives, or iron pills? In her purse? On a shelf? Your sister's thyroid medication? Your brother's diet pills? A friend's bottle of aspirin or prescription pain pills? Where are the deodorants, aerosols, fingernail polish and remover, and all the rest? Does the guest room door lock so everything can be secured behind it? If so, that might be your answer. If not, you should openly discuss the potential hazard of these substances with your guest(s) and establish secured (locked) areas to safeguard them.

Are there medications or other poisonous items in the glove compartment of your car? How about a desk in the house or at your place of work (if you take your children there to visit from time to time)? If you are a woman, what's in your purse? Where do you leave your purse when you're at home, at someone else's house, at the market, or in the car? Where do you put visitors' purses, jackets, coats, luggage? Do you put pills in the pockets of pants, jackets, or coats? Many men and some women do. Sometimes this can't be avoided because the medication must be immediately available. Ask yourself and your doctor whether a safety cap is possible (assuming you could still get to the medication quickly). If not, take great care to make sure you are always in possession of such medications and that they are not accidentally left in pockets or on nightstands.

Consider the last time when someone (even the child) was ill. Medicine may have been given. Was it then locked up, or was it left out until it was time for it to be given again? If you or another adult or an older child was sick, did you or someone else leave medicine(s) on the nightstand, the dresser, or the bathroom or kitchen sink? This would be a perfectly reasonable, convenient, and human thing to do—unless a small child (or even an inquisitive older one) is around. With this added ingredient (the child being there), seemingly convenient and safe actions can suddenly turn to tragedy. Remember, medicine encompasses an entire range of products, from over-the-counter drugs (aspirin, cold medications, acetaminophen, cough suppressants, and so on) to prescription drugs. All medicines should have safety caps, and care should be taken to properly replace the cap every time a medication is used.

There are other considerations to keep in mind that increase the risk for poisoning. Turmoil or change in the home or in the young person's environment encompasses a whole spectrum of possibilities. The risk for a poisoning incident is greater for children whose parents are just separated, going through a divorce, or having problems—or if there is *any type of family crisis* where emotions are stirred or heightened.

Don't forget that a family crisis could involve a whole range of possibilities! Someone in the family may be in the hospital; the family may be in the process of moving to a new home; another child in the family may be having trouble at school; there may be economic problems that increase the tension at home; or mom or dad may suddenly

184

LIFE-
THREATENING
EMERGENCIES:
ONLY A
MATTER OF
MOMENTS

be working quite late and experiencing enormous stress. The scenarios are endless—but in all situations, *the people involved are usually preoccupied, under pressure, less aware, and often more absentminded.*

Consider, too, that for some very bright children, it seems perfectly reasonable to get up when they are sick and take "some more of that stuff" that makes them feel better (particularly when it's easily accessible). Since they have no concept of danger and no idea what amount is safe—they take several pills and/or mouthfuls of liquids. Why not? If a little makes them feel better, just imagine what an entire bottle or two might do!

Putting something in the wrong container can also spell disaster. Ever put wood stain in a peanut butter jar or a cola bottle or can? How about gasoline or turpentine or a strong solvent or cleaner in a plastic milk jug? If the cough medicine bottle leaks after getting it home, would you transfer the medicine to a jelly jar (or other food container) or take it back to the store for a replacement?

The point is, we sometimes think nothing of putting potentially dangerous substances in food containers—because it's convenient, cost-effective, and seems reasonable! Remember, the child knows food is "good" to eat. Therefore, anything in a food container is fair game and safe. That's very logical! Putting poisonous substances in food containers is really not a safe practice for adults either. It's easy to grab a container, forget what is in it or not read the new label you put on it, get a mouthful, and swallow *before* you know what hit you. So it's best never to keep anything but food in any food container.

In fact, *it's best never to have any poisonous product in the kitchen at all!* The kitchen is the place where good food is made and often served. The kitchen (to the child) is a special place—where mom, dad, grandpa, grandma, or others prepare yummy food that makes him or her feel satisfied and good all over. The smell of cooking, the enjoyment of eating, and even the love and warmth that come with a good meal are what the kitchen is all about. To young people, then, everything in the kitchen is good for them—or it wouldn't be there! You should also keep in mind that research has shown that the peak time for poisoning with small children is one hour before dinner.

No one who really cares about children intentionally leaves out a poisonous substance or is intentionally less attentive to the children's needs. Things happen because of circumstances. If we are aware of the particular kinds of circumstances that set the stage for poisoning incidents, then we can avoid a potentially tragic situation. When a crisis or stressful situation arises in the home, we need to remember that a child's normal reaction is to seek more attention. He doesn't think, "I'll drink this poison, and someone will pay more attention to me!" In fact, he doesn't usually know that those pills or that liquid is "poisonous." The child may simply be aware that these are "no-nos." He also realizes that there is no better way to get attention than to get into the "no-nos"!

There have been situations where a little one has been told, "Don't touch that. It will make you sick." Ironically, an older brother or sister or someone else in the family may be sick and may rightfully be getting a lot of extra attention. It's perfectly logical, then, for the child to eat or drink an available "no-no" that will make people pay special attention to her, as well. Or if another child in the family is sick and that child "gets to" take this special stuff that makes him feel better, it's perfectly normal for the other child (or children) to want some, too. If the medicine is available to youngsters, they will simply take it—a lot of it!

Here's something that might surprise you. Did you know that *once a child has experienced accidental poisoning, she has a 30-percent to 50-percent chance of being poisoned again?* To most people, this *fact* seems almost inconceivable and preposterous. But think about it for a moment. A repeat poisoning may occur simply because of the child's personality and temperament. A curious, active, aggressive, determined, and inquisitive youngster is *not* going to change her whole personality and temperament *just* because she got awfully sick or even ended up in the hospital because of a previous poisoning incident. Again, never underestimate the strength and determination of a curious child who has no sense of danger.

At times, too, the situation or circumstances that led to the first poisoning incident *have not been remedied or have only partially been remedied!* For example, the stress, emotional tension, family crisis, turmoil, or change(s) may not yet be resolved. Or if lack of adequate supervision was the problem, it may still exist—particularly if the parents or others feel that *now* the child "knows better" than to do this again (either because he or she got so sick or because of the fear of punishment).

Repeat poisonings are also seen because many parents and others *make the mistake of removing only the specific poisonous substance(s)* that caused the last poisoning event. Others *only clean out that particular unsafe cupboard or cabinet implicated* in the poisoning incident—but do not poisonproof (and childproof) the rest of the house (which includes the garage and yard) and even the car and office (if the child visits there). Why? Because they really believe that the youngster won't do it again, that he or she has learned a valuable lesson, or that they will be more careful to watch the child from now on.

In summary, we need to be aware (and teach others to be aware) of the ages when children are at high risk for accidental poisoning and be sensitive to the kinds of circumstances or situations that set the stage for a poisoning incident. Each of us needs to be keenly conscious of the real threat of poisoning, be diligent about taking all possible preventive measures, and become extraordinarily vigilant when circumstances exist that heighten the risk for a poisoning.

Poisoning: Signs and Symptoms

Any discussion of the signs and symptoms of poisoning must be approached from a rather different perspective than other illnesses. With most medical problems, we learn to watch for early signs and symptoms—then take action. When it comes to poisoning,

186

LIFE-
THREATENING
EMERGENCIES:
ONLY A
MATTER OF
MOMENTS

the hope is to discover that poisoning has occurred long *before* the young person shows any physical signs and symptoms. That may sound absurd or impossible, but when you're dealing with poisoning, you're running a race against time. In fact, time (besides the amount and type of poison itself) can be the youngster's and your greatest ally or worst enemy. The sooner you can determine probable poisoning and take action, the better the odds that the poison can be stopped. As time goes by and a discovery is not made, the scale tips more toward serious illness, death, or lifelong disabilities if the youngster survives. Therefore, it is very important to know *when* to consider poisoning as the possible culprit and to take action immediately.

Often a young person gets into a poisonous substance, ingests or inhales it or makes skin contact—but does not show the effects (signs and symptoms) of being poisoned for several minutes to several hours. The onset and severity of symptoms will be determined by: the type of poison (slow-acting or fast-acting, very deadly or moderately poisonous); the amount of poison involved (a little bit, a moderate amount, or a great deal); and the systems of the body it attacks (brain and central nervous system, heart, lungs, liver, kidneys, and so forth).

Unfortunately, there are some poisons that are so fast-acting and deadly that the best medical care in the world may not be able to stop them. These poisons represent the exceptions, though, not the rule when it comes to treating poisoning. So your detective skills and quick action *can* make a very big difference the vast majority of the time. As we discussed in previous chapters, you can make that *big difference* and help the young person by staying calm and thinking on your feet whenever a medical emergency occurs.

Much of the time it is fairly obvious that a child has been poisoned, because he or she is found with the poison in his possession. At other times, the surrounding evidence strongly points to poisoning. For example, you find an opened or spilled container of pills or some other poisonous substance. You notice that a bottle of pills or another poisonous product is missing or that the amount left in the container is suddenly and unexplainably reduced. In all cases, you must consider the possibility that the child has been poisoned.

Even if you *know for sure* that a substance was carefully locked up—*do not* assume poisoning is ruled out. In each of these situations, it is vital that the missing container (or amount) be found or an absolutely verifiable explanation for its disappearance be discovered. (For example, your husband or wife or another person knows for sure that it was used, spilled, or he or she has it.) Never just put this off, assuming there must be a logical explanation. It is always best to *find* the logical explanation immediately and *know* the youngster could not have been involved.

If you see a poisonous substance on the young person—on her face, around her mouth or on her lips, on her hands, on other areas of the body, or even on her clothing—you must assume that poisoning has occurred and take action. If you smell a poisonous substance on the youngster's breath, on his skin, or on his clothing—again, the evidence points to probable poisoning. (Poisons that smell include gasoline, turpentine, alcohol, bleaches and strong cleaners, furniture polishes, and other such substances.) In each of these situations, you can't take the risk of waiting and doing nothing unless the youngster suddenly becomes sick.

If the young person suddenly starts vomiting and/or has diarrhea—*without* other signs of a common illness (such as fever, congestion, cough, rash)—you should consider the possibility of poisoning. Be suspicious, too, if he or she has any symptoms that *do not act like a common, explainable illness*. When situations like these arise, play detective as fast as you can. Other signs and symptoms of possible poisoning usually come on suddenly and without explanation. You might recognize that the youngster is sleepy, groggy, lethargic, delirious, excitable, irritable, irrational, or shows some other changes in his or her normal behavior that are rather perplexing. If the young person suddenly experiences convulsions, shock, or collapse, and there is no apparent cause for any one of these—then you need to suspect poisoning. If you see sudden sweating, flushing, and/or pale or rashy skin for no other reason—again, suspect poisoning. If the youngster suddenly starts gagging, choking, or coughing and you have ruled out airway obstruction and aspiration—once more, consider that a poisoning could have occurred.

Whenever poisoning is a possibility, you need to act very quickly. Check all rooms of the house for the possible culprit. Look under and on beds, on tabletops, sinks, floors, in cupboards and medicine cabinets—even in locked areas. See if any plants have bite marks or tears.

Find out if there is something missing from or open in your coat, jacket, other pockets, or purse. Check everything you can think of as quickly as possible. It's very important to find the poison and attempt to determine how much is missing. Do not forget to consider where else the youngster has been in the last few hours—outside; at a friend's, relative's, or neighbor's; in the grocery store; in the garage; and so on— where he or she might have unsuspectingly gotten into a poisonous substance or poisonous plant.

The important thing to remember when it comes to poisoning is *not to wait* until you see signs and symptoms before you take action. Anytime you suspect that poisoning may have occurred (and the child is conscious), it's time to do a thorough search. Most often, the opened or spilled poisonous substance can be found if poisoning has taken place.

A Word About Drugs

Drug. Standing alone, the word means something different to each of us. To some people, a drug is a substance used only in medicine. To others, a drug is an illegal substance bought on the streets. In reality, the word stands for a whole host of chemical agents—prescription drugs; over-the-counter drugs; illegal or street drugs; and even alcoholic beverages, nicotine, and vitamins.

The fact of the matter is—a young person can experience poisoning from any kind

188

LIFE-
THREATENING
EMERGENCIES:
ONLY A
MATTER OF
MOMENTS

of drug. Alcoholic beverages can cause a serious toxic reaction in toddlers and other young children even if no more than one ounce is ingested. Alcohol can cause liver problems, low blood sugar, and even a deadly coma if the youngster drinks enough of it. But we don't think of alcohol as a drug—and certainly not as a poison. If large amounts of cigarettes or other tobacco products are eaten (which happens commonly), a child or young person can experience vomiting and diarrhea or even excitement and delirium. Again, we forget that the nicotine in cigarettes is a drug and a poison if enough is ingested.

What we need to do, then, is not only safely lock up all prescription, over-the-counter, and illegal drugs, but alcohol and cigarettes, as well. Is your liquor cabinet locked? Are cigarettes, cigars, pipe tobacco, and chewing tobacco locked up, or do these sit around in drawers, on sinks, and on coffee tables? Are there filled ashtrays lying around the house, or are the contents safely disposed of immediately so the child cannot get to them? The easiest and safest way to discard these is to wrap them in aluminum foil, then take them outside to the trash container. The aluminum foil (if carefully sealed) protects against fire, and the outside trash can prevents the child from reaching them.

To some people, a discussion on illegal drugs may not seem valid here. However, health care professionals are seeing more and more cases of poisoning by illegal drugs each year. This problem is not confined simply to the teenager who curiously tries street drugs or alcohol. Babies and toddlers are also frequent victims. As with any other poisoning incident, curiosity leads them to eat or drink these drugs, if available. And even sadder, at other times, parents or older youngsters ''feed'' the drug to them! Cocaine, LSD, PCP (angel dust), marijuana, and other drugs can kill—just as any drug can kill if too much is taken.

It is imperative that immediate medical assistance be sought (poison control center, hospital emergency room, or family doctor) if you discover that a child has ingested any drug—legal *or* illegal. The youngster's life may well be in danger, and there is no time to hesitate and no time to hedge about the type of drug consumed. In order for professionals to take every step to halt the devastating effects of a drug, they must know the type and amount of the drug taken by the youngster. Honesty in these situations saves time and may even save the child's life. Therefore, when it comes to poisoning by drugs of any kind, act quickly and be absolutely honest.

Preventing Poisoning

It's a lot easier and less stressful to prevent poisoning than to go through the often frightening and harrowing experience. No one can be expected to be everyplace all the time. Parents, grandparents, relatives, friends, and baby-sitters are fooling themselves if they honestly believe they are capable of watching every move a child makes— every second of the day. There is, however, a very reasonable and practical solution to this problem. Poisonproofing your home, garage, garden, yard, car, and even office is the best way to *prevent* accidental poisoning. We still have to be diligent about watching our children even if our homes are poisonproofed, but it makes our jobs a great deal easier. We can't stress enough the importance of going through Chapter 2 (Safety: Preventing Accidents and Injuries) in careful detail. Those Safety Checklists were developed as ammunition for your fight against your children's unnecessary death or lifelong disability. By using the checklists as guidelines and taking all possible steps to poisonproof and childproof your home, garage, yard, garden, car, and office, you are better armed to battle the epidemic of childhood poisoning and other accidents. Your weapons are sound safety precautions, common sense, and the removal and locking up of all potentially hazardous substances.

THE DON'TS

Don't hesitate to call the poison control center, hospital emergency room, or family doctor—even if you only suspect poisoning. Remember, it's far better to be sure and cautious than to lose valuable time if poisoning did occur. Keep in mind that time can be your greatest ally or your cruelest enemy.

Don't hesitate to call the poison control center if you're not sure a substance is poisonous. The poison control center is a lifesaving and valuable resource for you and for medical professionals. Its staff is always willing to answer any question regarding poisoning—particularly if you know a child just ate, inhaled, or made skin contact with something you are not sure is poisonous. The sooner you call them, the faster they can assist you.

Don't induce vomiting unless the poison control center (or emergency room personnel or family doctor) instructs you to do so. However, if the product label directs you to induce vomiting (or if the poison was a medication or drug) and you are unable to reach medical help for instructions, then induce vomiting. (Do not be confused if you are told not to induce vomiting, then when the youngster is in the care of medical professionals, they decide to induce vomiting. In such cases, causing vomiting would be safe only under careful medical supervision and with special equipment available.)

Don't induce vomiting in these specific situations:
- The youngster is unconscious or not fully alert.
- The substance swallowed was an acid, a strong alkali (such as drain cleaner, dishwasher detergent, or a cleaning product), or contains a petroleum product (such as gasoline, kerosene, or furniture polish).
- The youngster is vomiting blood or having bloody diarrhea.
- The youngster is having convulsions.

Don't try to give liquids (or medications) to a child who is very sleepy or unconscious, even if he or she was poisoned. The risk for the youngster aspirating (inhaling) the liquid is very high under these circumstances.

190

LIFE-
THREATENING
EMERGENCIES:
ONLY A
MATTER OF
MOMENTS

Don't use the material called "the universal antidote." It is not effective and may be harmful.

Don't forget that a child can be poisoned during the most unexpected times. Whether you're changing a baby's diaper, taking a three-year-old to the store with you, or sitting talking to a friend, poisoning can occur—rapidly.

Don't forget to be sensitive to those ages and circumstances that create a high-risk environment for a poisoning incident.

Don't forget to encourage others (grandparents, other relatives, friends, and neighbors) to poisonproof and childproof their homes, yards, garages, cars, and other areas.

PLEASE NOTE: Now that you have a grasp of how to recognize and manage poisoning, it would be extremely helpful for you to go back to the Emergency Quick Reference With the Steps in Detail and review it carefully. The more familiar you are with that material, the more useful it will be to you when you need it.

CHAPTER 11

Drowning

EMERGENCY QUICK REFERENCE

With the Steps in Detail

Managing Drowning

Reviving someone from a drowning or near-drowning incident often involves some or all of the steps in CPR. If you are certified in CPR and are unable to remember the details of the procedure at any time while going through this Emergency Quick Reference, turn to the Emergency Quick Reference on page 113, entitled "A Review of the Six Steps of CPR."

▶ **GET THE YOUNG PERSON OUT OF THE WATER AS QUICKLY AS POSSIBLE.**

- If you are a long way from shore and the youngster is not breathing, begin rescue breathing while in the water if you can.

- If you think the youngster may have a head, neck, or back injury, move him or her with as much care as possible while in the water and be extraordinarily careful while moving the youngster out of the water.

192

LIFE-
THREATENING
EMERGENCIES:
ONLY A
MATTER OF
MOMENTS

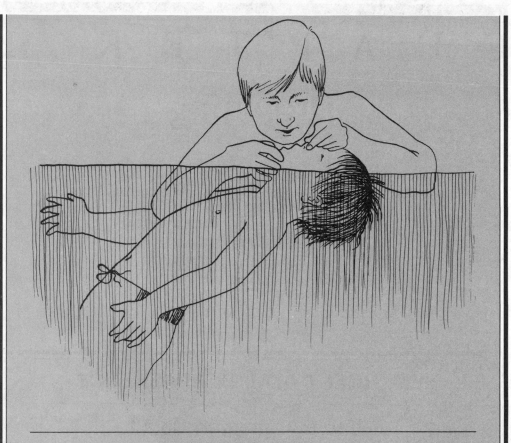

If you can, begin rescue breathing in the water when a youngster is not breathing and you are a long distance from land.

- If one or more people are with you, have them help you by lifting and moving the youngster as a unit—that is, keeping the head, neck, shoulders, back, and legs in a straight line, placing special emphasis on immobilizing the head and neck.

- If you must remove the youngster from the water yourself, do everything you can to support and immobilize the head, neck, and shoulders.

▶ **HAVE SOMEONE ELSE CALL THE PARAMEDICS WHILE YOU TREAT THE CHILD. IF NO ONE IS WITH YOU, CONTINUE TREATING THE CHILD WHILE YOU PERIODICALLY SHOUT FOR HELP. WHEN HELP ARRIVES, HAVE THAT PERSON CALL THE PARAMEDICS.**

▶ **PLACE THE YOUNGSTER ON HIS OR HER BACK ON A FLAT, SOLID SURFACE, SO YOU CAN BETTER ASSESS THE SITUATION.**

- When positioning her, please note the preceding information about moving a youngster when there is the possibility of a head, neck, or back injury.

- If the child is vomiting, turn him on one side or facedown, so the vomitus (vomited material) will drain out of his mouth. Take care in doing this if you suspect a head, neck, or back injury.

If the Youngster Is Unconscious

▶ **OPEN THE AIRWAY, AS YOU WERE TAUGHT IN CPR TRAINING.**

- Prop a towel, folded lengthwise, under the shoulders to keep the head tilted backward or use a folded towel under the base of the skull to tilt the head into the "sniffing" position.

- You may need to pull the tongue upward or lift the jaw forward by grasping the jaw and pulling it forward

▶ **CHECK TO SEE WHETHER THE YOUNGSTER IS BREATHING.**

- If the youngster is *not* breathing, begin rescue breathing.

- If the youngster *is* breathing, maintain an open airway and watch carefully for any change in breathing status.

- If at any point the youngster starts to vomit, turn her head to one side so she does not aspirate (inhale) the vomited material. Take care in doing this if you suspect a head, neck, or back injury.

▶ **CHECK TO SEE WHETHER THE YOUNG PERSON HAS A PULSE.**

- *If he or she does not have a pulse*, begin full CPR (rescue breathing with chest compressions), as you were taught in CPR training.

- Continue your rescue efforts until the paramedics or other trained help arrives and takes over performing CPR. ***Do not* give up.**

- If the youngster must be moved without professional assistance, make sure you continue your rescue efforts and CPR while en route.

- *If he or she has a pulse*, continue rescue breathing and reassess the pulse every five minutes.

194

LIFE-
THREATENING
EMERGENCIES:
ONLY A
MATTER OF
MOMENTS

▶ **IF THE YOUNGSTER STARTS BREATHING ON HIS OWN AND THE HEART BEGINS WORKING AGAIN, CONTINUE TO EVALUATE HIS STATUS, AND RENEW YOUR RESCUE EFFORTS IF BREATHING STOPS AGAIN OR BOTH LUNG AND HEART FUNCTIONS CEASE.**

If the Youngster Is Conscious

▶ **DO NOT INTERFERE WITH HIS OR HER ATTEMPTS TO COUGH AND BREATHE.**

- Try to keep the child calm and tell him to continue coughing if he feels the need. (Sometimes, people try not to cough.) Tell the youngster you are there to help and everything will be all right.

- If breathing is regular and the child is coughing, it is OK for her to rest on her abdomen if that is more comfortable.

▶ **IF THE YOUNG PERSON SEEMS FINE AFTER SEVERAL MINUTES, KEEP HIM CALM; THEN HAVE THE YOUNGSTER EVALUATED PROMPTLY BY HIS DOCTOR OR IN AN EMERGENCY ROOM.**

- If paramedics are on the scene, they will more than likely insist that the child be taken to a hospital.

- Hospitalization and observation may be recommended because of the risk of later complications from even momentary lack of oxygen or from aspirated (inhaled) water.

▶ **IF AT ANY TIME THE YOUNGSTER BECOMES UNCONSCIOUS, RE-FER TO PAGE 193 AND FOLLOW THE STEPS INDICATED UNDER THE HEADING "IF THE YOUNGSTER IS UNCONSCIOUS."**

Drowning: The Risks

When we think about drowning, we usually imagine a rough ocean, large lake, or fast-moving river—with a hopelessly fatigued youngster stranded far from the shore. This has certainly been the scenario many times. But we rarely think about the bathtub, hot tub or home spa, ornamental pond, quarry pit, well, iced-over pond or lake, wash, or riverbed—equally risky for children and teenagers.

We often forget about the danger a home swimming pool (even a small plastic one) represents. Water sports also must be added to the list: waterskiing, water polo, surfing, bodysurfing, windsurfing, sailing, diving, or even fishing. It doesn't occur to us to be concerned about the street sewage system—where a small child (or even a larger one) can be swept into the gutter and down the drain! Drainage ditches and flood-control channels are also high-risk areas for drowning—but we don't think much about them either.

The point is, drowning can occur almost anyplace at any time—even in a puddle—where there is as little as one or two inches of water. Of course, the more water involved and the more water movement, the greater the risk. But crawlers and toddlers have drowned in bathtubs, toilets, cleaning pails, buckets, planter boxes, and rain puddles. Anything that can collect a few inches of water poses a potential hazard. Those in the crawler and toddler stages are curious enough to get into, but often do not have the strength, coordination, or "know-how" to get out of a dangerous predicament. If they fall headfirst into a toilet or bucket of water (or other fluid), they simply cannot throw their weight backward to free themselves or push (or pull) themselves out. At other times they slip, fall, or hit their heads—and drowning occurs, partly because they are stunned or unconscious.

The problem with drowning is that the risk factors vary depending on the youngster's age. Children at certain ages are more prone to drown in a particular way or place. Therefore, if you have children of different ages, then you must be even more aware of the potential risks for each child (as well as sensitive to changes in risk factors for each child as he or she grows older).

For example, infants don't usually drown in the ocean or lake—they drown in the sink, bathtub, or bathing basin. Toddlers drown in the bathtub, too—often when left alone "only for a second" or when left in the care of a sibling too young to safeguard them. Toddlers also drown in home swimming pools. Those most vulnerable to accidental drowning—particularly in the bathtub or swimming pool—are youngsters under three years old. In fact, children from birth to four years of age are involved in a significant proportion—40 percent—of all swimming pool deaths.

Crawlers and toddlers are curious, intrigued by water, or sometimes even oblivious to its existence. Most drowning or near-drowning incidents do not occur when adults are playing with these children in the water or attentively supervising them around the pool. Often unattended children ride their tricycles or other wheeled toys into the pool; fall in while playing around the pool; slip and hit their heads, then fall or roll into the pool; or slide onto the shallow steps to play but slip and go under. Toddlers must also be carefully watched at lakes, ponds, and other bodies of water where it is easy to have a false sense of security because the water is calm.

Once children reach school age—although many by then know how to swim or float—they still drown in pools and lakes. They are also attracted to drainage ditches, which are especially hazardous after storms. Often parents and other adults feel the children are now old enough to take care of themselves in the water (that is, they have a false sense of security about the youngsters' ability to swim) or that they have the

196

LIFE-
THREATENING
EMERGENCIES:
ONLY A
MATTER OF
MOMENTS

common sense to stay out of dangerous situations. For those who live near or vacation at the ocean, their children are at risk for drowning there, as well.

Teenagers are natural risk-takers and tend to drown in oceans, lakes, and rivers. Teenagers have the highest death rate for drowning—even though they are only the second largest age group involved in swimming accidents, not the first. They are often involved in water sports such as surfing, sailing, waterskiing, windsurfing, water polo, diving, fishing, long-distance swimming, or even challenging rough surf or running rapids. Drowning can occur as a result of injury (usually head or neck injury, which paralyzes youngsters or knocks them unconscious) or fatigue. In swimming pools, many teenagers drown after diving into a too shallow area or after excessive hyperventilation (to allow them to swim underwater for long periods of time).

Studies have shown that, unfortunately, a great many teenage drowning victims had been drinking alcohol. One study found that 20 percent to 30 percent of teenage and adult drowning victims had significant blood–alcohol levels. Another study of teenagers who had drowned showed that 50 percent had alcohol in their blood when autopsies were performed. These findings are significant and point to the need for teenagers to be better educated about the risks for drowning when drinking. These same cautions also apply to the use of other drugs that influence the level of awareness or judgment.

Drowning and Near-Drowning: The Problem

The terms *drowning* and *near-drowning* often confuse or mislead people. Technically speaking, *drowning* means that a person was immersed in water, causing suffocation and resulting in death. To be classified as a drowning, death must take place within twenty-four hours of the immersion incident. *Near-drowning*, on the other hand, means that a person was immersed in water but survived, at least initially. If death takes place later (more than twenty-four hours after the immersion incident), then the cause of death would be classified as "near-drowning," not drowning.

The basic problem experienced in all drowning incidents is that the body (as well as the brain) is deprived of oxygen.

When water fills the lungs (which occurs in about 90 percent of drowning cases), oxygen cannot be absorbed into the lungs. Lack of oxygen causes body cells to burn fuel inefficiently, leading to acid buildup, a process that further poisons the cells. Carbon dioxide, the waste product of respiration, also builds up in the body. This built-up carbon dioxide also acts like a poison. In the other 10 percent of drowning cases, the culprit is not water in the lungs. Instead, water irritates the windpipe, and it closes off (shuts) as a defense mechanism. Unfortunately, the body's attempt to protect itself in this way also results in suffocation—because the airway is blocked.

The type of drowning—"wet" (where the lungs fill with water) or "dry" (where the windpipe closes off)—makes little difference, nor does the type of water involved (salt water or fresh water). The basic problem remains the same—lack of adequate oxygen to the body. When the body experiences lack of oxygenation, one of the first things to occur is a disturbance in heart function. The heart begins to pump less effectively, leading to shock. This lack of oxygen (called hypoxia) in turn leads to other serious problems and eventually death.

As we discussed in Chapter 9 (Unconsciousness), lack of oxygen to the brain, even for a short period of time, leads to several predictable events—no matter what caused the hypoxia. If the person survives the initial physical insult, changes in behavior and unconsciousness may be seen as a result of the hypoxia. Within minutes to hours, the damaged brain cells begin to swell. This swelling (called cerebral edema) increases intracranial pressure (that is, pressure inside the head). This increased pressure causes further problems, such as a reduction in consciousness, changes in blood pressure, and problems with the functioning of other organs. It's simply a vicious circle.

Current therapy for near-drowning victims is targeted primarily at managing and treating cerebral edema (brain swelling) while supporting breathing and heart function. Space-age technology allows for vigorous monitoring of intracranial pressure (remember, as the brain swells, the pressure inside the skull increases, causing more damage). This constant and specialized monitoring, coupled with dramatic measures to keep the pressure under control, is an attempt to allow the brain cells to recover (if they can) from the damage they sustained from lack of oxygenation. Usually, initial recovery takes three to five days but may continue for seven or more days.

Because of the resiliency of most youngsters and today's advanced technology, full recovery is now common. Even if the youngster has been unconscious and submerged for five minutes (sometimes even longer if the water is very cold), complete recovery is possible. Therefore, it is vital that rescue efforts *not* be stopped if you are performing CPR—even if the situation looks hopeless. However, the faster you get to the youngster and the sooner you initiate CPR—the better are his or her chances for full recovery.

One note of caution: When near-drowning occurs, many other problems can arise—even days later. The lungs can experience damage. Direct damage to the lining of the lungs, leading to pneumonia and fluid buildup, is common. This can be worsened if the youngster vomited and aspirated (inhaled) stomach contents. Also, the debris and bacteria in the inhaled water can pose a problem. Many youngsters who suffer immersion require vigorous respiratory treatment—mechanical respirators, antibiotics, oxygen, and treatment to drain the lungs of fluid and debris and to reduce inflammation.

Other organs of the body can be damaged by lack of oxygen and the shock that results from poor or absent blood circulation. The heart muscle can be damaged, causing ineffective pump action. Shock then follows. This shock—circulatory failure—is the factor primarily responsible for damage to other organ systems. The kidneys are especially vulnerable to temporary or permanent damage. The intestines and liver can also experience temporary or permanent damage. While many of these problems can be serious and result in lifelong disabilities, they can often be temporary and can repair themselves with excellent medical support and treatment.

It is important for everyone to understand these many possible complications and complexities of near-drowning, because it is easy to become confused and frustrated

198

LIFE-
THREATENING
EMERGENCIES:
ONLY A
MATTER OF
MOMENTS

by events after a near-drowning incident. For example, a young person may wake up shortly after an immersion incident and appear fine. He or she may then deteriorate several hours later. This so-called secondary drowning is the manifestation of the tissue damage and brain swelling that resulted because of the initial lack of oxygen. Brain swelling and lung complications are the most common "later" manifestations of near-drowning and must be vigorously treated.

Because of this frequently experienced delay in the onset of problems, it is imperative that *all* youngsters who have experienced even a short and seemingly uneventful near-drowning episode (where breathing stopped or may have stopped even momentarily) be evaluated medically. The risk for these complications makes a short (twenty-four- to seventy-two-hour) hospital stay a good idea for almost all near-drowning victims. This period of close observation may make a major difference in the long-term results.

One further note: Parents and others should remember that they will not really know how well a youngster will do until at least a three- to ten-day period has passed. All too often we read in the newspapers or hear on the television or radio that a miracle has taken place—a young person was revived after his lung and heart functions had ceased for some time. (In other words, the youngster was clinically dead when rescuers reached him.) These situations sometimes receive headline coverage but may be misleading. Everyone is then shocked when the youngster dies two or three days later, or even months later, after being in a coma all that time. The reverse is also possible. The youngster may look hopelessly damaged but, with vigorous treatment, may improve days later and ultimately recover. Some young near-drowning victims end up with mild to severe brain damage and other chronic problems that require intensive, long-term rehabilitation.

The point is, near-drowning is a complex problem whose end results cannot be second-guessed. The process of treatment often has many ups and downs—things look good, then look bad, then look good again. But one thing is certain: the sooner someone can get to the young person and begin CPR—the greater the odds that the youngster will experience a full recovery.

How Prevalent Are Drowning and Near-Drowning?

Most people do not realize how prevalent drowning is, and few recognize that the number of "near-drowning" incidents is virtually incalculable. Statistics are rather sketchy because there are flaws in the reporting system. For example, a death certificate in some states may read "respiratory and cardiac failure" or "hypoxic encephalopathy" (brain damage due to oxygen lack) rather than "death due to near-drowning." This makes it difficult to establish the actual number of people who drown each year in the United States.

We do know that in 1980 seven thousand drowning deaths were reported, which made it the third leading cause of death from accidental injury. For those between five and forty-four years old, drowning was the second leading cause of death from accidental injury—taking a backseat only to death from motor vehicle accidents. It is also a fact that for youngsters between the ages of five and fourteen, drowning is the second leading cause of accidental death. Furthermore, falls on board and falls overboard from boats were the cause of 20 percent to 30 percent of water-related deaths. And many of these occurred when people were involved in a passive activity, such as fishing.

The incidence of near-drowning is even more difficult to calculate than the incidence of drowning. But think about it for a moment. Chances are, you or someone you know has been in a very touchy situation (at least once) where drowning could easily have occurred. How many times has a youngster fallen into a pool, slipped in the bathtub, or been knocked over by a wave—thankfully to be grabbed so quickly that no harm took place? At other times, the determined efforts of those trained in both water rescue and CPR made the crucial difference. Their quick, skilled action converted a certain tragedy into a rather uneventful dunking or a serious but treatable near-drowning incident.

Injuries also play a significant role in water deaths or lifelong disabilities. It is estimated that approximately 140,000 injuries that are directly related to swimming activities take place each year in the United States alone. The Centers for Disease Control estimate that 700 spinal cord injuries occur each year, and the majority of these are serious enough to result in permanent paralysis. One study pointed out that diving, waterskiing, and surfing accounted for 77 percent of all reported spinal cord injuries. In fact, the number of spinal cord injuries due to diving alone far exceeds those experienced in all other sports combined. We also know that approximately 1,100 people required emergency room treatment in 1980 because of injuries sustained in hot tubs and home spas.

Ninety-five percent of all reported drownings or near-drownings in children take place when they are not watched carefully. This includes incidents in bathtubs, as well as in swimming pools, at beaches, and at swimming holes, where supervision is inadequate and/or there are many children in the water who cannot swim or swim very poorly. Fifty percent of all residential swimming pool deaths take place in neighbors' pools.

What You Can Do to Prevent Drowning

A fact: Most accidental drowning can be prevented—if safety measures are diligently enforced and proper adult supervision is guaranteed. It is certain that neither you nor any other adult can control every move your children (particularly teenagers) make, but you can provide a safe environment, teach water safety, and ensure excellent supervision during water activities.

200

LIFE-
THREATENING
EMERGENCIES:
ONLY A
MATTER OF
MOMENTS

BATHTUBS, SINKS, AND BABY BATH BASINS

Proper and constant supervision is the key to preventing drowning in bathtubs, sinks, and baby bath basins. The usual scenario goes something like this: mother, father, grandmother, grandfather, another relative, a friend, or a baby-sitter is giving the infant crawler, toddler, or preschooler a bath. Something takes the adult's attention away from the child for a few seconds or minutes (like the phone, a doorbell, something boiling over on the stove, or another child requiring assistance). While the adult is gone, the youngster slips under the water or hits his head on the tub or faucet and submerges. This occurs in seconds—and unless someone is right there to intervene, drowning results. Therefore, it is imperative that a child never be left—even for a second—in a bathtub or sink. Let the phone ring, or pick up the youngster and take him with you.

There have also been cases where an older sibling was left with a younger brother or sister, either to give the bath or to watch the child for a moment. Young people asked to help or supervise should be mature enough for this responsibility, strong enough to handle the child and avert a possible tragic situation, and old enough to understand the seriousness of maintaining undivided and constant attention on the child. Often in drowning situations, a four-, five-, or six-year-old has been left in charge of a one- or two-year-old. *All are children* and hence incapable of being responsible for the life and safety of another.

In keeping with recent reports of toddlers' drowning in toilets, buckets, and other unlikely spots, take particular care with these kinds of containers. Keep the toilet lid down in all bathrooms. Teach toddlers not to play in the toilet or lift the lid, and turn buckets and other containers upside down when not in use. Do not leave pails of water where curious toddlers could fall in while you are cleaning. And finally, start to empty the bathtub or sink even before you remove the youngster from it. In this way, you are assured that the drain has been opened. It eliminates the risk of youngsters' getting into a tub or sink that was unknowingly left full of water.

SWIMMING POOLS

Swimming pool deaths are so prevalent because many pools are not fenced properly, and supervision is often inadequate. Many people assume that a swimming pool is safely fenced if there is a fence around the three exposed sides of the pool, with a side of the house acting as the fourth side. If there are *no openings* in the house wall, this may be adequate, but all too often there are sliding doors, pet doors, or windows for access. Crawlers and toddlers in particular can slip by unsuspecting adults and fall into the pool—most often while playing. They "escape" through these openings, and the next thing you know, they are in the water.

Making a swimming pool (whether in the ground or above ground) safe requires a fence around all four sides; a gate that is self-closing and has a self-latching mechanism far beyond the reach or climbing ability of small children; and a lock that ensures that no one can enter without your being aware. Make the fence *at least* five feet tall (higher is probably better) and from material that cannot be climbed. Be sure horizontal fence pieces are on the pool side of the fence, so youngsters cannot use them as ladders for climbing in.

Consider using a sturdy, properly secured pool cover. However, be aware that a cover can also entrap a child beneath it—making it a hazard. A high-quality pool alarm to alert you if someone (or something) has entered the pool is also very helpful.

Every pool should be equipped with usable and sturdy safety equipment, such as life preservers, a long pole, and a float attached to a rope. Lifesaving procedures (CPR, how to pull someone out, and so on) should be posted next to the pool and easily visible.

Children who cannot swim should always be required to wear life jackets (properly secured) when around the pool. Do *not* use toy rings or flotation devices as safety equipment, because they are not safety equipment. Be sure that children are taught to swim early (by people who are qualified to teach swimming and water safety to youngsters). Classes are available for infants as young as six months. These classes teach floating and such, which may help an infant somewhat if he or she falls into a pool. All youngsters should be taught to float on their backs if they fall into water or get tired while swimming. Practice this technique as a drill or game, so they can and will float on command or if they accidentally fall in. (However, having provided this training should never lead to your having a false sense of security that the baby or child is now "poolsafe" or "watersafe"—because young children can't be counted on to *use* these skills if they get into trouble. It just means that they may have a little more time to spare in which you can reach and rescue them.)

Every single person who has a swimming pool should be certified in CPR. Classes are available for anyone age eleven years and older. Water safety classes that teach rescue techniques are also a must for those who have pools or who spend any time at all around water (for recreation or on vacations). The few hours it takes to complete these courses may make the difference between life and death for a family member or even a stranger.

To protect the life and well-being of your own children and other youngsters, there should always be an adult (who swims well, knows rescue techniques, and is certified in CPR) supervising all pool activities. Provide proper supervision at public pools even if a lifeguard is on duty. If you have teenagers who are excellent swimmers, then obviously it would be difficult to insist that an adult be by the pool whenever they use it. However, you can and should insist that no one swim alone, regardless of the time of day. With young children, who move quickly, be sure that there is a *particular person* who is assigned to watch each youngster. Many toddlers drown when adults are in the vicinity because each person thought someone else was watching.

A word about small wading pools and fish ponds. Be sure that any permanent wading pool is covered by a standard pool cover that cannot be removed or lifted by a child (so he or she cannot crawl under it and into the water), or drain it after each use.

202

LIFE-
THREATENING
EMERGENCIES:
ONLY A
MATTER OF
MOMENTS

Inflatable pools should be emptied and deflated after youngsters are finished using them. Fence fish ponds and waterfall areas to prevent youngsters from getting in or falling in. And, again, be sure that you don't expect children under the age of ten or so to supervise their younger siblings—they too easily get distracted and forget to watch those in their charge. They most often do not have the capacity to rescue a youngster in trouble either. The older and more mature the person is who is supervising, the safer the environment is for your children.

HOT TUBS AND SPAS

When it comes to hot tubs and spas, there is an obvious drowning risk to small children—since for them, any amount of water is a potential hazard. Beyond this, there is a further concern about the severe heat of the water and its effects on very small youngsters, who are unable to maintain a steady body temperature.

Do not allow young children in a spa without constant adult supervision, and do not allow infants, toddlers, or young children in at all if the temperature is above 104 degrees. Be sure the spa has a sturdy cover that cannot be lifted by children—again, to prevent them from crawling under the cover and into the water.

There is yet another risk of which few people are aware. The suction created at the bottom by the jets can pull a child underwater and hold him or her there. There are reports of children's long hair being caught in the bottom outlet—dragging them underwater. Children have also been found at the bottom held down by suction of the drain against their abdomens. In addition, the risk of drowning is greater in warm water than in cold—at high temperature, there is less "protection" of the brain and other body tissues from lack of oxygen. Also, it appears that certain bacteria that are commonly found in hot tubs cause severe pneumonia in young near-drowning victims rescued from these tubs.

If you have teenagers, you should be aware that there is a direct correlation between drowning in spas (and all other bodies of water) and the use of alcohol. But especially when hot water and alcohol mix—tragedy often results. Therefore, you should be careful to explain this very *real* risk to your teenagers and make it clear that drinking alcohol is not allowed when they intend to use the spa (or the pool).

OCEANS, RIVERS, AND LAKES

Teenagers are at greatest risk for drowning in oceans, rivers, and lakes—in fact, all large bodies of water. This is true in part because of their great involvement in water sports and also because, as noted earlier, they are particularly daring and prone to taking risks. It is difficult for parents to control their teenagers' actions. However, early safety training can pay off here, as can insistence that youngsters learn how to swim, know water safety principles, and be trained in how to perform CPR. All young people who swim in oceans, rivers, and lakes should also know how to handle heavy surf, riptides, currents, rough rapids, and other such hazards.

Junior lifeguard programs and the like are particularly valuable—for training in safety and responsibility, as well as for socialization. These rigorous programs combine fun with teaching water safety skills and activities. And the young people who have completed such programs tend to have a sense of accomplishment, self-respect, and confidence in what they know. Because of this, they are likely to be cautious themselves and to warn their friends to have respect for water. They do not need to be daring in order to prove themselves—to themselves or to others—and they do not tend to buckle under to peer pressure and take unnecessary risks when it comes to water. Most often they feel they are skilled and knowledgeable and have already "proved" themselves in rigorous and prestigious training programs.

With younger children, parents and others must exercise extreme caution about watching them carefully. It's easy to forget that a riptide can pull a youngster out into the ocean from an area that is only ankle or knee deep. Don't forget, too, that youngsters can be swept out into the rapids or into the rushing water of a drainage ditch or flood-control channel so quickly that adults may not be able to reach them fast enough. And don't feel overly secure when a lifeguard is present at a pool, river, lake, or beach. Lifeguards have important skills but a hard job, watching so many people at once. Your attention to your own child may save his or her life.

It is always best to go into the water with young children, even if they are playing only in ankle-deep water. Make the very young ones wear life jackets (which should be *safety equipment*, not toys) if they cannot swim. These will give you a certain advantage in terms of time if a youngster does get away from you. Floats, in general, are not safe because youngsters have a tendency to slip out of them.

BOATING, WATER SPORTS, AND FISHING

All children, no matter how well they swim, should be required to wear a life jacket whenever they are on any boat. (This is also imperative for teens and adults, especially when weather is even a little threatening.) Flotation seats should be available on every boat, and all those aboard should be required to sit on seats, not move around or sit on the bow or elsewhere. Drinking alcohol should be restricted, since it is constantly implicated in boating accidents.

Safety rules for any water sport should be strictly enforced. Life jackets are a must for all waterskiers, and surfers should never surf alone. They must be on the lookout for heavy surf warnings and dangerous riptides. Be aware of approaching weather conditions whenever you will be on the water, and heed any warnings.

The bottom line in preventing drowning is close supervision, abiding by safety rules, and being skilled in rescue techniques and CPR. If these steps were followed, the vast majority of drownings could be prevented.

204

LIFE-
THREATENING
EMERGENCIES:
ONLY A
MATTER OF
MOMENTS

THE DON'TS

Don't forget to take a CPR certification course, as well as water safety and rescue training. Everyone in the family should have formal training in all these areas by the teenage years.

Don't forget to have each of your children given formal swimming lessons. Children can be taught to float and swim at very young ages. Classes are available at public pools and private swimming centers.

Don't ever leave a child unattended in or near a bathtub, pool, sink, or any body of water. Remember, virtually all drownings of young children could be prevented if proper and constant supervision were available and if other safety measures were followed.

Don't ever give up on a drowning victim. Continue your rescue efforts until the paramedics or other medical personnel take over.

Don't forget to educate your teenagers about the dangers of combining alcohol and water activities.

Don't allow anyone to swim without another qualified swimmer in attendance. Be sure that person knows rescue techniques and CPR.

Don't leave young children in charge of younger brothers or sisters—whether in a bathtub or swimming pool or at the beach. Too many times this situation results in tragedy.

Don't fail to fence your pool properly and safely. This step alone can mean the difference between life and death for a youngster.

PLEASE NOTE: Now that you have a grasp of how to recognize and manage drowning, it would be extremely helpful for you to go back to the Emergency Quick Reference With the Steps in Detail and review it carefully. The more familiar you are with that material, the more useful it will be to you when you need it.

Illness in Infants, Children, and Adolescents

Question: What do you think is the one overriding concern of parents (and others) about their children's health? If you gathered together a stadium full of parents, grandparents, and baby-sitters, then asked them, "What worries you the most and makes you most insecure?" what do you think the vast majority would say? The fear expressed most often (to doctors and other health-care professionals) is this: "How will I know if my child is really sick and needs immediate attention? What if I make a mistake?"

Don't let anyone fool you. Every parent—*every parent*—worries about this. Even doctors and other health-care professionals have the same concern when it comes to their own children. Why? Because it's very difficult to be objective when it's *your* child who is hurting. And it's important to remember that it's just as easy to *underreact* as to *overreact*—whether you're involved in health care in some capacity or not. It's a universal concern and a very real one. No matter if you already have five children or if this one is your first—it's the same scary feeling, and it will plague you at some time.

What can make the difference, however, is knowledge. The more you know, the better equipped you are to make sound judgments. In fact, by learning all you can about how to recognize symptoms that point to a potentially serious problem and distinguish them from symptoms that are less worrisome—the more self-confidence you will have.

Trusting one's judgment is not built on faith—it's built on facts. Knowing the facts and looking at the situation as objectively as possible are the keys to evaluating illness and injury.

Parents and others who panic at every sign of a possible illness and call their doctor **205**

206

ILLNESS IN
INFANTS,
CHILDREN,
AND
ADOLESCENTS

constantly for reassurance are *not* trying to be difficult. To them, the symptoms they see are frightening because they simply aren't sure what the symptoms mean. Rather than risk their child's health or well-being, they call for advice or make an appointment. One mother put it this way: "I'm just afraid I'll make a mistake. And if I do make a mistake, it's not like buying the wrong-sized dress on sale and not being able to take it back. I'm talking about my child's life, and I can't afford to make a serious mistake. That would be a lot of sorrow, guilt, and 'what ifs' to have to live with."

Throughout childhood and adolescence, youngsters experience countless minor illnesses, and some may even face a serious or potentially serious problem, as well. That adds up to a great deal of decision making for parents, grandparents, relatives, friends, and even baby-sitters. Section 3 (Chapters 12, 13, and 14) will better equip you to make informed judgments about the significance (or relative lack of significance) of symptoms and illnesses. Some of the most common minor illnesses and more serious ones are covered.

Most important, you will have the information you need to recognize a symptom (or set of symptoms) that points to the need for immediate medical evaluation and treatment. You will also know what steps you can take to treat common, minor illnesses and know when a common problem has advanced to the point where medical intervention is necessary or desirable.

Chapter 12 is, in essence, a pivotal chapter in this book—because it teaches you how to better recognize and assess potentially serious illness by recognizing and assessing symptoms only. By reviewing the information in Chapter 12 a few times and using it as a resource when a youngster is ill, you will be able to recognize those signs and symptoms that point to potentially serious illness or to mild or moderate illness. By understanding the information in this chapter, you will be able to optimally use the Emergency Quick Reference guides in Chapter 12, as well as those in Chapter 1 (How and When to Get Help).

Still, whenever in doubt, call your doctor for advice. That's part of trusting your own judgment, too. If you're not sure about the significance of a problem—then your judgment is to call the doctor. In this case, that's a very reasonable and responsible decision!

Recognizing and Assessing Serious or Potentially Serious Illness

The following ten assessment areas are keys to determining whether a young person has a serious or potentially serious illness, or a moderate to mild problem. Essentially, a doctor assesses a youngster in a similar manner—by asking questions (called the present medical history) and by looking at the child (performing a physical examination).

The ten assessment areas are listed at the front of the chapter (with corresponding page numbers), so they will be readily accessible to you, if you need them.

208

ILLNESS IN
INFANTS,
CHILDREN,
AND
ADOLESCENTS

The Problem

Caitlin's mother and father were perplexed and worried. For the last eight days, their twelve-month-old daughter had been experiencing diarrhea. She was irritable and crying a lot, waking up every two hours at night. She wasn't eating as usual and simply "wasn't herself." They had changed her diet five days earlier—removing all milk products, fruit juices, and fruit. The only exception was bananas, which help control diarrhea, as well as rice cereal and soy milk. After five days of a changed diet, Caitlin's diarrhea seemed to be worsening—not getting better.

The point is, Caitlin's parents had no idea what illness their daughter had or might have. All they had to go on was the set of symptoms Caitlin was exhibiting. Was this a serious problem? Did they need to call the paramedics or an ambulance? No, they knew her symptoms didn't warrant that response. Then, should they take their daughter to the emergency room, call her doctor immediately, wait a few more hours to see how she was doing and then call the doctor, or wait until the doctor's regular office hours tomorrow and call for an appointment? Or should they continue to treat Caitlin's symptoms at home (and if so, for how long)?

Each of us has faced this same dilemma countless times. Think about it. Have there been times when you just knew your child had a cold, the flu, or croup and other times

209

RECOGNIZING
AND ASSESSING
SERIOUS OR
POTENTIALLY
SERIOUS
ILLNESS

when you suspected strep throat or an ear infection, for example, and found out you were right? But think, too, about the times you were able to recognize the symptoms your child was experiencing (or one symptom standing alone) but had no idea what illness the symptoms pointed to. And even more significant—with only symptoms to guide you, were you able to assess the child and determine the seriousness or lack of seriousness of the problem and what action to take?

The fact is, probably in eight out of every ten illnesses a youngster experiences, you will not know what illness is causing the symptoms and must be able to take action based on your ability to both recognize and assess the symptoms the child exhibits.

Symptoms, in reality, are excellent measuring sticks for determining if an illness is serious or potentially serious, or is a moderate or mild problem. In most situations, it is the *set of symptoms, as well as the intensity and longevity of those symptoms*, that is the keys to determining the seriousness of the problem and thereby the action(s) to take. Now and then, however, one symptom standing alone is significant enough to require an immediate response. Therefore, your ability to recognize and assess symptoms is vital.

The Formula

In order to effectively assess symptoms, you need to know what you're looking for. In this chapter, we do *not* discuss the treatment and/or management of problems— *but* rather how to recognize and assess symptoms only. Chapters 13 and 14 describe how to treat and/or manage serious and minor symptoms and illnesses. However, even though this chapter does not discuss the details of how to treat and/or manage problems, the Emergency Quick Reference guide found at the start of each assessment category will help you to determine when you should get help for the youngster—by, for example, calling the paramedics, calling the doctor immediately (or taking the child to an emergency room), calling the doctor within an hour or two, or calling the doctor for an appointment (as one or more of these apply to each assessment category).

At the start of this chapter, you will find an overview discussion about symptoms— the body's special communications system. This short discussion is followed by the ten areas of assessment. Each assessment category begins with an Emergency Quick Reference guide, followed by what we have called an Assessment Checklist for that specific area of assessment. An in-depth discussion of that assessment area follows each checklist, and is broken down by age group—*infants and toddlers, young children*, and *older children and teenagers*.

You've probably noticed immediately that the Assessment Checklists are new items that haven't appeared in previous chapters—items, in fact, that are found only in this chapter. Why have we included *two types of tools*—Emergency Quick Reference guides

210

ILLNESS IN
INFANTS,
CHILDREN,
AND
ADOLESCENTS

and Assessment Checklists—to help you better evaluate symptoms? Simply, they serve different yet complementary functions.

By now, you are quite familiar with the Emergency Quick Reference guides—how they work and how best to use them. There is only one difference between the Emergency Quick Reference guides in this chapter and those you've already encountered and will find after this chapter. *In other chapters you have known what the problem is* (for example, serious bleeding, shock, cardiopulmonary arrest, unconsciousness, poisoning, and drowning). In all chapters that follow this one (excluding Chapter 15, "Assessing Injury"), the Emergency Quick Reference guides refer to a specific illness, problem, or injury (such as croup, pneumonia, fracture, shin splints, abdominal injury, and so on).

In this chapter, the Emergency Quick Reference guides deal with symptoms only (for example, fever, breathing difficulty, dehydration, neck stiffness, pain, general behavior, and so on). These Emergency Quick Reference guides will assist you in your decision making, based on the symptoms the child has, as well as their intensity and duration.

The Assessment Checklist found in each assessment category is designed to help you better evaluate your child when he or she is ill and you have no idea what illness or disease the youngster has. At times, you will have only the youngster's symptoms to guide you. In this situation, the ten Assessment Checklists may be very helpful to you.

The best way to use an Assessment Checklist is to go through it with the youngster right in front of you. You can then look at the youngster, ask him questions (if he can talk), and evaluate him in a step-by-step manner as you go down the checklist. Each checklist helps you assess a different, major symptom area—for the presence, as well as the severity and duration, of symptoms.

Keep in mind that you may be able to understand symptoms and what they mean so well that you may not need to use the Assessment Checklists after reviewing them and the information in this chapter the first time. However, there may be times when one or more of the Assessment Checklists will be invaluable to you.

The information from one or more of the Assessment Checklists can also help you if you need to talk to your child's doctor—since you will be able to tell the doctor in an organized fashion exactly what symptoms the youngster has (including their intensity and duration) and what symptoms she doesn't have.

As noted previously, *Should I Call the Doctor?* was designed with many backup systems. The ten Emergency Quick Reference guides and the ten Assessment Checklists in this chapter were developed as part of this backup system. The following, then, is a rundown—or formula—developed to help you better recognize and assess symptoms in a step-by-step manner, as well as identify a symptom that, even when it stands alone, signals the need for medical evaluation. With this information, you will better understand the symptoms in each assessment area that point to serious or potentially serious illness, in contrast to those that signal moderate to mild illness. A grasp of

211

RECOGNIZING
AND ASSESSING
SERIOUS OR
POTENTIALLY
SERIOUS
ILLNESS

this information will enable you to respond more quickly and confidently when necessary.

Therefore, if your child becomes ill and you have no idea what is wrong and/or what action to take—you can use this assessment chapter to help you. How you use the information should depend on your own personal preference and what works best for you. The following are a few ideas you might consider.

- You may want to go directly to the *Emergency Quick Reference guide for a specific assessment area*—based on the most obvious or severe symptom the youngster is exhibiting. For example, if she is having breathing difficulty, you would turn to the Emergency Quick Reference guide for Breathing Difficulty and Breathing Pattern and review it. (Or, you may choose to use the Emergency Quick Reference guides in Chapter 1.)

- You may want to go directly to the *Assessment Checklist for a specific assessment area*—based on the most obvious or severe symptom the youngster is exhibiting. For example, if he is experiencing pain, then you would turn to the Assessment Checklist for Assessing the Presence and Degree of Pain and complete the checklist. Once you have completed the checklist, you would turn to the Emergency Quick Reference guide for that assessment area.

- *You may want to evaluate the youngster overall*. Using the list of the ten assessment areas at the start of the chapter, you would first go quickly down the list to rule out those symptoms you know the youngster doesn't have and note those you should review closely. For example, the child may not be having any breathing difficulty; the soft spot may not apply; you have checked for neck stiffness, and there is none; and so on. After quickly moving down the list, you decide to review one or several Assessment Checklists that you think might apply (for example, Presence and Degree of Dehydration, Appetite and Feeding Behavior, Level and Length of Fever, and Presence and Degree of Pain). After completing those checklists, you would then turn to the Emergency Quick Reference guides for each of the assessment areas completed. Or you may wish to go directly to the Emergency Quick Reference guides for those areas identified if you feel you are quite aware of the intensity and duration of the symptoms the child is experiencing. (Again, you may also use the broad-based Emergency Quick Reference guides in Chapter 1 instead.)

In other words, you can use the Emergency Quick Reference guides and Assessment Checklists for each assessment area in the manner in which you would feel most comfortable. By reading the entire chapter, then reviewing the Emergency Quick Reference guides and Assessment Checklists, you will not only have an excellent grasp of how to recognize and assess symptoms—but will also feel comfortable and confident in using the Emergency Quick Reference guides and/or Assessment Checklists in the

212

ILLNESS IN
INFANTS,
CHILDREN,
AND
ADOLESCENTS

way most helpful to you. You will feel more confident in using the broad-based Emergency Quick Reference guides in Chapter 1, as well.

Again, the information found in this chapter *should be used as a guideline only*. If you are not quite sure of the significance of the symptoms you see, always call the doctor for advice. Also, *if your child has a chronic illness or disability*, it is vital that you talk to the child's doctor about the specific symptoms that would signal a serious or potentially serious problem for your child, and what action you should take if the youngster ever experiences these symptoms.

Symptoms: The Body's Way of Communicating

Do you understand this sentence: ··· ···· --- ··- ·-·· -·· ·· -·-· ·- ·-·· ·-·· - ··· · -·· --- -·· - --- ··-·? Of course not, unless you were trained in Morse code! Can you imagine how frustrating and difficult it would be to have someone communicate with you by tapping out Morse code—if you didn't know how to translate the series of dots and dashes into letters, words, and sentences? (It means, by the way, "Should I Call the Doctor?")

For example, if you had asked for a weather report, you would not know if the person was trying to warn you that a tornado was looming, that a short but not dangerous storm was about to break, or simply that a little light rain was on its way. You would feel confident, however, if you knew how to receive and interpret the information transmitted. With this knowledge, you could take appropriate action (as necessary) whenever weather information was communicated to you.

In reality, there is very little difference between Morse code and the information our body sends us through physical symptoms. Both are special means of communication, and both require translation. Essentially, then, symptoms are actually our body's way of telling us something—its way of talking to us. Our body sends us signals, and we must then know how to interpret them.

To take this one step further, an expert in Morse code could send and receive information at the same speed he or she could have exactly the same verbal conversation with someone. A doctor (an expert at interpreting the body's communications) is able to translate a specific set of symptoms (special communications) into a diagnosis (what is wrong) or at least obtain enough information to point him or her in the right direction. From here, special tests can either verify or rule out the various possibilities.

However, you do not have to be an "expert" at Morse code for it to be useful and helpful to you—just as you need not be an "expert" at interpreting symptoms for the information to be invaluable to you. Just as you can learn Morse code, you can learn a great deal about the body's communications system. By knowing about illness and having a better understanding of symptoms, you can recognize a symptom or set of symptoms that warn you of a potentially serious problem (a tornado looming); a problem that requires medical evaluation and possible treatment (a short but not dangerous storm); or an illness easily treated and managed at home (a little light rain on its way).

Infants and Not-Yet Talking Toddlers

It's a terribly helpless feeling. Your infant or not-yet-talking toddler appears to be sick. How in the world can you be expected to know what's wrong or how minor or serious the problem might be—when the child can't even tell you what's bothering her? It's very painful and frustrating to hear a child cry or whimper—or watch him crawl into your arms and hold on tight or just lie there looking at you. It's a universal sentiment expressed by all parents (and other care-givers): "If only the youngster could tell me where it hurts or what's the matter!"

What you can do, however, is become keenly aware of the *overt symptoms* your child is exhibiting—in other words, how he or she is acting. The nonverbal child "tells" you what's the matter through his or her actions. Translated: Actions are essentially symptoms. This is where a doctor starts questioning parents—asking them *how* the child is acting.

In young infants and toddlers, however, it is easy to misinterpret the signals the little one gives. Misinterpretation of symptoms occurs because we very often base our opinions on incorrect assumptions or because we don't look at all the possibilities. It is important that we look at *what* the youngster is specifically doing and describe exactly that—before trying to interpret it. For example, it's easy to assume that an infant who is not eating or is refusing to drink liquids has a stomachache or an upset stomach. But this same symptom (not eating or drinking) can mean such things as sore mouth, sore throat, lack of appetite, or even more serious, that the little one is too weak to suck at the breast or bottle. By keeping an open mind and by being more keenly aware, we can more successfully decide what is likely going on—or equally important, what is *not* going on.

The Verbal Child

The problem with the young verbal child is that he is still *too young* and *inexperienced* (with illness) to distinguish between major symptoms and minor ones. Therefore, you still have to be keenly aware of how the child acts, as well as what he says. For example, a four-year-old may complain about a stomachache, but when he's seen by the doctor, you find out he has a throat infection. Why didn't he complain of a sore throat? Perhaps because it didn't bother him as much as his stomach did, or maybe because he didn't know exactly how to tell you his throat hurt so you'd understand.

214

ILLNESS IN
INFANTS,
CHILDREN,
AND
ADOLESCENTS

And even with an older child, it's possible for us to misinterpret what the youngster says—because of our own experience and expectations.

As a child grows older (into early school years), she acquires more experience with illness and can communicate her feelings better. In fact, she is now more able to help in the reasoning process. Therefore, she will be better equipped to describe her symptoms and let you know which are the major symptoms and which are the more minor ones. For example, a young child might complain that her joints and muscles ache (often associated with a fever) and may not mention the sore throat that caused the fever. In contrast, an older child may tell you, "I have a terrible sore throat, my head hurts, and I feel really hot" (the major symptoms). "The hotter I get, the worse my arms and legs ache" (the minor symptom).

The Teenager

When a youngster reaches the teenage years—depending on what he was taught, his maturity and awareness, as well as his past experiences with illness—he will probably *tell* you what he thinks is wrong with him. Most often, you will hear things like: "I think I have the flu"; "I have a really bad sore throat. Do you think I have strep throat, Mom?"; or, "I don't think this is a pulled muscle in my side, Dad. Do you suppose it could be appendicitis?"

When the teenager isn't quite sure what might be wrong, she can usually describe her symptoms in detail and tell you how often they occur and how severe they are. She may even ask to see the doctor—or may at other times seem very reluctant to go to the doctor or call for advice. These young people need you to be understanding about their reluctance. *But* you will also need to either coax the teenager to see the doctor or step in to make sure she is seen by a physician if the problem warrants evaluation.

Misinterpreting Symptoms

A mother called one day because she was very concerned about her year-old son. Teddy had a runny nose, wasn't eating well, was quite irritable, and had been running a fever of 102 degrees for twenty-four hours. Her husband gave Teddy children's Tylenol four hours earlier, but it had not reduced the fever, she said. A fever that cannot be reduced *is* a signal for concern. However, after further questioning, it became clear that the parents had not given the correct dose of Tylenol—based on Teddy's weight. The mother was told to give Teddy the correct dose at proper intervals and to call back if the temperature did not return to normal after another two days or call sooner if other serious symptoms appeared. From all indications, Teddy had a cold.

215

RECOGNIZING
AND ASSESSING
SERIOUS OR
POTENTIALLY
SERIOUS
ILLNESS

The mother did call back—the next morning. She said the correct dose had lowered the fever within a few hours and that the youngster was fine. They had continued to give the medication at the intervals recommended, and Teddy's temperature had been normal most of the night and this morning. He, of course, still had a runny nose and other symptoms of a cold—which take time to resolve.

A concerned father called one day because his three-year-old had "severe diarrhea," wasn't eating much, and was quite cranky. He and his wife feared little Carolyn had some terrible disease. After further questioning, it became obvious that the parents did not really know what severe diarrhea was. Why should they? No one had ever told them what severe diarrhea was and wasn't!

Carolyn did have loose stools (bowel movements). Of course, when you have to keep cleaning that up, it sure seems like severe diarrhea! Carolyn had a viral intestinal flu and would be fine in a few days. She did not have serious enough problems to even modify her diet very much. Her parents were given information about what to feed her to make her more comfortable (and not make her loose stools worse), as well as what medicine to use to reduce her fever. They were also told what symptoms to look for that would signal pending dehydration and to call back for an appointment if these signs appeared.

There are countless other examples of how we misinterpret signs and symptoms. Misinterpretation is usually the result of misunderstanding, misinformation, or lack of information. Think about it. We learn about illness as we are growing up. Our information is based on what we *hear* and are *told*. We therefore base our judgments on information that is often not particularly precise. We hear that fever, vomiting, diarrhea, pain, nausea, dizziness, and bleeding (to name a few) are cornerstones of illness and should be respected and feared. But no one tells us how high a fever is high. No one says how long a fever must continue to be "prolonged" and what level of fever (if any) heralds serious or potentially serious illness. No one explains what "severe" diarrhea is, or how much nausea or what degree of dizziness points to a more serious problem.

For you (or anyone) to really understand warning signs, you need to know more about the significance of these symptoms (or when these symptoms become significant). Again, we must better understand the body's special code. We also need to keep in mind the perspective from which we are judging these symptoms. This is always a bit difficult to do.

For example, when *we* get a cold, we know we will be miserable for three or four days. We may have a cough, congestion, and a fever. We also know we may not feel like "ourselves" for another week or so, but we don't worry about it. We may have a cough that lasts throughout the night, but we aren't concerned that it's anything serious. We may not even be particularly aware that we also have loose stools, ache all over, aren't eating much, and are irritable. These symptoms are not worrisome to us because we *know* we have a cold and accept all these things as part of the illness.

But when one of our children gets a cold, we forget *all* those things that come with it. We are concerned because we hear the youngster cough off and on throughout the

216

ILLNESS IN
INFANTS,
CHILDREN,
AND
ADOLESCENTS

night. (Coughing usually doesn't keep the child up—but it keeps the parents up!) We are worried about severe diarrhea, when what he or she really has is loose stools. We are fearful that something terrible is wrong because the youngster just won't eat well. We're nervous about the fever. We spend a lot of time worrying.

We often worry, not because we are overreactive, panicky people, but because we have frequently heard that so many diseases have symptoms in common. In fact, some illnesses do exhibit only very subtle differences—and this problem rightfully makes many parents nervous. Is it an infection or cancer, the mumps or meningitis, an allergic rash or measles? Is this only a cold, or could it be the start of pneumonia or a serious ear infection? However, the complex diagnostic puzzle is not as scary as it seems. There *are* distinct differences between illnesses.

For the nonphysician, the distinction between a minor versus a potentially more serious illness is based on the *intensity and/or duration of the symptoms*. Also, there are certain very specific symptoms that signal a serious situation and require immediate action if they occur. Therefore, what you need to know is the basic significance of various symptoms (or in some situations, how severe or prolonged these symptoms must become in order to be significant). With this information in hand, you will be able to assess your child when he or she is sick and feel more confident about the action you take. You will also know *where* to look for information when you need it—particularly when you have no idea what disease the child has. In essence, then, you will be able to respond by recognizing and interpreting the body's special means of communicating with you—symptoms of illness.

217

RECOGNIZING
AND ASSESSING
SERIOUS OR
POTENTIALLY
SERIOUS
ILLNESS

EMERGENCY QUICK REFERENCE

With the Steps in Detail

Breathing Difficulty and Breathing Pattern

When to Call the Paramedics or an Ambulance

In the following situations, have someone else call the *paramedics* or an *ambulance* (if there are no paramedics in your area) while you treat the youngster. If no one else is with you, continue treating the child while you periodically shout for help. When help arrives, have that person call the paramedics or an ambulance.

▶ **BREATHING AND/OR PULSE HAVE STOPPED (FOR ANY REASON).** (If you are certified in CPR and are unable to remember the details of the procedure, turn to the Emergency Quick Reference on page 113, entitled "A Review of the Six Steps of CPR.")

▶ **THE YOUNGSTER IS STRUGGLING FOR BREATH—BUT YOU CANNOT HEAR OR FEEL AIR ENTERING THE LUNGS.** (If you are unable to remember the details of managing this problem, turn to the Emergency Quick Reference on page 127, entitled "Managing Airway Obstruction/ Choking," for a review.)

▶ **THE CHILD IS STRUGGLING FOR BREATH—AND HAS EXTREMELY BLUE, PURPLE, OR PALE SKIN.**

▶ **THE YOUNGSTER IS STRUGGLING FOR BREATH, IS ANXIOUS AND EXCITED *OR* VERY LISTLESS AND LETHARGIC—AND IS MAKING NOISE WHEN HE OR SHE INHALES (STRIDOR) OR EXHALES (WHEEZING).**

▶ **THERE ARE SIGNS OF BREATHING DIFFICULTY—ALONG WITH HIVES AND/OR SWELLING OF THE TONGUE, LIPS, OR FACE.** (If you are unable to remember the details of managing this problem, turn to the Emergency Quick Reference on page 324, entitled "Anaphylaxis," for a review.)

218

ILLNESS IN
INFANTS,
CHILDREN,
AND
ADOLESCENTS

▶ **A YOUNG PERSON IS UNCONSCIOUS OR VERY LETHARGIC—AND HIS OR HER BREATHING IS SLOWER THAN FIFTEEN BREATHS PER MINUTE AND/OR VERY IRREGULAR.**

▶ **AFTER A NEAR-DROWNING EPISODE, A YOUNGSTER IS NOT FULLY ALERT AND/OR IS COUGHING AND GAGGING.** (If you are unable to remember the details of managing this problem, turn to the Emergency Quick Reference on page 191, entitled "Managing Drowning," for a review.)

▶ **A CHILD HAS THE FOLLOWING SYMPTOMS, AND YOU ARE UNABLE TO REACH YOUR DOCTOR OR GET THE CHILD TO AN EMERGENCY ROOM SAFELY *WITHIN FIFTEEN MINUTES*: SEVERE DIFFICULTY WHEN INHALING (BREATHING IN)—ALONG WITH REFUSAL TO SWALLOW ANYTHING (EVEN SALIVA), DROOLING, FEVER, AND ANXIETY.**

- Stay calm and try to keep the child as calm as possible while you wait for the paramedics.

- Do not try to look into the child's throat or put anything into his mouth.

When to Go to an Emergency Room

▶ **A CHILD HAS THE FOLLOWING SYMPTOMS, AND YOU ARE UNABLE TO REACH YOUR DOCTOR *WITHIN FIFTEEN MINUTES*: SEVERE DIFFICULTY WHEN INHALING (BREATHING IN)—ALONG WITH REFUSAL TO SWALLOW ANYTHING (EVEN SALIVA), DROOLING, FEVER, AND ANXIETY.**

- Stay calm and try to keep the child as calm as possible.

- Do not try to look into the child's throat or put anything into her mouth.

When to Call the Doctor Immediately

The following symptoms and signs are serious enough that your infant, child, or teenager will usually need to be evaluated *within an hour or so*. Call your child's doctor for advice *immediately*. If you are unable to reach the doctor within fifteen to thirty minutes, take the youngster to an emergency room for evaluation.

219

RECOGNIZING
AND ASSESSING
SERIOUS OR
POTENTIALLY
SERIOUS
ILLNESS

▶ THERE IS MODERATE TO SEVERE BREATHING DIFFICULTY (DIFFICULTY CATCHING BREATH—WITH RETRACTIONS BUT WITHOUT BLUENESS).

▶ BREATHING IS VERY LABORED—AND/OR THE YOUNGSTER COMPLAINS OF PAIN OR DISCOMFORT WITH EACH BREATH.

▶ BREATHING IS VERY RAPID (BREATHING MORE THAN SIXTY TIMES A MINUTE IN YOUNG INFANTS, TODDLERS, AND YOUNG CHILDREN OR MORE THAN FORTY TIMES A MINUTE IN OLDER CHILDREN AND TEENAGERS).

▶ BREATHING IS VERY SHALLOW, SLOW (FEWER THAN FIFTEEN TIMES A MINUTE)—OR IRREGULAR IN A YOUNGSTER WHO IS ILL OR MAY HAVE BEEN INJURED OR POISONED.

▶ THE YOUNGSTER MAKES GRUNTING SOUNDS WITH BREATHING.

▶ THERE IS SEVERE STRIDOR OR SEVERE WHEEZING.

▶ THERE IS SEVERE DIFFICULTY WITH BREATHING IN, ASSOCIATED WITH ANXIETY, FEVER, REFUSAL TO SWALLOW ANYTHING (EVEN SALIVA), OR DROOLING. (IN THIS SITUATION, TAKE THE YOUNGSTER TO AN EMERGENCY ROOM IF YOU ARE UNABLE TO REACH THE DOCTOR *WITHIN FIFTEEN MINUTES*.)

▶ THE YOUNGSTER HAS EXPERIENCED A NEAR-DROWNING EPISODE BUT IS AWAKE AND BREATHING WITH LITTLE OR NO DIFFICULTY.   Remember, a youngster should *always* be evaluated by a doctor after a near-drowning episode because of the possibility of later serious complications.

When to Call the Doctor Within an Hour or Two

In the following situations, an infant, child, or teenager may require evaluation *within a few hours*. Call your doctor for advice or arrange for the youngster to be seen in an emergency room (if you have no doctor or are not near or cannot reach your doctor).

▶ MODERATE BREATHING DIFFICULTY—WITH OR WITHOUT FEVER.

220

ILLNESS IN
INFANTS,
CHILDREN,
AND
ADOLESCENTS

▶ **THERE IS WHEEZING—WITHOUT OTHER SIGNS OF DISTRESS.**

▶ **THE CHILD HAS MODERATE OR MILD STRIDOR—WITHOUT SKIN COLOR CHANGE OR OTHER SIGNS OF DISTRESS.**

▶ **THE YOUNGSTER'S BREATHING RATE IS SLIGHTLY OR MODER-ATELY INCREASED.** (An infant or young child is breathing more than forty times per minute but fewer than sixty times per minute, or an older child or teenager is breathing between thirty times per minute and forty times per minute.)

▶ **A YOUNGSTER HAS A HIGH FEVER—ALONG WITH EVEN MILD BREATHING DIFFICULTY.**

▶ **AN INFANT, TODDLER, OR YOUNG CHILD HAS UNUSUALLY SE-VERE, PROLONGED COUGHING SPELLS.**

- There are repeated coughing spells during which the little one is unable to catch his or her breath, turns blue, or vomits.

When to Call the Doctor for an Appointment

In the following situations, an infant, child, or teenager requires evaluation *within a day or two.* Call your doctor's office to arrange an appointment.

▶ **A YOUNG INFANT'S NOSE CONGESTION IS SEVERE—ESPECIALLY IF IT INTERFERES WITH FEEDING OR SLEEPING.**

▶ **COUGHING IS PROLONGED OR SEVERE.**

▶ **A YOUNGSTER HAS A "RATTLING CHEST," AND YOU ARE UN-CERTAIN IF THE RATTLING IS COMING FROM THE NOSE AND THROAT OR FROM THE CHEST.**

▶ **BREATHING PROBLEMS DO NOT SEEM PARTICULARLY SEVERE BUT PERSIST FOR LONGER THAN A WEEK OR TWO OR SEEM TO RECUR FREQUENTLY.**

221

RECOGNIZING
AND ASSESSING
SERIOUS OR
POTENTIALLY
SERIOUS
ILLNESS

ASSESSMENT CHECKLIST

Breathing Difficulty and Breathing Pattern

OBSERVE THE YOUNGSTER CAREFULLY FOR SIGNS OF SEVERE BREATHING DIFFICULTY.

yes no Is air moving in and out of the lungs? (Can you see the youngster's chest rise
☐ ☐ and fall, or hear or feel air moving in and out of his nose or mouth?)

yes no Does his breathing appear to be labored?
☐ ☐

yes no Is she fighting for breath?
☐ ☐

yes no Is breathing uncomfortable?
☐ ☐

yes no Is her color blue, deep purple, gray, very pale, or mottled?
☐ ☐

yes no Are there any retractions (sucking in of the spaces between the ribs or above
☐ ☐ the breastbone or below the rib cage when the youngster breathes in)?

CHECK THE YOUNGSTER'S PULSE (HEARTBEAT), AS YOU WERE TAUGHT
IN CPR TRAINING.

yes no Is the heartbeat strong and steady?
☐ ☐

yes no Is the heartbeat weak and thready?
☐ ☐

IS THE YOUNG PERSON'S BREATHING PATTERN ABNORMAL?

yes no Is he or she breathing very irregularly?
☐ ☐

222

ILLNESS IN
INFANTS,
CHILDREN,
AND
ADOLESCENTS

yes no Are the breaths very shallow or very deep?
☐ ☐

yes no Is the breathing pattern normal?
☐ ☐

COUNT THE YOUNGSTER'S RESPIRATORY (BREATHING) RATE.

yes no Is a young infant, toddler, or young child breathing very rapidly—more than
☐ ☐ sixty times per minute?

yes no Is an older child or teenager breathing very rapidly—more than forty times
☐ ☐ per minute?

yes no Is the sick youngster breathing fewer than fifteen times per minute?
☐ ☐

LISTEN FOR ANY UNUSUAL NOISES.

yes no Can you hear a harsh, crowing noise when the youngster breathes in (called
☐ ☐ stridor)?

yes no Can you hear a whistling, musical noise when the youngster breathes out
☐ ☐ (called wheezing)?

yes no Can you hear snorting, gurgling, or rattling noises?
☐ ☐

yes no Is the child coughing?
☐ ☐

yes no Is the youngster's voice or cry hoarse?
☐ ☐

PAY ATTENTION TO OTHER SYMPTOMS THAT CAN OCCUR WITH SOME BREATHING PROBLEMS.

yes no Is there swelling of the lips, face, and/or tongue, with or without hives?
☐ ☐

yes no Is the youngster showing signs of anxiety, restlessness, or agitation?
☐ ☐

223

RECOGNIZING
AND ASSESSING
SERIOUS OR
POTENTIALLY
SERIOUS
ILLNESS

yes no Is he unconscious?
☐   ☐

yes no Is he difficult to arouse?
☐   ☐

yes no Is she drooling or refusing to swallow?
☐   ☐

yes no Does she have a fever?
☐   ☐

Assessing Breathing

"I've always been frightened that one of my children would get pneumonia, because my mother always talked about her older brother who died from it when he was a little boy. When my sister and I were young, my mother always hovered over us whenever we had a cough or cold. You couldn't blame her! Unfortunately, I find myself doing the same thing now with my children. I guess it's because I don't understand what kinds of things really mean a serious breathing problem. To me, a cough or congestion equals panic."

Most children who are ill have some change(s) in the way they breathe. Because of this, it is important that you be able to distinguish the breathing changes that would signal serious illness, in contrast to those usually seen with mild to moderate problems. Most parents feel unsure about their ability to tell the difference between serious and nonserious breathing symptoms. This feeling is certainly justifiable if no one has ever explained the difference to them. Again, it's like Morse code—you need to be taught or teach yourself how to interpret signals correctly. Here are a few facts.

Normally, a young infant breathes through her nose when resting. If the nose is congested or has mucus in it (because of a cold or dryness in the air), the little one may be fussy. She has trouble with feeding, because it is difficult for her to breathe through her nose and suck at the same time. But when she is quiet, she breathes comfortably. The same stuffy, runny nose in an older youngster is bothersome, but not as much of a problem for the youngster.

On the other hand, a baby or child who has a serious breathing problem *looks* as if he is in trouble. Breathing is *labored* and usually *rapid*, even when he is trying to rest. His color may be poor—*pale, grayish, or bluish*, especially around the mouth and under the fingernails or toenails. He looks as if he *cannot catch his breath* and may have a *cough* or *noisy breathing*. All of these point to the real difficulty: the youngster cannot get enough air to move into and out of his lungs.

Obviously, the major risk with breathing problems is lack of oxygen. Normally, air moves easily in and out of the lungs. Oxygen passes through the lungs into the blood and is carried around the body to all the organs and tissues. Carbon dioxide (the waste product of cell function) is carried back to the lungs from the tissues and organs and expelled from the lungs during normal breathing. Ineffective breathing leads to inefficient expulsion of the carbon dioxide, as well as lack of oxygen. If not enough oxygen is supplied to the tissues and organs, they function ineffectively. As a response, excessive acids are produced and build up in the body. The combination of lack of oxygen (called hypoxia) along with the buildup of carbon dioxide and acids acts as a poison to the cells and tissues. This initially causes temporary damage—and if not reversed, permanent damage to cells, tissues, and organs will occur. The cells of the brain, kidneys, and heart muscle are especially vulnerable to this kind of damage.

Because of this potential risk, it is important for each of us to learn how to distinguish between the life-threatening types of severe breathing difficulty and mild to moderate problems. Knowing this, you can make intelligent, appropriate decisions about when your child needs to be evaluated by the doctor, taken to an emergency room, or the paramedics must be called.

Evaluation of Breathing Pattern and Breathing Difficulty

One of the first (and sometimes only) signs of serious illness is a change in the breathing pattern. *Rapid breathing* is one of the changes most commonly seen. This is the body's attempt to increase the amount of oxygen delivered to the lungs and/or get rid of carbon dioxide. Generally, breathing speeds up not only with lung problems but also when a youngster has a fever, is experiencing pain, or is dehydrated, to name a few other causes.

Slow or irregular breathing can also be a signal of serious illness. Breathing normally slows down during sleep or when a youngster is resting quietly. It also slows with certain drugs or poisons and with some forms of brain injury. Irregular breathing can be normal, especially in some infants during sleep, but can also signal serious diseases.

It's important to remember that the normal breathing rate *differs* with age: young infants usually breathe faster than older children, teenagers, and adults. The number of times a youngster breathes each minute is called the *respiratory rate*. The first step in evaluating a youngster's breathing pattern is to have him or her be as quiet as possible. Watch the chest rise and fall. Using a watch with a second hand, count the number of times the youngster breathes for one minute (sixty seconds). Every time you see the chest rise (the child inhales), you count "one" breath. If the breaths are regular and even, you can count for thirty seconds and multiply that number by two. If breathing is irregular (some irregularity can be normal, as mentioned earlier—especially in very young babies), then count for a full minute.

Infants under two months of age may breathe as fast as fifty or sixty times a minute for short periods of time but settle down to rates slower than forty breaths per minute most of the time. Infants and toddlers under two years old usually breathe fewer than thirty times a minute, and six-year-olds (and other school-aged children) ordinarily have a respiratory rate under twenty-five per minute. Teenagers and adults usually breathe fewer than twenty times a minute. High fever increases the respiratory rate, so take that into account before you become overly concerned. However, a *breathing rate of over forty times a minute* in a child who is sick (has other symptoms of illness), regardless of age or level of fever, should signal the need for medical evaluation.

After you know how many breaths (respirations) the youngster takes per minute, look at the *youngster's chest to see how it moves.* Is his breathing labored? Are there any unusual movements of the chest? For example, do the areas between the ribs suck in when she inhales? Does the area above the collarbone suck in when he inhales? Does the abdomen—under the ribs—suck in with each breath? These are called *retractions* and are associated with a wide variety of respiratory diseases, nearly all of them potentially serious.

Next, *listen for any unusual sounds or noises* when the youngster breathes. *Grunting* and *gasping* noises may mean there is a problem within the lung or that the youngster is in severe pain. If these are associated with retractions, they can signal a serious problem. A harsh, crowing noise when the youngster inhales (called *stridor*) means partial blockage/obstruction or swelling in the upper airway (at or around the voice box or in the windpipe). You may hear this noise either with each breath or only when the child is upset. A hoarse cry and/or hoarse voice are often associated with stridor, as is a barking, croupy cough. The noise is made by air being forcefully sucked past a now-narrowed area of the large upper airway.

A soft, sometimes musical whistling noise heard when the youngster breathes out (exhales) is called a *wheeze.* This noise is made when air is forced out through too-narrow breathing tubes (called bronchioles and bronchi) in the lungs. This wheezing can occur because of asthma, certain lung infections, and when there is a small foreign object caught in the small airways of the lungs, as well as in other less common situations. If there is drastic narrowing of the airways, musical wheezes may turn into squeaking and might be heard with inhalation, as well as exhalation. A tight cough is often associated with wheezing.

A word about *"rattling chest"*: Many parents are worried when they notice that their infant or child's chest "rattles" or vibrates during breathing. Most often, the youngster is not distressed by the rattling and is in the recovering stage of an illness. This rattling (and gurgling noises that are sometimes associated with it) usually arises from the throat—not the chest. Don't be concerned unless the youngster is also experiencing breathing difficulty or other symptoms that point to a serious respiratory

226

ILLNESS IN
INFANTS,
CHILDREN,
AND
ADOLESCENTS

problem. However, don't hesitate to talk to your doctor about rattling chest if you are worried or not sure whether a more serious problem may be involved.

If a child has a *cough*, listen to it carefully and try to determine its major characteristic, its frequency, and how bothersome it is. A dry, hacking cough is most often due to irritation of the throat and airways. A harsh, barking cough (that may have an almost metallic sound to it) can result from inflammation or partial blockage of the windpipe. Unusually severe or prolonged coughing spells, especially in very young infants and children, can indicate potentially serious problems. A wet, loose cough helps clear the airways of mucus and often signals that the youngster is improving. Some infants and children cough so hard they vomit. This often results from the combination of forceful coughing and irritating mucus in the stomach. As long as the vomiting is only occasional, this alone should not concern you excessively.

Try to distinguish between true breathing difficulty and the snorting, noisy sounds a baby or child may make with *nose congestion*. With nasal congestion, mucus partially or completely blocks the nasal passages, leading to unusual (and sometimes comical) noises, especially during feeding. This occurs because the little one (who must suck to drink) tries to suck and at the same time breathe through the blocked nose. This kind of congestion and breathing difficulty is almost never serious, although it is bothersome.

Infants and Toddlers

BREATHING DIFFICULTIES: WHEN SERIOUSLY OR POTENTIALLY SERIOUSLY ILL

''Michelle didn't seem so sick at first. She got what looked like her first cold at three months old. She had a little runny nose and cough and didn't eat as well as usual. But then on the second day, I became more and more worried. She really looked pale and was breathing so fast. When I took her nightie off, her little chest was heaving very fast, and the skin between her ribs was really sucking in a lot. I knew there was trouble when she seemed too tired to eat, and then I noticed that her lips looked just a little blue. By this time, I could hear her wheeze with every breath.''

Rapid breathing is one of the first signs of a serious lung problem in anyone, including a young infant. Other signs of serious or potentially serious illness in infants and toddlers are: labored breathing; persistent breathing rates faster than forty per minute in babies over a few days old up until about two years old; grunting sound when

227

RECOGNIZING
AND ASSESSING
SERIOUS OR
POTENTIALLY
SERIOUS
ILLNESS

breathing; stridor or wheezing, especially if associated with other symptoms of serious illness; and unusual chest motion or retractions (the spaces between the ribs and under the rib cage suck in when the baby breathes in). Call the doctor and have the little one evaluated as soon as possible if any of these symptoms occur.

Poor color is also a sign of potentially serious respiratory difficulty. A youngster with serious breathing problems may be pale or blue (called cyanosis). This poor color indicates that not enough oxygen is being exchanged in the lungs. Bluish or grayish lips or nailbeds are early warning signs and occur before the baby's or youngster's skin color becomes totally blue (a very serious sign). Take the youngster to an emergency room if you can get there within five to ten minutes, or call the paramedics for help.

Some types of cough signal serious illness, especially in infants and toddlers. With certain diseases (such as one form of pneumonia caused by a germ called chlamydia, and pertussis, or whooping cough), the little one may have severe coughing spells. If she has trouble catching her breath after a spell or makes a loud "whooping" noise at the end of a spell, have her promptly evaluated by the doctor.

BREATHING DIFFICULTIES:
WHEN MODERATELY OR MILDLY ILL

> "Joey really seems miserable with this cold. I always knew colds were difficult for little babies, but he has this awful rattling in his chest and has such a terrible time eating. He hardly seems interested in food at all and takes a long time to drink his bottle."

In an infant or toddler, it's always hard to know when a cold is more than just a cold. We tend to forget that the baby's or toddler's nasal passages are smaller than ours and that he must breathe through his nose while he nurses. Therefore, if there is a lot of nasal congestion, the little one will often struggle and seem miserable, especially when feeding. He will also tend to have noisy, snorting breathing because of the swelling and mucus in the nose and throat. Sometimes, breathing is slightly faster than usual, especially if there is a fever, but the breathing rate is still under forty per minute. In mild to moderate illness, coughing is not severe and tends not to even keep the youngster awake. When you *really* look at the baby or toddler, you can see that there is not very much difficulty with breathing—even if there is a lot of noise. There is no sure treatment for this misery, but call the doctor for advice if the baby seems unusually congested or unhappy or if she is totally unable to drink.

Sometimes, it's easy to become overly concerned about noisy breathing and a wet, loose cough. The wetness, especially when it appears after two to three days of congestion, actually means the cold is getting better. Call the doctor for advice if you're concerned, but remember to look at the entire youngster for other signs of a serious problem, as well.

228

ILLNESS IN
INFANTS,
CHILDREN,
AND
ADOLESCENTS

Young Children

BREATHING DIFFICULTIES:
WHEN SERIOUSLY OR POTENTIALLY SERIOUSLY ILL

"Johnny looked as if he was having his usual asthma attack, but I started to get worried when the problem didn't seem to be clearing up. Even the extra things his doctor prescribed didn't help. At first, I thought it was a good sign that he was falling asleep, but then I realized that he was having an awful lot of trouble breathing and his color was really bad."

In young children, as in young infants, breathing difficulties can worsen quickly. The signs of trouble are the same, although in small children, breathing rates are normally a little slower. In young children, be concerned if the breathing rate is faster than thirty to thirty-five times a minute. Youngsters who can talk can also tell you they feel short of breath and may complain of pain or discomfort in the chest, particularly if they are wheezing. Other signs of serious problems include: grunting sound when breathing; stridor or wheezing; and coughing that occurs in prolonged bouts, followed by a loud, harsh "whoop" as the youngster catches his or her breath. If a child has any of these symptoms, call your doctor promptly for advice, or go to an emergency room if you don't have a doctor or can't reach your doctor. If a child has stridor along with fever, sore throat, and drooling, go calmly but quickly to an emergency room, while trying to keep the youngster calm. If you cannot get to an emergency room within ten to fifteen minutes, call the paramedics.

Youngsters with severe lack of oxygen show signs of mental irritation or alteration—for example, severe anxiety, delirium, irritability, or extreme sleepiness. Buildup of carbon dioxide leads to excessive sleepiness or drowsiness and is a danger signal when there is a lot of breathing trouble. If these signs occur in a youngster with breathing difficulty, get help immediately.

BREATHING DIFFICULTIES:
WHEN MODERATELY OR MILDLY ILL

"We were awakened in the night to the sound of a barking cough and ran to the children's room. There was Matthew, sitting up and crying. Every few minutes, his crying was interrupted by this terrible cough. He seemed very upset and out of control. After a few minutes, we got him calmed down a little and found that he seemed fine except that his voice was hoarse and he seemed to have a very slight fever."

229

RECOGNIZING
AND ASSESSING
SERIOUS OR
POTENTIALLY
SERIOUS
ILLNESS

As with young infants and toddlers, young children can make a lot of noise with mild to moderate respiratory problems. While noisy breathing and scary coughs are common, there is a key to deciding whether the underlying illness is serious or not: if the youngster seems otherwise quite healthy (has no other serious symptoms), then more than likely the illness is not serious. For example, if there is no real breathing difficulty associated with the cough and congestion—then it is probably a minor illness. Also, a cough that is *not* associated with trouble catching the breath or repeated vomiting usually signals a mild problem—as long as it does not persist beyond several weeks and seems to improve gradually. Call the doctor if there is no improvement or if other symptoms warrant it.

Older Children and Teenagers

BREATHING DIFFICULTIES: WHEN SERIOUSLY OR POTENTIALLY SERIOUSLY ILL

"For a week or so, I had been wondering whether Amy was sick or not. She had been complaining about being tired and looked pale and thinner to me. Since her appetite had been voracious, it didn't make sense. Neither did the fact that she complained of extreme thirst and dry mouth—even though she had been drinking more than ever before and urinating almost constantly. But at first, I put this off as part of growing up. She was starting into puberty, and I had heard young girls tend to eat more. Then I noticed that she seemed to be breathing so deeply and fast. Now I knew what it was! It had to be pneumonia! I was shocked when the doctor said Amy had diabetes."

As with other age groups, changes in color, stridor or wheezing, complaints of chest pain, or difficulty breathing can signal potentially serious illness in older children and teenagers. While changes in breathing pattern and rapid breathing (over thirty breaths a minute in older youngsters and teenagers) can mean pneumonia and lung problems, they can also signal other serious diseases. In addition to diabetes, poisoning or over-dosing on certain drugs needs to be considered when an older youngster breathes more rapidly or slower than usual (especially when there are changes in alertness or behavior).

BREATHING DIFFICULTIES: WHEN MODERATELY OR MILDLY ILL

"Sarah had not been acting like herself for several days before we really suspected she might be sick. She then developed a little fever and came

230

ILLNESS IN
INFANTS,
CHILDREN,
AND
ADOLESCENTS

home from junior high ready to 'lie down for a few minutes,' she said. Then she began coughing. We knew she was congested but were surprised when the doctor said she had a mild viral pneumonia. She really wasn't having any difficulty breathing that we could see.''

In older children and teenagers, an infection or inflammation of the lungs needs to be really severe in order to cause breathing difficulty. Mild to moderate illness should be suspected if a youngster has any of the following: mildly noisy breathing; congestion of the nose, windpipe, or lungs that doesn't cause the young person trouble when trying to catch his or her breath and is not associated with rapid breathing (breathing more than twenty-five times a minute should prompt concern if there is also fever); mild hoarseness and cough; and coughing that does not prevent the youngster from sleeping.

THE DON'TS

Don't forget to evaluate a youngster's breathing difficulty and breathing pattern systematically. It is easy to assume either that he or she is ''fine'' or that there is a very serious problem unless you look carefully at specific signs and symptoms of trouble.

Don't hesitate to call your doctor for advice if you are unsure whether or not your child really has a serious breathing problem. The doctor can often help you make further observations or will ask you to bring the child in for evaluation.

PLEASE NOTE: Now that you have a grasp of how to assess breathing pattern and recognize breathing difficulty, it would be extremely helpful for you to go back to the Emergency Quick Reference With the Steps in Detail and the Assessment Checklist and review them carefully. The more familiar you are with that material, the more useful it will be to you when you need it.

231

RECOGNIZING
AND ASSESSING
SERIOUS OR
POTENTIALLY
SERIOUS
ILLNESS

EMERGENCY QUICK REFERENCE

General Behavior (Including Level of Activity, Responsiveness, and Irritability)

When to Call the Paramedics or an Ambulance

In the following situations, have someone else call the *paramedics* or an *ambulance* (if there are no paramedics in your area) while you treat the youngster. If no one else is with you, continue treating the child while you periodically shout for help. When help arrives, have that person call the paramedics or an ambulance.

▶ **THE YOUNGSTER IS UNCONSCIOUS, OR VERY DIFFICULT OR IMPOSSIBLE TO AROUSE.**   (If you are unable to remember the details of managing this problem, turn to the Emergency Quick Reference on page 160, entitled "Managing Unconsciousness," for a review.)

▶ **THE CHILD IS EXTREMELY AGITATED OR EXTREMELY LETHARGIC—AND IS HAVING DIFFICULTY BREATHING (WITH OR WITHOUT BLUE, PURPLE, OR GRAY SKIN).**

▶ **THE CHILD IS AGITATED OR EXTREMELY LETHARGIC—AND HAS SIGNS OF SHOCK:**   pale, pasty, or mottled skin; cool, clammy skin; severe weakness, dizziness, or light-headedness; rapid, weak, thready heartbeat; poor circulation. (If you are unable to remember the details of managing this problem, turn to the Emergency Quick Reference on page 152, entitled "Managing Shock," for a review.)

When to Call the Doctor Immediately

The following symptoms and signs are serious enough that your infant, child, or teenager will usually need to be evaluated *within an hour or two.* Call your child's doctor for advice *immediately.* If you are unable to reach the doctor within fifteen to thirty minutes, take the youngster to an emergency room for evaluation.

▶ **THE CHILD IS LETHARGIC AND/OR EXTREMELY IRRITABLE—AND HAS SIGNS OF SERIOUS INFECTION:**   high fever, bulging soft spot if an infant, stiff neck, a rash that looks like tiny blood spots, and so on.

232

ILLNESS IN
INFANTS,
CHILDREN,
AND
ADOLESCENTS

▶ **THE YOUNGSTER IS LETHARGIC AND/OR EXTREMELY IRRITA-BLE—AND HAS SIGNS OF DEHYDRATION:** very dry mouth, extreme thirst, sunken eyeballs, doughy skin, poor urine production, and so on. (If you are unable to remember the details of managing this problem, turn to the Emergency Quick Reference on page 352, entitled "Dehydration," for a review.)

▶ **AN INFANT OR TODDLER IS EXTREMELY LETHARGIC AND/OR IR-RITABLE—*AND* REFUSES TWO OR MORE CONSECUTIVE FEED-INGS.**

▶ **THE YOUNGSTER IS IRRATIONAL, INCOHERENT, AND "OUT OF TOUCH."**

When to Call the Doctor Within an Hour or Two

In the following situations, an infant, child, or teenager may require evaluation *within a few hours*. Call your doctor for advice or arrange for the youngster to be seen in an emergency room (if you have no doctor or you cannot reach or are not near your doctor).

▶ **YOUR *INFANT* OR *TODDLER* "JUST DOESN'T SEEM RIGHT" OR "DOESN'T SEEM HERSELF."**

▶ **THE YOUNGSTER CRIES CONSTANTLY—WITH OR WITHOUT OTHER SYMPTOMS.**

▶ **THE YOUNGSTER HAS UNUSUAL LISTLESSNESS OR WEAKNESS THAT IS OUT OF PROPORTION TO WHAT APPEAR TO BE OTH-ERWISE MILD SYMPTOMS OF AN ILLNESS.**

▶ **THE CHILD IS SLEEPING ALL THE TIME, REFUSES ALL ACTIVITY—AND/OR REFUSES TO EAT OR DRINK AT ALL.**

When to Call the Doctor for an Appointment

In the following situations, an infant, child, or teenager requires evaluation *within a day or two*. Call your doctor's office to arrange for an appointment.

▶ **THE CHILD HAS PERSISTENT LISTLESSNESS OR APATHY—OR REFUSES TO PLAY OR TAKE PART IN HIS NORMAL ACTIVITIES.**

233

RECOGNIZING
AND ASSESSING
SERIOUS OR
POTENTIALLY
SERIOUS
ILLNESS

▶ **THE YOUNGER CHILD, OLDER CHILD, OR TEENAGER "JUST DOESN'T SEEM RIGHT" OR "DOESN'T SEEM HIMSELF."**

▶ **THE YOUNGSTER HAS REDUCED ACTIVITY OR DISTURBED SLEEP OUT OF PROPORTION TO WHAT APPEAR TO BE OTHERWISE MILD SYMPTOMS OF AN ILLNESS.**

▶ **YOU ARE UNABLE TO DETERMINE THE CAUSE OF CONSTANT CRANKINESS.**

ASSESSMENT CHECKLIST

General Behavior (Including Level of Activity, Responsiveness, and Irritability)

Infants and Toddlers

ASSESS THE INFANT'S OR TODDLER'S LEVEL OF ACTIVITY.

yes no Are the little one's activity level and responsiveness normal or near normal?

yes no Does she sleep much more than usual?

yes no Is she lethargic (very inactive, apathetic)?

yes no Does he have only short periods of activity or play interspersed with unusually inactive times?

yes no Is he weak, floppy, and moving very little?

ASSESS THE GENERAL LEVEL OF AWARENESS AND RESPONSIVENESS OF THE INFANT OR TODDLER.

yes no Is he difficult or impossible to arouse?

yes no Does she respond to you at all?

234

ILLNESS IN
INFANTS,
CHILDREN,
AND
ADOLESCENTS

yes no Is she "spacey," or does she seem out-of-touch?

yes no Is the little one apathetic about strangers or about being handled?

yes no If she is crying constantly, can you get her to quiet down or relax?

yes no Does he pay attention to you and to his surroundings?

yes no Is he sleeping more than usual but easy to arouse?

yes no Will she remain alert for periods of time?

ASSESS THE INFANT'S OR TODDLER'S DEGREE OF IRRITABILITY.

yes no Does he cry or whimper constantly even when you try to comfort him?

yes no Does his cry sound normal?

yes no Does extreme irritability alternate with extreme lethargy?

yes no Does she act as if everything hurts or as if she doesn't want to be touched?

yes no Is he mildly cranky, as opposed to inconsolably irritable?

yes no Does she seem agitated or panic-stricken?

Young Children, Older Children, and Teenagers

ASSESS THE YOUNG CHILD'S, OLDER CHILD'S, OR TEENAGER'S LEVEL OF ACTIVITY.

yes no Does she refuse to play or move around at all?

yes no Does he sleep nearly all the time, arousing only briefly?

yes no Is she lethargic?

yes no Can she be enticed to play quietly or to read, listen to music, or watch television for part of the day?

yes no Is he able to take part in some or all of his usual activities?

yes no Does he object to resting or taking a nap?

ASSESS THE YOUNG CHILD'S, OLDER CHILD'S, OR TEENAGER'S LEVEL
OF AWARENESS AND RESPONSIVENESS.

235

RECOGNIZING
AND ASSESSING
SERIOUS OR
POTENTIALLY
SERIOUS
ILLNESS

yes no Is he difficult or impossible to
☐ ☐ arouse?

yes no Does he seem interested in fam-
☐ ☐ ily events or things happening
with friends or at school?

yes no Does she recognize you and make
☐ ☐ sense in conversation?

ASSESS THE YOUNG CHILD'S, OLDER CHILD'S, OR TEENAGER'S DEGREE
OF IRRITABILITY.

yes no Does the youngster complain or
☐ ☐ whine constantly?

yes no Is she more "cooperative" or
☐ ☐ submissive than usual?

yes no Is he unusually demanding, an-
☐ ☐ gry, or uncooperative? Is he
cranky or unable to be pleased?

Assessing General Behavior

"I just can't explain why I feel this way, but something is wrong with Billy.
He's just not himself!"

You've probably heard others say this very thing or have said it yourself. There are
thousands of jokes, cartoons, and funny stories about parents' "intuition." The fact
of the matter is—there's nothing funny about it. Parents, on the whole, do an excellent
job of practicing "gut medicine." What many people don't realize is that their gut
feelings are actually based on their observations of the youngster.

Think about it. You know how your child normally acts; the amount of energy he
usually expends at play; how responsive he is when first awakened or when being
talked to or played with; and you are keenly aware of his normal personality and
disposition. A parent's "gut feeling" that a child is sick or something is wrong actually
comes from seeing *changes from the norm* in a youngster's general behavior, level of
activity, responsiveness, and irritability. Therefore, your "gut feeling" is based much
more on fact and very little on fiction—if you are or can learn to be a sensitive
observer.

The truly sick infant or child will tell you—by her actions—that she is sick. The
older child or teenager may also verbally tell you she doesn't feel well—but her actions

236

ILLNESS IN
INFANTS,
CHILDREN,
AND
ADOLESCENTS

will talk to you, too. How much a youngster's overall general behavior differs from normal *is one of the most useful and sensitive gauges* as to whether she is getting sick, is sick (and how sick), is staying at the same level of sickness, is getting worse, or is getting better.

Infants and Toddlers

GENERAL BEHAVIOR: WHEN SERIOUSLY OR POTENTIALLY SERIOUSLY ILL

"Susie just seems to lie there. When I pick her up, her body seems floppy, like a rag doll. If she's not sleeping, she seems to be crying. I know she's only four months old, but I feel like she's trying to tell me to leave her alone."

One of the clearest indications of serious illness in infants and toddlers is lethargy. Lethargy is an abnormal state where there is overpowering sluggishness, apathy, drowsiness, and sleepiness. An infant who is lethargic is *very* inactive—even when stimulated or bothered. He is very difficult to awaken and continues to go back to sleep if not stimulated to stay awake. When awake, he will not move his arms and legs much, if at all, and does not move around. Usually, he does not coo and gurgle. In fact, when seriously ill, a baby may not return to his regular level of awareness even with the most vigorous attention and no matter how long you have been able to keep him awake. Some people say the infant seems almost "spacey"—not alert and difficult or impossible to arouse. Often, lethargy alternates with irritability when the infant feels bothered or is bothered. You might notice that the baby's arms and legs and entire body might be unusually weak or floppy—or even seem stiffer than usual.

A strange or unusual cry may also herald serious illness in infants and toddlers. The cry is very different—weak, whimpering, or high-pitched. It's something most parents immediately recognize as "not normal" for their child. Crying or whining, in fact, may be nearly constant and follow almost any stimulation or bother. The baby may act as if everything hurts (and indeed, it may) and she *doesn't* want you to bother her. This unusual crying may alternate with periods of lethargy.

Seriously ill babies and toddlers also seem to sleep all the time. They are usually very difficult to awaken and, once awakened, are not fully responsive (no matter how you try to stimulate them). Even with a great deal of stimulation, they seem to fall asleep again. Sleepiness goes hand in hand with lethargy.

An infant or toddler who is normally fearful of strangers and most often clings to a parent may be apathetic, uninterested, and even nonobjecting if a stranger picks him up. Or the little one may show some signs of displeasure but not to the degree that he usually displays.

GENERAL BEHAVIOR:
WHEN MODERATELY OR MILDLY ILL

237

RECOGNIZING
AND ASSESSING
SERIOUS OR
POTENTIALLY
SERIOUS
ILLNESS

> "Teddy seems very crabby and demanding. He's sleeping a little more than usual, but once up, he wants almost constant comforting and attention. Frankly, he's driving us crazy!"

In contrast to the seriously ill little one, the mildly to moderately ill infant or toddler will often be listless—less active than usual—but able to be aroused to his normal state of awareness and attentiveness. He is able to play and pay attention to his surroundings for short periods of time—but will then be less attentive and often cranky.

When mildly or moderately ill, an infant or toddler will cling even more than usual to her parents and be especially wary of strangers. She may become more upset than she normally is when picked up by either a stranger or someone other than her parents.

The baby or toddler may have short bursts of playing interrupted by quiet times where he requires comforting (often insisting on being comforted). He will most likely sleep more than usual—but will have *definite* awake periods. Most parents (and others) when describing a moderately or mildly ill baby or toddler say he is cranky or crabby but can be comforted (most successfully by his mother). All agree that the little one is very demanding and the experience very frustrating. This is in great contrast to the seriously ill baby or toddler—who most often cannot be calmed, comforted, or encouraged to be responsive.

Young Children

GENERAL BEHAVIOR:
WHEN SERIOUSLY OR POTENTIALLY SERIOUSLY ILL

> "In the past, when Jimmy was sick, he loved to watch television or listen to a story. Most six-year-olds do. This time, we can't seem to get him to do anything. He wants to sleep all the time, and he's almost impossible to wake up. This is really starting to scare us."

Many of the same basic behavioral principles we discussed in regard to the infant apply to the seriously ill young child, as well. He will often be truly lethargic—just lie around without playing at all. He cannot be enticed to watch television, listen to a story, or be involved with his favorite quiet activities. He will sleep more than usual and be very difficult or impossible to arouse.

When the child talks to you, she might not make sense, may not even remember the things you've told her, or might not even seem to know who you are. She will

238

ILLNESS IN
INFANTS,
CHILDREN,
AND
ADOLESCENTS more than likely be extremely irritable. No matter what you do, she will not be comforted and may seem distant. The child may act as if everything hurts when you try to cuddle or hug her and may cry very easily.

GENERAL BEHAVIOR:
WHEN MODERATELY OR MILDLY ILL

> "I was getting concerned until I saw Katie go out in the backyard and start swinging. So I put it off as moodiness until she was right back inside within fifteen minutes. She followed me around the house—right on my heels—until I finally picked her up and sat down in my chair. It was obvious she wasn't feeling well. She had refused to be held and cuddled like this since she was a baby."

As with the mildly or moderately ill infant, the young child who is mildly or moderately ill will be less active than usual but will be able to play with short bursts of energy. She may be more content to play quiet, less active games, read or be read to, watch television, or listen to music. And she may follow you around a lot, because she doesn't feel very well. Often, the child acts as if she is insecure and wants to keep you "in sight."

Remember, too, that a young child will often become more infantile and revert to those things that were comforting earlier in his life. A special blanket, a pacifier, a favorite stuffed animal, being held and cuddled for longer periods of time mean security and comfort. Let the little child have these "special" things and don't make him feel foolish for wanting or needing them to feel better.

As is true with youngsters of other ages, the small child who is moderately or mildly ill will sleep more than usual and more fitfully. When awakened, she will seem more like herself (will be responsive) but will probably be more irritable and whiny than you would normally expect.

Older Children and Teenagers

GENERAL BEHAVIOR:
WHEN SERIOUSLY OR POTENTIALLY SERIOUSLY ILL

> "It just isn't like Christine to fall asleep in the middle of a conversation. She doesn't even object to being told to go to bed—she just goes. That's just not like a teenager."

The seriously ill older child or teenager's general behavior is very consistent with that of the infant or small child. She will also be lethargic and completely unable to take part in normal activities. Often, the youngster will drift off to sleep in the middle of conversations or activities. Most telling is the fact that she will not object to your insistence that she rest—no matter what "fun" activity may be going on at school or after school.

239

RECOGNIZING
AND ASSESSING
SERIOUS OR
POTENTIALLY
SERIOUS
ILLNESS

The seriously ill older child or teenager just doesn't seem himself when you try to awaken him. He may seem to sleep continuously and often restlessly. Besides all these behavioral differences, the youngster may be quite irritable—suddenly hostile, yelling, whining, or crying for the simplest of reasons or for no reason at all! He will generally be "out of sorts," as most parents describe it.

When you talk to or do things for her, the very ill youngster may be terribly uncooperative. She may sound irrational and agitated and even fight against you and others who are trying to help or be comforting. On the other hand, often youngsters who are seriously ill are so lethargic and out of touch that they do not even object to the most painful things being done to them.

So you need to recognize not only the infant, toddler, small child, older child, or teenager who is totally lethargic and totally unresponsive –but the one who alternates between lethargy and outbursts of rage, crying, irrationality, and other changes in behavior that seem totally unreasonable.

GENERAL BEHAVIOR:
WHEN MODERATELY OR MILDLY ILL

"Eric kept pushing and pushing himself at baseball practice but continued to play poorly. It was really unlike him to get so angry and frustrated. Once we got home, he threw his mitt on his bedroom floor and flopped down on his bed. At first, we thought he was just having one of those bad days when you can't seem to do anything right. Later, it became obvious that he was sick."

Unlike the infant or small child, the mildly to moderately ill older child or teenager will push himself to do the things he most enjoys doing—even though he is feeling poorly. Often, he will be frustrated with himself for being sick when he has so many important and better things to do. At times, he will even deny not feeling well, until his symptoms are such that it is obvious he is sick.

Although the older child or teenager may sleep more than usual, she can also entertain herself for short periods of time—usually in quiet activities, such as reading, watching television, playing home video games, or talking to friends (especially on the telephone).

That is not to say that the older child or teenager won't be cranky. She usually will

240

ILLNESS IN
INFANTS,
CHILDREN,
AND
ADOLESCENTS

be but will alternate cranky times with periods where she will act more like herself. Most often, the older child or teenager feels miserable and is frustrated and angry about feeling this way. This often leads to irritability and sarcasm even with those trying to help. You should also keep in mind that the older child or teenager may revert to more childish behavior when mildly to moderately ill. Even though it is *difficult* at times, you should try not to make fun of the youngster's regression or get too angry when he or she is stubborn, a bit obnoxious, irritable, or sarcastic. The youngster has lost some control—gotten sick—and it's always difficult to relinquish the control you want to have over your physical being.

THE DON'TS

Don't delay in getting medical help if a youngster is extremely lethargic or difficult to arouse, regardless of other symptoms. True lethargy, while having many causes, can signal a very serious, life-threatening illness.

Don't forget that changes in a youngster's general behavior can have many causes. However, often the presence or absence of behavior change is one of the most important clues as to whether a youngster has a mild, moderate, or serious illness (when coupled with other symptoms of illness).

PLEASE NOTE: Now that you have a grasp of how to assess general behavior, it would be extremely helpful for you to go back to the Emergency Quick Reference and the Assessment Checklist and review them carefully. The more familiar you are with that material, the more useful it will be to you when you need it.

241

RECOGNIZING
AND ASSESSING
SERIOUS OR
POTENTIALLY
SERIOUS
ILLNESS

EMERGENCY QUICK REFERENCE

The Soft Spot (in Infants and Some Toddlers)

When to Call the Paramedics or an Ambulance

In the following situations, have someone else call the *paramedics* or an *ambulance* (if there are no paramedics in your area) while you treat the youngster. If no one else is with you, continue treating the child while you periodically shout for help. When help arrives, have that person call the paramedics or an ambulance.

▶ **AN INFANT OR TODDLER HAS A BULGING SOFT SPOT—ALONG WITH DIFFICULT OR IRREGULAR BREATHING.**

▶ **HE HAS A BULGING SOFT SPOT—ALONG WITH POSSIBLE OR KNOWN HEAD INJURY.** (If you are unable to remember the details of managing this problem, turn to the Emergency Quick Reference on page 573, entitled "Head, Neck, and Back Injuries," for a review.)

▶ **THE LITTLE ONE HAS SIGNS AND SYMPTOMS OF SHOCK—ALONG WITH A BULGING OR SUNKEN SOFT SPOT.** (If you are unable to remember the details of managing this problem, turn to the Emergency Quick Reference on page 152, entitled "Managing Shock," for a review.)

▶ **SHE IS UNCONSCIOUS OR VERY DIFFICULT TO AROUSE—ALONG WITH A BULGING OR VERY SUNKEN SOFT SPOT.** (If you are unable to remember the details of managing this problem, turn to the Emergency Quick Reference on page 160, entitled "Managing Unconsciousness," for a review.)

▶ **HE HAS HAD A CONVULSION/SEIZURE THAT LASTED LONGER THAN FIVE MINUTES—*AND* ALSO HAS A BULGING SOFT SPOT.** (If you are unable to remember the details of managing this problem, turn to the Emergency Quick Reference on page 337, entitled "Convulsions/Seizures," for a review.)

242

ILLNESS IN
INFANTS,
CHILDREN,
AND
ADOLESCENTS

▶ **THE PUPILS OF THE INFANT OR TODDLER'S EYES ARE NOT EQUAL IN SIZE OR DO NOT REACT NORMALLY WHEN YOU SHINE A LIGHT INTO THEM—** *AND* **THE SOFT SPOT IS TENSE OR BULGING.**

When to Call the Doctor Immediately

The following symptoms and signs are serious enough that your infant or toddler will need to be evaluated and treated *within an hour*. Call your child's doctor for advice *immediately*. If you are unable to reach the doctor within fifteen to thirty minutes, take the little one to an emergency room for evaluation, or call the paramedics or an ambulance if you cannot get to an emergency room promptly.

▶ **THE INFANT OR TODDLER HAS SYMPTOMS OF INFECTION—ALONG WITH A TENSE OR BULGING SOFT SPOT.** These include: fever; listlessness or irritability; a rash that looks like broken blood vessels or bruises; neck stiffness; refusal to eat or drink; vomiting.

▶ **THE INFANT OR TODDLER HAS SIGNS OF SEVERE DEHYDRA-TION—ALONG WITH A VERY SUNKEN SOFT SPOT.** Signs of dehydration include: little or no urine for twelve or more hours; sunken eyeballs; dry mouth; dry, doughy skin; listlessness and/or irritability. He or she usually has also been vomiting and/or had severe diarrhea.

243

RECOGNIZING
AND ASSESSING
SERIOUS OR
POTENTIALLY
SERIOUS
ILLNESS

ASSESSMENT CHECKLIST

The Soft Spot (in Infants and Some Toddlers)

ASSESS THE SOFT SPOT BY HOLDING THE SICK INFANT OR TODDLER IN
A SITTING OR UPRIGHT POSITION AND QUIET HIM BEFORE YOU CHECK
THE SOFT SPOT.

yes no Is the soft spot open? (If not,
☐ ☐ then this Assessment Checklist
will not assist you in assessing
the infant or toddler.)

yes no Is his soft spot sunken very
☐ ☐ deeply?

yes no Is her spot bulging above the
☐ ☐ surface of her skull and tense or
hard?

DOES THE INFANT OR TODDLER HAVE ANY OTHER SYMPTOMS THAT
OFTEN OCCUR ALONG WITH A BULGING SOFT SPOT?

yes no Is the infant or toddler having
☐ ☐ difficulty breathing, or breathing
slowly or irregularly?

yes no Is his neck stiff?
☐ ☐

yes no Is she unconscious?
☐ ☐

yes no Has she had a fever or other signs
☐ ☐ of infection?

yes no Is she very lethargic, irritable,
☐ ☐ or difficult to arouse?

yes no Do the pupils of the infant or
☐ ☐ toddler's eyes look normal and
react to light normally?

yes no Has he had a convulsion?
☐ ☐

yes no Does he have a skin rash—es-
☐ ☐ pecially one that looks like broken blood vessels or bruising?

yes no Has he been vomiting or refus-
☐ ☐ ing feedings?

yes no Did the infant or toddler fall, or
☐ ☐ was he or she shaken hard?

244

ILLNESS IN
INFANTS,
CHILDREN,
AND
ADOLESCENTS

yes no Has he had severe or persistent
☐ ☐ vomiting and/or diarrhea?

yes no Are there signs of shock (skin
☐ ☐ color that is pale, pasty, or mottled; cool, clammy skin; severe
weakness; weak, rapid, thready
pulse; anxiety or extreme listlessness)?

yes no Are there signs of serious de-
☐ ☐ hydration (little or no urine for
twelve or more hours; very dry
mouth; sunken eyeballs; weak
cry; dry, doughy skin; severe
listlessness)?

Assessing the Soft Spot

"I never really knew why an infant was born with a soft spot on his or her
head. I was really amazed to find out that this same soft spot could tell me
that my child had a serious illness or problem."

The "soft spot" (fontanel) is an area on
top of an infant or toddler's head that feels
softer than the surrounding bones. It usually
feels round or diamond-shaped and can range
in size from as small as ¼ inch across to
as large as 1½ inches across. The fontanel
is actually an area between the bones of the
skull. This space allows the brain to grow
rapidly within the expanding skull. Essentially, then, it gives the brain leeway to
expand. The normal soft spot closes over
(with bone) after the major part of brain
growth has occurred. This is usually when
the baby or toddler is between twelve months
and eighteen months of age. The brain will
continue to grow, but more slowly, after
the fontanel closes.

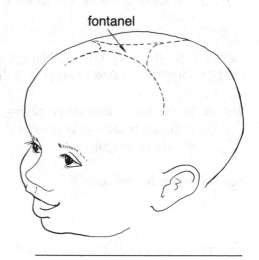

The fontanel (soft spot) is a diamond-shaped area between the bones of
the skull.

Normally, the soft spot is flat (level with the surface of the skull) or slightly sunken
(depressed) when an infant or toddler is sitting up and is quiet. It will *normally* bulge
out and become hard if the baby cries and may bulge a little when he or she is lying
down. (It will not be hard, however.) When the baby is quiet, you might even be able
to feel the fontanel pulsate with the baby's heartbeat.

Even though the fontanel feels soft, the brain underneath is actually well protected
by very tough membranes. Therefore, you don't need to worry about hurting the baby

by gently pushing on the soft spot to check it (or by washing the baby's head, even quite vigorously—something some parents are fearful to do).

It's important for you to feel your baby's soft spot occasionally when he is not sick—so you know what's normal for him. Make sure you check the soft spot when the baby is sitting up and is quiet. In this way, you will know what it feels and looks like when normal and be able to compare this to times when the baby is sick. Obviously, once the fontanel is closed, it is no longer a valuable evaluation tool. By periodically checking the soft spot, you will also know when it has closed and can no longer be used in your evaluation efforts.

Infants and Some Toddlers

THE SOFT SPOT: WHEN SERIOUSLY OR POTENTIALLY SERIOUSLY ILL

"My eleven-month-old seemed very lethargic and nonresponsive this morning. Last night she had a fever of 104 degrees, which we were able to reduce to 102, but it hasn't seemed to make much difference in how she feels. I don't know if this means anything, but when I sat Carrie up, I noticed that her soft spot seemed to be bulging and hard. At first, I wondered if she had hit her head. But then I realized that there was no way she could have bounced on her head right there."

The fontanel is useful in signaling potentially serious illness in infants and some toddlers in whom the soft spot is still present. With some serious illnesses (and injuries), the brain itself swells or there is increased pressure inside the skull. When either of these occur, the soft spot bulges above the surface of the skull and is firm—when the baby is quiet (not crying or screaming) and is sitting (or propped) up. With some other serious illnesses or problems, the fontanel will become *very* sunken (depressed). A depressed fontanel along with vomiting, diarrhea, or both, signals severe dehydration (a very serious situation for an infant or toddler).

Bulging or *deep* depression of the soft spot requires an immediate call to the doctor for advice. Determine what other symptoms the baby or toddler has before calling the doctor, so you can give him or her this information, as well.

THE SOFT SPOT: WHEN MODERATELY OR MILDLY ILL

The soft spot is usually *normal* in infants and toddlers who are mildly or moderately ill. It may be normal in some serious illnesses, as well. If you check the soft spot and

246

ILLNESS IN
INFANTS,
CHILDREN,
AND
ADOLESCENTS

it appears to be normal, continue to look at the infant or toddler for other signs of illness.

THE DON'TS

Don't hesitate to react quickly if your infant or toddler has a tense or bulging soft spot. Problems that cause increased pressure around the brain, and therefore lead to bulging of the soft spot, are very serious and potentially life-threatening.

Don't wait for neck stiffness to appear in an infant or toddler whose soft spot is bulging. In infants and toddlers whose soft spot is open, neck stiffness may not appear until some time after the pressure inside the head is higher than normal.

Don't overreact to a sunken soft spot if your infant or toddler is not ill. It is normal for the soft spot to be somewhat sunken at times in healthy infants. Check your baby's soft spot a few times when he or she is well, so you know how it normally feels.

Don't hesitate to call your child's doctor if you are not sure whether to worry about your sick baby's soft spot. It is better to ask how you can tell for sure whether there is a problem than to misread this important sign of illness.

PLEASE NOTE: Now that you have a grasp of how to assess the soft spot, it would be extremely helpful for you to go back to the Emergency Quick Reference and the Assessment Checklist and review them carefully. The more familiar you are with that material, the more useful it will be to you when you need it.

247

RECOGNIZING
AND ASSESSING
SERIOUS OR
POTENTIALLY
SERIOUS
ILLNESS

EMERGENCY QUICK REFERENCE

Neck Stiffness·

When to Call the Paramedics or an Ambulance

In the following situations, have someone else call the *paramedics* or an *ambulance* (if there are no paramedics in your area) while you treat the youngster. If no one else is with you, continue treating the child while you periodically shout for help. When help arrives, have that person call the paramedics or an ambulance.

▶ **THE YOUNGSTER HAS A STIFF NECK AND IS UNCONSCIOUS OR EXTREMELY DIFFICULT TO AROUSE.** (If you are unable to remember the details of managing this problem, turn to the Emergency Quick Reference on page 160, entitled "Managing Unconsciousness," for a review.)

▶ **HE HAS SEVERE BREATHING DIFFICULTY—ALONG WITH A STIFF NECK.**

▶ **SHE HAS SYMPTOMS AND SIGNS OF SHOCK—ALONG WITH A STIFF NECK.** (If you are unable to remember the details of managing this problem, turn to the Emergency Quick Reference on page 152, entitled "Managing Shock," for a review.)

▶ **THE CHILD SEEMS EXTREMELY ILL, AND YOU ARE UNABLE TO GET HIM TO THE DOCTOR OR AN EMERGENCY ROOM QUICKLY.**

When to Call the Doctor Immediately

The following symptoms and signs are serious enough that your infant, child, or teenager will usually need to be evaluated *within an hour or two*. Call your child's doctor for advice *immediately*. If you are unable to reach the doctor within fifteen to thirty minutes, take the youngster to an emergency room for evaluation.

▶ **THE YOUNGSTER HAS SYMPTOMS AND SIGNS OF INFECTION** (FEVER; LETHARGY; SEVERE HEADACHE; SENSITIVITY OF THE EYES TO LIGHT; AND/OR RASH, ESPECIALLY A RASH THAT LOOKS LIKE SMALL BROKEN BLOOD VESSELS OR BRUISING)—**ALONG WITH THE STIFF NECK.** (If you are unable to remember the details of managing

248

ILLNESS IN
INFANTS,
CHILDREN,
AND
ADOLESCENTS

this problem, turn to the Emergency Quick Reference on page 360, entitled "Meningitis," for a review.)

▶ **THE CHILD SEEMS LISTLESS, IRRATIONAL, OR EXTREMELY IRRITABLE—ALONG WITH HAVING A STIFF NECK (WHETHER OR NOT THERE ARE SYMPTOMS AND SIGNS OF INFECTION).**

When to Call the Doctor Within an Hour or Two

In the following situations, an infant, child, or teenager may require evaluation *within a few hours*. Call your doctor for advice or arrange for the youngster to be seen in an emergency room (if you have no doctor or are not near your doctor).

▶ **THE CHILD HOLDS HER HEAD TO ONE SIDE OR THE OTHER SIDE AND REFUSES TO MOVE HER HEAD FREELY IN ALL DIRECTIONS.**

▶ **HE HAS SWELLING IN THE NECK—ALONG WITH NECK STIFFNESS AND PAIN WHEN HE BENDS OR TURNS HIS NECK.**

When to Call the Doctor for an Appointment

In the following situation, an infant, child, or teenager requires evaluation *within a day or two*. Call your doctor's office to arrange for an appointment.

▶ **A YOUNGSTER MAY HAVE HAD A MILD INJURY AND IS COMPLAINING OF A STIFF NECK—WITHOUT OTHER SIGNS OF INFECTION OR SERIOUS ILLNESS.**

249

RECOGNIZING
AND ASSESSING
SERIOUS OR
POTENTIALLY
SERIOUS
ILLNESS

ASSESSMENT CHECKLIST

Neck Stiffness

TO ASSESS YOUR SICK YOUNGSTER FOR NECK STIFFNESS, HAVE HER TRY TO TOUCH HER CHIN TO HER CHEST.

yes no Can the youngster easily touch
☐ ☐ her chin to her chest?

yes no Does bending his head forward
☐ ☐ cause severe pain in the back of
his neck or head?

IF YOU ARE UNABLE TO ENTICE YOUR CHILD TO TRY TO BEND HIS NECK FORWARD (OR HE IS TOO YOUNG TO UNDERSTAND DIRECTIONS), ATTEMPT TO GENTLY BEND HIS NECK FORWARD.

yes no Can you touch his chin forward
☐ ☐ onto his chest without difficulty?

yes no If the child resists your attempts,
☐ ☐ do you notice that she draws up
her legs and bends her knees
every time you try to bend her
head forward?

ASSESS THE YOUNGSTER FOR OTHER SYMPTOMS COMMONLY ASSOCIATED WITH TRUE STIFF NECK.

yes no Does the youngster have a fe-
☐ ☐ ver?

yes no If the soft spot is open (in an
☐ ☐ infant or toddler), is it tense or
bulging?

yes no Is he unconscious, very difficult
☐ ☐ to arouse, extremely listless, or
very irritable?

yes no Does the youngster object to you
☐ ☐ moving him in any way, even
when you try to comfort him?

yes no Is she complaining of a severe
☐ ☐ headache?

yes no Are there signs of shock (skin
☐ ☐ color that is pale, pasty, or mottled; extreme weakness; dizziness or light-headedness; weak,
thready pulse; cool, clammy
skin)?

yes no Does bright light bother her eyes?
☐ ☐

yes no Is there a rash, especially one
☐ ☐ that looks like tiny broken blood
vessels or bruising?

yes no Is she having any difficulty
☐ ☐ breathing?

250

ILLNESS IN
INFANTS,
CHILDREN,
AND
ADOLESCENTS

ASSESS THE YOUNGSTER FOR OTHER SYMPTOMS THAT COMMONLY POINT TO A MINOR ILLNESS OR INJURY.

yes no Does her pain seem more severe
☐   ☐   or equally severe when she turns
          to one side or the other or looks
          upward?

yes no Do you see any swelling in his
☐   ☐   neck? (Look for enlarged lymph
          nodes on the side or back of the
          neck.)

yes no Has he experienced a possible
☐   ☐   neck injury?

yes no Does he hold his head stiffly—
☐   ☐   especially tilted to one side or
          the other?

Assessing Neck Stiffness

"I've always been confused about what kind of 'neck stiffness' means a serious illness or problem. I mean it's scary to hear that a stiff neck can equal meningitis or other serious problems, but you don't know exactly *what* anyone means by that. So every time one of our children says his or her neck hurts or feels stiff, I get this sick feeling in my stomach and wonder whether I should be rushing to the doctor instead of just standing here worrying if this time it is *the* time and the *for real* stiff neck."

Neck stiffness *is* an important symptom because it can mean serious inflammation or infection of the coverings of the brain and spinal cord (an infection called meningitis). Although neck stiffness can represent other problems, as well, meningitis is such a serious problem that it must be considered first and hopefully ruled out.

As you can imagine, there are many kinds of neck stiffness, but the kind you are looking for is quite specific. Here, neck stiffness means tightness and spasm of the muscles of the neck and back—where the youngster (of any age) *can't or won't be able to bend the neck forward* because of severe pain or muscle stiffness. Essentially, any movement that *stretches* the membranes covering the spinal cord and brain causes spasm and pain. That is why bending the head to touch the chin to the chest (which stretches these membranes) is the best test. Most often, this kind of stiff neck is accompanied by a severe headache, as well.

With stiff necks due to "sleeping wrong," athletic injury, mild flulike illnesses, sore throat, sore neck lymph nodes (called "swollen glands" by some people), pulling a muscle in the neck, and so on, pain and discomfort are often found even when you move the head and neck from side to side or bend the head backward. This is usually not the case when the stiff neck is due to meningitis or other serious illness until the stiffness is really severe. Also, the sensation is more one of discomfort than of really severe pain or true stiffness with these milder problems.

251

RECOGNIZING
AND ASSESSING
SERIOUS OR
POTENTIALLY
SERIOUS
ILLNESS

To check for this kind of neck stiffness, ask the *youngster* to bend her head forward and touch her chin to her chest. If there is *true* neck stiffness, the youngster will *not* be able to do this or will be in severe pain attempting to do so. With a *very young child*, you may have to play a "game" to get him to try this. Have him sit up with his legs stretched out in front of him. Try to get him to look downward at his belly button or at a toy held there. Check to see that the little one bends his head all the way down so his chin touches his chest *without pain or crying*.

An *infant or child* who is too young to play the "game" or who refuses to do so needs to be checked for neck stiffness in a different way. Have her lie flat on her back and put your hand under her head. *Gently* try to bend her head forward and try to touch her chin to her chest. The little one's neck is not stiff if you are able to do this without her crying; drawing up her knees, as well; or stiffening up in an attempt to stop you from causing pain. Be aware that sometimes this test is confusing, because it can be hard to tell if the little one is objecting to your bending the neck forward because it truly hurts or because she just doesn't want to be touched. If you have any questions or concerns about whether there is a potential problem, promptly call your doctor for advice.

Infants and toddlers with stiff necks hold their heads *very still* and try not to move at all. They often cry or fuss if you try to move their heads or even attempt to change their position (for example, turn them on their sides or back). In babies whose soft spots (fontanels) haven't closed, neck stiffness occurs much later than the soft spot's bulging, so be sure always to check the soft spot first (since it would be an earlier sign of a serious problem in these little ones).

Even though mild pain and fussiness upon bending or turning the head can mean mild to moderate illness or injury, it is important that the doctor evaluate the youngster with a stiff neck to rule out the possibility of serious illness.

THE DON'TS

Don't hesitate to get help immediately if a child seems moderately or seriously ill and also has a stiff neck (cannot or will not touch her chin to her chest). Stiff neck, along with other signs of infection, can signal meningitis—a serious infection of the coverings and linings of the brain and spinal cord.

Don't assume a youngster has meningitis if his "stiff neck" means pain only when turning the head to one side or the other. This kind of pain usually means muscle inflammation or injury.

PLEASE NOTE: Now that you have a grasp of how to assess neck stiffness, it would be extremely helpful for you to go back to the Emergency Quick Reference and the Assessment Checklist and review them carefully. The more familiar you are with that material, the more useful it will be to you when you need it.

252

ILLNESS IN
INFANTS,
CHILDREN,
AND
ADOLESCENTS

EMERGENCY QUICK REFERENCE

With the Steps in Detail

Presence and Degree of Dehydration

When to Call the Paramedics or an Ambulance

In the following situations, have someone else call the *paramedics* or an *ambulance* (if there are no paramedics in your area) while you treat the youngster. If no one else is with you, continue treating the child while you periodically shout for help. When help arrives, have that person call the paramedics or an ambulance.

▶ **THE YOUNGSTER SHOWS SIGNS OF SHOCK** (collapse; pale, blue, purple, gray, or mottled skin; weak, rapid, thready heartbeat; cool, clammy skin; severe weakness, dizziness, or light-headedness; anxiety or listlessness)—**ALONG WITH SIGNS OF DEHYDRATION:** very dry mouth; sunken eyeballs; dry, doughy skin that has lost its elasticity; little or no urine for eight to twelve hours. (If you are unable to remember the details of managing this problem, turn to the Emergency Quick Reference on page 152, entitled "Managing Shock," for a review.)

▶ **THE YOUNGSTER IS HAVING SEVERE DIFFICULTY BREATHING, AND HIS SKIN COLOR IS BLUE, PURPLE, OR GRAY—ALONG WITH SIGNS OF DEHYDRATION.**

When to Call the Doctor Immediately

The following symptoms are serious enough that your infant, child, or teenager will usually need to be evaluated *within an hour or two*. Call your child's doctor for advice *immediately*. If you are unable to reach the doctor within fifteen to thirty minutes, take the youngster to an emergency room for evaluation.

▶ **THE YOUNGSTER HAS SIGNS OF SEVERE DEHYDRATION—BUT IS NOT HAVING DIFFICULTY BREATHING AND IS NOT IN SHOCK. THE SIGNS OF SEVERE DEHYDRATION INCLUDE THE FOLLOWING:**

- Very dry, sticky mouth.

- Sunken eyeballs.

253

RECOGNIZING
AND ASSESSING
SERIOUS OR
POTENTIALLY
SERIOUS
ILLNESS

- Very sunken soft spot (in an infant or toddler whose soft spot is open).

- Doughy, wrinkled skin that does not have its usual elasticity.

- Extreme irritability and extreme listlessness.

- Failure to urinate for more than eight hours for an infant, toddler, or young child or twelve hours for an older child or teenager, when there are other signs of dehydration.

When to Call the Doctor Within an Hour or Two

In the following situations, an infant, child, or teenager may require evaluation *within a few hours*. Call your doctor for advice or arrange for the youngster to be seen in an emergency room (if you have no doctor or you are not near or cannot reach your doctor).

▶ **A YOUNGSTER SHOWS SIGNS OF MODERATE DEHYDRATION, IN-CLUDING:**

- Very dry mouth.

- Dry-looking, dull eyes, with few or no tears when the little one cries.

- Extreme thirst.

- Failure to urinate for more than eight hours for an infant or twelve hours for an older child, with small, concentrated amounts of urine, when there are other signs of dehydration.

- Slightly sunken soft spot (in an infant or toddler whose soft spot is open).

▶ **THE YOUNGSTER HAS VOMITING AND/OR DIARRHEA, OR FEVER— ALONG WITH SIGNS OF MILD DEHYDRATION, INCLUDING:**

- Fewer wet diapers in infants or toddlers, or the diapers are just damp rather than wet.

- Urinating fewer times than normal in children and older youngsters.

- Urine that is dark and strong smelling.

- More thirst than usual.

- Refusal to drink more than sips of water or other liquids.

- Dry lips.

254

ILLNESS IN
INFANTS,
CHILDREN,
AND
ADOLESCENTS

- Sticky or "tacky" tongue and mouth.

- Mild listlessness or irritability.

▶ **A YOUNGSTER SEEMS TO BE DEVELOPING SIGNS OF DEHYDRATION IN SPITE OF DRINKING LARGE QUANTITIES OF LIQUIDS AND IS PASSING LARGE AMOUNTS OF PALE, DILUTE URINE.** (If you are unable to remember the details of managing this problem, turn to the Emergency Quick Reference on page 356, entitled "Diabetes Mellitus," for a review.)

When to Call the Doctor for an Appointment

In the following situation, an infant, child, or teenager requires evaluation *within a day or two*. Call your doctor's office to arrange an appointment.

▶ **THE YOUNGSTER IS HAVING SYMPTOMS THAT OFTEN LEAD TO DEHYDRATION** (PERSISTENT VOMITING AND/OR DIARRHEA, PERSISTENT HIGH FEVER, DRINKING OF LESS LIQUID THAN YOU WOULD EXPECT)—**BUT IS NOT SHOWING OBVIOUS SIGNS OF DEHYDRATION.**

255

RECOGNIZING
AND ASSESSING
SERIOUS OR
POTENTIALLY
SERIOUS
ILLNESS

ASSESSMENT CHECKLIST

Presence and Degree of Dehydration

ASSESSING FOR THE PRESENCE AND DEGREE OF DEHYDRATION RE-
QUIRES BEING KEENLY AWARE OF HOW MUCH FLUID THE YOUNGSTER
IS TAKING IN (DRINKING) AND HOW MUCH BODY FLUID HE OR SHE IS
LOSING.

yes no Has the youngster been vomit-
☐ ☐ ing? (If so, how much and for
how long?)

yes no Has the youngster been refusing
☐ ☐ to drink water or other "clear"
liquids for longer than eight to
twelve hours?

yes no Has she had diarrhea? (If so, how
☐ ☐ much and for how long?)

yes no Has he had a fever?
☐ ☐

yes no Does she have both vomiting and
☐ ☐ diarrhea?

ASSESS THE YOUNGSTER FOR SIGNS AND SYMPTOMS OF DEHYDRATION.

yes no Has the infant or toddler had a
☐ ☐ wet diaper in the past eight hours?
(Was the diaper very wet or just
damp?)

yes no Does the infant, toddler, or young
☐ ☐ child produce tears when he cries?

yes no Has the younger child, older
☐ ☐ child, or teenager urinated in the
past twelve hours? (Was there a
large amount of urine or just a
few drops?)

yes no Is she complaining of severe thirst
☐ ☐ (or, if an infant or toddler, acting
thirsty)?

yes no Is the urine very dark in color
☐ ☐ and/or strong smelling?

yes no Are the youngster's eyeballs
☐ ☐ sunken?

yes no Is the inside of his mouth dry or
☐ ☐ sticky?

yes no Is the soft spot deeply sunken (in
☐ ☐ an infant or toddler with an open
soft spot)?

256

ILLNESS IN
INFANTS,
CHILDREN,
AND
ADOLESCENTS

yes no Is his skin dry and doughy or wrinkled?

yes no Does her skin feel as firm and elastic as usual?

yes no Is the youngster very listless?

yes no Is she irritable when you disturb her?

ASSESS THE YOUNGSTER FOR PROBLEMS THAT CAN BE ASSOCIATED WITH DEHYDRATION.

yes no Are there signs of shock (pale or mottled skin; severe dizziness or weakness; rapid, weak, and thready heartbeat; cool, clammy skin; extreme anxiety or irritability; severe listlessness or inability to be aroused), along with signs of dehydration?

yes no Does she complain of severe or persistent pain, particularly in the abdomen?

yes no Is there fever? (If so, how high is it, and for how long has it been a problem?)

yes no Does he appear dehydrated, in spite of drinking large amounts of liquids and urinating in large quantities?

yes no Has the youngster been exercising or playing hard without drinking liquids, especially if the weather is extremely warm?

yes no Does she have sores in her mouth or complain of a sore throat and refuse to drink even sips of liquids?

Assessing Dehydration

"I've always thought that you would look skinny, you know, if you were dehydrated. I've always thought, too, that it was a simple matter of drinking a glass of water or something and the problem would be easily remedied. I guess I never understood it or saw it as a serious thing. I found out . . . with one of my children . . . that I sure was wrong."

Dehydration *is* a serious problem that occurs when an infant or youngster (or an adult, for that matter) loses more body fluids (water) than he or she is able to replace by drinking liquids. Dehydration, then, is simply a reduction in the amount of fluid

257

RECOGNIZING
AND ASSESSING
SERIOUS OR
POTENTIALLY
SERIOUS
ILLNESS

in the body. But there's nothing else simple about it. Dehydration is a serious problem because of the domino effect it can have on the body's organs, systems, and functions—damaging *or* destroying one right after the other as the severity of the dehydration worsens. And dehydration can be a viciously rapid problem and become totally out of control.

Most people do not fully appreciate what an important role water plays in the human body. Did you know that, at birth, water makes up 75 percent to 85 percent of the baby's body weight? In the childhood years, water (although less than at birth) totals 65 percent to 70 percent of the child's weight. And nearly 60 percent of an older youngster's or teenager's weight is composed of water. All in all, that's a lot of water and points to the importance that it plays in human existence.

Did you know that every cell in the body has water as one of its vital components? Not only is water vital to the life of every cell—water also surrounds the cells as a special protective cushion. In addition, a good deal of our blood is composed of water. Water is also found in bone and connective tissue (muscles, ligaments, tendons) and is an important component of the fluid that surrounds the brain and spinal cord. Without water, waste products could not be purged from the body. The list goes on and on, but the point is that water is an *essential* component of life!

There's another aspect of this, as well. When dehydration occurs, the sensitive chemical balance of the body is disrupted. Special chemicals called electrolytes (composed of potassium, sodium, magnesium, chloride, bicarbonate, calcium, and organic phosphates, to name a few) are vital to maintaining water volume and balance in the body. This is accomplished by a very complex and sophisticated biochemical process.

When dehydration takes place, abnormal amounts of electrolytes, as well as water, are lost in the process. We naturally lose fluids *and* electrolytes through perspiration, urination, respiration, and the gastrointestinal system. Electrolytes and fluids can also be decreased through burns and through blood loss—for example, due to a wound. Vomiting and diarrhea are further ways of losing fluids and electrolyes.

When more fluids are lost than are taken into the body, a "thirst" mechanism is automatically tripped, and the fluid is replaced by drinking water or other beverages. In fact, partial dehydration is a natural daily occurrence. The process is actually finely tuned. We lose water, get thirsty, and replace the water lost (and stop drinking when the balance is regained). Notice how thirsty children get after vigorous exercise or when out in the hot weather. That's because they have lost a lot of fluid through perspiration and respiration (the harder you breathe, the more water is used). But it's usually a simple matter of having a few glasses of water, juice, cola, or another drink to replenish the fluids lost.

When fluids are *not* replaced, however, the domino effect begins. To protect and maintain remaining fluids and electrolytes, blood flow to the kidneys is reduced, and a special mechanism in the kidneys diminishes the amount of urine released. This is the body's "automatic fluid-conservation system"—less water is lost to the outside of the body through the urine. Less saliva and fewer tears are produced to further

258

ILLNESS IN
INFANTS,
CHILDREN,
AND
ADOLESCENTS

conserve fluid. The water that cushions the cells is reduced, making the skin look dry and doughy and lose its elasticity. When water loss becomes greater, waste chemicals accumulate in the body fluids (they are not processed through the kidneys and released through the urine). As the cells of the body get sicker and the tissues have less fluid, the cells burn fuel (glucose) less efficiently. This inefficient metabolism leads to a buildup of excess acid (known as acidosis). Acidosis itself leads to further "poisoning" of the cells, and the domino effect proceeds.

One of the most serious consequences of dehydration is a reduction in blood volume. The body's protective mechanisms keep the blood flow and pressure as close to normal as possible—for as long as possible. If the dehydration is not treated, blood volume becomes critically low, and blood flow becomes inadequate. The body then goes into shock. The heartbeat can become rapid and irregular. The person becomes weak and eventually drops into coma. What all of this means is that when severe dehydration occurs, it can cause kidney failure and heart failure and can damage or destroy other organs and systems. Ultimately, the brain can be damaged or die from lack of oxygen (due to inadequate blood flow to the brain).

Each of us has a special "thirst mechanism" that tells us we are thirsty—so we drink something. Infants, however, present a unique problem. They cannot say, "Hey, mom or dad, I'm thirsty!" Because of this, infants and nonverbal toddlers are at greater risk for dehydration than other age groups. Small and even older children who are sick must also be watched carefully to ensure that they are drinking an adequate amount of fluids. This is particularly important if the infant or youngster is experiencing severe diarrhea and vomiting or has a prolonged high fever. In fact, the infant or child with *severe* diarrhea (watery and frequent) or *severe* vomiting (where he or she just can't keep much [or anything] down) is at great risk for dehydration.

However, the possibility of dehydration should *not* alarm you—if you know the infant or child is drinking an adequate amount of liquids. Also, by knowing the *warning signs* of dehydration, you can take appropriate action early—long before the problem becomes serious or critical. Even if severe dehydration occurs rapidly (it can be a gradual or more rapid process), you can take immediate action because you *know* what the problem is and can get the youngster prompt medical attention. The fact of the matter is, there is no reason to overreact to the potential for dehydration. It is much more important to know what it is, the symptoms it displays, and what to do if mild, moderate, or severe dehydration does occur. Most often, people just don't know what is happening to the child. By knowing the warning signs, people can frequently recognize dehydration before it becomes severe and dangerous.

One note: An often-asked question is why an IV (intravenous) solution is started before someone goes into surgery or when he or she is seriously ill. These special solutions provide the necessary fluids for the body to function normally, electrolytes to maintain the correct chemical balance, and a sugar for fuel. An IV in place also provides a "direct" line for medications to be administered rapidly. IVs are also inserted whenever people are unable to drink enough liquids (because they are either too sick, too weak, experiencing severe vomiting and diarrhea, or unconscious).

All Ages

DEHYDRATION: WHEN SERIOUSLY OR POTENTIALLY SERIOUSLY ILL

"I think something is terribly wrong. Bobby is just thirteen months old and has never been really sick before. For the last twenty-four hours, though, he's been vomiting and having diarrhea. I really didn't feel worried until this morning. He was very hard to wake up and keeps going back to sleep. His body seems limp and floppy. He seems pale to me, and his eyes look strange . . . sort of sunken or dark. As I think about it, he's only wet his diaper once in the last fourteen hours, and it was more damp than wet."

The symptoms of severe dehydration apply to all age groups. If an infant, toddler, young child, older child, or teenager experiences severe dehydration, you would see some or all of the following symptoms. The youngster would be extremely lethargic, and his body would feel limp and weak. He may also be quite irritable and appear anxious, and (if he is little) his cry would be weak. He may have very sunken eyeballs and dark circles under his eyes. These, however, would look different from the dark circles we usually think of as meaning lack of sleep. The dark circles associated with dehydration arise because of the sunken eyeballs. His skin may be very dry and feel doughy or wrinkled. When you stretch it or pinch up a small amount of skin, it would not be as elastic as normal (not bounce back to its usual place and shape quickly).

With severe dehydration, you will notice that the youngster has had no or little urine production in over twelve to twenty-four hours. Obviously, it's easier to pinpoint this in infants and children still in diapers! But if you're worried about dehydration, watch the youngster to see how often she goes to the bathroom and tell an older youngster to let you know when she goes to the bathroom.

A very depressed (sunken-in) soft spot is a sign of severe dehydration in infants and toddlers with soft spots (fontanels) still present. However, this is a late sign of severe dehydration and requires a rapid response.

When dehydration becomes life-threatening and there is no longer enough water to allow the blood to circulate properly, the youngster might go into shock. You should have had ample warning that there was a problem before this, but once in a while, dehydration happens so rapidly that it might sneak up on you. With shock, the skin may be very pale and mottled, or even bluish. If you press on the skin, the color will not return rapidly. The youngster will have a very fast, thready pulse and will show signs of deepening lethargy. Breathing is rapid or irregular, and the youngster eventually loses consciousness. If emergency intervention does not occur immediately, the child could die from the shock.

260

ILLNESS IN
INFANTS,
CHILDREN,
AND
ADOLESCENTS

When symptoms of severe dehydration occur, it is vital that you *take the child to an emergency room immediately*. If the child is having any trouble breathing, shows signs of shock, is unconscious because of dehydration, or you cannot make it to the emergency room within five to ten minutes, then *call the paramedics for assistance*.

If you must go to the emergency room, call your doctor (if possible) and either talk with him or her or leave a message that you are taking the child to the emergency room. (Make sure you tell the answering service *which* hospital is your destination and why you are going there.)

When dehydration occurs (particularly moderate to severe dehydration), the youngster is most often hospitalized, and an IV (intravenous solution) is started to replace fluid and electrolyte losses. It usually takes twelve to twenty-four hours of IV therapy to replace the fluids and electrolytes lost.

DEHYDRATION:
WHEN MODERATELY OR MILDLY ILL

"I'm not sure if I should be concerned or not. My seven-year-old has been sick with the stomach flu, or at least she's been vomiting a lot. Karen keeps saying she's thirsty but just can't keep much of anything down. Her lips are now very dry, and she says her mouth feels funny. I've noticed that she hasn't been going to the bathroom much. Most of the time, when I ask her if she'd like some help in getting to the bathroom, she says, 'Mommy, I don't have to go.' The last time she went, I was surprised that her urine was dark yellow and smelled strong. There wasn't much there, either."

One of the earliest signs of dehydration is a decrease in urine production and output. In other words, you will notice that when the infant, child, or older youngster urinates, the amount of urine is reduced, the urine becomes more concentrated (stronger), and the young person urinates less often than usual. As noted previously, this is the body's automatic fluid-conservation method—its way of trying not to lose too much fluid.

With *mild dehydration*, you will notice: fewer wet diapers in infants and toddlers (damp rather than the normally soaked diaper); urinating fewer times a day in children and older youngsters; urine that is strong smelling and dark yellow in color; dry lips; greater thirst than normal; and sticky or "tacky" dry tongue and mouth. There will be no drooling in infants and younger children, and you won't see much (if any) saliva in all age groups. The amount of tears a little one has gets less and less. When the tongue and mouth (of any age youngster) become sticky or "tacky" dry—that means that mild dehydration is moving into moderate dehydration.

When the infant, toddler, young child, older child, or teenager reaches the sticky mouth and tongue stage, it's important to call the doctor and get advice within two to three hours. The doctor may want to suggest further home treatment, see the child, or begin IV (intravenous) treatment immediately (but this will depend on the individual child and specific circumstances). Home care can be very successful in treating a youngster who is mildly dehydrated, but this needs to be done with the doctor's supervision, so you'll know how to gauge your success. This is especially true with very young infants, whose condition can change rapidly with only small variations in the amount of body water.

When the body's automatic fluid-conservation methods stop working and the mild dehydration has not been successfully treated, mild dehydration progresses to moderate dehydration, and other symptoms begin to appear.

With *moderate dehydration*, you may see all or some of the following symptoms: no wet diapers for more than eight to twelve hours in infants and toddlers; urinating less often than every twelve hours in small children, older children, and teenagers (with small, concentrated amounts of urine); very dry mouth; extreme thirst; irritability and listlessness; dry-looking, dull eyes, with no tears; and *slightly* sunken soft spot (fontanel) in infants and toddlers who still have an open soft spot.

When moderate dehydration occurs, it is important to call the doctor *and* get help within an hour or so. If you cannot reach the doctor or he or she does not return your call within about forty-five minutes, call or take the young person to the emergency room. Make sure you tell the emergency-room personnel that you tried to reach your doctor, so they can call and advise him or her of the situation.

One note: If severe diarrhea and/or severe vomiting continue for over twenty-four hours, you must assume dehydration is progressing to a stage where medical intervention may be necessary. Check for signs and symptoms to verify this, but also call the doctor for advice. Obviously, if signs of moderate to severe dehydration occur before the twenty-four-hour period is up—then take the action recommended for moderate or severe dehydration right away. (Since vomiting and diarrhea are very common problems, they are described and discussed in detail in Chapter 14.)

THE DON'TS

Don't delay in getting immediate medical care for your youngster if he or she has signs of severe or moderate dehydration. The situation can worsen quickly, leading to shock and potentially serious or life-threatening problems.

Don't hesitate to contact your doctor if you are unsure about whether or not your youngster is becoming dehydrated. The doctor can help you to determine whether or not you should be concerned and can tell you what steps to take to prevent dehydration if your youngster is at risk for developing problems.

PLEASE NOTE: Now that you have a grasp of how to assess the presence and degree of dehydration, it would be extremely helpful for you to go back to the Emergency Quick Reference With the Steps in Detail and the Assessment Checklist and review them carefully. The more familiar you are with that material, the more useful it will be to you when you need it.

262

ILLNESS IN
INFANTS,
CHILDREN,
AND
ADOLESCENTS

EMERGENCY QUICK REFERENCE

With the Steps in Detail

Level and Length of Fever

When to Call the Paramedics or an Ambulance

In the following situations, have someone else call the *paramedics* or an *ambulance* (if there are no paramedics in your area) while you treat the youngster. If no one else is with you, continue treating the child while you periodically shout for help. When help arrives, have that person call the paramedics or an ambulance.

▶ **THE INFANT OR YOUNG CHILD HAS A FEVER—AND IS HAVING A CONVULSION THAT HAS LASTED FOR LONGER THAN FIVE MINUTES.** (If you are unable to remember the details of managing this problem, turn to the Emergency Quick Reference on page 337, entitled "Convulsions/Seizures," for a review.)

▶ **THE YOUNGSTER HAS A FEVER, IS HAVING DIFFICULTY BREATHING—AND HIS SKIN COLOR IS BLUE, PURPLE, OR GRAY.**

▶ **THE CHILD HAS A RASH CAUSED BY BROKEN BLOOD VESSELS** (tiny red dots that don't disappear when you press on the skin or larger blood spots that look like bruises)—**AND SHOCK** (collapse; pale, blue, or mottled skin; a weak, rapid, thready heartbeat; severe anxiety, listlessness, or agitation; cool, clammy skin)—**ALONG WITH FEVER.**

When to Call the Doctor Immediately

The following symptoms are serious enough that your infant, child, or teenager will usually need to be evaluated *within an hour or two*. Call your child's doctor for advice *immediately*. If you are unable to reach the doctor within fifteen to thirty minutes, take the youngster to an emergency room for evaluation.

▶ **AN INFANT, TODDLER, OR YOUNG CHILD HAS HAD A CONVULSION THAT HAS STOPPED BY ITSELF WITHIN FIVE MINUTES—AND HAS A FEVER.**

263

RECOGNIZING
AND ASSESSING
SERIOUS OR
POTENTIALLY
SERIOUS
ILLNESS

- Take steps to reduce the fever while you wait to talk to the doctor and/or before you go to the emergency room.

- Remove the child's clothing.

- Give the little one the correct dose of acetaminophen (Panadol, Tylenol, or similar medication).

- Sponge her with lukewarm water, or put her into a bathtub containing lukewarm water.

▶ **HE HAS A STIFF NECK—ALONG WITH A FEVER.**

▶ **AN INFANT OR TODDLER HAS A TENSE OR BULGING SOFT SPOT—WITH A FEVER.**

▶ **THE YOUNGSTER HAS A RASH CAUSED BY BROKEN BLOOD VESSELS** (tiny red dots that don't disappear when you press on the skin or larger blood spots that look like bruises)—**ALONG WITH A FEVER (WITH OR WITHOUT A STIFF NECK OR A BULGING SOFT SPOT).**

▶ **THE YOUNGSTER IS HAVING DIFFICULTY BREATHING—ALONG WITH A FEVER, OR HE IS EXPERIENCING RAPID BREATHING AFTER THE FEVER HAS BEEN REDUCED.**

▶ **SHE HAS SIGNS OF MODERATE OR SEVERE DEHYDRATION ALONG WITH A HIGH FEVER.** (If you are unable to remember the details of managing this problem, turn to the Emergency Quick Reference on page 352, entitled "Dehydration," for a review.)

When to Call the Doctor Within an Hour or Two

In the following situations, an infant, child, or teenager may require evaluation *within a few hours.* Call your doctor for advice or arrange for the youngster to be seen in an emergency room (if you have no doctor or you are not near or cannot reach your doctor).

▶ **THE CHILD (OF ANY AGE) SEEMS VERY ILL OR MUCH SICKER THAN YOU WOULD EXPECT, REGARDLESS OF THE DEGREE OF FEVER HE HAS.**

264

ILLNESS IN
INFANTS,
CHILDREN,
AND
ADOLESCENTS

➤ **THE YOUNGSTER HAS SEVERE PAIN** (for example, severe sore throat, difficulty swallowing, abdominal pain, back pain, and so on)—**ALONG WITH A FEVER.**

➤ **AN INFANT YOUNGER THAN TWO MONTHS OF AGE HAS A FEVER OVER 101 DEGREES—WITH OR WITHOUT OTHER SIGNS OF IN-FECTION.**

➤ **THE TODDLER OR YOUNG CHILD'S FEVER IS OVER 105 DE-GREES—REGARDLESS OF HER OTHER SYMPTOMS.**

- Take steps to reduce the fever while you wait for the doctor to reach you or before you go to the emergency room.

When to Call the Doctor for an Appointment

In the following situations, an infant, child, or teenager requires evaluation *within a day or two.* Call your doctor's office to arrange an appointment.

➤ **A YOUNGSTER HAS HAD FEVER FOR LONGER THAN TWENTY-FOUR TO FORTY-EIGHT HOURS—AND SEEMS MODERATELY UN-COMFORTABLE OR ILL.**

➤ **HE HAS MILD SYMPTOMS ALONG WITH A LOW FEVER—AND THE FEVER HAS LASTED FOR LONGER THAN FORTY-EIGHT HOURS.**

➤ **YOU ARE UNSURE ABOUT WHETHER THE YOUNGSTER HAS A PROBLEM THAT REQUIRES TREATMENT.**

➤ **YOUR CHILD SEEMS TO GET FREQUENT FEVERS WITHOUT AP-PARENT CAUSE.**

265

RECOGNIZING
AND ASSESSING
SERIOUS OR
POTENTIALLY
SERIOUS
ILLNESS

ASSESSMENT CHECKLIST

Level and Length of Fever

ASSESS THE YOUNGSTER FOR THE PRESENCE AND LEVEL OF FEVER.

yes no Does the youngster feel hot to the touch? (Check his forehead and abdomen, in particular.)

yes no Is the temperature over 101 degrees (if the baby is under two months old)?

yes no Does she feel warmer than usual, but not hot?

yes no Is the temperature over 105 degrees (for children older than two months)?

yes no Have you taken her temperature with a thermometer? How did you check the temperature (by mouth, by rectum, or in the armpit)?

DETERMINE HOW LONG THE YOUNGSTER HAS HAD THE FEVER.

yes no Did the fever just start?

yes no Has the fever persisted for longer than twenty-four to forty-eight hours?

yes no Has the youngster had the fever for less than twenty-four hours?

ASSESS THE PATTERN OF THE FEVER.

yes no Does the fever come and go on its own, without any treatment?

yes no Is the fever present or at its highest in the late afternoon and evening hours, and is the fever low or the temperature normal during the daytime?

yes no Does the fever go down when you treat the youngster with acetaminophen, then go up again after a few hours?

266

ILLNESS IN
INFANTS,
CHILDREN,
AND
ADOLESCENTS

ASSESS THE YOUNGSTER BOTH WHEN THE FEVER IS HIGH AND AFTER THE FEVER HAS COME DOWN.

yes no Does she seem very ill (very listless or lethargic or very irritable) when she has the fever?

yes no Does he improve a great deal after you have been successful in lowering his fever?

yes no Is he very active in spite of the fever?

yes no Does the youngster seem hungry?

yes no If she is not hungry, will she drink liquids?

ASSESS THE YOUNGSTER FOR OTHER SYMPTOMS OR SIGNS THAT COMMONLY OCCUR WITH A FEVER.

yes no Has the child had a convulsion? If so, for how long did it last?

yes no Are there any obvious signs of infection (for example, congestion, cough, earache, sore throat)?

yes no Does the youngster have a stiff neck and/or severe headache?

yes no Is the infant or toddler's soft spot bulging above the surface of the skull?

yes no Is he experiencing severe pain or continuously whimpering or crying?

yes no Has she experienced any vomiting or diarrhea?

yes no Are there any signs of dehydration?

yes no Does he or she have a rash?

yes no Has the youngster been exposed to anyone who has had a similar problem?

Assessing Fever

267

RECOGNIZING
AND ASSESSING
SERIOUS OR
POTENTIALLY
SERIOUS
ILLNESS

"Even the word *fever* frightens me. It always has! When I was a child, the minute I didn't look right or said I didn't feel well, the first thing my parents and other adults would whisper was, 'Oh dear, I hope she doesn't have a fever!' Then out would come all the hands pressing against my forehead and under my chin. They always had such worried looks on their faces. If they didn't like what they felt, the frowns would deepen, and out would come the thermometer.

"By the time I was a teenager, every time I didn't feel well, the first thing I'd think was 'Oh dear, I hope I don't have a fever.' What's funny about this is that I've *never* really understood what a fever is and what it really means when you're sick. To me, it was and still continues to be something to fear. So every time one of my small children doesn't feel well . . . guess what? Yup, I whisper, 'Oh dear, I hope . . .' Well . . . you know the rest!''

Sound familiar? Even if you don't feel this way, you probably know countless other people who do. To them, fever is frightening, and most were taught to see fever as some ominous, unexplainable phenomenon. Some people think fever causes illness, while others think fever is a disease. The fact is, there is a great deal of misunderstanding when it comes to what fever is and isn't. Understanding fever, knowing when it is significant and when it should concern you, not only would be useful to you—but also would help you avoid undue concern and fear when you have little to worry about.

Essentially, fever is merely an abnormal rise in body temperature. It is not a disease. It does not cause illness. Most often, a fever *signals* the presence of an illness (but sometimes, a rise in body temperature can be perfectly normal, too). It is simply a symptom, usually of illness—one of the many indicators that helps point to a possible cause of the problem, and one of many gauges that helps determine the possible seriousness of a problem.

Usually, fever tells us that there is an infection in the body. But other things can cause a rise in body temperature, as well. For example, if you took a youngster's temperature after vigorous exercise on a hot day—you might find his or her temperature as high as 101 degrees. Some metabolic (general bodily function) problems such as overactive thyroid gland cause a rise in body temperature. Some people have "heat intolerance" and experience a rise in body temperature just by being out in the sun. Still others who have defects in their ability to sweat cannot keep their body temperature regulated in extreme heat. And there are many other noninfectious causes of fever, too. *Fever standing alone—no matter how high—does not point to a specific illness. Nor does fever standing alone—no matter how high—necessarily signal serious illness.* It's important to remember that *the level of fever that may signal a potentially serious*

268

ILLNESS IN
INFANTS,
CHILDREN,
AND
ADOLESCENTS

illness varies from age group to age group. The fact is, it's all the symptoms that occur *with* a fever that really tell us how sick a youngster may actually be.

You should also know that there is a *normal variation* in body temperature throughout the day. The body temperature is at its lowest in the early morning hours and rises as the day progresses. That means the body's temperature will be higher in the late afternoon or early evening and highest in the evening hours. This variation in range (usually a matter of tenths of degrees when a youngster is well) often frightens parents when a youngster is sick.

For example, a child's temperature will be slightly higher at 9:00 P.M. than when a parent took it that same afternoon. Many parents call the doctor late at night, embarrassed and frustrated—embarrassed because they feel they should have caught this earlier and frustrated because they thought this fever was under control! Of course, parents call because they fear the problem is getting worse and will be out of control by morning. Unless the fever has jumped dramatically (over 104 degrees) and cannot be reduced, a rise of one to three degrees at night should actually be expected during an illness.

There is also a *range* in the so-called normal temperature. The traditional 98.6 degrees is not the magical number people are led to believe it is. In some youngsters, their *normal* temperature is slightly higher than 98.6 degrees, and in others, their *normal* temperature is lower than 98.6 degrees. Knowing this, you will be much less worried when the thermometer registers 99 or 100 degrees.

How you take a youngster's temperature can make a difference in the reading, as well. Many people try to "guess" how high the temperature is without actually measuring it. While it is very true that most people can tell that a child has an elevated body temperature because he or she "feels" warmer than usual or even downright hot, *no one* can accurately measure how high a fever is without a thermometer.

As noted, most often parents (and others) suspect a fever when a child's skin feels warmer than usual. The best areas of the body to feel for a fever are the forehead and/ or the abdomen. Use the back of your hand rather than your palm, or the tops of your fingers. Your skin is thinner in these areas and more sensitive to slight temperature changes than the thicker palm side of the hand or even the fingertips. Touch the skin lightly rather than pushing hard against it.

If you suspect a high fever or you are not sure if a sick youngster has a mild fever, measure the temperature. It's the only way to know for sure if the youngster has a fever and how high it is. An infant or toddler's temperature is usually measured in the rectum, using a rectal thermometer (it has a blunt end). Lubricate the mercury-containing end (silver color) with petroleum jelly or a similar lubricant and gently insert it into the rectum about one inch. You'll have to hold the child still so he or she doesn't roll around or kick and risk getting hurt. Most children are more easily held still while on their tummies rather than lying on their backs. Be sure to hold the thermometer at all times.

Wait for two to three minutes, then gently remove the thermometer. To read the temperature, roll the thermometer back and forth slowly, until you can see the level

269

RECOGNIZING
AND ASSESSING
SERIOUS OR
POTENTIALLY
SERIOUS
ILLNESS

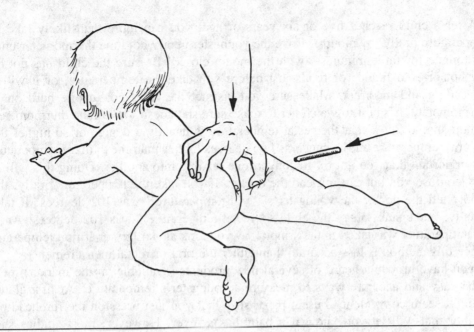

Rectal temperatures are most reliable in infants and young children, and are not difficult to measure.

of the mercury. You'll need to read the temperature in degrees. (Each of the tiny lines is equal to 0.2 degree.) So if the mercury reads one tiny line past 98.6 degrees—the youngster's temperature is 98.8 degrees. If two tiny lines past 100 degrees, the youngster's temperature is 100.4 degrees (called "one hundred point four" or "one hundred and four-tenths"). The rectal method is the most accurate way to measure body temperature until your child is five to six years old.

If a young child does not cooperate when you try to take the temperature rectally and is too young for you to use an oral thermometer, you can measure what is called the axillary temperature (which is taken in the armpit). All you need to do is gently place the mercury end of the thermometer high up in the armpit and hold the child's arm down against his or her side for five minutes. The trick here, as you can imagine, is holding the child's arm to his or her side for five minutes—which seems like an eternity to young children! Read the thermometer as usual.

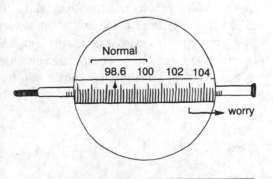

It's important to learn to read a thermometer correctly.

270

ILLNESS IN
INFANTS,
CHILDREN,
AND
ADOLESCENTS

After a child reaches five or six years of age, you can more than likely take her temperature orally (by mouth). Have the youngster gently hold the thermometer under her tongue for three minutes—with the mouth closed! Be sure the child has not had any hot or cold liquids or foods just before you take the temperature, or it will be misleading and incorrect. Make sure you instruct the child not to bite hard on the thermometer. (It's best to watch her to make sure she doesn't break the thermometer.)

You should know that the rectal temperature is usually a degree or so higher than the oral temperature and as much as two degrees higher than the axillary temperature. It's important that you not try to convert one reading into another. Doing this will not only confuse you but can mislead the doctor. If you take the temperature orally, then simply tell the doctor the youngster's ''oral temperature'' was 102 degrees. If taken rectally, make sure to say the child's ''rectal temperature'' was 102 degrees. And if the temperature was taken in the armpit, say you took an axillary or armpit temperature (since this method is less accurate than either the oral or rectal measurement).

You have probably heard of several new products (available on the market) meant to be easy and accurate ways to measure a youngster's temperature. At first glance, it might seem convenient to use a paper strip that you just press on the forehead or a pacifier that will let you know if a baby has a fever. However, most studies show these new products to be quite unreliable, and relatively expensive at that. It is always best to use the good ''old-fashioned'' standard mercury thermometer if you are going to measure the temperature at all.

By the way, you can use the blunt-ended ''rectal'' thermometer for any method of measurement. This is the type to have in your ''mini–medicine center,'' and you don't need to buy an ''oral'' thermometer once a child reaches five or six years old. As long as you leave the blunt thermometer in the mouth for three minutes, it will have time to register the correct temperature. Just be sure you wash the thermometer *well* (with soap and *cold* water) before and after every use.

If you feel the child is only mildly warm and is not showing other signs that worry you, it is not necessary to measure his or her temperature. Likewise, it is perfectly reasonable to feel the youngster's skin periodically during a known illness to see if fever is still a problem, rather than taking the temperature repeatedly. You will be able to tell the difference between ''a little warmer than usual'' and ''burning up.'' Once you know that fever is or is not present, and approximately how high the temperature is, you don't need to be compulsive about using the thermometer. (This is particularly true if a youngster fights you when you try to measure the temperature.)

Infants and Toddlers

271

RECOGNIZING
AND ASSESSING
SERIOUS OR
POTENTIALLY
SERIOUS
ILLNESS

FEVER: WHEN SERIOUSLY OR POTENTIALLY SERIOUSLY ILL

"I picked up Jacob to give him a hug, when I realized he was very hot. He was so little, only six weeks old, that I just felt panic-stricken. His temperature was 101.5 degrees, which was a relief, since I had heard children usually have very high fevers when they're sick. So I decided not to call the doctor. By the next morning, Jacob seemed so spacey and distant, but really irritable when I tried to change him or play with him. I called the doctor immediately. I didn't know a slight fever in very young infants was a potential danger signal."

As noted previously, when you are trying to determine the potential significance of a fever, you need to remember that the level of fever that signals a possible problem *varies from age group to age group*. It's also vital for you to determine if there are any other symptoms (besides the fever), because a set of symptoms will tell you (and the doctor) more about how serious the problem might be than the height and length of the fever alone.

A fever over 101 degrees in *an infant under two months old* is often significant and can indicate a *potentially serious illness*. Even though this is a relatively low fever (for other age groups), with these tiny babies, any fever over 101 degrees should prompt a call to the doctor for advice.

In contrast, *babies older than two months of age* can have significantly higher fevers before you should be concerned about the fever alone. If a baby or toddler has a 105-degree fever—with or without other symptoms—it's important to begin home treatment immediately (including medication to reduce fever, sponging the child with lukewarm water, and/or placing him or her in a tub of lukewarm water). Most doctors would like a call within an hour or two when this level of fever has been reached.

If a baby over two months old or a toddler experiences a fever of 103 degrees or 104 degrees (with no other serious symptoms) and you cannot reduce it with home treatment within twenty-four hours, or the fever lasts off and on for longer than twenty-four hours—it is important to call the doctor. These specific situations do not always point to serious illness, but they can.

Again, it's important to evaluate all other indicators of potentially serious illness before you call the doctor. If an infant or toddler has a fever *with* other symptoms that signal potentially serious illness, then begin treating the fever, but call the doctor promptly.

272

ILLNESS IN
INFANTS,
CHILDREN,
AND
ADOLESCENTS

FEVER: WHEN MODERATELY OR MILDLY ILL

''Danny had been running a 104-degree fever for a while, but we were finally able to get it down to 100.4 degrees and keep it there. He has a stuffy nose, some diarrhea, and is very cranky. He seems so miserable to me. He's only fourteen months old, and I just can't believe this could only be a cold or the flu.''

Between two months and two years of age, infants and toddlers tend to run rather high fevers—sometimes even over 104 degrees—with many kinds of illnesses (the vast majority being mild or moderate). Fevers between 101 degrees and 104 degrees, without other symptoms, most often point to a mild to moderate viral infection or illness. Although fever at this level can be a signal of a more severe disease, it is usually not the fever that will tip you off that the problem is more serious.

Again, it is the other symptoms that the infant or toddler experiences along with the fever that point either to a serious illness or to a mild to moderate problem. In babies and toddlers over six months old, temperatures between 100 degrees and 102 degrees are not only common but also most often do *not* mean serious disease (and for that matter, may not signal any worrisome disease).

Young Children

FEVER: WHEN SERIOUSLY OR POTENTIALLY SERIOUSLY ILL

''My five-year-old had a 104-degree fever. At first, I thought he was sleepy because of it. I gave Benjamin Tylenol and got his temperature down to 102 degrees, but he didn't seem much better. Four hours later, his temperature went back up to 104 degrees, and he vomited, too. I was able to get the fever down again, but Benjamin didn't seem much better at all.''

Since young children tend to run much higher temperatures than older youngsters with the *same illness*, it's nearly impossible to give an absolute ''worry level'' that would apply to children of all ages. Therefore, different age groups have to be handled separately. When it comes to young children, most doctors want to know about fevers of 105 degrees or higher (even when there are *no other symptoms*) within an hour or two from the time you have recognized the fever and taken the temperature. But it's important to start home treatment first (including medication to reduce fever, sponging the child with lukewarm water, and/or placing him or her in a tub of lukewarm water).

If your young child has a fever of 103 degrees or 104 degrees (but no other symptoms) and you cannot reduce the fever over a twenty-four-hour period (or it keeps coming

273

RECOGNIZING
AND ASSESSING
SERIOUS OR
POTENTIALLY
SERIOUS
ILLNESS

back off and on for more than twenty-four hours), then it is important to call the doctor. Also, any fever over 101 degrees lasting more than four days, even if there are no other symptoms, should prompt a call to the doctor for advice.

It's vital to remember that when fever stands alone, it is usually not a worrisome problem—unless it cannot be reduced with home treatment. On the other hand, *any level of fever* that occurs with *other* symptoms of serious illness should prompt you to call the doctor for advice.

The point is, most of the time a young child with high fever (because of a mild illness) feels and looks better once the fever is treated and reduced. But a young child with a potentially serious illness will not look, feel, or act significantly better once the fever is treated and reduced. Essentially, the higher the fever goes, the sicker the child looks (from the fever alone). But once the fever is treated and reduced, the youngster should look and feel much better. If not, it is not the fever alone that is causing the discomfort. It's vital, then, to look for other symptoms that point to serious illness.

A word about fever and convulsions: Although relatively uncommon, convulsions occur in some children with fevers over 103 degrees. These are called febrile seizures and are seen in one in every twenty to twenty-five children, usually between the ages of six months and four years. More than half the children who experience a febrile seizure never have another one, and nearly all the children who have febrile seizures are otherwise completely normal. The fear of febrile seizures is much greater than the actual incidence of them.

If your young child has had a temperature of 103 degrees or 104 degrees and has not experienced a febrile seizure, the chance that he or she will with another fever is quite low. Most children who experience febrile seizures have a rapid increase in their body temperature (in other words, the temperature shoots up so quickly that often the seizure is the first indicator to a parent that the child has a fever).

A fever over 103 degrees is treated *mostly* for the comfort of the child and also to reduce the risk of a febrile seizure's occurring. (For more on febrile seizures, see Chapter 13.)

FEVER: WHEN MODERATELY OR MILDLY ILL

"All I've ever heard about is how children have convulsions when they get a high fever. So when my six-year-old woke up one morning with a 102.5-degree temperature, I just jumped in the car and took her to the doctor. I found out I had overreacted! They gave her some Tylenol and removed the layers of clothing I had bundled her up in the minute I realized she had a fever. Within two hours, her temperature was near-normal."

Of all symptoms, fever is the one that most people overreact to and don't understand. We have been led to believe that young children should be bundled up and the doctor called at the first sign of a fever. You do want to keep the child from getting chilled (because it's uncomfortable and is the body's way of actually getting the temperature

274

ILLNESS IN
INFANTS,
CHILDREN,
AND
ADOLESCENTS

higher). However, you only increase his discomfort by bundling him up so he feels even hotter. Dress him in light clothing and give him aspirin substitute if he is uncomfortable.

Especially in young children, high fevers of 103 degrees to 104 degrees most often mean mild viral infections, as long as the little one looks and feels otherwise well. These fevers should not cause you undue concern if they last less than three or four days. Fevers lower than 102 degrees (that last less than three or four days) and not associated with other symptoms of illness also usually mean the child is experiencing a viral infection.

As with all age groups, the height of a fever is not as significant as the length of the fever, as well as the other symptoms that occur at the same time. They will be the *real* clues about what might be wrong and how serious the problem might be.

Older Children and Teenagers

FEVER: WHEN SERIOUSLY OR POTENTIALLY SERIOUSLY ILL

"I'm really concerned about Mary. Because she's never been sick much, I wasn't sure if a 103-degree fever was something to worry about in a twelve-year-old. I've tried to get it down and keep it down for the last three days using Panadol. But it keeps going up and down, up and down. Now I've noticed that she just isn't herself at all. She seems irritable, hard to wake up, and vomited once this morning."

Temperatures over 102 degrees are rather unusual in older children and teenagers and may signal a serious illness. However, here, too, the symptoms that occur along with the fever are very important in determining how serious the problem is or isn't. If a youngster experiences a fever of 102 degrees (or greater) with no other symptoms and you are unable to reduce it after forty-eight hours, it's important to call the doctor for advice.

As is the case with all other age groups, it's important to notice whether the youngster looks and feels better once a fever is reduced. Most youngsters look, feel, and even act greatly improved once a fever is reduced—if the problem is mild to moderate. If more serious, the youngster may not look or feel substantially better nor act much like his or her usual self—even once the fever is reduced.

Most often, with older children and teenagers, there will be other symptoms besides fever that will signal the problem as being more serious or less worrisome. It's important to remember that the presence of a fever by itself doesn't tell you very much. When it comes to fever, what is important to recognize is the set of symptoms. Therefore, if the youngster has fever and other signs of serious illness, then call the doctor immediately for advice.

FEVER: WHEN MODERATELY OR MILDLY ILL

''I just couldn't understand it. Bill would come home after high school and just didn't look quite himself. He seemed really tired, more than I'd expect. After a few days of this, I took his temperature. It was 101.5 degrees. Later that evening, it was normal again. This went on for a week. He'd come home with a temperature of 101 or 102 degrees and looking tired. The fever was always gone by evening, and he said he was fine. I finally took Bill to the doctor fearful of some terrible disease like cancer. He came out smiling. It seems that football practice in the heat was the culprit. I never knew vigorous exercise and heat could make anyone's temperature rise.''

When it comes to older children and teenagers, you really have to be aware of the other things besides illness that can raise the body temperature. Calls are made to doctors each year because a youngster is experiencing an off-and-on fever. With further questioning, it becomes obvious that the youngster's problem is not really a problem at all, but a normal rise in body temperature due to vigorous exercise—especially when the weather is hot.

Fevers under 102 degrees in older children and teenagers, associated with other mild symptoms, usually mean mild to moderate illness. However, as noted previously, fevers over 102 degrees in the older child or teenager can signal serious illness, or at least illness that requires detection and treatment. Therefore, it is best to call the doctor for advice whenever an older child or teenager experiences a fever higher than 102 degrees for over forty-eight hours. Again, look for other symptoms that point to serious illness, since these—and not the fever alone—are the best clues as to the severity of the problem.

THE DON'TS

Don't delay in getting immediate medical help (by calling either the paramedics or your doctor) if an infant, toddler, young child, older child, or teenager seems very ill with a fever. In other words, the youngster is truly lethargic, unresponsive, and has other symptoms of serious illness—along with a fever. Take steps to start reducing the fever while you wait.

Don't hesitate to call your doctor if you are unsure about whether or not a youngster with a fever needs to be evaluated by the doctor.

Don't overreact to a fever in an infant over two months old, a toddler, a young

276

ILLNESS IN
INFANTS,
CHILDREN,
AND
ADOLESCENTS

child, an older child, or a teenager if the youngster seems otherwise mildly or moderately ill. Children run higher fevers than adults with most illnesses and are able to tolerate fevers much better. Be sure, however, to take steps to treat the fever if it is over 103 degrees or if the youngster seems uncomfortable with the fever.

PLEASE NOTE: Now that you have a grasp of how to assess the level and length of fever, it would be extremely helpful for you to go back to the Emergency Quick Reference With the Steps in Detail and the Assessment Checklist and review them carefully. The more familiar you are with that material, the more useful it will be to you when you need it.

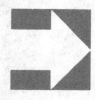

EMERGENCY QUICK REFERENCE

With the Steps in Detail

Appetite and Feeding Behavior

When to Call the Paramedics or Ambulance

In the following situations, have someone else call the *paramedics* or an *ambulance* (if there are no paramedics in your area) while you treat the youngster. If no one else is with you, continue treating the child while you periodically shout for help. When help arrives, have that person call the paramedics or an ambulance.

▶ **THE YOUNGSTER IS REFUSING TO DRINK ANY LIQUIDS AT ALL—AND HAS SIGNS OF SHOCK:** collapse or extreme lethargy; rapid, weak, thready heartbeat; agitation or irritability; cold, clammy skin. (If you are unable to remember the details of managing this problem, turn to the Emergency Quick Reference on page 152, entitled "Managing Shock," for a review.)

▶ **SHE HAS BEEN REFUSING TO DRINK—AND IS NOW DIFFICULT OR IMPOSSIBLE TO AROUSE.**

▶ **HE HAS NOT BEEN DRINKING AT ALL—AND NOW HAS SEVERE DIFFICULTY BREATHING, OR SLOW, IRREGULAR BREATHING—AND A BLUE, PURPLE, OR GRAY SKIN COLOR.**

277

RECOGNIZING
AND ASSESSING
SERIOUS OR
POTENTIALLY
SERIOUS
ILLNESS

When to Call the Doctor Immediately

The following symptoms are serious enough that your infant, child, or teenager will usually need to be evaluated *within an hour or two*. Call your child's doctor for advice *immediately*. If you are unable to reach the doctor within fifteen to thirty minutes, take the youngster to an emergency room for evaluation.

▶ **THE YOUNG INFANT APPEARS SICK IN ANY OTHER WAY** (fever, constant or unusual crying, lethargy or listlessness, and so on) **AND— COMPLETELY REFUSES TWO CONSECUTIVE FEEDINGS.**

▶ **THE YOUNGSTER REFUSES TO DRINK EVEN SMALL AMOUNTS OF LIQUIDS—AND HAS SIGNS OF MODERATE OR SEVERE DEHYDRA-TION:** little or no urine, very dry mouth, poor skin elasticity, sunken eyeballs, listlessness, severe weakness, dizziness, irritability. (If you are unable to remember the details of managing this problem, turn to the Emergency Quick Reference on page 352, entitled "Dehydration," for a review.)

▶ **HE REFUSES TO DRINK EVEN SMALL AMOUNTS OF LIQUIDS—AND IS VOMITING A GREAT DEAL AND/OR HAVING SEVERE DIARRHEA.**

▶ **SHE IS NOT DRINKING LIQUIDS—AND IS COMPLAINING OF SE-VERE PAIN** (for example, abdominal pain, sore throat, and so on).

▶ **THE INFANT APPEARS TO HAVE BREATHING DIFFICULTY THAT IS SEVERE ENOUGH TO MAKE IT IMPOSSIBLE OR VERY DIFFICULT FOR HER TO NURSE OR DRINK FROM A BOTTLE.**

When to Call the Doctor Within an Hour or Two

In the following situations, an infant, child, or teenager may require evaluation *within a few hours*. Call your doctor for advice or arrange for the youngster to be seen in an emergency room (if you have no doctor or are not near or cannot reach your doctor).

▶ **THE YOUNGSTER IS DRINKING VERY LITTLE—AND HAS MODER-ATE OR SEVERE DIARRHEA.** (If you are unable to remember the details of managing this problem, turn to the Emergency Quick Reference on page 399, entitled "Diarrhea," for a review.)

278

ILLNESS IN
INFANTS,
CHILDREN,
AND
ADOLESCENTS

▶ **SHE IS DRINKING ONLY SMALL AMOUNTS OF LIQUIDS—AND HAS SIGNS OF MILD DEHYDRATION** (little or no urine, dry mouth, and listlessness).

When to Call the Doctor for an Appointment

In the following situations, an infant, child, or teenager requires evaluation *within a day or two*. Call your doctor's office to arrange an appointment.

▶ **THE YOUNGSTER IS EATING AND/OR DRINKING VERY LITTLE (FOR MORE THAN TWENTY-FOUR HOURS)—AND IS HAVING OTHER SYMPTOMS THAT POINT TO A MILD OR MODERATE ILLNESS** (such as mild or moderate breathing difficulty, fever, pain, and so on)—**EVEN IF SHE HAS NO SIGNS OF DEHYDRATION.**

▶ **HE HAS HAD LITTLE OR NO APPETITE FOR MORE THAN ONE WEEK—WITH OR WITHOUT OTHER SYMPTOMS.**

▶ **THE CHILD HAS HAD A NORMAL OR INCREASED APPETITE FOR FOOD OR LIQUIDS—BUT APPEARS TO BE LOSING WEIGHT.**

279

RECOGNIZING
AND ASSESSING
SERIOUS OR
POTENTIALLY
SERIOUS
ILLNESS

ASSESSMENT CHECKLIST

Appetite and Feeding Behavior

Infants, Toddlers, and Small Children Who Do Not Talk

ASSESS THE APPETITE AND FEEDING BEHAVIOR OF THE INFANT, TODDLER, OR SMALL CHILD, PAYING PARTICULAR ATTENTION TO WHAT HE WILL EAT AND HOW MUCH HE WILL DRINK.

yes no Is he eating and drinking normally or nearly normally?

yes no Is she refusing all or most of her solid foods (if she usually takes them), accepting only small amounts of her favorite foods?

yes no Will he nurse for short periods of time, or take small amounts of his regular formula or milk?

yes no Does she drink water, fruit juice, or commercial electrolyte solution (such as Pedialyte or Gatorade)? If so, how much?

yes no Has he completely refused to drink anything? For how long?

yes no If a young infant, has he refused more than two consecutive feedings?

yes no Does she seem interested in eating or drinking at all?

yes no Does he suck as vigorously as usual when nursing or taking a bottle?

IF THE INFANT, TODDLER OR SMALL CHILD IS REFUSING ALL LIQUIDS, ASSESS WHETHER HE HAS OTHER SYMPTOMS THAT POINT TO A SERIOUS OR POTENTIALLY SERIOUS ILLNESS.

yes no Is he very lethargic, or difficult to arouse?

yes no Is she having enough breathing difficulty to interfere with sucking?

yes no Are there any signs of dehydration (little or no urine, dry mouth, sunken eyeballs, weakness, listlessness, poor skin elasticity)?

yes no Does she gag or spit out the liquids you offer her?

280

ILLNESS IN
INFANTS,
CHILDREN,
AND
ADOLESCENTS

yes no Has he been vomiting?

yes no Does she have diarrhea?

yes no Does he cry, whimper, or act as if he is in pain?

yes no Is his abdomen swollen, hard, or tender if you press on it?

yes no Are there any signs of serious infection (fever, lethargy, irritability, bulging soft spot, stiff neck, rash, and so on)?

yes no Does she look as if she has lost weight?

Small Children Who Talk, Older Children, and Teenagers

ASSESS THE APPETITE AND FEEDING BEHAVIOR OF THE CHILD OR TEENAGER, PAYING PARTICULAR ATTENTION TO WHAT SHE WILL EAT AND HOW MUCH SHE WILL DRINK.

yes no Does she say she is hungry? (If so, for what?)

yes no Is he thirsty? (If so, for what?)

yes no Is she eating any solid foods? (If so, how much and how often?)

yes no Have you been able to entice him to eat his favorite foods?

yes no Will he drink liquids? (If so, is he drinking more than usual, or less than usual? How much at a time?)

yes no Has she refused to drink anything? (For how long?)

yes no Do you have to constantly encourage or nag the youngster to drink more than a few sips of water, juice, or other liquid?

ASSESS THE YOUNGSTER FOR OTHER SYMPTOMS THAT POINT TO A SERIOUS OR POTENTIALLY SERIOUS PROBLEM.

yes no Is the youngster lethargic or extremely listless?

yes no Is he showing signs of a serious infection (high fever, stiff neck, headache, rash, shock, and so on)?

yes no Does she complain of severe pain anywhere? (If so, where?)

yes no Has he lost weight?

ASSESS THE CHILD TO HELP YOU DETERMINE WHAT MIGHT BE CAUSING HIS APPETITE PROBLEM OR HIS REFUSAL TO EAT.

yes no Is he experiencing nausea (feel-
☐ ☐ ing sick to his stomach)?

yes no Is he having pain? (If so, where
☐ ☐ and how severe is it?)

yes no Has she vomited?
☐ ☐

Assessing Appetite and Feeding Behavior

"He's always had such an excellent appetite. Something just has to be wrong if he won't even touch his most favorite foods!"

A child's appetite is *one of the most sensitive indicators of how sick* he or she is or isn't. The fact of the matter is, very few infants, toddlers, children, or teenagers who are seriously ill eat much of anything. And more important, a seriously ill youngster will usually not readily drink enough liquids—which is a much more serious symptom.

However, it is vital that parents and others take careful note of *exactly* what an infant, child, or older youngster *eats and drinks* over a period of time. Parents often misinterpret the problem because they really don't know how much food or how much liquid a youngster has actually consumed. Therefore, if you feel your child is not eating or drinking adequately and wish to determine the seriousness of the problem, then it is best to write down exactly what and how much he or she ate or drank and the time it was consumed. In this way, you can more precisely determine the *overall amount* of foods and/or liquids consumed over a period of time.

What you need to pay particular attention to is if the child is getting *enough liquids*. This is much more important than how much or how little a youngster eats. It is important to write the information down, because most people judge what a youngster eats or drinks by what he or she consumes during the three major meals of the day— and forget about what the child may be snacking on throughout the day and night. The time to really worry is when an infant, toddler, small child, older child, or teenager won't drink any liquids at all. This leads to very serious problems and in itself may signal serious illness.

282

ILLNESS IN
INFANTS,
CHILDREN,
AND
ADOLESCENTS

Infants and Toddlers

APPETITE AND FEEDING BEHAVIOR: WHEN SERIOUSLY OR POTENTIALLY SERIOUSLY ILL

"Blair seemed to have a little diarrhea, so I wasn't surprised when she refused to breast-feed and wouldn't take water either. I figured if I wouldn't eat with an upset stomach and diarrhea—why should a five-month-old! My problem was, I didn't know how long to allow this to go on. She always seemed to be such a hardy baby that I decided twenty-four hours wouldn't make much difference. By morning, she was very sick, and now I feel horrible that I waited so long."

A seriously ill infant or toddler will most often refuse several feedings. She may not only refuse solid foods (if she already takes them) but will also refuse liquids. Most parents find it difficult to judge "how long" to wait to see if this is a momentary problem due to a mild or moderate illness or a warning sign of a potentially serious disease.

A rule of thumb to follow is this: If a *baby under six months of age completely refuses more than two consecutive feedings and won't take water or juice either*—it is important to contact the doctor. Similarly, if a sick baby over six months of age or a toddler refuses to drink at least half of her usual amount of liquid in a twenty-four-hour period, contact the doctor. This rule is especially vital if the infant or toddler is also vomiting and/or having diarrhea. Of course, act more quickly if there are any other signs of obviously serious illness.

APPETITE AND FEEDING BEHAVIOR: WHEN MODERATELY OR MILDLY ILL

"Sara isn't taking much when she's breast-feeding and is only drinking about half her bottle of juice. She won't even touch solid foods or water but did have about two ounces of apple juice this afternoon. At this rate, she'll starve to death, won't she?"

Unlike a seriously ill infant who will not eat or drink, an infant or toddler who is mildly to moderately ill will continue to eat and drink, but in lesser amounts than usual. She may tolerate only small amounts of food or refuse most (or all) solid foods but will drink some liquids—sometimes more than usual for her. It's as if food just doesn't taste good to her, but liquids can be tolerated or might even be refreshing.

283

RECOGNIZING
AND ASSESSING
SERIOUS OR
POTENTIALLY
SERIOUS
ILLNESS

The best way to put this into perspective is to think of how *you* usually feel when you have a cold, flu, or other mild to moderate illness. Food just isn't very appealing, although you might have a few favorite foods you eat "a little of" when you're sick (chicken soup, hot cereal, mashed potatoes, Jell-O, pudding, and so on). However, unlike an older child or adult, a baby is very limited in the number of solid foods he is able to eat normally. If the baby enjoys pudding or yogurt, then keep to those foods when he's feeling poorly, and emphasize liquids for the most part.

If possible, try to determine the cause of his poor appetite. Does he have a fever? Is his throat red, or are there patches or sores in his mouth, making it painful to swallow or even have food or certain liquids in his mouth? Does she appear to be nauseated or experiencing abdominal pain (pulling her legs up to her stomach, objecting when you move her or touch her stomach)? Is she just too weak or listless to eat much? Having some idea as to the cause will help you determine whether you need to call the doctor or can treat the baby at home.

Young Children

APPETITE AND FEEDING BEHAVIOR: WHEN SERIOUSLY OR POTENTIALLY SERIOUSLY ILL

"We knew it couldn't just be the flu when Theresa opened her eyes just long enough to look at her favorite grape juice and close her eyes again. Even though we pleaded for just a few little sips, she moaned that she was sleepy."

Young children who are seriously ill usually totally refuse to eat solid foods. Most often, they must be forced to drink even small amounts of liquid but may become upset when forced to do so. Others may be just too lethargic and sleepy to even try to drink. Often, they act as if they don't even care whether they eat or drink anything and are not in touch with their parents' pleas for even a few sips of juice, soda, or water. Some children will tell you why they can't eat or drink (no appetite, stomachache, and so on), but most will simply say they "can't" or just turn their heads away.

284

ILLNESS IN
INFANTS,
CHILDREN,
AND
ADOLESCENTS

Older Children and Teenagers

APPETITE AND FEEDING BEHAVIOR:
WHEN SERIOUSLY OR POTENTIALLY SERIOUSLY ILL

''You may laugh, but we didn't know John was really sick until he refused
to take more than one sip of his favorite cola. It was always the thing we
could count on when he was sick. This time, it was different.''

Even though seriously ill, the older child or teenager will usually understand why
it is important to eat and drink something. Parents can often reason with these youngsters
but will find themselves having to constantly encourage the youngsters to drink enough
fluids. Most will refuse to eat food and only take a sip or two of a liquid.

Parents surprisingly find that it takes a great deal of time and lots of coaxing to get
the youngster through one glass of even his or her favorite soda or juice. Most older
children and teenagers will volunteer an explanation for their behavior—they have no
appetite, feel nauseated, have a sore throat, nothing tastes good, they're too tired, it's
too much trouble, or it takes too much of an effort.

Young Children, Older Children, and Teenagers

APPETITE AND FEEDING BEHAVIOR:
WHEN MODERATELY OR MILDLY ILL

''I'm really concerned that Jeremy's health and well-being are being jeopardized. He'll eat only chocolate pudding and popsicles. He's drinking a lot
of grape juice, too. I'll tell you, the combination of chocolate pudding,
popsicles, and grape juice sounds just horrible! This can't be good for someone who's sick!''

Mildly to moderately ill young children, older children, and teenagers will usually
have reduced appetites but can be enticed to eat their favorite foods—unless they are
very nauseated. Many parents worry that because their children are not eating whole-
some, well-balanced meals, their health will be impaired or their recovery from illness
prolonged.

If a youngster has been healthy before experiencing a mild to moderate illness,
eating relatively poorly will *not* damage his health or slow down the healing process—

285

RECOGNIZING
AND ASSESSING
SERIOUS OR
POTENTIALLY
SERIOUS
ILLNESS

if the poor nutritional habits do not persist longer than a week or two. Although it would be better if the youngster would eat well-balanced meals—you just can't expect this when he is ill. Unless the illness itself requires a special diet (which the doctor would give you to follow) or the illness is expected to be prolonged beyond several weeks, it is better to let the young person eat and drink what tastes the best to him and in the amounts he can tolerate. When we worry about how much a youngster eats (or refuses to eat), we tend to overlook how many calories are in the drinks he takes or the "snacks" he nibbles on. We also forget that he is not as active as usual and so doesn't need quite as much food for "fuel." We fear that the youngster will starve. Not so (and force-feeding the "good" foods is not the answer either)!

As noted previously, a youngster's appetite is an excellent gauge of the degree of his or her illness. Therefore, a sick youngster who has a normal appetite is almost always mildly ill. In the same sense, you can use the reappearance of a good appetite as an excellent indicator that a youngster is returning to normal health.

THE DON'TS

Don't delay in calling the doctor if an infant under six months of age who appears to be ill completely refuses more than two consecutive feedings. This can be a symptom of serious illness, and the baby needs to be evaluated promptly.

Don't forget that a child's appetite can be a very good indicator of the seriousness of an illness. Children who are seriously ill usually will eat very little or nothing (and may need to be forced to drink liquids). On the other hand, a youngster who has a normal appetite is usually only mildly ill.

Don't worry excessively about a youngster who will drink normal or large amounts of liquids when sick, but will not eat solid foods. This is very common—and is not harmful. He will not suffer from malnutrition if this goes on for as long as a week! (However, after that length of time, it's a good idea for the youngster to be evaluated by the doctor.)

Don't forget that the return of a child's normal appetite is an excellent indicator that she is getting well.

PLEASE NOTE: Now that you have a grasp of how to assess appetite and feeding behavior, it would be extremely helpful for you to go back to the Emergency Quick Reference With the Steps in Detail and the Assessment Checklist and review them carefully. The more familiar you are with that material, the more useful it will be to you when you need it.

286

ILLNESS IN
INFANTS,
CHILDREN,
AND
ADOLESCENTS

EMERGENCY QUICK REFERENCE

The Skin (Including Color, Temperature, Texture, and Rash)

When to Call the Paramedics or Ambulance

In the following situations, have someone else call the *paramedics* or an *ambulance* (if there are no paramedics in your area) while you treat the youngster. If no one else is with you, continue treating the child while you periodically shout for help. When help arrives, have that person call the paramedics or ambulance.

▶ **THE YOUNGSTER'S SKIN IS BLUE, PURPLE, OR GRAY ALL OVER, (INCLUDING THE INSIDE OF HIS MOUTH)—AND HE IS HAVING DIFFICULTY BREATHING.**

▶ **THE YOUNGSTER'S SKIN IS VERY PALE, PASTY, OR MOTTLED, AND COLD AND CLAMMY—ALONG WITH OTHER SIGNS OF SHOCK, SUCH AS WEAKNESS, DIZZINESS, AND A WEAK, RAPID, THREADY PULSE.** (If you are unable to remember the details of managing this problem, turn to the Emergency Quick Reference on page 152, entitled "Managing Shock," for a review.)

▶ **SHE HAS A RASH CAUSED BY BROKEN BLOOD VESSELS** (tiny red dots that don't disappear when you press on her skin, or larger blood spots that look like bruising)—**ALONG WITH SIGNS OF SHOCK, ESPECIALLY IF AN INFANT OR TODDLER HAS A BULGING SOFT SPOT AND/OR A CHILD OF ANY AGE HAS A TRUE STIFF NECK, AND/OR HAS HAD A CONVULSION.**

▶ **THE YOUNGSTER HAS SUNKEN EYEBALLS, WRINKLED SKIN, AND DRY MOUTH—ALONG WITH SIGNS OF SHOCK, ESPECIALLY IF SHE HAS HAD VOMITING AND/OR DIARRHEA.** (If you are unable to remember the details of managing this problem, turn to the Emergency Quick Reference on page 352, entitled "Dehydration," for a review.)

▶ **HE HAS SWELLING AROUND THE EYES AND FACE, ITCHING, AND DIFFICULTY BREATHING—WITH OR WITHOUT HIVES (A RED, BLOTCHY RASH).** (If you are unable to remember the details of managing this problem, turn to the Emergency Quick Reference on page 324, entitled "Anaphylaxis," for a review.)

287

RECOGNIZING
AND ASSESSING
SERIOUS OR
POTENTIALLY
SERIOUS
ILLNESS

When to Call the Doctor Immediately

The following symptoms are serious enough that your infant, child, or teenager will usually need to be evaluated *within an hour or two*. Call your child's doctor for advice *immediately*. If you are unable to reach the doctor within fifteen to thirty minutes, take the youngster to an emergency room for evaluation.

▶ **THE CHILD HAS SUNKEN EYEBALLS, DRY MOUTH, AND WRINKLED SKIN WHICH DOES NOT HAVE ITS USUAL ELASTICITY—ALONG WITH OTHER SIGNS OF SEVERE DEHYDRATION** (listlessness, poor urine output, weak cry, and/or a very sunken soft spot in an infant or toddler), **ESPECIALLY IF SHE HAS HAD VOMITING AND/OR DIARRHEA.** (If you are unable to remember the details of managing this problem, turn to the Emergency Quick Reference on page 352, entitled "Dehydration," for a review.)

▶ **SHE HAS A RASH CAUSED BY BROKEN BLOOD VESSELS** (tiny red dots that don't disappear when you press on the skin, or larger blood spots that look like bruises) **AND APPEARS ILL—ESPECIALLY WITH SYMPTOMS OF A FEVER, WITH OR WITHOUT A TRUE STIFF NECK AND/OR BULGING SOFT SPOT IN AN INFANT OR TODDLER.**

▶ **HE HAS HIVES** (red, blotchy rash that itches), **WITH OR WITHOUT PUFFINESS AROUND THE FACE—BUT IS HAVING NO DIFFICULTY BREATHING.** (If you are unable to remember how to manage this problem, refer to the Emergency Quick Reference on page 324, entitled "Anaphylaxis," for a review.)

▶ **THE CHILD HAS HOT, FLUSHED OR PALE SKIN—ALONG WITH A FEVER OVER 105 DEGREES (OR AN INFANT UNDER TWO MONTHS OF AGE HAS A FEVER OVER 101 DEGREES)—AND ANY OTHER SIGNS OF SERIOUS ILLNESS.**

When to Call the Doctor Within an Hour or Two

In the following situations, an infant, child, or teenager may require evaluation *within a few hours.* Call your doctor for advice or arrange for the youngster to be seen in an emergency room (if you have no doctor or are not near or cannot reach your doctor).

288

ILLNESS IN
INFANTS,
CHILDREN,
AND
ADOLESCENTS

▶ **THE YOUNGSTER HAS A NEW RASH—ALONG WITH OTHER SIGNS OF POTENTIALLY SERIOUS ILLNESS** (fever over 103 degrees, dramatic changes in behavior, persistent crying, persistent or recurring pain, mild to moderate vomiting and/or diarrhea, refusal to drink liquids, and so on).

▶ **HIS MOUTH AND LIPS ARE VERY DRY—ALONG WITH OTHER SIGNS OF DEHYDRATION** (reduced urine, listlessness, irritability, severe thirst)— **AND HE HAS HAD VOMITING AND/OR DIARRHEA, OR REFUSES TO DRINK LIQUIDS.**

▶ **A YOUNG INFANT HAS VERY YELLOW SKIN—ALONG WITH YELLOW COLOR OF THE WHITES OF HER EYES.**

▶ **AN OLDER CHILD'S EYES ARE YELLOW—WITH OR WITHOUT APPARENT YELLOW SKIN.**

▶ **YOU NOTICE ANY CHANGES IN SKIN COLOR, TEMPERATURE, OR TEXTURE—ALONG WITH OTHER SIGNS OR SYMPTOMS THAT MAKE THE YOUNGSTER APPEAR QUITE ILL.**

When to Call the Doctor for an Appointment

In the following situations, an infant, child, or teenager requires evaluation *within a day or two*. Call your doctor's office to arrange an appointment.

▶ **A CHILD APPEARS QUITE PALE—WITH OR WITHOUT OTHER SYMPTOMS OF ILLNESS.**

▶ **SHE HAS A RASH THAT YOU ARE UNABLE TO EXPLAIN OR UNDERSTAND—BUT DOES NOT APPEAR SERIOUSLY ILL.**

▶ **HE APPEARS TO HAVE DARK CIRCLES UNDER HIS EYES—OR PERSISTENT OR REPEATED PUFFINESS OF THE EYES, HANDS, OR FEET.**

289

RECOGNIZING
AND ASSESSING
SERIOUS OR
POTENTIALLY
SERIOUS
ILLNESS

ASSESSMENT CHECKLIST

The Skin (Including Color, Temperature, Texture, and Rash)

ASSESS THE COLOR OF THE YOUNGSTER'S SKIN BY LOOKING CAREFULLY AT HIS ENTIRE BODY, AS WELL AS IN HIS MOUTH.

yes no Is the child's overall color blue, purple, or gray? (Be sure to check his body, fingertips, face, lips, and inside his mouth.)

yes no Is her skin flushed or more red than usual?

yes no Is her skin mottled (speckled with blue, pink, purple, and white spots)?

yes no Is his skin yellow? (If so, are the whites of his eyes also yellow?)

yes no Is he more pale than usual?

PRESS ON THE YOUNG PERSON'S SKIN, THEN RELEASE THE PRESSURE AND WATCH WHAT HAPPENS TO THE COLOR.

yes no Does the color return quickly after you release the pressure on the child's skin?

ASSESS THE TEMPERATURE OF THE YOUNGSTER'S SKIN, ESPECIALLY ON THE FOREHEAD AND THE ABDOMEN.

yes no Does her skin feel normal in temperature?

yes no Is his body dry?

yes no Is his skin very hot?

yes no Is her body moist or clammy?

yes no Is her skin much cooler than usual?

290

ILLNESS IN
INFANTS,
CHILDREN,
AND
ADOLESCENTS

ASSESS THE TEXTURE OF THE YOUNGSTER'S SKIN BY LOOKING AT AND FEELING THE SKIN.

yes no Does he look swollen or more "puffy" than usual? (Check his eyes, hands, and feet.)

yes no Is her skin rough and dry?

yes no Do her eyes look sunken?

yes no Does her skin feel "doughy," or does it stay tented up when you gently pinch it?

yes no Are there dark circles under the youngster's eyes?

yes no Does his skin feel as firm and elastic as usual?

yes no Is his skin dry and wrinkled?

LOOK CAREFULLY FOR A RASH THAT YOU MAY NOT HAVE SEEN BEFORE. MAKE A NOTE OF THE COLOR OF ANY RASH, AS WELL AS WHERE YOU FIRST NOTICED IT.

yes no Does the youngster have a rash? (If so, where is it located?)

yes no Are there any blisters? (If so, how big are they? Where are they?)

yes no Does the rash look like small red or purple spots of blood, or like bruising?

yes no Does the rash itch? (Is he scratching or rubbing the rash?)

yes no Can you feel the rash? (It might feel bumpy, rough like sandpaper, or like welts.)

yes no Is her skin peeling or cracking?

ASSESS THE YOUNGSTER FOR OTHER SYMPTOMS THAT CAN BE ASSOCIATED WITH CHANGES IN SKIN COLOR, TEMPERATURE, TEXTURE, AND RASH.

yes no Does the youngster have a fever?

yes no Is the soft spot bulging (in an infant or toddler) or is there neck stiffness in a youngster of any age?

yes no Is she having trouble breathing?

291

RECOGNIZING
AND ASSESSING
SERIOUS OR
POTENTIALLY
SERIOUS
ILLNESS

yes no Is he lethargic or difficult to
☐ ☐ arouse?

yes no Is she experience vomiting and/
☐ ☐ or diarrhea?

yes no Has she had a seizure?
☐ ☐

yes no Is he urinating normally?
☐ ☐

yes no Does he have signs of shock
☐ ☐ (weak, rapid, thready pulse; dizziness; weakness and so on)?

yes no Is she eating and/or drinking
☐ ☐ normally?

Assessing the Skin

"I've heard over and over again to look for changes in skin color or see if
I can find a rash. So I look and I look and I look. The problem is, I'm not
really sure what I'm looking for—and even if I find 'it,' I have no idea what
it means. There's just got to be some method to this madness."

The skin and the tissue right under it—called the subcutaneous ("under the skin")
tissue—make up the largest organ of the body. Yes, the skin is considered an "organ"!
Skin protects the underlying organs and structures from countless insults and plays a
role in temperature regulation. As the largest organ, it is also the most visible. Any
change or "blemish" is readily apparent to all who look closely. Because of this, the
skin and its changes during certain illnesses can provide clues to what might be wrong
and how serious the problem might be.

This easy visibility has its drawbacks, as well. Many of us tend to overreact to
things we see on our skin—and that of our children. This, in part, is the result of
what we've heard or been taught. But another factor is also important—especially
when it comes to rashes and blemishes. How our skin looks is really part of our
identity—our "image." If there is a serious problem with the skin—particularly a
disfiguring or scarring one—this can have an impact on us for a long time, sometimes
even for a lifetime. We are therefore naturally very protective and concerned when
we or one of our children has a skin problem. But the kind of skin problems most
people are concerned with (rashes, birthmarks, acne, and so on) are not the same
things (other than newly appearing rashes) that we need to talk about here.

Skin evaluation can be a vital way of determining the presence or absence of serious
illnesses or problems. Essentially, when you are evaluating the skin, you are actually
looking for signs and symptoms of dehydration, fever, shock, oxygen deprivation, and
rashes that would herald serious or potentially serious illness. The skin is therefore
evaluated in four areas: (1) color, (2) temperature, (3) texture, and (4) rash. *Your
assessment is basically the same for all age groups*, although the key symptoms that
point to problems vary slightly from age group to age group.

292

ILLNESS IN
INFANTS,
CHILDREN,
AND
ADOLESCENTS

Skin Color: What You Should Know

The color of the skin is determined by both the pigments found in its cells and the blood flowing beneath it. Normally, each individual has a specific color and complexion that is determined by his or her genes. This skin coloring results from the number and location of granules of melanin pigment—which are plentiful in dark-skinned people and relatively few in fair-skinned people. The type of complexion a person is born with tends to stay the same throughout his or her life. Changes in skin pigmentation (tanning or darkening or freckling) are almost always caused by exposure to sunlight rather than by illness.

However, minute-to-minute and hour-to-hour changes in skin color occur for different reasons. The pink or "flesh" color of the skin is the result of blood flowing under and through the skin and its underlying tissue. Blood carrying oxygen is bright red, while blood that has little or no oxygen in it appears deep purple or blue. For example, you can see the veins close to the skin. They appear bluish because they carry nonoxygenated blood back to the lungs to pick up oxygen. Arteries, which are deep inside the tissues, would appear redder if they could be seen, because they carry oxygenated blood from the lungs to the tissues. The tiny blood vessels in the skin (called capillaries) carry blood that is mostly oxygenated and give the skin its usual pink or "flesh-colored" look.

If nonoxygenated blood is flowing in the tiny blood vessels as well as the veins, the skin will appear bluish. The most serious cause of this kind of overall blueness is lack of oxygen in the blood. This can occur because there is something wrong with the lungs (they are not able to get enough oxygen to the blood) or because there is not enough air being moved into and out of the lungs to supply the blood with adequate oxygen.

The more blood there is flowing through the skin—and the more rapidly it flows— the more pink or "rosy" the skin will appear. (The pink color, which reflects the red color of oxygen-carrying blood, is modified in people with a great deal of melanin pigment, but they still have a "rosy" look, and their lips and mouth linings are pink.) When blood flows sluggishly, more and more oxygen is removed by the surrounding tissues, so the blood will also appear more blue. Therefore, if blood flow is slower than normal, the skin in that area will look bluish.

The amount of blood flowing through the skin depends on many things and is regulated by reflexes that cause the small arteries, veins, and capillaries to either dilate (open wider) or constrict (become narrower). For example, when the weather is hot or a person is exercising, the skin is usually very pink or red (and warm). Blood is shunted through the skin so that the cooler air can cool it down. In contrast, when it is very cold, the body's reflexes cause the arteries to narrow down in order to keep the blood nearer the interior of the body (so it does not cool down too far). This makes the skin appear to be pale, or even bluish and mottled (speckled with blue, pink, purple, and white).

Likewise, when there is not enough blood to circulate effectively—as is the case

293

RECOGNIZING
AND ASSESSING
SERIOUS OR
POTENTIALLY
SERIOUS
ILLNESS

when a person is in shock—the reflexes go into action and narrow the blood vessels to the skin. The purpose is to divert all possible blood to the vital organs rather than "wasting" it on the skin. Here again, the skin will appear pale and even bluish. In addition, because the blood flow is so sluggish, the skin "color" will not return quickly (as it usually does) after you press or push on the skin. Other aspects of the skin's reflex actions cause sweating to occur or not occur and sometimes lead to the production of "goose bumps." Most people don't know that "goose bumps" are a reflex mechanism that is meant to increase body heat. (In other words, they do not make you feel cold but rather occur in response to your feeling cold.)

A third factor that influences skin color (when both healthy and ill) is the presence of unusual pigments in the blood or in the skin itself. Jaundice, which manifests itself by turning the color of the skin and mucous linings yellow, is caused by an abnormal amount of a yellow pigment called bilirubin. This pigment can build up when certain liver diseases occur and also is found in high levels in newborn infants for many reasons. There is another cause of yellow color of the skin, called carotenemia, that always has to be differentiated from jaundice. Carotenemia usually occurs in children who eat large quantities of vegetables that contain orange pigments (for example, carrots, squash, tomatoes). Certain medications and dyes will also cause skin discoloration (although this is most often temporary).

Assessment of Skin Color

Start by looking at the youngster's face. Is his skin color normal for him, or is he *pale, bluish, or yellow?* Is he flushed? Is there any blueness around his mouth? Now look inside the young person's mouth. Are the inside of the mouth and tongue their usual pink, "healthy" color, or are they pale or blue? Now examine the rest of his body. Does his skin have its usual healthy look? Again, is he pale, bluish, or flushed? Are his hands and feet a different color than they normally are? Is there any blueness under the fingernails or toenails?

The next step is to press firmly on the youngster's skin. Press hard enough to make the skin underneath your fingers pale. Watch to see how quickly the color returns to the youngster's skin after you stop pushing. Does the color return as quickly as it does when you do the same thing to yourself? Now do this one more time and look carefully at the skin where you pressed. Is there a yellow color left, or is there a rash present that you can't make disappear by pressing on the area?

Skin Temperature: What You Should Know

Like skin color, skin temperature can be influenced by several factors. Obviously, one important determinant is the temperature of the environment the youngster is in. In very cold environments, the skin will be cool or cold, even when the body's reflexes

294

ILLNESS IN
INFANTS,
CHILDREN,
AND
ADOLESCENTS

shunt extra blood to the surface. The hands and feet are especially likely to feel cold. When the weather is hot or a youngster has been exercising, the skin feels hot and moist. Here, the body is widening the surface blood vessels to allow more and more blood to circulate to the surface. In this way, heat can be eliminated from the skin, and the cooler air on the surface can help to reduce body temperature.

When a youngster is ill, the skin temperature can be warm, cool, or normal. With fever, the skin usually feels hot and dry, especially on the chest and abdomen. The hands and feet might feel quite cool, because the body's reflex actions narrow the blood vessels in an attempt to keep the temperature up. With shock, the skin also feels cool and often clammy or moist. In this case, the small blood vessels are also constricted, but for a different reason. Here, the body is attempting to shunt the blood to vital organs, as would also happen with dehydration.

Assessment of Skin Temperature

The second step in skin evaluation is determining its temperature. Babies will usually have pink, warm skin everywhere but can also have cold, bluish hands and feet (which is normal). When a baby is cold, the skin not only feels cold but looks pale, bluish, and mottled (speckled with blue, pale, and pink areas). An infant who is cold is also usually fussy. When an infant gets too hot (especially when he or she has too many clothes on), the skin is red and hot. This makes for a cranky baby who may breathe faster than usual (pant). Some small babies do not sweat when very warm, while others do.

If a fever is involved, the baby, toddler, small child, or older child's forehead and body will feel very warm, while the arms and feet (and sometimes nose) will feel cool or cold. You may notice a slight bluish tinge to his or her fingernails, toenails, and around the lips. This happens because the blood vessels of the hands and feet constrict (narrow).

Skin Texture: What You Should Know

Most infants and children have smooth, warm skin with good elasticity. It has few if any wrinkles and feels firm and "healthy" underneath when you press on it or squeeze it. There may be a small amount of fat under the skin, and the muscles feel strong and firm. When you pinch up a small amount of skin and tissue between your fingers, then let go, the skin will spring back into its normal shape and place. Several factors are responsible for the skin's feeling normal: the amount of water in the cells and between the cells of the skin and subcutaneous tissue; the amount of fat; the amount of muscle and how well it has developed and been used; and whether or not the subcutaneous tissue is healthy.

The most common abnormalities in skin texture result from either abnormalities in the water and electrolyte (salt) content of the body or poor nutrition. Sudden changes in the skin texture are most often caused by abnormalities in the water content—either too much (which is called edema) or too little (which is called dehydration). More chronic, long-standing abnormalities in skin texture and elasticity usually result from malnutrition—regardless of the cause of the malnutrition (such as poor nutrition, malabsorption of food in the intestine, and many other chronic diseases).

Assessment of Skin Texture

Feel the skin first to tell if it is dry or rough to the touch. Look at the entire youngster. Is he or she unusually puffy? Check for puffiness especially around the eyes and face, then check the hands, ankles, and feet. These are signs of excess water in the tissues (edema).

To check for skin elasticity, pinch up a small piece of the skin over the youngster's abdomen. When you let it go, does it stay "tented up," or does it immediately fall down into place again? If it stays "tented up," it means the skin has lost its elastic ability. Does the skin feel "doughy"? If so, the youngster is probably seriously dehydrated. Sometimes, in seriously malnourished youngsters, the skin is quite wrinkled. A youngster's eyeballs may also appear sunken—because of lack of water in the tissues or due to lack of fat behind the eye.

Rashes and Skin Eruptions: What You Should Know

Rashes are very common among infants and children. They can result from infections and other illnesses or can merely be the result of irritation from or sensitivity to something in the environment. While most rashes signal mild disease, a few of them herald the need for prompt medical attention.

Rashes are among the hardest things for parents (and others) to evaluate. Worse yet, most people find that trying to describe a rash they see is even more difficult than trying to evaluate it in the first place. For this reason, the doctor might want to see the youngster with a rash if there is any question as to whether or not the rash is one that signals a serious disease.

Rashes and irritations of the skin can have both internal and external causes. For example, an external cause of a rash or skin irritation can be direct injury to the skin, whereas internal causes may be infections and other conditions. What a rash looks like—whether flat or bumpy, wet or dry, bumpy or blistery—depends on what caused

296

ILLNESS IN
INFANTS,
CHILDREN,
AND
ADOLESCENTS

the rash, as well as what layers of the skin have been damaged or affected. (Common rashes are discussed in more detail in Chapter 14.)

Rashes that signal true emergencies are usually caused by generalized infections—and require prompt action. One of these serious rashes is called a petechial rash—that results from actual bleeding under the skin. The little blood spots can be tiny, or there can be so much bleeding under the skin that the rash runs together, looking much like large bruises. This kind of rash does not disappear momentarily when you press the skin. There is almost always *no doubt* that a youngster with this kind of rash is critically ill—that he or she may be in shock (or soon will be) and is often lethargic and almost in coma. *The presence of a petechial rash in a sick youngster is an emergency.* Call the doctor immediately or get him or her to an emergency room right away. If you cannot do so within ten to fifteen minutes, call the paramedics.

Assessment of Rashes and Skin Eruptions

The fourth step in your evaluation of the skin is to check for rashes and skin eruptions. Are there spots, irritations, or eruptions on the skin—or anywhere on the body? As noted, although some rashes are associated with serious diseases, most represent less serious problems. Some rashes mean the youngster has an infection, while others are caused by various kinds of irritation.

When you find a rash—look at it carefully and feel it. The doctor will probably ask you the following questions. Where and when did the rash first appear? Where is it located now (what areas has it spread to)? What does it look like exactly? Is it getting better or worse? Have you ever seen anything like this rash before? Has your child ever had a rash like this before?

Infants and Toddlers

THE SKIN: WHEN SERIOUSLY OR POTENTIALLY SERIOUSLY ILL

"David's skin just didn't seem right. It had a blue tinge to it, and he seemed rather pale. You know, for a toddler, he didn't have that rosy, healthy look. Then I realized he wasn't acting like himself. He seemed very tired, almost too weak to even get up."

Signals for concern in infants and toddlers, particularly when there are other signs of serious illness, are: the skin is very pale, blue, or mottled; the color does not return quickly if you press firmly on the skin; or the skin has lost its elastic ability (when you pinch it, it stays "tented up" for longer than normal). If any of these symptoms

297

RECOGNIZING
AND ASSESSING
SERIOUS OR
POTENTIALLY
SERIOUS
ILLNESS

appear, you should *take the youngster to an emergency room promptly, or call the paramedics if it would take you longer than ten to fifteen minutes to get to the emergency room*.

You should also promptly check with your doctor if the infant or toddler experiences: persistent blueness around the lips, fingernails, or toenails (even when she is not cold and particularly if there are other symptoms that concern you); wrinkling of the skin or lack of skin elasticity, but she does not seem particularly sick; persistent pale or yellow color of the skin; and/or puffiness or swelling of the skin (around the face, the eyes, or the rest of the body). These symptoms can also signal potentially serious illness, but you will usually have enough time to make an appointment to see the doctor within a day or so.

As previously noted, a rash caused by bleeding under the skin—called a petechial rash—is also a symptom that points to serious illness. *This rash signals an emergency and requires that you call the doctor or take the youngster to the nearest emergency room immediately (or that you call the paramedics if you cannot make it to the emergency room within ten to fifteen minutes).* A petechial rash most often looks like tiny red dots (there may be just a few red dots or many close together). Again, you check for this kind of rash by pushing on the skin where you see red dots or spots. If the rash is *not* a petechial rash, the rash will *disappear* momentarily when you release your fingers from pressing on the skin. If the rash *is* a petechial rash or other serious rash caused by bleeding into the skin, the rash will *not* momentarily disappear when you press on the skin, then release the pressure. As mentioned, when the bleeding under the skin is severe, the rash may actually look like rapidly appearing bruises.

Also, a blistering rash in an infant under two months old—a form of infection called *bullous impetigo*—is a signal for concern. This problem causes blisters (up to one-half inch in size) to appear and break quickly. It leaves raw, red skin beneath the area where the blister once was. Most often, this rash starts in the diaper area or lower abdomen.

Hives, although rare in young infants, can be associated with breathing problems when they occur in infants and toddlers. This rash has various-sized and -shaped red or white welts. The welts are *very* itchy. If an infant or toddler gets hives, you should call the doctor for advice.

Young Children, Older Children, and Teenagers

THE SKIN: WHEN SERIOUSLY OR POTENTIALLY SERIOUSLY ILL

"Heather just wasn't herself when she came home from school. She seemed distant and aloof, not like the vivacious seven-year-old I was used to hearing nonstop chatter from. Her skin was hot except for her hands, which were

298

ILLNESS IN
INFANTS,
CHILDREN,
AND
ADOLESCENTS

icy. She went to lie down. About an hour later, I checked on her. I went to give her a hug and was shocked. Her skin felt clammy and very cold. When I turned her around and looked carefully at her face, I realized she was pale and seemed to have dark circles under her eyes. Then I noticed that the color had not returned to the areas where I had held her shoulders and arms. It was almost as if I had left my hand and fingerprints right there on her skin.''

If the following symptoms occur in a young child, older child, or teenager, the youngster would require immediate medical evaluation: very pale, cold, clammy skin (which suggests shock); blue or mottled skin (which also suggests shock); skin whose color does not return quickly after you press on it firmly (another symptom of shock); skin that has lost its elastic ability (it stays ''tented up'' after pinching it); a petechial rash (caused by bleeding under the skin) or severe, unexplainable bruising; hives along with lip and/or tongue swelling or any breathing difficulty.

Jaundice (yellow color of the skin), persistent or severe paleness, and persistent or severe puffiness of the eyelids or the hands and feet are other symptoms that point to potentially serious illness. These require you to call the doctor and receive advice within a day.

All Ages

THE SKIN: WHEN MODERATELY OR MILDLY ILL

''Jonathan seemed fairly active, but cranky and a little more tired than he usually gets. After playing outside for a half hour, he came in saying he was thirsty. I realized he was a bit pale and had dark circles under his eyes. He just sat there for a while, then decided to watch television rather than join the other children in the backyard.''

Changes in skin color, temperature, texture, or the presence of a rash can also mean mild or moderate illness in *infants and toddlers*. A warm body and cold, pale hands and feet are usually little to worry about if the infant or toddler does not seem to have any other symptoms that point to serious illness. In fact, this is common with a fever and quite normal in very young infants who are not sick.

Mild paleness is seen with many mild or moderate illnesses in *youngsters of all ages*, as are dark circles under the eyes. Again, if the youngster does not have any other symptoms of serious illness, you should not be too concerned. Cracked, dry lips—without changes in the texture of the skin—most often mean the infant or toddler has a mild or moderate illness or has even had too much exposure to the sun or wind.

299

RECOGNIZING
AND ASSESSING
SERIOUS OR
POTENTIALLY
SERIOUS
ILLNESS

Although many people fear rashes and believe all signal serious illness—most in fact are more bothersome and frustrating than serious. A diaper rash (except for the blistering diaper rash seen in very young infants, as previously discussed) is most often a mild problem. Some diaper rashes can get out of control but can be treated quite successfully and are never life-threatening. Scaly, itchy rashes are unpleasant for a child, especially if they are extensive, but do not pose a serious hazard to health or well-being.

This is also the case when it comes to the many red, dotted, bumpy rashes people so often think of as "measles." Most of these rashes are not measles (but are often a skin response to an infection, virus, and so on). These are also fairly harmless and should not worry you. Again, more than a rash itself, the presence or absence of other symptoms will tell you about the seriousness or lack of seriousness of a youngster's problem—unless the rash is the kind that suggests bleeding into the skin (a petechial rash, for example).

THE DON'TS

Don't delay in calling the paramedics if a young person has blue skin, especially if he or she is having difficulty breathing. A blue color means that he is not getting enough oxygen.

Don't hesitate to call your doctor immediately or go to an emergency room if a youngster has a rash caused by broken blood vessels. This kind of rash usually signals serious, potentially life-threatening infection or a bleeding disorder.

Don't delay in calling the doctor if an infant, toddler, young child, older child, or teenager has dramatic changes in skin color, temperature, or texture—or has a rash, along with other signs of serious illness. The doctor can help you to determine what further action to take.

Don't overreact to dark circles under a youngster's eyes if she does not appear otherwise seriously ill. This is a common problem and usually does not signal serious illness. Do, however, make an appointment for the youngster to be evaluated by the doctor, if you are worried.

PLEASE NOTE: Now that you have a grasp of how to assess the skin, it would be extremely helpful for you to go back to the Emergency Quick Reference and Assessment Checklist and review them carefully. The more familiar you are with that material, the more useful it will be to you when you need it.

300

ILLNESS IN
INFANTS,
CHILDREN,
AND
ADOLESCENTS

EMERGENCY QUICK REFERENCE

The Eyes

When to Call the Paramedics or Ambulance

In the following situations, have someone else call the *paramedics* or an *ambulance* (if there are no paramedics in your area) while you treat the youngster. If no one else is with you, continue treating the child while you periodically shout for help. When help arrives, have that person call the paramedics or an ambulance.

▶ **A YOUNGSTER'S EYELIDS ARE VERY PUFFY OR SWOLLEN SHUT (WITH OR WITHOUT ITCHING)—AND HE IS HAVING TROUBLE BREATHING.** (If you are unable to remember the details of managing this problem, turn to the Emergency Quick Reference on page 324, entitled "Anaphylaxis," for a review.)

▶ **A CHILD'S EYEBALLS ARE VERY SUNKEN—AND SHE HAS SIGNS OF SEVERE DEHYDRATION WITH SHOCK** (very dry mouth, little or no urine; poor skin elasticity; pale, blue, gray, or mottled skin; weak, fast, thready heartbeat; severe listlessness or anxiety). (If you are unable to remember the details of managing this problem, turn to the Emergency Quick Reference on page 152, entitled "Managing Shock," for a review.)

▶ **THE PUPILS ARE VERY LARGE (WHETHER OR NOT THEY ARE EQUAL)—AND THE YOUNGSTER IS DIFFICULT OR IMPOSSIBLE TO AROUSE.** (If you are unable to remember the details of managing this problem, turn to the Emergency Quick Reference on page 160, entitled "Managing Unconsciousness," for a review.)

▶ **THE YOUNGSTER'S PUPILS ARE UNEQUAL OR DO NOT REACT TO LIGHT—AND SHE HAS HAD A CONVULSION THAT LASTED LONGER THAN FIVE MINUTES.** (If you are unable to remember the details of managing this problem, turn to the Emergency Quick Reference on page 337, entitled "Convulsions/Seizures," for a review.)

When to Call the Doctor Immediately

The following symptoms are serious enough that your infant, child, or teenager will usually need to be evaluated *within an hour or two*. Call your child's doctor for advice

301

RECOGNIZING
AND ASSESSING
SERIOUS OR
POTENTIALLY
SERIOUS
ILLNESS

immediately. If you are unable to reach the doctor within fifteen to thirty minutes, take the youngster to an emergency room for evaluation.

A CHILD HAS ONE EYE WHICH IS VERY SWOLLEN, WITH A VERY RED- OR PURPLE-COLORED EYELID, WITH OR WITHOUT PUS IN THE EYE.

A YOUNGSTER'S PUPILS ARE UNEQUAL OR DO NOT REACT TO LIGHT—AND HE HAS SIGNS OF SERIOUS INFECTION (high fever, bulging soft spot and/or stiff neck, severe headache, with or without a rash that looks like tiny blood spots).

THE YOUNGSTER'S PUPILS ARE NOT EQUAL OR DO NOT REACT TO LIGHT—AND SHE HAS HAD A CONVULSION WHICH LASTED LESS THAN FIVE MINUTES.

THE CHILD'S PUPILS ARE NOT EQUAL OR DO NOT REACT TO LIGHT—AND THERE WAS OR COULD HAVE BEEN A HEAD INJURY.

THE CHILD'S EYEBALLS ARE VERY SUNKEN—AND HE HAS SIGNS OF DEHYDRATION (little or no urine, dry mouth, poor skin elasticity, listlessness), **ESPECIALLY IF HE HAS HAD VOMITING OR SEVERE DIARRHEA.**

THE YOUNGSTER'S EYE(S) APPEAR TO TURN IN OR OUT SUDDENLY—ESPECIALLY WITH OTHER SIGNS OF ILLNESS OR INJURY.

When to Call the Doctor Within an Hour or Two

In the following situations, an infant, child, or teenager may require evaluation *within a few hours.* Call your doctor for advice or arrange for the youngster to be seen in an emergency room (if you have no doctor or are not near or cannot reach your doctor).

ONE OR BOTH OF A CHILD'S EYES LOOKS INFECTED (the whites of the eye[s] are very red and sore, the eyelid[s] are slightly swollen, and there is pus in the eye[s], with or without a fever).

▶ **ONE OR BOTH OF HER EYES HAVE BECOME VERY PUFFY, WITH OR WITHOUT OTHER SYMPTOMS.**

302

ILLNESS IN
INFANTS,
CHILDREN,
AND
ADOLESCENTS

▶ **THE CHILD'S EYEBALLS LOOK SOMEWHAT SUNKEN OR THERE ARE DARK CIRCLES UNDER THEM—AND HE HAS SIGNS OF MILD DEHYDRATION** (less urine than usual; dry, sticky mouth; no tears).

When to Call the Doctor for an Appointment

In the following situations, an infant, child, or teenager requires evaluation *within a day or two.* Call your doctor's office to arrange an appointment.

▶ **A YOUNG INFANT HAS MATTER WHICH APPEARS IN THE COR-NER(S) OF THE EYE(S) WITHOUT REDNESS OR SWELLING OF THE EYELID(S).**

▶ **THE CHILD HAS MILD INFLAMMATION OF THE EYES** (redness, mild puffiness, matter in the eyes)—**AND OTHER SIGNS OF MILD INFEC-TION** (for example, congestion, mild fever, cough, and so on).

▶ **A YOUNGSTER HAS PERSISTENT OR REPEATED PROBLEMS WITH RED, ITCHY EYES.**

▶ **THE CHILD HAS PERSISTENT OR REPEATED PROBLEMS WITH PUFFY EYES, ESPECIALLY IF THERE IS ALSO PUFFINESS OF THE HANDS OR FEET.**

▶ **YOU ARE CONCERNED ABOUT PERSISTENT OR REPEATED "DARK CIRCLES" UNDER THE YOUNGSTER'S EYES.**

▶ **ONE OR BOTH OF THE YOUNGSTER'S EYES ARE SUDDENLY TURNED IN OR OUT—BUT THERE ARE NO OTHER SIGNS OF SE-RIOUS ILLNESS OR INJURY.**

▶ **A YOUNGSTER DOES NOT APPEAR TO SEE AS WELL AS USUAL, OR COMPLAINS OF TROUBLE SEEING, WITH OR WITHOUT OTHER SIGNS OF IRRITATION OF HER EYES.**

303

RECOGNIZING
AND ASSESSING
SERIOUS OR
POTENTIALLY
SERIOUS
ILLNESS

ASSESSMENT CHECKLIST

The Eyes

LOOK CAREFULLY AT THE YOUNGSTER'S EYES TO SEE IF THEY WILL GIVE YOU CLUES ABOUT THE ILLNESS.

yes no Do the child's eyes look as bright
☐ ☐ and "alive" as usual?

yes no Are there tears when he cries?
☐ ☐

yes no Do her eyes look dull or lack
☐ ☐ sparkle?

yes no Do her eyes seem to tear more
☐ ☐ than you would expect?

yes no Do his eyes appear "vacant" or
☐ ☐ "spacey"?

yes no Does light bother his eyes?
☐ ☐

yes no Can the youngster focus her eyes
☐ ☐ on you?

yes no Does she blink or squint a great
☐ ☐ deal?

yes no Do his eyes appear straight when
☐ ☐ he looks at you?

yes no If he is old enough to tell you,
☐ ☐ can he see the same as usual?

LOOK TO SEE IF THE YOUNGSTER'S EYELIDS ARE SWOLLEN.

yes no Is there swelling of the eye(s)?
☐ ☐ (If so, can the youngster still open
them?)

yes no Does his swollen eye appear to
☐ ☐ bulge out from the eye socket?

yes no Is only one eye puffy or swol-
☐ ☐ len? (If so, is the eyelid very red
or purple?)

yes no Do her eyelids seem puffier than
☐ ☐ usual? (If so, does the puffiness
disappear during the daytime,
then reappear the next day?)

yes no If only one eye is swollen, is
☐ ☐ there a deep red or purple color
to the eyelid?

304

ILLNESS IN
INFANTS,
CHILDREN,
AND
ADOLESCENTS

CHECK TO SEE IF THE EYES ARE SUNKEN.

yes no Do the child's eyes appear to have
☐ ☐ dark circles under them?

yes no Are his eyes sunken deep in the
☐ ☐ socket?

LOOK FOR SIGNS OF INFLAMMATION OR INFECTION OF THE EYE(S).

yes no Is there any redness of the eye(s)?
☐ ☐ (If so, where? Just the eyelid[s],
the linings of the eyelid[s], or
the white part of the eye[s]?)

yes no Does the child rub his eyes, or
☐ ☐ complain that they hurt?

yes no If only one eye is red, is the eye-
☐ ☐ lid swollen shut (or nearly so),
and very red or purple?

yes no Have you looked into the eye(s)
☐ ☐ to see if there is anything stuck
there that could be irritating her
eyes (an eyelash, particle of dirt,
and so on)?

yes no Is there ''matter'' or pus in the
☐ ☐ eye(s)? (If so, what color is it?
How often do you have to wipe
it away?)

CHECK THE PUPILS OF THE CHILD'S EYES.

yes no Are both pupils the same size?
☐ ☐

yes no Do both pupils work together?
☐ ☐

yes no Do the pupils respond nor-
☐ ☐ mally—that is, get smaller in
bright light and larger when it's
darker?

LOOK FOR OTHER SIGNS OF A SERIOUS OR POTENTIALLY SERIOUS ILLNESS.

yes no Does the youngster seem very ill
☐ ☐ (high fever, lethargic, refusing
to eat, and so on)?

yes no Is he having any breathing dif-
☐ ☐ ficulty?

yes no Has she had a convulsion?
☐ ☐

yes no Has she been vomiting or having
☐ ☐ severe diarrhea?

305

RECOGNIZING
AND ASSESSING
SERIOUS OR
POTENTIALLY
SERIOUS
ILLNESS

yes no Are there signs of dehydration ☐ ☐ (little or no urine, dry mouth, poor skin elasticity, listlessness, and so on)?

yes no Could he have gotten into any ☐ ☐ medication or other poison? (This often causes changes in the eyes, so it's important to carefully check around the house, garage, and so on, to see if there are any signs that the youngster got into something and got it into his eyes or ingested it. Be sure to ask the talking child if she put something into her eyes or ate anything unusual.)

Assessing the Eyes

"Every time my baby gets sick, I worry about him because his eyes always look so bad. They usually look sort of glassy and bloodshot and tend to get matted shut. I wonder if this should worry me."

It has been said that our eyes are the windows of the world. They are, indeed—in many ways. In medicine, the eyes can tell us a great deal, and changes in the eyes can give clues to both serious and mild to moderate illness. Not only do the eyes show changes in their outer appearance, but they may also change in their function, especially with serious or potentially serious problems. Because of the eyes' ability to tell us so much, it's important that they be part of the overall assessment process. Your assessment of the eyes should be performed in a systematic way—so you don't miss some of the clues they offer. In a sense, each assessment area adds information to the diagnostic puzzle and helps put the pieces of the puzzle together—so you know what actions to take.

Many people think only about looking at the pupils of the eyes—the black openings in the middle—when they are worried about illness or injury. In fact, the eyes can give you much more information if you look at them carefully.

You may not be aware of exactly *how* a child's eyes change with illness, but their general appearance will often give you your first clue that a youngster is not feeling quite himself. A baby or child who is simply not feeling well or is "not herself" will often have eyes that are just not as "bright" and alert as usual. It is not at all uncommon for a sick child's eyes to seem darker than normal or to have dark circles under them. With some illnesses (even mild ones), a little puffiness of the eyelids and even mild redness of the "whites" of the eyes are common.

True puffiness and inflammation of one or both eyes can point to either mild to moderate problems or serious illnesses. You will need to look closely to try to make

306

ILLNESS IN
INFANTS,
CHILDREN,
AND
ADOLESCENTS

the distinction between mild and worrisome puffiness and between mild redness and true inflammation. In either case, it's a question of degree. And while "dark circles" are common, truly "sunken" eyeballs signal a serious problem—dehydration.

Many people do not understand how the pupils of the eyes work, and this leads to confusion and frustration when they try to determine if the pupils are normal or not. In essence, the pupils change in size—dilate (open wider) or constrict (become smaller)—in response to the amount of light. The pupils constrict in order to protect the sensitive retina (at the back of the eye) from too much light. This essentially dims bright light so vision is better. The pupils dilate to allow more light into the eye when it is darker, and this, too, improves vision. The pupils work together. That is, normally both pupils should be the same size. When light is shined into one, both should get smaller. When there is less light, both should dilate.

Many problems and conditions influence the size of the pupils and how they react when light is shined into them. The muscles that control the pupil reflexes are controlled by certain nerves from the brain. They can malfunction for a number of reasons, including: inflammation of the nerves that control them, infection of the brain itself, direct injury to the eye, increased pressure inside the skull, and certain drugs and medications—to name a few. Abnormal pupils react to light incorrectly. They may not react at all, or one pupil might not act the same way the other one does.

The Eyes: What You Should Know

Your assessment procedure applies to children of all ages. As noted, when you are looking at the eyes of a sick child, try to look systematically. First, consider the overall appearance of the eyes. Do they look the way they normally do, or are they dull or less alert? This is common with any illness. Check to see if the eyelids are unusually puffy or unusually sunken. Both of these symptoms suggest that there may be a problem with water and salt balance or that there is inflammation of the area around the eyes. If the child is crying, does he have tears? Is there any redness of the eyeball itself or any discharge or secretion in the eyes?

Do the youngster's eyes seem to be bothering him? Ask the older child if she can see or has any pain in her eyes. A younger infant or toddler may rub the eyes or seem bothered by the light when his or her eyes hurt.

After you have evaluated the overall appearance of the eyes, look at how the eyes move. They should move as a unit. Do both eyes seem straight when the child looks straight ahead? Check to see if one eye seems to be turned in or out. If the child's eyes are normally straight, this would signal a potentially serious problem. With an older child, ask if it hurts to move the eyes or to look at light. This can be a clue to inflammation and infection.

Checking the pupils is next. You will need a flashlight or other similar light for part of your check. Do these tests in a slightly darkened room without a light shining

307

RECOGNIZING
AND ASSESSING
SERIOUS OR
POTENTIALLY
SERIOUS
ILLNESS

directly on the child. First look at the pupils. They should both be the same size. Now shine your light directly into *one* eye. Watch the pupil get smaller, then enlarge again as you remove the light. Now shine the light into the eye again and watch the *other* eye. The opposite pupil should also get smaller when you shine the light, then enlarge when you remove the light. Do the same thing with the other eye. Shine the light into the youngster's eyes enough times that you are sure the pupils work together—getting larger when the light is dim and smaller when the light is bright.

All Ages

THE EYES: WHEN SERIOUSLY OR POTENTIALLY SERIOUSLY ILL

"At first, I thought Johnny had just scratched his eye while he was playing. But then he developed a fever of 103 degrees, and his eye began to look just terrible. The eyelid got very swollen and deep red. He couldn't even open his eye because it was so swollen, and he got very upset when I tried to touch it."

Serious infections of the eyes not only cause swelling of the eye and surrounding tissue but also are usually associated with high fever, behavior and activity changes, and other symptoms of serious illness. In other words, the child looks really sick. While most eye infections are mild (there is only mild eye puffiness, slight redness, or small amounts of discharge), a deep infection of the tissues around the eyeball can occur—especially in infants, toddlers, and small children. With a serious eye infection, there is a great deal of swelling of the infected eye and a deep red, almost purple or violet discoloration of the eyelid and skin surrounding the eye. The eye may look very swollen and appear to be bulging out. Serious infections of the eye can be associated with generalized, or systemic, infection (sepsis) and should be treated immediately. (Sepsis is discussed in detail in Chapter 13.) Contact the doctor or take the youngster to an emergency room for evaluation if you see signs of a serious eye infection.

Other clues the eyes give us about the presence of serious or potentially serious illness include: severe puffiness of the eyes after an insect sting somewhere else on the body or when you suspect an allergy (especially if these signs are associated with any trouble breathing); yellow color of the white parts of the eyes (except in a newborn infant when the doctor has already told you about the jaundice); sudden turning in or out of one eye in a child whose eyes were straight; eyes that appear very sunken in a youngster who is at risk for dehydration; and persistent, definite puffiness of the eyes, especially in the morning, even if the puffiness disappears during the day.

Most of these eye changes are accompanied by *other* signs of potentially serious illness and signal the need to immediately take the youngster to the doctor or an

308

ILLNESS IN
INFANTS,
CHILDREN,
AND
ADOLESCENTS

emergency room for evaluation. If, however, you see any of these symptoms (by itself) in a youngster who does not seem ill—call the doctor for advice. Each is sufficiently serious that the child will most likely need prompt medical evaluation.

Several types of pupil abnormalities can signal potentially serious illness. You may notice that one pupil is definitely larger than the other, even when you don't shine a light into the eyes. While this is occasionally normal, check with your doctor promptly if it is associated with any other symptoms of illness or follows an injury. You should also be concerned if one pupil doesn't get smaller if light is shined into either eye. These situations suggest serious problems with the nerves or muscles controlling the eyes.

In addition, if the pupils do not react at all when you shine light into them, there may be a serious problem. (It doesn't matter if they remain very large, very small, or somewhere in between. The point is, they do *not* respond to direct light.) Certain medicines make the pupils not react to light. If you cannot make the pupils change in size by shining a light into them in a darkened room (and no injury is involved), it is best to check to see whether a toddler or child got into a medicine or poison, or whether an older youngster or teenager took a drug or medication. This is especially important if the child's behavior is also abnormal.

All Ages

THE EYES: WHEN MODERATELY OR MILDLY ILL

> "I've been concerned about Kim for a long time. She seems to always have dark circles under her eyes, and she rubs them a lot. I was really relieved when the doctor said she probably had an allergy."

Dark circles under the eyes, *without* any other really obvious changes in the eyes themselves, are common in many youngsters. No one is sure exactly why this occurs, but most parents think it means lack of sleep. (It may in some youngsters—try an extra hour or so for a few days.) It can be seen with a multitude of problems. In certain youngsters, however, dark circles are associated with allergies—to inhalants (things in the air) and even to foods.

Mild puffiness of the eyelids that is temporary and not associated with other signs of serious illness should not cause you undue concern. However, if this puffiness increases or lasts for longer than a few days, call the doctor for advice.

Other signs of usually mild or moderate illness include: slight redness of the eyelids or eyes, with small amounts of discharge or crusting; itching or rubbing of the eyes; and yellowness of the eyes in a newborn who is otherwise healthy (and the doctor is already aware of the jaundice). You should not be unduly concerned by the *size* of the pupils as long as they react to light and work together.

309

RECOGNIZING
AND ASSESSING
SERIOUS OR
POTENTIALLY
SERIOUS
ILLNESS

THE DON'TS

Don't forget to look carefully at a sick youngster's eyes to assist you in deciding whether or not she might have a serious or potentially serious problem. Her eyes can give you clues about serious infection, dehydration, allergy, poisoning, as well as about more mild problems.

Don't overreact to "dark circles" under a youngster's eyes unless he has other signs of a problem. Children who have repeated dark circles under their eyes usually are not seriously ill.

Don't overlook signs of vision problems in your youngster. Repeated eye rubbing, blinking, headaches, and mild redness may be clues that she is not seeing as well as she should be.

PLEASE NOTE: Now that you have a grasp of how to assess the eyes, it would be extremely helpful for you to go back to the Emergency Quick Reference and the Assessment Checklist and review them carefully. The more familiar you are with that material, the more useful it will be to you when you need it.

310

ILLNESS IN
INFANTS,
CHILDREN,
AND
ADOLESCENTS

EMERGENCY QUICK REFERENCE

Presence and Degree of Pain

When to Call the Paramedics or Ambulance

In the following situations, have someone else call the *paramedics* or an *ambulance* (if there are no paramedics in your area) while you treat the youngster. If no one else is with you, continue treating the child while you periodically shout for help. When help arrives, have that person call the paramedics or an ambulance.

▶ **THE YOUNGSTER COMPLAINS OF SEVERE PAIN ANYWHERE OR APPEARS TO BE IN SEVERE PAIN—AND HAS SIGNS OF SHOCK** (pale, blue, gray, or mottled skin; weak, fast, thready pulse; cool, clammy skin; severe weakness; dizziness; lethargy or agitation). (If you are unable to remember the details of managing this problem, turn to the Emergency Quick Reference on page 152, entitled "Managing Shock," for a review.)

▶ **THE YOUNGSTER HAS OR SEEMS TO HAVE PAIN—AND IS HAVING DIFFICULTY BREATHING AND/OR HAS BLUE, GRAY, PALE, OR MOTTLED SKIN COLOR.**

When to Call the Doctor Immediately

The following symptoms are serious enough that your infant, child, or teenager will usually need to be evaluated *within an hour or two*. Call your child's doctor for advice *immediately*. If you are unable to reach the doctor within fifteen to thirty minutes, take the youngster to an emergency room for evaluation.

▶ **AN INFANT OR YOUNG CHILD IS CRYING OR MOANING CONTIN-UOUSLY AS IF IN PAIN—AND HAS OTHER SIGNS OF SERIOUS OR POTENTIALLY SERIOUS INFECTION** (high fever, bulging soft spot and/or stiff neck, a rash caused by broken blood vessels, and so on).

▶ **AN OLDER CHILD COMPLAINS OF SEVERE HEADACHE—AND HAS FEVER, STIFF NECK, AND/OR A RASH THAT IS CAUSED BY BRO-KEN BLOOD VESSELS.**

311

RECOGNIZING
AND ASSESSING
SERIOUS OR
POTENTIALLY
SERIOUS
ILLNESS

▶ A YOUNGSTER HAS OR SEEMS TO HAVE SEVERE PAIN IN THE ABDOMEN—AND A SWOLLEN, HARD, TENDER ABDOMEN.

▶ THE CHILD COMPLAINS OF SEVERE SORE THROAT—AND REFUSES TO SWALLOW EVEN SIPS OF WATER—ALONG WITH FEVER AND/OR DIFFICULTY BREATHING.

When to Call the Doctor Within an Hour or Two

In the following situations, an infant, child, or teenager may require evaluation *within a few hours.* Call your doctor for advice or arrange for the youngster to be seen in an emergency room (if you have no doctor or are not near or cannot reach your doctor).

▶ A YOUNGSTER HAS OR APPEARS TO HAVE SEVERE OR PERSISTENT PAIN ANYWHERE—AND ANY OTHER SIGNS OF ILLNESS.

▶ THE CHILD HAS ENOUGH PAIN THAT HE IS NOT ABLE TO BE COMFORTED FOR ANY PERIOD OF TIME.

When to Call the Doctor for an Appointment

In the following situations, an infant, child, or teenager requires evaluation *within a day or two.* Call your doctor's office to arrange an appointment.

▶ AN INFANT, TODDLER, OR YOUNG CHILD SEEMS UNUSUALLY FUSSY, BUT NOT IN SEVERE PAIN—WITH OR WITHOUT SYMPTOMS OF A MILD TO MODERATE ILLNESS.

▶ AN OLDER YOUNGSTER HAS PERSISTENT OR RECURRENT MILD TO MODERATE PAIN, ESPECIALLY IF THE PAIN INTERFERES WITH HIS OR HER USUAL ACTIVITIES.

312

ILLNESS IN
INFANTS,
CHILDREN,
AND
ADOLESCENTS

ASSESSMENT CHECKLIST

Presence and Degree of Pain

Infants, Toddlers, Small Children, as well as Youngsters of Any Age Who Do Not Talk

ASSESS THE INFANT, TODDLER, SMALL CHILD OR YOUNGSTER FOR SIGNS THAT HE IS EXPERIENCING PAIN.

yes no Is he crying much more than usual?

yes no Is he moaning, sighing, or grunting as if he is in pain?

yes no Is she whimpering a great deal, or crankier than usual?

yes no Is she rubbing, holding, or "favoring" one part of her body?

yes no If she seems uncomfortable, can you comfort her? (If so, what seems to make her feel better?)

yes no Does one part of his body seem sore or tender if you touch or move it?

yes no Does the little one object, cry, or cringe if you pick him up or move him?

yes no Is she moving much less than normal, or much more slowly than usual?

TRY TO DETERMINE HOW SEVERE THE PAIN IS.

yes no Can you comfort the infant, toddler or small child (who does not talk) by holding him or distracting him?

yes no Does the crankiness or crying improve if you give him the correct dose of aspirin substitute/acetaminophen (like Panadol or Tylenol)?

yes no Does she seem uncomfortable all the time?

yes no Will she play or pay attention to her surroundings some or nearly all of the time?

313

RECOGNIZING
AND ASSESSING
SERIOUS OR
POTENTIALLY
SERIOUS
ILLNESS

LOOK FOR OTHER SIGNS OF A SERIOUS OR POTENTIALLY SERIOUS ILLNESS.

yes no Does the little one have a fever? (If so, how high is it and how long has it been this high?)

yes no Is she lethargic or listless?

yes no Is he refusing to eat?

yes no Will he drink liquids, even in small amounts?

yes no Is there any breathing difficulty?

yes no Is her soft spot bulging (if it is open)?

yes no Is his neck stiff?

yes no Has she been vomiting and/or having severe diarrhea?

yes no Do you see any swelling or redness (for example, of a lymph node in the child's neck, or an arm or leg)?

yes no Is his abdomen swollen or bloated and hard?

yes no Does she seem to be belching a great deal or having excessive gas?

yes no Does the little one cry or complain when she urinates?

Small Children, Older Children, and Teenagers Who Can Talk

ASK THE YOUNGSTER WHETHER OR NOT SHE IS EXPERIENCING ANY PAIN.

yes no Does he hurt anywhere? (If so, what hurts?) (Have the youngster point or touch the exact spot that hurts.)

yes no Does she hurt all the time?

yes no Does anything make the pain go away (eating, walking, urinating, having a bowel movement, lying down, moving around, and so on)?

yes no Does anything make it hurt more (coughing, moving around, walking, eating, lying down, urinating, having a bowel movement, and so on)?

314

ILLNESS IN
INFANTS,
CHILDREN,
AND
ADOLESCENTS

TRY TO DETERMINE THE SEVERITY OF THE PAIN AND WHAT IT FEELS LIKE.

yes no Has the pain immobilized the youngster? (Does he say it is unbearable or severe?)

yes no Does it help her to lie very still?

yes no Does the youngster say the pain is more like a dull ache? (Can she describe the pain in any way?)

yes no Does the pain hurt more when you push on the area that hurts?

yes no Does the pain make him want to cry or scream?

yes no Does he hurt more when you release the pressure, then let go?

LOOK AT THE YOUNGSTER TO DETERMINE HOW THE PAIN IS AFFECTING HER.

yes no Does the young person *look* sick?

yes no Will she or can she take part in her normal activities (school, play, interacting with friends and family) in spite of the pain?

yes no Does she prefer to lie quietly in bed—refusing all activities?

yes no Is he moaning, crying, or otherwise showing you that he hurts?

ASSESS THE YOUNG PERSON FOR OTHER SIGNS OF A SERIOUS OR POTENTIALLY SERIOUS ILLNESS.

yes no Does he have a fever? (If so, how high is the fever, and how long has he had the fever?)

yes no Have there been any changes in his appetite, bowel habits, or urination? (For example, is he eating more or less than usual, drinking more or less than usual, or urinating more or less than usual?)

yes no Does she seem lethargic, listless, or out of sorts?

yes no Do you see any swelling or any other abnormality in the area that the youngster says hurts?

yes no Is she experiencing any breathing difficulty?

yes no Is the young person refusing to drink even small amounts of liquids?

315

RECOGNIZING
AND ASSESSING
SERIOUS OR
POTENTIALLY
SERIOUS
ILLNESS

Assessing Pain

''She's only a tiny baby. How can I be expected to tell if she is in pain and where she hurts? Parents aren't mind readers, and we don't have any special magic to help us out. I've worried about this from the minute I was pregnant. How dreadful to think that I might allow my helpless child to suffer because I don't know she's hurting. That's just the most unnerving thought!''

Think about it for a moment. Have you ever been in pain—really hurting—yet never said a word to anyone? If so, what happened? Did someone ask you if you were feeling all right? Did anyone notice you were more quiet than usual, or even aloof or preoccupied, or just not ''yourself'' today? Did someone notice that you seemed kind of ''stiff'' or that you seemed to be moving very slowly or not at all? When at lunch or dinner—were you asked why you didn't seem hungry or weren't eating your food? Did anyone say you seemed more tired than usual or looked ''worn out''?

If your arm was hurting (let's say), did you jump or gasp when someone grabbed your arm to say hello? Did anyone ask you why you were favoring a part of your body or why you weren't moving that part? Did anyone say you looked pale, pasty, or sickly? Were you asked if you thought it was too hot in a room—since someone noticed you were perspiring and uncomfortable? Did someone ask you why you were frowning, grimacing, or seemed tense or stressed? Were you told you looked anxious or overly worried about something?

The point is, the human body shows signs and symptoms of pain—even if the person hurting *says* nothing. Basically, your body speaks *for* you. The ability to be perceptive and sensitive to the body's communications system is particularly important when it comes to infants, nonverbal children, and small children (because they cannot always be specific about what's happening to them or how much they really hurt).

Feeling pain, although very unpleasant, is our body's way of telling us *something is wrong*. The ''something'' may be little more than eating too-spicy foods that gave you a stomachache. It may, on the other hand, indicate a much more serious problem— like the pain that tells you something is wrong with your heart. The same premise holds true with children—pain can signal a minor problem or a very serious and potentially life-threatening illness or condition.

Pain can be sharp, dull, stabbing, boring, burning, cramping, throbbing, intermittent, or constant. It can become worse when moving a certain way (or when moving at all). Pain can be felt right at the place from which it originates or at another area (or other areas) served by the same nerves where the problem exists. (This is called referred pain.) It's helpful in infants, toddlers, and small children to try to determine the presence, intensity, and possible location of pain. In order to do this, you'll have to carefully watch the infant, toddler, or small child to see how he or she looks and acts. Small children may also tell you that they hurt and ''sort of'' where they hurt.

On the other hand, older children and teenagers are more capable of describing:

316

ILLNESS IN
INFANTS,
CHILDREN,
AND
ADOLESCENTS

where the pain is located; what it feels like (steady, sharp, dull, burning, stabbing, constant, and so on); what makes it feel better or worse; if they have ever had any pain like this before; and what other symptoms (if any) they are also experiencing.

In addition to trying to determine the location and severity of pain, take into account your own youngster's usual response to pain or illness. Some youngsters are very stoical—they seem to be less bothered by pain or illness than others. If this type of youngster complains, be sure to take notice. On the other hand, if your youngster tends to be "sensitive" or a complainer, take that into account also. This child's "severe" pain may be quite different from the other more stoic child's pain. That is not to say they both don't hurt—it's just a matter of degree.

Like all other assessment categories, one symptom standing alone is usually not as significant as a set of symptoms in pointing you in the right direction. However, *the intensity, duration, and/or location of pain* can (without other symptoms) herald a serious problem. Therefore, when it comes to pain, what you really want to know is: from where is the pain originating (as specifically as possible); how intense is the pain (unbearable, debilitating pain; intense but bearable pain; discomfort; and so forth); and how long does the pain last (minutes, hours, days, weeks).

Sometimes, it's not possible to find the answers to all of those questions (particularly in infants, nonverbal toddlers, and small children), but you can get important clues to these answers by watching how a child acts and by paying attention to how he looks and feels. In older youngsters and teenagers, it's obviously much easier to get this information, since the youngster can also *tell* you how he feels.

Infants and Toddlers

PAIN: WHEN SERIOUSLY OR POTENTIALLY SERIOUSLY ILL

"Michael just hasn't been himself for the last twenty-four hours. He has been pale, cranky, and cries every time I pick him up. He also has had a very low-grade temperature—ranging between 99.5 and 100 degrees. He seems to grimace when I move him at all and appears to stay very still even when he is awake. When I was changing his diaper this morning, I noticed that his knee was very swollen. That must have happened overnight! He's only six months old, but when I touched his knee, he really let me know what he thought of that. He screamed like I've never heard before and then whimpered for a long time."

Essentially, an infant or toddler who can't verbally tell you she hurts will tell you by her behavioral changes. She may cry easily, be very fussy and cranky, refuse to

317

RECOGNIZING
AND ASSESSING
SERIOUS OR
POTENTIALLY
SERIOUS
ILLNESS

eat much or at all, and seem very unhappy and anxious. She may also be pale; have moist/sweaty skin; have dull, lackluster eyes; and develop a fever.

However, there is a test you can perform that is fairly accurate in determining if an infant or toddler may be in pain. It is not normal for a baby or toddler to fuss and cry (even scream) when you pick him up and to quiet and calm down when you put him back into his crib and leave him alone. All children like to be comforted, held, cuddled, and loved—particularly when not feeling well. But when it comes to pain, movement is just too painful, and the baby (to everyone's surprise) seems more miserable and unhappy when you try to comfort, cuddle, or move him in any way. You will also notice that when the baby is put back in his crib, he tries to lie very still and moves carefully and slowly.

Look to see if you can find any swollen glands, swollen joints, or a body part or area that appears to be more sensitive to the touch (the baby cries or flinches). Of course, look for any other symptoms of serious illness, too. If there are other symptoms of serious illness, then call the doctor immediately or take the little one to the emergency room if you cannot reach the doctor quickly.

Of course, your actions must be based on the severity of the other symptoms. If you first recognize that an infant or toddler is in pain and then he or she has severe breathing trouble, collapses, or becomes unconscious—then calling the paramedics is the action to take. If the baby has no other symptoms that point to serious illness, then call the doctor for advice. Usually, the doctor will want to examine a baby who appears to be in severe pain.

PAIN: WHEN MODERATELY OR MILDLY ILL

"Beth had a cold for about two days and a little fever. Nothing actually to get concerned about. We were perplexed when she woke up in the middle of the night screaming and crying. When we went into her bedroom, she was rubbing her ears and hitting her head on the mattress. We had never seen or heard anything like this before. An hour later, she seemed much better. We had no idea she had an ear infection."

Infants and toddlers with mild to moderate illness may show you signs of discomfort or pain by their actions. You may notice irritability or a change in their cry—they *do* let you know that they hurt. In contrast to a little one with serious illness, they remain quite active and can be comforted somewhat by your efforts. Their pain can often be lessened by a mild pain reliever such as Tylenol—and they seem more comfortable. They may be able to play for short periods of time, although not as much as usual.

Here again, the other associated symptoms are helpful. One of the most common causes of crying as if in pain in young infants and children is earache—and ear infection is one source of pain that should be detected and treated. Treatment is quite easy, but the consequences of ignoring the infection can be severe. If you have questions about whether a small infant or toddler has pain, call your doctor for advice or an appointment.

318

ILLNESS IN
INFANTS,
CHILDREN,
AND
ADOLESCENTS

Young Children

PAIN: WHEN SERIOUSLY OR POTENTIALLY SERIOUSLY ILL

"Stephanie first complained of a headache. We thought it was from playing so long in the heat and weren't surprised when she didn't eat much of her dinner and went to bed early. This morning was a different story. She didn't look right and felt as if she had a fever. It was 102 degrees. She seemed to be holding her head stiffly, so we asked if her head still hurt. She's a very uncomplaining six-year-old, so we knew she was really hurting when she suddenly started crying. Her head still hurt, she said, but now her neck hurt, too. When we asked her to try to touch her chin to her chest, she just couldn't do it, and just cried and cried. As you can imagine, we're absolutely panic-stricken."

Young children will usually tell you that they hurt. If you ask them "where" they hurt the most, though, you may not get an exact answer (either because they are not sure or because they don't quite know how to explain what's happening). If you ask "how much" they hurt—again, you may not get a precise answer. This is a judgment call and asks what degree of pain the youngster is in—which is difficult to answer if he or she hasn't experienced different types of pain.

Pain is *pain* to young children. They often have little or no frame of reference from which to judge the degree of pain. If it's the most intense pain they have ever felt—like all of us, they will say it hurts very badly. Later, you may find out the problem was indigestion. In these situations, you must pay attention not only to *what* the child says but also to *how* he or she acts.

If the young child ceases his normal activities, decreases his food intake or won't eat at all, refuses to move or moves very little, and prefers to lie still instead of sitting up—then more than likely the pain is quite intense. If the child continues most of his usual activities, eats normally, and moves around fairly easily—the pain is probably less intense or is uncomfortable only. In this case, you would want to keep an eye on the child to see if the problem progresses.

So that the information you have is more precise, it is best to ask the child to touch the spot that hurts the most. Then ask her if she hurts anywhere else. If so, have her touch that spot also. Gently push on the spot(s) she identified. Does it hurt more when you push on it, or when you let go? Does she jump or cry when you gently press on a certain area? Then ask her how long has this been hurting—was it just now or this morning, or was it yesterday? Always look for other signs of serious illness.

If pain is the only symptom, but it seems to be fairly intense and lasts more than an hour or two, call the doctor (or go to the emergency room if you are not able to reach the doctor within an hour). Again, if the symptoms are life-threatening, then call the paramedics for assistance.

PAIN: WHEN MODERATELY OR MILDLY ILL

"Paul came home from kindergarten acting very cranky and irritable. When the baby-sitter asked what was wrong, he said his body hurt everywhere. Within a couple of hours, she was on the phone with me. Paul now had a terrible tummyache, she said, and was crying. When I got home, he felt very warm, so I took his temperature. It was 103 degrees, but I was able to reduce it to 101 degrees fairly quickly with children's Panadol. It became more and more obvious that he probably had a viral flu. The tummyache continued for twenty-four hours with an off-and-on fever. Within forty-eight hours, he was just fine."

Most mild to moderate illnesses in young children have some pain or discomfort associated with them. Aching all over, headache, and tummyache can all be the result of fever, a viral illness (such as the flu or a cold), or some other mild but unidentifiable bug!

Again, what you really want to do is look at the overall picture. If the young child has no symptoms of serious illness (as specified in the various assessment categories in this book), then more than likely the child is experiencing a mild to moderate illness. If, however, even minor symptoms persist, then you should call your doctor for advice. Also, since such things as ear infections and strep throat in children can cause serious, long-lasting problems if not treated, anytime symptoms point to either of these, you should call the doctor for advice. Most often, the child should be seen so the problem can be identified and treatment can begin. If at any time you are unsure of the significance of a symptom or set of symptoms, call the doctor for advice.

A word about "growing pains": Many young children (and older children and teenagers), especially the very active ones, complain of various aches and pains, especially in their legs. These leg pains may wake them at night and seem very severe. They usually pass after a few minutes of rubbing on the legs or after a warm bath. They are probably muscle cramps, at least in some children, and are a mild (though bothersome) problem. If you have questions about this kind of pain, have the youngster evaluated by his or her doctor.

Older Children and Teenagers

PAIN: WHEN SERIOUSLY OR POTENTIALLY SERIOUSLY ILL

"Wayne has always been so active in athletics that we were fairly sure he had pulled a muscle in his side. When he came home from high school track practice, he was favoring his right side and said it was just aching. After a

320

ILLNESS IN
INFANTS,
CHILDREN,
AND
ADOLESCENTS

while, though, he decided to lie down but got up saying he was a little nauseated and his side ached a bit more. He seemed pale and warm, so I took his temperature. It was only 100.5 degrees, so I didn't worry much. Even though he said he didn't feel like eating, he tried a little food and vomited soon afterward. He went to bed early but woke us up in the middle of the night. He had never done that before. At this point, he was really hurting and said he felt just terrible. The pain had localized in the right lower side, and he felt more comfortable lying on his side with his knees bent. All symptoms now pointed to appendicitis.''

The older child or teenager usually has had enough experience with illness and is mature enough to be fairly exact in describing his or her symptoms. The same is true when it comes to pain. Obviously, because of age and experience, the youngster will be able to answer many more questions and describe the problem in greater detail.

When an older child or teenager is in pain, you should ask the following questions: Where exactly is the pain located? What does the pain feel like? Is it dull, sharp, throbbing, aching, burning, boring, or shooting? Is the pain constant? If off and on, how often does it happen? Does it hurt more when you move or are in a certain position? Is there any position or movement that makes it feel better? Does the pain occur only when you do certain things (like run, bend over, stretch, go to the bathroom)? How long have you been hurting like this? Is the pain getting worse, better, or staying the same? Have you ever had any pain like this before? Do you have any other symptoms besides the pain?

Even with all of this information, visually assess the youngster yourself. Sometimes, an older child or teenager will say he's OK (because he either has things he wants to do and hopes the pain will go away or is frightened and doesn't want to go to the doctor).

Again, if the youngster decreases her normal activity, isn't eating much or eats nothing at all, and prefers to lie down or hold still—then the pain is probably intense enough to warrant evaluation or at least a call to the doctor, even if the youngster says she's fine. If, however, the youngster does not change her behavior and seems active and well, most often the pain is more like discomfort and she is telling the truth about how she feels. Still, watch the young person to see whether the problem is progressing so you can take action, if necessary.

As with all other age groups, when a youngster is experiencing pain but has no other symptoms of serious illness, it's best to call the doctor for advice. If, on the other hand, other symptoms of serious illness are present, then call the doctor promptly, or take the youngster to the emergency room if you cannot reach the doctor within an hour or two. If any symptoms are life-threatening, immediately call the paramedics for help.

PAIN: WHEN MODERATELY OR MILDLY ILL

321

RECOGNIZING
AND ASSESSING
SERIOUS OR
POTENTIALLY
SERIOUS
ILLNESS

"Terra first said her throat felt scratchy. By the next morning, she said she was too sick to go to school. Since she always loved school, particularly the seventh grade, I knew she must be feeling poorly. Her throat was burning, and it hurt to swallow. I checked her temperature and it was 101.5 degrees, and the glands in her neck were a little swollen and tender. I really felt this would turn out to be a cold, so I gave her plenty of liquids and two aspirins to reduce her fever and throat pain. By early afternoon, however, Terra said her throat hurt so much she could hardly swallow. Even though her temperature was now 99.8 degrees, she didn't feel much better. I called the doctor, who said to bring her in for a throat culture and examination. She ended up having strep throat."

As with most age groups, the older child or teenager will most often have a mild or moderate illness when he or she complains of pain. Some of these, however, will require medical attention, while others can be cared for at home.

Again, the *most important* part of assessment is to put the pieces of the puzzle together and then determine if the symptoms warrant medical evaluation and treatment or if the problem is mild enough to be treated at home. Most pain that is experienced in mild to moderate illnesses is joined by other mild symptoms of illness. In other words, the entire set of symptoms will be mild and treatable at home, or the entire set of symptoms will point to the need for medical evaluation within a day or so, so treatment can occur.

Problems that require medical evaluation are those that point to infection. If you feel the symptoms (along with pain) herald possible strep throat, urinary tract infection, lung infection, or systemic or other infection, then call the doctor for an appointment. In addition, prolonged or recurring pain is unusual in young people and should be evaluated.

THE DON'TS

Don't hesitate to contact your youngster's doctor for advice if you are not sure about the significance of a youngster's pain or apparent pain. The doctor will be able to help you with deciding about if and when the youngster should be seen.

Don't overreact to a child's complaint of pain if she seems as active as usual or is able to be comforted. However, a youngster with persistent or recurrent pain should be evaluated by the doctor.

PLEASE NOTE: Now that you have a grasp of how to assess the presence and degree of pain, it would be extremely helpful for you to go back to the Emergency Quick Reference and the Assessment Checklist and review them carefully. The more familiar you are with that material, the more useful it will be to you when you need it.

322

ILLNESS IN
INFANTS,
CHILDREN,
AND
ADOLESCENTS

Assessment: Putting It All Together

Your first impression may be that there is no way you can remember all the assessment categories and the key points from each. Not true! Assessing how ill an infant, toddler, young child, older child, or teenager is *requires having an overall grasp of how the body communicates—and knowing where to find the information you want when you need it!*

The most important thing to remember is that you can recognize and assess your child's symptoms and you do know where you can find the information you want when you need it. Whether you use the ten Assessment Checklists or the ten Emergency Quick Reference guides in this chapter or prefer to use the broad-based Emergency Quick Reference guides in Chapter 1—these and other tools throughout the book will assist you in your decision making.

Assessment is not difficult if you have a "feel" for what signals a serious illness and the need for immediate medical evaluation and treatment. When you're not sure, turn to one or more of the Assessment Checklists or Emergency Quick Reference guides (based on the child's most obvious or severe symptom) for assistance.

Finally, it is always helpful to periodically review the Emergency Quick Reference guides and the Assessment Checklists in this chapter, as well as the broad-based Emergency Quick Reference guides in Chapter 1. Remember, these various tools are readily accessible for you and can be consulted whenever you're not sure what action to take. If ever in doubt—call your doctor for advice.

CHAPTER 13

Recognizing and Managing Serious or Potentially Serious Illness

Included in this chapter is information on how to recognize and manage the serious or potentially serious illnesses listed below. The page numbers in parentheses indicate where the Emergency Quick Reference for each illness can be found.

324

ILLNESS IN
INFANTS,
CHILDREN,
AND
ADOLESCENTS

EMERGENCY QUICK REFERENCE

With the Steps in Detail

Anaphylaxis
(Overwhelming Allergic Reaction)

*If the Youngster Is Unconscious
or Has Collapsed*

▶ **HAVE SOMEONE ELSE CALL THE PARAMEDICS WHILE YOU TREAT THE CHILD. IF NO ONE IS WITH YOU, CONTINUE TREATING THE CHILD WHILE YOU PERIODICALLY SHOUT FOR HELP. WHEN HELP ARRIVES, HAVE THAT PERSON CALL THE PARAMEDICS. IF THERE ARE NO PARAMEDICS IN YOUR AREA, GET THE CHILD TO THE NEAREST EMERGENCY ROOM IMMEDIATELY.**

▶ **LAY THE YOUNGSTER DOWN ON HIS BACK.**

▶ **CHECK TO SEE WHETHER THE CHILD IS BREATHING.**

- If not, begin rescue breathing. (If you are unable to remember the details of performing rescue breathing, turn to the Emergency Quick Reference on page 113, entitled "A Review of the Six Steps of CPR.")

- If he is breathing, watch him carefully for a change in his breathing status.

▶ **CHECK FOR A PULSE.**

- If there is no pulse, perform full CPR (rescue breathing combined with chest compressions), as you were taught in your CPR certification training course. (If you are certified in CPR and are unable to remember the details of the procedure, turn to the Emergency Quick Reference on page 113, entitled "A Review of the Six Steps of CPR.")

- If there is a pulse, watch the child carefully for a change in his status.

▶ **IF THE ANAPHYLAXIS IS DUE TO A VENOMOUS INSECT STING OR A MEDICATION INJECTED *INTO AN ARM OR LEG*:**

325

RECOGNIZING
AND
MANAGING
SERIOUS OR
POTENTIALLY
SERIOUS
ILLNESS

- Fasten a constricting tie (such as a belt, scarf, tie, or piece of cloth) between the sting or injection site and the rest of the body. This tie should be snug but not so tight that it cuts off all blood flow.

- Look for the stinger (if an insect sting) and remove it if you can. Do this by scraping across it with your fingernail or a knife blade. *Do not try to pull it out with tweezers, since you may squeeze more venom into the skin.*

- Apply ice or cold compresses to the sting or injection site, if you can.

▶ **IF THE DOCTOR HAS PRESCRIBED A SPECIAL EMERGENCY KIT FOR THE TREATMENT OF INSECT STINGS OR SEVERE ALLERGIC REACTIONS TO OTHER MATERIALS, FOLLOW THE INSTRUCTIONS IN THE KIT OR THOSE GIVEN YOU BY THE DOCTOR WHO PRE-SCRIBED IT.**

▶ **FOLLOW ANY OTHER INSTRUCTIONS YOUR YOUNGSTER'S DOC-TOR MAY HAVE GIVEN YOU FOR SUCH EMERGENCIES (FOR EX-AMPLE, SOME ASTHMATIC CHILDREN REQUIRE SPECIAL BREATHING TREATMENTS OR ADMINISTRATION OF SPECIAL MEDICATIONS).**

▶ **TREAT FOR SHOCK.** (If you are unable to remember the details of managing this problem, turn to the Emergency Quick Reference on page 152, entitled "Managing Shock," for a review.)

If the Youngster Is Conscious and Alert

▶ **HAVE HER LIE DOWN AND TRY TO KEEP HER CALM.**

▶ **CALL THE PARAMEDICS IF THE PROBLEM IS PROGRESSING (WORSENING).**

▶ **TAKE THE YOUNGSTER TO THE NEAREST EMERGENCY ROOM IMMEDIATELY IF SHE SEEMS TO BE STABLIZED** (THE REACTION IS NOT PROGRESSING ANY FURTHER), **BUT WATCH HER CARE-FULLY FOR SIGNS OF BREATHING DIFFICULTY (OR BREATHING SUDDENLY STOPPING) AND CONTINUE TO CHECK TO SEE IF SHE HAS A PULSE.**

326

ILLNESS IN
INFANTS,
CHILDREN,
AND
ADOLESCENTS

> ➤ **IF YOUR DOCTOR HAS PRESCRIBED A SPECIAL EMERGENCY KIT FOR THE TREATMENT OF INSECT STINGS OR SEVERE ALLERGIC REACTIONS TO OTHER MATERIALS, FOLLOW THE INSTRUCTIONS IN THE KIT OR THOSE GIVEN TO YOU BY THE DOCTOR WHO PRESCRIBED IT.**

> ➤ **IF THE PROBLEM IS DUE TO AN INSECT STING OR A MEDICATION INJECTED INTO AN ARM OR LEG, FOLLOW THE INSTRUCTIONS PREVIOUSLY GIVEN IN THIS EMERGENCY QUICK REFERENCE.**

> ➤ **FOLLOW ANY OTHER INSTRUCTIONS YOUR YOUNGSTER'S DOCTOR MAY HAVE GIVEN YOU FOR SUCH EMERGENCIES.**

Serious Allergic Reactions

Anaphylaxis is a serious, immediate allergic reaction that can rapidly lead to collapse, shock, and even death if not treated. It most commonly occurs in youngsters who have asthma or are known to be allergic to one or more things but can happen suddenly and without warning in any youngster.

An anaphylactic reaction is basically a bodily defense reaction that has gone too far. Our immune systems are designed to recognize "foreign" materials as dangerous and mount a defense—with antibodies—against them. Even though this reaction is meant to be protective, it "backfires" in some situations, leading to life-threatening complications.

When an allergic child is exposed to a "foreign" material (by eating it, inhaling it, touching it, or being injected with it), special cells within the body may begin to make antibodies against that material. Each time the youngster is exposed to that same material (after these antibodies have been made), the antibodies gather together to destroy the "foreign" material. Each time she is exposed to the material, she becomes more and more sensitive to it. And the reaction to the material becomes more dramatic and severe with each exposure. Finally, an immediate, life-threatening reaction—the anaphylactic reaction—can occur.

One of the most disturbing things about anaphylaxis is that no one can predict when, if ever, such a reaction will take place in someone who has never before had an anaphylactic reaction. Although a person has to have been exposed to the offending material *at least once in the past* (to produce antibodies), often that exposure may not be remembered—because no reaction occurred.

For example, a youngster may have been stung by a bee and you thought little of it, since there was no sign of a problem. There wouldn't have been, because—never having been stung by a bee before—the youngster could not have produced antibodies. An allergic reaction can only occur at the second or subsequent exposure to bee stings. But no one is prepared for an overwhelming allergic reaction (anaphylaxis) because there is no warning! In other children (or adults), there is some warning because you will see increasingly severe reactions with each exposure to the same material—for example, first mild swelling, then swelling and itching, then severe hives, and finally anaphylaxis.

Anaphylaxis: Signs and Symptoms

The earliest symptoms of a severe allergic reaction are usually very subtle but may be severe. The type of symptoms a child experiences depends on what is causing the reaction and the physical idiosyncrasies of each individual child. We are all different genetically, chemically, and physiologically. Symptoms also depend on how much of the allergen (the material to which he is sensitive) he was exposed to and how the exposure occurred (ingestion, inhalation, skin contact, or injection). However, there is one vital aspect in your favor. Each child tends to have the *same* type of reaction to a specific substance, so if she had a previous reaction (for example, itching and redness after eating fish), you can expect to see the same thing—most likely with greater speed or severity—with another exposure. (Don't forget, though, that an anaphylactic reaction can take place.)

One of the most common things to which youngsters are sensitive is the venom of stinging insects of the bee and wasp family. With stings, the venom is injected under the skin. The earliest sign of a problem is what is called a local reaction—sudden, very painful swelling at the sting site. This reaction is more severe than the usual tenderness and pain of a sting in a nonsensitive individual. The child may then develop one or more of the symptoms listed below within seconds or minutes. (These same symptoms occur with exposure to all other materials—foods, plants, inhalants, medications—to which a youngster is severely allergic, except there would be no sting site.)

- Severe pain, redness, swelling, and/or itching at the sting (or injection) site. This may be the first sign of a problem or may occur along with the following more serious symptoms.

- Sudden, severe swelling of the lips, tongue, eyes, and entire body.

- Generalized (all over) itching, with or without a rash, redness, or hives.

- Hives (blotchy red areas with raised white or pink irregularly shaped centers that usually itch terribly).

328

ILLNESS IN
INFANTS,
CHILDREN,
AND
ADOLESCENTS

- Minor to severe breathing difficulty (due to upper airway blockage from swelling at the vocal cords) or wheezing (due to asthma).

- Sudden coughing.

- Dizziness, light-headedness, anxiety, overall weakness.

- Severe nausea, vomiting, and/or diarrhea.

- Collapse, with or without stoppage of breathing and heartbeat (this can be slow in occurring or can happen suddenly and unexpectedly).

Similar types of reactions occur whenever a sensitizing material is injected into the body. Penicillin and its relatives cause this kind of allergic reaction in some people, although this is seen more commonly in adults than in children. However, it is one of the reasons why many doctors prefer to give oral medicines instead of "shots," especially to children prone to be "allergic"—unless there is no alternative to the injectable medication. Other antibiotics, as well as materials containing iodine (for example, "dyes" used in certain X-ray tests) and "allergy shots" given to youngsters to desensitize them to certain materials, are also common culprits. However, *any* injected material can cause this kind of reaction in a sensitive person. Less common but possible culprits are materials, such as plants and flowers, whose chemicals get into the body through breaks in the skin (often scratches or cuts).

Certain foods or drugs (taken by mouth) can cause immediate allergic reactions in some people. When eating the food or taking the drug by mouth is the cause of the reaction, hives or skin itching or rash, as well as breathing problems, may occur. Nausea, vomiting, diarrhea, or abdominal cramping may also result if the child eats a substance to which he or she is allergic. Suspect such foods as strawberries or other berries, fish or other iodine-containing foods or medications, tomatoes, citrus fruits, nuts, and chocolate.

Inhaling sensitizing materials (called inhalants) usually causes breathing problems in those who are allergic. Most often, asthmatic youngsters develop asthmatic symptoms (shortness of breath, coughing, and wheezing) when they are exposed to inhalants and may show the same symptoms in response to certain materials if injected or eaten. Swelling of the voice box and resultant upper airway blockage is also possible and *is immediately life-threatening*.

THE DON'TS

Don't delay in treating known or possible anaphylactic reactions. They can worsen rapidly, leading to disaster.

Don't forget to talk to your youngster's doctor if you feel your child has had an allergic reaction to a material (even if it was mild).

329

RECOGNIZING
AND
MANAGING
SERIOUS OR
POTENTIALLY
SERIOUS
ILLNESS

Don't hesitate to ask your youngster's doctor for information about special medications or anaphylaxis kits if your child has had a serious allergic reaction to a specific material. You can begin treatment no matter where you happen to be if you have this kind of kit with you. It is especially helpful if a youngster is seriously allergic to stinging insects and is often in the woods or where he is at special risk for being stung or if the youngster has serious food allergies and you can't be sure about what is in everything he eats (no matter how careful you are).

Don't forget to inform others who spend a great deal of time with your youngster about his or her potential allergic reaction(s), and tell them what to do if a reaction occurs. Teachers, relatives, baby-sitters, neighbors, and others should know not only how to recognize and manage your child's problem, but also what they can do to avoid a reaction.

PLEASE NOTE: Now that you have a grasp of how to recognize and manage anaphylaxis, it would be extremely helpful for you to go back to the Emergency Quick Reference With the Steps in Detail and review it carefully. The more familiar you are with that material, the more useful it will be to you when you need it.

330

ILLNESS IN
INFANTS,
CHILDREN,
AND
ADOLESCENTS

EMERGENCY QUICK REFERENCE

With the Steps in Detail

Asthma

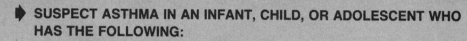

▶ **SUSPECT ASTHMA IN AN INFANT, CHILD, OR ADOLESCENT WHO HAS THE FOLLOWING:**

- Wheezing and dfficulty breathing with a cold (except for the first episode in a young infant).

- Repeated bouts of coughing and/or wheezing with colds, with exposures to specific things to which the child is allergic (such as pollens), or with exercise.

- Repeated episodes of pneumonia.

- Wheezing or difficulty breathing if there is known hay fever, eczema, or asthma in the family.

- Wheezing, difficulty breathing, or night cough in a youngster who has known allergies.

▶ **CHILDREN WITH ASTHMA SHOULD BE UNDER THE CARE OF A DOCTOR WHO KNOWS THEM AND THEIR DISEASE. CALL THE DOCTOR FOR ADVICE AND PROMPT EVALUATION IF:**

- The youngster is having difficulty breathing and is not under a routine asthma treatment program.

- The youngster's usual treatment is not effective this time.

- The youngster is vomiting her usual medication.

▶ **TAKE THE YOUNGSTER TO AN EMERGENCY ROOM FOR PROMPT EVALUATION AND TREATMENT IF:**

- You don't have a doctor or can't reach your doctor, and a youngster has symptoms suggesting asthma.

- The youngster is having great difficulty breathing, is very anxious and agitated, and is/was not helped by his usual treatment.

331

RECOGNIZING
AND
MANAGING
SERIOUS OR
POTENTIALLY
SERIOUS
ILLNESS

▶ **IF THE YOUNGSTER HAS ASTHMA AND STARTS WHEEZING, BEGIN HER USUAL TREATMENT WITHOUT DELAY.** DO NOT WAIT UNTIL SYMPTOMS BECOME SEVERE. THE EARLIER TREATMENT BEGINS, THE MORE SUCCESSFUL IT IS LIKELY TO BE.

▶ **DO NOT USE OVER-THE-COUNTER INHALERS OR MEDICATIONS FOR ASTHMA WITHOUT A PHYSICIAN'S SUPERVISION.** IMPROPER USE OF THESE MEDICATIONS CAN LEAD TO SERIOUS PROBLEMS OR EVEN DEATH.

Asthma: A Chronic Problem

Asthma is a chronic disease that affects many more children and adults than most people realize. It has several possible causes and can vary in its seriousness. While it cannot really be "cured," it *can* be controlled in the vast majority of people who have it. If left untreated and/or uncontrolled, it can lead to permanent lung damage.

Asthma is basically a disease in which there is partial, reversible blockage of the small airways of the lungs (the bronchi and bronchioles). During an asthma attack, the muscles that surround the small airways spasm. Sometimes, the attack is worsened by an accumulation of mucus and secretions that partially block the small airways. As you can imagine, narrowing of these small air passages leads to difficulty breathing—with breathing out (exhaling) being more difficult than breathing in (inhaling). Wheezing—a whistling noise caused by the narrowing of the small airways—is the symptom you can *hear* when partial obstruction occurs.

Common consequences of an asthmatic attack are mucous production, varying degrees of shortage of oxygen, collapse of small areas of the lung—and pneumonia. Less commonly, a severe asthmatic attack can result in such a significant lack of oxygenation that the youngster can become unconscious and stop breathing.

Some children have their first asthma attack during infancy, while others have no problems until adolescence. Most often, however, the first asthma attack is experienced in the preschool years, usually appearing to be a respiratory infection. Parents and doctors are tempted to call this infection bronchitis, until another attack occurs. After several attacks, it generally becomes clear that the problem is asthma. In others, the first attack looks like (and may be) bronchiolitis (due to respiratory syncytial virus, as discussed later in this chapter). Some youngsters have only one or two mild asthma attacks, while others have such severe asthma that, without medication, they would wheeze every day.

You should know that there is a great deal of debate about the causes of asthma.

332

ILLNESS IN
INFANTS,
CHILDREN,
AND
ADOLESCENTS

In certain youngsters, there is little doubt that allergy to known or unknown substances is the culprit. In others, it is not so clear, and no particular sensitivity can be detected. In still other youngsters, another underlying chronic disease may be to blame. Determining the causes of an individual child's asthma requires careful medical evaluation and often long-term care and reevaluation. At times, no clear-cut cause and effect can be pinpointed.

Asthma: Signs and Symptoms

The hallmark of asthma is *wheezing*—a whistling or musical sound a youngster makes when he or she breathes out. Wheezing may also be heard when a youngster with asthma breathes in, but this often signals more severe airway obstruction. Asthma is almost always associated with a tight *cough* that is most pronounced when the child is excited, agitated, or exercising. The youngster usually complains of *shortness of breath* (or looks and sounds breathless when talking, eating, or playing). Older youngsters tend to complain of a "tight" feeling in the chest, as well. In the early stages of an asthma attack or when there is just mild wheezing, the youngster normally has no fever, but a youngster with severe or prolonged wheezing may develop a *low-grade fever* (under 101 degrees).

If the partial blockage of the airways (caused by muscle spasm) is not relieved or becomes much worse, there is a tendency for *mucus* and *secretions* to build up and further block the airways. When this happens, wheezing can get worse, and infection can occur. Airway spasm can become so severe that there is not even enough air moving in and out to cause wheezing. If blockage is severe, lack of oxygen can make a youngster very anxious and agitated, then progressively pale, blue, and sleepy. At this point, the youngster is in serious danger. The effort to breathe can cause severe fatigue, and this in turn may result in the youngster's stopping breathing. It is important that a youngster who is experiencing severe wheezing be seen and treated immediately.

How Asthma Is Treated

Asthma is a serious chronic disease that requires medical evaluation and treatment. Mild cases of asthma normally respond to an oral (taken by mouth) medication that relaxes the muscle spasm in the bronchi and controls the wheezing within a few hours from the time it was taken. Most commonly, a drug called theophylline or one of several adrenalinelike drugs is used to treat mild cases of asthma—and in some children, this only needs to be taken during an acute attack.

More severe attacks of asthma may require injections of adrenaline, the use of theophylline, as well as special breathing treatments. Sometimes, doctors prescribe

333

RECOGNIZING
AND
MANAGING
SERIOUS OR
POTENTIALLY
SERIOUS
ILLNESS

antibiotics (if there is an infection involved) and cortisone-related drugs. If wheezing does not progressively improve with treatment, or if the youngster vomits medications, then hospitalization and more intensive treatment are necessary.

Youngsters with severe asthma require daily medications and breathing treatments in order to control their wheezing and prevent serious asthma attacks. These youngsters need frequent medical attention—with the treatment goal being the control of wheezing and the management of the asthma—so the youngsters can lead as normal a life as possible. With good control, most asthmatics can be fully active and participate in all activities and sports. They may have very little, if any, chronic lung disease.

You should know that the medicines used for the control of asthma are excellent but very strong and *can* be dangerous if misused. These medications work when there is a steady and specific level of the drugs in the blood. Therefore, the proper dose of each drug needs to be taken on a *very* specific schedule—not more and not less, not sooner and not later. Often, blood tests are used to monitor the drug levels in the blood. Likewise, aerosol (breathing) treatments can unintentionally be abused—which can be particularly dangerous and at times deadly.

One note: You've probably seen or heard about the many over-the-counter medications and inhalers that are marketed to control asthma. These should not be used— especially by children. The use of the portable, hand-held nebulizers has been associated with sudden death when they are accidentally abused. If a child (or adult) has asthma, he or she should be under a doctor's care and taking only the medications prescribed (in the amounts and on the time schedule prescribed).

THE DON'TS

Don't try to treat an asthma attack with over-the-counter medications. Asthma is a serious chronic disease that requires medical supervision and treatment if long-term disability and even death are to be avoided.

Don't use more than the prescribed doses of medication or alter the schedule without contacting the youngster's doctor and receiving his or her approval. The doses needed for most asthma medications are very specific. Giving too much may put the youngster at risk for serious side effects. Giving too little may not control the asthma, and the youngster will suffer needlessly.

Don't allow a youngster to use a doctor-prescribed hand-held inhaler or nebulizer without your supervision or that of another adult who clearly understands the dose, time schedule, and proper use of the inhaler.

Remember, don't use over-the-counter inhalers at all without medical approval!

PLEASE NOTE: Now that you have a grasp of how to recognize and manage asthma, it would be extremely helpful for you to go back to the Emergency Quick Reference With the Steps in Detail and review it carefully. The more familiar you are with that material, the more useful it will be to you when you need it.

334

ILLNESS IN
INFANTS,
CHILDREN,
AND
ADOLESCENTS

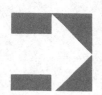

EMERGENCY QUICK REFERENCE

With the Steps in Detail

Bronchiolitis

▶ **SUSPECT BRONCHIOLITIS IN AN INFANT OR TODDLER WHO HAS TROUBLE BREATHING AND IS WHEEZING.**

▶ **CALL THE DOCTOR FOR AN APPOINTMENT TODAY OR HAVE THE INFANT OR TODDLER SEEN IN AN EMERGENCY ROOM IF:**

- He is taking more than forty breaths per minute.

- Wheezing is severe or can be heard when the child is breathing both out and in.

- She is pale or bluish.

- He seems very tired or listless.

- She is too tired or distressed to drink from the breast or bottle.

▶ **FOR MILD BRONCHIOLITIS, THE FOLLOWING MIGHT BE HELPFUL:**

- Use a cool-mist vaporizer in the baby's room to make the air more moist (and more comfortable to breathe).

- Prop the baby in a partially sitting position or use an infant seat (or even a car restraint seat). The sitting position is usually the most comfortable position for the baby. Tilt the head of her mattress up slightly.

- Encourage the little one to take extra liquids, especially "clear" liquids (dilute juices and other liquids that you can see through).

- If the doctor has prescribed or recommended any medication(s), use it (them) only as directed. Be sure you understand the purpose and exact dosage (amount and time intervals) of the medication(s) prescribed or recommended.

335

RECOGNIZING
AND
MANAGING
SERIOUS OR
POTENTIALLY
SERIOUS
ILLNESS

Bronchiolitis: What Is It?

A common viral infection of young infants, bronchiolitis causes inflammation of the very tiny airways in the lungs (called bronchioles). Swelling of these little structures, along with mucous production, leads to narrowing and partial blockage of these airways. The result? Wheezing and trouble breathing.

Bronchiolitis is caused by what is called respiratory syncytial virus—which is most often active in the winter months. This virus usually strikes infants under a year old but can affect toddlers if they haven't yet developed immunity to it. It is quite contagious and spreads easily among young, susceptible infants. However, once a child has had bronchiolitis, he or she is immune to the virus.

Because bronchiolitis is a viral infection, there is no cure for it—and the virus must simply run its course. Most cases of bronchiolitis are moderate in their severity, some are mild, and a few are very serious. Some infants (one-third to half) who have had bronchiolitis later develop asthma.

Bronchiolitis: Signs and Symptoms

The first symptoms of this viral disease are usually those of an ordinary cold—stuffiness, runny nose, and a cough. Then you will notice that a baby has a tight, hacking cough and is breathing fast. These symptoms get progressively worse over three to four days—then gradually improve.

Usually, babies have a respiratory rate (frequency of breathing in and out) of forty to sixty times a minute, but they can breathe up to eighty to one hundred times a minute with this disease. You may also notice retractions of the chest and hear a whistling, musical noise (a wheeze) when the baby breathes out and/or in. Some babies with bronchiolitis have a low fever (up to 102 degrees is not unusual), and most look pale and listless. Babies can be so breathless that they cannot even suck well, and they tire easily when they must work so hard to breathe. Some sleep more than usual, while others have trouble sleeping and are cranky and irritable. Coughing is common and can be very bothersome for the baby.

Bronchiolitis usually lasts about seven to ten days. It gets progressively worse over the first three to four days, then gradually improves. You will notice that the cough changes from a hacking one to wet and loose. This signals that the baby is getting progressively better.

Bronchiolitis: When to Worry

As previously noted, bronchiolitis usually worsens gradually over three to four days—then gets steadily better. A baby who is in the early stages of the disease and is breathing very fast can sometimes get progressively fatigued as the disease worsens.

336

ILLNESS IN
INFANTS,
CHILDREN,
AND
ADOLESCENTS

The baby may be so distressed that he cannot suck (eat) and breathe at the same time. At this point, the baby may need to be hospitalized. Here he can be observed, given oxygen, if needed—along with other special treatments that will make him more comfortable until the virus has run its course. Sometimes, the baby must be fed intravenously.

Unfortunately, there is no cure for bronchiolitis except "time." Most medicines for wheezing and cough are not very effective and can sometimes even be dangerous for very young infants who get this disease. Again, because this is a viral disease, antibiotics are of no help. However, sometimes doctors may recommend certain drugs to treat wheezing and congestion, in the hope that they may help. Fluids, comfort, and careful watching for signs of oxygen shortage, severe tiring, or inability to drink are the mainstays of treatment. Other measures are not nearly as important.

THE DON'TS

Don't give an infant under one year of age medicine without a doctor's recommendation, and be sure to ask what is the correct dose to be given. Young infants are especially susceptible to the side effects of over-the-counter drugs.

Don't overlook the signs of serious trouble in an infant. Call the doctor and have the little one evaluated if he or she seems particularly ill or distressed.

Don't assume that a child who wheezes with more than one illness is having bronchiolitis repeatedly. After once having had the viral disease (respiratory syncytial virus), a youngster is resistant to it for the rest of her life. If a youngster continues to wheeze with subsequent illnesses, then she probably has asthma or another lung disease and requires evaluation by your doctor.

PLEASE NOTE: Now that you have a grasp of how to recognize and manage bronchiolitis, it would be extremely helpful for you to go back to the Emergency Quick Reference With the Steps in Detail and review it carefully. The more familiar you are with that material, the more useful it will be to you when you need it.

337

RECOGNIZING
AND
MANAGING
SERIOUS OR
POTENTIALLY
SERIOUS
ILLNESS

EMERGENCY QUICK REFERENCE

With the Steps in Detail

Convulsions/Seizures

▶ **IF A CHILD IS HAVING A CONVULSION—MOVE HER TO A SAFE PLACE WHERE SHE CANNOT HURT HERSELF.**

- Put her on the floor or on a wide bed, where she cannot hurt herself if she thrashes around.

- If you cannot move her, then move any furniture or other items that she might roll against or hit and hurt herself.

▶ **MAKE SURE THE AIRWAY IS OPEN.**

- Put the youngster on his side, so any mucus, vomit, or other secretions drain out of the mouth. (This is done so he will not choke or aspirate— inhale vomited material.)

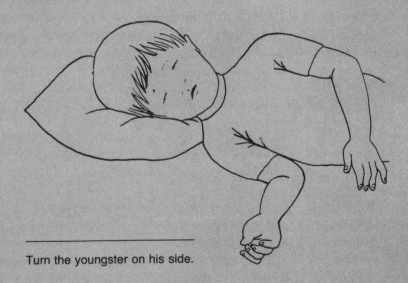

Turn the youngster on his side.

- Tip the head back a bit so the jaw is jutted slightly forward.

- Clear the mouth of any debris if you can, but *don't* try to pry the mouth

338

ILLNESS IN
INFANTS,
CHILDREN,
AND
ADOLESCENTS

open or push a stick between the teeth. This is futile and can injure the youngster and you.

▶ **LOOK AT YOUR WATCH OR A CLOCK (IF YOU CAN), SO YOU CAN TIME HOW LONG THE CONVULSION LASTS.**

- Most convulsions stop by themselves in less than five minutes.

▶ **WATCH THE CHILD FOR THE FOLLOWING:**

- Extreme blueness. If this occurs, readjust the airway and try to give rescue breaths, as you learned in CPR training. (If you are unable to remember the details of rescue breathing, turn to the Emergency Quick Reference on page 113, entitled "A Review of the Six Steps of CPR.")

- What parts of the body are affected by the seizure and what the seizure looks like.

▶ **IF THE SEIZURE LASTS LONGER THAN FIVE MINUTES OR THE YOUNGSTER BECOMES VERY BLUE, HAVE SOMEONE ELSE CALL THE PARAMEDICS WHILE YOU TREAT THE CHILD. IF NO ONE IS WITH YOU, CONTINUE TREATING THE CHILD WHILE YOU PERIODICALLY SHOUT FOR HELP. WHEN HELP ARRIVES, HAVE THAT PERSON CALL THE PARAMEDICS.**

▶ **AFTER THE SEIZURE IS OVER, CHECK THE YOUNGSTER TO SEE IF SHE HAS A FEVER. IF HER TEMPERATURE IS OVER 103 DEGREES, TAKE STEPS TO LOWER THE TEMPERATURE.**

- Take her clothing off.

- Give an appropriate dose of acetaminophen (such as Tylenol, Datril, or Tempra) by mouth—but *only* if the youngster is awake.

- Sponge the child with cool, wet cloths and let her air-dry.

- Do *not* give anything by mouth if the youngster is still unconscious.

▶ **CALL YOUR DOCTOR TO DISCUSS FURTHER EVALUATION AND TREATMENT.** UNLESS THE YOUNGSTER IS KNOWN TO HAVE SEIZURES/CONVULSIONS, HE WILL NEED TO BE EVALUATED IN THE DOCTOR'S OFFICE OR EMERGENCY ROOM.

What You Should Know About Convulsions (Seizures)

A convulsion (or *seizure*, as it is more correctly called) occurs when there is abnormal electrical activity in the brain. A seizure is most often generalized (involves the whole body) in infants and young children but can, in some cases, involve only a part of the body. There are many possible causes of seizures, including fever, brain injury, and disturbances in body chemistry and water balance. In many children (and adults), the cause is never really found. While some youngsters with seizure problems are obviously handicapped, the vast majority of them (especially those who have seizures only with fever) are otherwise completely normal.

It is always imperative that an infant, child, or older person who has had a seizure be evaluated carefully to try to determine its cause. This involves not only a careful medical history and physical examination but also certain laboratory tests. Often, the doctor will want to do an electroencephalogram (EEG)—a brain-wave test—to see if there might be an abnormality on the surface of the brain that could explain the seizure. The doctor may also recommend certain special X rays and other studies, depending on what he or she thinks the cause of the seizure is likely to be. The tests recommended may differ, depending on whether or not the seizure was associated with fever.

Most *seizure disorders* (a term preferred over the older term, *epilepsy*) can be controlled with medications so a young person does not have further convulsions. This is always the goal of treatment. Some children can be taken off medication after only a few years, while others must take it for life. This depends on the cause of the seizures.

Recognizing a Seizure

There are many myths about seizures, but one thing is true—they are very frightening. With the most common type, the youngster becomes unconscious and usually falls down if he is not already lying down. He becomes stiff and begins jerking in a rhythmic way. There may be mucus and saliva in the mouth and throat, and sometimes he becomes pale or even blue. It always seems as if the convulsion is lasting forever—but in fact, most last for less than five minutes and stop all by themselves.

Many children wet themselves and/or lose control of their bowels during the seizure. Afterward, the youngster is not able to be fully awakened for five to thirty minutes and prefers to sleep for a short time. He usually is confused and does not remember what happened. Sometimes, there is temporary overall weakness or weakness of one side of the body.

340

ILLNESS IN
INFANTS,
CHILDREN,
AND
ADOLESCENTS

Febrile Seizures: A Special Problem

Certain infants and children between the ages of six months and four years are susceptible to convulsions when they run very high fevers. When their temperatures rise high enough—usually above 103 degrees—they may have a convulsion. About one in twenty or twenty-five children will experience this kind of seizure. Only half of the children who have had a febrile seizure ever experience more than one, and this tendency stops after the preschool years. While some youngsters go on to have a chronic seizure disorder, the vast majority of them are perfectly normal and have no other problems with seizures.

Febrile convulsions usually are generalized—they cause jerking of the whole body and loss of consciousness. They rarely last more than five minutes or need special medications to stop them. Control of high fever is the key both to controlling febrile seizures and to preventing them in the future.

If a youngster obviously has a fever and has had a convulsion, it is important to try to lower her fever before rushing to the doctor or emergency room. Take her temperature and begin to cool her—using cool, wet cloths and lukewarm baths. If the youngster is arousable, give acetaminophen (aspirin substitute) by mouth (in the correct dose). If the youngster is not able to be awakened, you can use an acetaminophen suppository (in the correct dosage) if you have one, but don't give an unconscious youngster anything to eat or drink. Try to reduce the temperature below 103 degrees if you can.

A few infants and children who have seizures when they have fever also have a serious underlying infection of the brain—called meningitis. Because of this uncommon but real possibility, it is vital that any infant who has a seizure when he has had a fever be evaluated by a doctor afterward, unless there has been a seizure in the past and the doctor has evaluated the youngster and told you what to do in the event another occurs. This evaluation will almost always include a spinal tap (also called a lumbar puncture) to be sure there is no meningitis. (It is often difficult to be sure there is no brain infection after a seizure by physical examination only, because the child is so sleepy or hard to arouse, and relaxed or limp.) A spinal tap is the only way to verify or rule out meningitis.

Treatment of Seizures

Most children with seizure disorders can be effectively treated with one or more medications. These medications reduce the sensitivity of the brain to abnormal electrical activity. The most commonly used drug (prescribed initially) is phenobarbital. Most youngsters need take only this drug for seizure control. If the youngster experiences extreme hyperactivity or excessive sleepiness, another drug might be prescribed. A

341

RECOGNIZING
AND
MANAGING
SERIOUS OR
POTENTIALLY
SERIOUS
ILLNESS

few youngsters, especially those with underlying brain damage, require several drugs to control their seizures.

Because of the potential side effects and to be sure seizure control is the best it can be, youngsters who are taking medications for seizures must be monitored carefully by their doctors. As part of this management, sometimes blood tests are done to measure the blood levels of the drugs and ensure correct dosages. Periodic EEGs are also performed to help the doctor decide if and when a youngster can stop taking medication.

You should know that there is considerable controversy about whether or not infants and children who have had febrile seizures (those that occur only with fever) should be given medication to prevent further convulsions. While the best preventive measure for febrile seizures is controlling the fever, certain children benefit from preventive use of phenobarbital for several years. Most doctors recommend this only after a youngster has had more than one seizure when he or she has a fever, but there may be a few situations in which medication would be suggested after the first such seizure. Most children with febrile seizures have normal EEGs and are taken off phenobarbital around the age of four years.

There is no logical reason for a youngster with febrile seizures to start taking phenobarbital at the first sign of a fever. The medicine is ineffective if given in this way—because it cannot build up in the bloodstream fast enough to have any preventive effect.

It is vital for a youngster who is prescribed a seizure-control drug to take this medication exactly as recommended—no more and no less. *The most common cause of seizures in a youngster who has had a seizure disorder diagnosed and medication prescribed is FAILURE TO TAKE THE MEDICATION.*

Other Precautions to Take

Many people feel that youngsters with seizure disorders must be kept from many normal activities. However, when seizures are under control, this is not true—with a few commonsense exceptions.

The major risk to a youngster who has a seizure is injury (due to loss of consciousness). Because of this, any activity in which a child or others would be in danger if he or she were to suddenly lose consciousness is potentially hazardous. A child with seizures should not be allowed to swim alone, climb trees, be involved in other dangerous physical activities without another person around, or be placed in potentially hazardous situations—*especially if the convulsions are not fully controlled by medication.* Likewise, teenagers and adults with seizure problems are not permitted to operate motor vehicles or dangerous equipment. Certain restrictions (for children and adults) can generally be removed if and when they have been without seizures for a number of years. If your child has a seizure disorder, it is vital to discuss any limitations

342

ILLNESS IN
INFANTS,
CHILDREN,
AND
ADOLESCENTS

or recommendations with his or her doctor. *Do not unnecessarily limit the youngster, but don't put him or her into jeopardy either*. In other words, be careful to follow the doctor's safety recommendations, but it is not necessary or even fair to a child to go beyond those recommendations.

Breath-Holding Spells: A Confusing Problem

Many older infants and toddlers have a breath-holding spell once or twice, and the effect on their parents can be dramatic—because the spell can be so impressive and frightening. It's important to understand the difference between this kind of spell and a convulsion.

Most children are between one and two years old when they have their first breath-holding spell, although a few will start at a younger age. This is a time when they are trying to assert themselves and often are frustrated easily—because you set limits on what they can do and their curiosity overwhelms them, or because they cannot communicate with you very well, for example. Some youngsters have only one spell, while others have many.

With a typical breath-holding spell, a toddler is very upset and crying, sometimes having a temper tantrum. As he is crying, he takes a deep breath and screams loudly, then holds his breath after he has completely exhaled. His face turns red, then purple, and then blue, and he stops breathing. After what seems like an eternity, he gets very limp and may even have a few jerking or convulsive movements. Then he looks peaceful, starts breathing again, and his color returns to normal. He may be slightly sleepy when he wakes up.

These spells are especially confusing when there are jerking movements, and some parents think they are convulsions. They are also worried because the little one turns so blue and becomes unconscious for a short time. Most often, these spells are not at all serious, and youngsters stop having them after one or two, especially if they learn that a temper tantrum like this still doesn't get them what they wanted.

The easiest way to tell the difference between this kind of tantrum and a seizure is to think about what was happening before the little one lost consciousness. With a temper tantrum/breath-holding spell, the child is *upset and crying* (whether because of a tantrum or because she hurt herself, for example), and she turns blue *before* she passes out and starts jerking. With a seizure, the little one is usually not upset but rather is doing normal activity. The loss of consciousness and jerking come "out of the blue," and the paleness and blueness of the skin come *after* the unconsciousness.

Try to stay calm if you think your little one is having a breath-holding spell. Calmly lay the child down on the floor so he can't hurt himself, and stand back and watch. Be sure the episode follows the general pattern discussed previously. When the little one wakes up, try to comfort him, but let him know by your actions that this kind of spell won't get him what he wanted (if the spell resulted from a temper tantrum).

343

RECOGNIZING
AND
MANAGING
SERIOUS OR
POTENTIALLY
SERIOUS
ILLNESS

If it happens in a public place, you will undoubtedly be embarrassed and concerned. Again, try to stay calm and not overreact. After the spell is over, pick the youngster up and go to an area where you can comfort the child and talk to her privately and let her regain her composure.

Most often, breath-holding spells are a passing fancy and don't require any action other than your staying calm. If you are having an ongoing problem, or the little one has repeated episodes with twitching and jerking, make an appointment with your doctor for an evaluation and discussion. He or she may have some additional strategies to suggest for curtailing the spells.

THE DON'TS

Don't try to put something in the mouth or between the teeth of a child who is having a convulsion. It is unnecessary and can even be damaging.

Don't fail to have an infant or toddler who has had a convulsion with fever (for the first time) examined by the doctor, even if he or she seems fine afterward. A few infants will have an underlying serious infection that needs prompt identification and treatment.

Don't stop seizure medications abruptly without your doctor's recommendation. The most common cause of seizures in children (and adults) whose seizures have been under control is failure to take the prescribed medication (or in young, growing children, "outgrowing" their dose—getting so large that they need more medication).

Don't expose a youngster with an uncontrolled seizure problem to unnecessary risk, but don't unnecessarily limit his or her activities either. If you have questions about certain activities, then speak with the youngster's doctor about any specific recommendations.

Don't forget to tell others who spend a great deal of time with your child about the possibility of her having a convulsion, especially if her seizures have not been completely controlled through medication. The normal panic that people feel can be lessened tremendously if they know what they might expect, and what they can do to help. Be sure to caution them about unnecessary risks, but emphasize that the child can take part in normal activities without undue concern.

PLEASE NOTE: Now that you have a grasp of how to recognize and manage convulsions/seizures, it would be extremely helpful for you to go back to the Emergency Quick Reference With the Steps in Detail and review it carefully. The more familiar you are with that material, the more useful it will be to you when you need it.

344

ILLNESS IN
INFANTS,
CHILDREN,
AND
ADOLESCENTS

EMERGENCY QUICK REFERENCE

With the Steps in Detail

Croup

▶ **SUSPECT CROUP IF A YOUNG CHILD WHO HAS SOME COLD SYMP-TOMS DEVELOPS A HARSH, BARKING COUGH; STRIDOR** (HARSH, CROWING NOISE WHEN BREATHING IN); **AND HOARSENESS, WITH OR WITHOUT A FEVER.**

- In mild croup, you may notice the loud breathing noise only when the little one is upset and crying.

- Croup most often first appears during the night and improves during the daytime.

▶ **IF THE CHILD IS BLUE AND ANXIOUS:**

- Call the paramedics or an ambulance (or go quickly [but safely] to an emergency room if you think you can get there within five to ten minutes).

- Have the little one sit up, or hold him upright, and try to calm him down.

- If you have called the paramedics and are waiting for assistance, take the child outside, if the air is cooler there.

- Continue to observe him carefully for signs of complete airway blockage. If these occur, try to open the airway and begin rescue breathing (as you were taught in CPR class). (If you are unable to remember the details of performing rescue breathing, turn to the Emergency Quick Reference on page 113, entitled "A Review of the Six Steps of CPR.")

▶ **IF THE CHILD HAS A HIGH FEVER, IS VERY ANXIOUS AND IS DROOLING OR REFUSES TO SWALLOW, AND HAS DIFFICULTY BREATHING IN (INHALING):**

- Go directly (but safely) to an emergency room if you can get there within ten minutes, or call the paramedics or an ambulance.

345

RECOGNIZING
AND
MANAGING
SERIOUS OR
POTENTIALLY
SERIOUS
ILLNESS

- Try to keep the youngster calm.

- Do *not* attempt home treatment. This may not be croup.

▶ **IF THE YOUNGSTER IS MAKING A LOT OF NOISE WITH BREATHING BUT IS NOT BLUE:**

- Try to calm him down. Crying and fussing further irritate the swollen voice box (remember how you feel with laryngitis) and are painful.

- Go into a steamy bathroom and stay there, calming the child, for twenty to thirty minutes. Be sure to shut the door. It is easier to make a lot of steam with your shower if the air in the bathroom is quite cool or cold, so don't be tempted to use a heater or heat lamp. You might find it comfortable to take a chair with you and even read the little one a book.

- If you cannot get much steam in your bathroom, go outside (if the air is cooler there) for twenty to thirty minutes. In most climates, the night air is moist and cool. This will often result in a miraculous improvement in the croup (and will *not* lead to further "cold" symptoms). Many a youngster who is being taken to an emergency room for croup is cured on the way!

- If there is no improvement, call your child's doctor or go to an emergency room.

▶ **IF THE SYMPTOMS ARE MILD, OR THE CHILD IMPROVED WITH THE STEAM TREATMENT, YOU MAY ALSO FIND THE FOLLOWING HELP-FUL FOR THE NEXT FEW HOURS AND DAYS:**

- A vaporizer in the child's room while he or she sleeps. Use a cool-mist vaporizer if you can, since it will keep the air cool and moist and will not pose the burn hazard of a steam vaporizer.

- A cough-suppressant medicine if your doctor recommends it. The cough of croup is very irritating to the swollen airways and is not effective in expelling mucus, so the cough can safely be suppressed.

- Encourage the little one to drink plenty of liquids. Usually, there is some soreness to the throat, so cool or cold, nonacid, noncarbonated liquids are generally very acceptable. Don't worry if the child won't eat solid foods.

- Use aspirin substitute for comfort and fever control. Be sure you use the correct dosage for your child's size.

346

ILLNESS IN
INFANTS,
CHILDREN,
AND
ADOLESCENTS

▶ **CALL THE DOCTOR FOR ADDITIONAL ADVICE IF THE SYMPTOMS LAST FOR LONGER THAN THREE DAYS OR IF YOU HAVE OTHER CONCERNS.**

● Be aware that croup is caused by a virus and therefore is not helped by antibiotic treatment.

● A few youngsters get ear infections when they have croup. If you are concerned about this, or your youngster is prone to ear infections, call your doctor.

● Certain youngsters are prone to get croup with any respiratory infection or for other unknown reasons. If this occurs, you will become an expert in recognizing and treating it—and will not panic when you hear your youngster's characteristic "bark."

Croup: What You Should Know

Croup is a frightening problem for many parents—partly because they don't really understand it and mostly because of the incorrect information they have heard about it. The fact of the matter is, the croup cough is scary and would frighten anyone who did not know what was going on and what to do about it. You should try to remember that most often croup is a mild disease, although there are a few situations in which it can be dangerous. By knowing what to do and learning what danger signs to look for, you will feel less fearful if your child gets croup.

Essentially, croup is usually a viral infection that causes sudden swelling (inflammation) of the upper airway, including the vocal cords, larynx, trachea, and sometimes the bronchi. The medical term for croup is a mouthful, but it actually pinpoints the inflamed areas. It's called *laryngotracheobronchitis*.

Croup most often affects little ones between six months and three years of age, although it can occur a bit earlier than that or a bit later. Younger infants (under six months) with croup symptoms need to be seen by a doctor so he or she can determine if they need to be evaluated for *other problems* of the airway. Some children have croup only once, if at all, while others seem to get it with almost all respiratory infections. Older children who get "croupy" with colds and other respiratory infections usually had their first attack of croup as infants or toddlers.

347

RECOGNIZING
AND
MANAGING
SERIOUS OR
POTENTIALLY
SERIOUS
ILLNESS

Croup: Signs and Symptoms

Croup most often starts out looking like a *usual cold*. An infant or toddler seems to have nose congestion, perhaps a little cough, and a slight fever. You might notice that his voice seems a bit *hoarse* or his cry a little more hoarse or raspy than usual. Then, during the first night or two of the cold, the child is suddenly awakened by a harsh, barking (*croupy*) *cough*, which may sound like a seal bark. He makes a loud, crowing noise (called *stridor*) when breathing in, especially when he is upset and crying. He will usually have a fever—even as high as 103 degrees. If you take off his pajamas, you'll notice that when he breathes in, his chest sucks in below the rib cage, above the collarbone, and between the ribs (these are called *retractions*). Because these symptoms are uncomfortable and the cough frightening, the child is rightfully very upset.

No one knows why, but most croup attacks occur at night. Children usually improve with home treatment, only to have another croup attack the next night. During the day, they may seem fine, except for some hoarseness and a barking cough, but there is no stridor with breathing. Then, at night, the stridor and difficult breathing start again, and the cough gets worse. This pattern (better in the daytime, worse at night) goes on for three or four days. Then the hoarseness improves, and the cough gradually gets better. However, the youngster may continue to have some coughing for as long as two weeks.

Occasionally, an attack of croup will be severe enough to require medical attention. When the airway blockage is severe enough that a baby *has extreme difficulty breathing and is making only a little noise, or when there is extreme paleness or any blueness of the skin*, then go to an emergency room without delay (within five to ten minutes), or call for paramedic or ambulance assistance. (Remember, you can often get to an emergency room with a "portable" infant faster and more safely than if you call an emergency vehicle. Save this for when you have no other alternative or when you need professional assistance.) If the infant or toddler is still breathing very noisily or having a lot of discomfort after you have tried home treatment, call your doctor for advice (or go to an emergency room if you have no doctor or are unable to reach your doctor).

When "Croup" Is Not Croup

Epiglottitis and *foreign body in the airway* are two serious problems that need to be considered when "croup" does not behave like croup!

Epiglottitis is a serious bacterial infection of the epiglottis—a structure in the back of the throat that covers the airway when we swallow. This infection usually strikes

348

ILLNESS IN
INFANTS,
CHILDREN,
AND
ADOLESCENTS

children between two and six years old, although it can affect younger and older children, as well. With this problem, a child becomes *suddenly (over hours) very ill, has a high fever (often over 103 degrees), very sore throat, and increasing difficulty breathing.* Her voice may seem muffled or unusual, and *she will avoid talking or coughing,* if possible. As the epiglottis becomes more and more swollen, the youngster will have difficulty when breathing in—but *makes much less noise than with croup.* She prefers to sit up to breathe, looks very sick, and shows signs of true anxiety (almost panic). She may refuse to swallow water or even her own saliva (and because of this may even drool). Skin color may be pale, flushed, or increasingly blue.

This is a true emergency, since the swollen epiglottis may block the airway at any time. Keep yourself and the youngster calm and go to an emergency room, or call the paramedics for assistance if it would take you longer than five or ten minutes to get there.

A *foreign body* caught in the upper airway can also masquerade as "croup." In this situation, however, the barking cough and stridor usually start while a youngster is awake and playing—and you may be able to tell that he or she choked on something. There is *no fever,* and there are *no other signs of respiratory infection.* If you suspect a foreign object in the airway, call your child's doctor or go to an emergency room for evaluation. For further information about this problem, refer to Chapter 6.

THE DON'TS

Don't panic when you hear the characteristic "bark" of croup. Even the loudest noise can mean mild croup.

Don't hesitate to get emergency help if the symptoms are NOT what you'd expect for croup. Since epiglottitis and foreign body in the airway can to a certain extent mimic croup, the minute you feel this may not be croup, call your doctor for advice.

Don't expect that viral croup should be treated with an antibiotic. Time and nature's healing process are all that will help. Direct your attention to helping the little one feel better.

PLEASE NOTE: Now that you have a grasp of how to recognize and manage croup, it would be extremely helpful for you to go back to the Emergency Quick Reference With the Steps in Detail and review it carefully. The more familiar you are with that material, the more useful it will be to you when you need it.

349

RECOGNIZING
AND
MANAGING
SERIOUS OR
POTENTIALLY
SERIOUS
ILLNESS

EMERGENCY QUICK REFERENCE

Cystic Fibrosis

Suspect cystic fibrosis in an infant or child who shows one or more of the following symptoms:

▶ **REPEATED LUNG INFECTIONS (PNEUMONIA) OR WHEEZING.**

▶ **EXCESSIVE SWEATING AND SKIN THAT TASTES SALTY.**

▶ **LARGE, FATTY BOWEL MOVEMENTS.**

▶ **FAILURE TO GAIN WEIGHT AT THE NORMAL RATE.**

Make an appointment with your youngster's doctor if you notice one or more of the symptoms of cystic fibrosis.

Cystic Fibrosis: What You Should Know

Cystic fibrosis is one of the most common of the genetic (inherited through the genes) diseases of children. It occurs in 1 out of every 1,500 to 1,600 births. While some of its more obvious and serious effects are on the lungs, it is a chronic disease that affects nearly all systems of the body and can worsen quickly or very slowly. While there is no cure for this disease, which often leads to death in childhood, modern treatment can prolong life well into the adult years, and many children with cystic fibrosis lead full, productive, and nearly normal lives. In general, the earlier the disease is recognized and treated, the better.

Cystic fibrosis is inherited as an autosomal recessive trait—that is, the youngster receives one abnormal gene from each parent. His parents appear completely normal but have a one-in-four chance that each of their children could have the disease because each carries the abnormal recessive gene for cystic fibrosis. If the child receives one abnormal gene for cystic fibrosis from one parent and a normal gene from the other parent, then she would not have cystic fibrosis but would be a ''carrier'' of the gene. There are a few tests being developed and studied for detecting cystic fibrosis before or at birth, but these tests are not as yet practical except in families in which there is known cystic fibrosis.

350

ILLNESS IN
INFANTS,
CHILDREN,
AND
ADOLESCENTS

While cystic fibrosis cannot be cured, it can be successfully treated in most young-sters. The treatment is best carried out or supervised through special pulmonary (lung) treatment centers.

Cystic Fibrosis: Signs and Symptoms

In children with cystic fibrosis, the glands secrete abnormally thick, sticky mucus. In the respiratory system, this leads to frequent lung infections (pneumonia) and chronic lung damage. In the digestive system, the pancreas does not produce digestive enzymes, so food is not properly absorbed. Bowel movements are abnormal, and the youngster does not gain weight normally. In addition, the thickness of the secretions can lead to obstruction (blockage) in the bowel, as well as prolapse (protrusion) of the rectal lining. Youngsters with cystic fibrosis sweat profusely and lose excessive amounts of salt in their sweat.

Sometimes, cystic fibrosis is suspected in newborn infants who have a particular type of bowel blockage called meconium ileus. However, more often it is suspected when a young infant does not gain weight as well as expected and has frequent or severe lung infections and excessive amounts of salty sweat. Some infants or young children show signs of serious malnutrition with few if any lung symptoms, while others have serious lung problems without many signs of intestinal malfunction.

The most telltale sign of cystic fibrosis is excessive loss of salt (sodium chloride) in the sweat. This fact is the basis for the diagnostic test for cystic fibrosis—a sweat analysis in which sweat is collected, then analyzed for its salt content. You can do a quick home test for this disease by tasting your youngster's sweat. Kiss the youngster, then lick your lips. Ordinarily, the infant will not "taste" excessively salty. However, with cystic fibrosis, your lips will taste salty consistently. If you detect this sign, contact your child's doctor for an appointment.

Cystic Fibrosis: What to Expect

Your child's doctor will want the child to have a sweat test if there is any suspicion of cystic fibrosis—no matter how remote the suspicion. If the salt content is abnormally high, the youngster may need to be in the hospital for a week or so to determine how advanced his disease is and treat him vigorously with pancreatic enzymes (to help digestion), as well as to administer antibiotics and provide other needed treatment for his lungs.

Most often, children with cystic fibrosis require hospitalization at first, then peri-odically if the disease is to remain under control. These youngsters will need to take substitutes for the missing pancreatic enzymes, have frequent chest therapy (done by slapping the back in a specified way in order to loosen the thick secretions within the respiratory tract), and take antibiotics most of the time. Most children with cystic fibrosis are hospitalized periodically for so-called tune-ups—the goal of which is to keep their functioning at or near normal. The antibiotics that are most successful in treating the bacteria that complicate cystic fibrosis must be given intravenously or by intramuscular injection.

THE DON'TS

Don't panic if your youngster's doctor recommends that your youngster have the sweat test for cystic fibrosis. While the disease is not rare, many youngsters who have some of the symptoms of cystic fibrosis do not, in fact, have the disease.

Don't panic if your child is diagnosed as having cystic fibrosis. Great strides have been made over the past several years in treating this disease, and new modes of treatment are being successfully developed all the time. If cystic fibrosis is diagnosed and treated early, and you and your doctor "stay on top" of the disease, your child has a chance of living a long, productive life—well into adulthood.

PLEASE NOTE: Now that you have a grasp of how to recognize and manage cystic fibrosis, it would be extremely helpful for you to go back to the Emergency Quick Reference and review it carefully. The more familiar you are with that material, the more useful it will be to you when you need it.

352

ILLNESS IN
INFANTS,
CHILDREN,
AND
ADOLESCENTS

EMERGENCY QUICK REFERENCE

With the Steps in Detail

Dehydration

▶ **CALL THE DOCTOR OR GO TO AN EMERGENCY ROOM PROMPTLY IF A CHILD (ESPECIALLY A YOUNG INFANT OR TODDLER) SHOWS ONE OR MORE SIGNS OF DEHYDRATION:**

- Little or no urine over an eight- to twelve-hour period.

- Dry, sticky mouth.

- Dry, sunken eyeballs.

- Severe thirst.

- Lethargy and irritability, along with weakness and weak cry.

- Skin that feels doughy in consistency or that stays "tented" up when you pinch it up.

- Signs of shock, with evidence of dehydration (cool, clammy skin; pale, gray, mottled, or bluish color; rapid or irregular breathing; rapid, weak pulse; collapse).

▶ **IF A YOUNGSTER HAS SIGNS OF SEVERE DEHYDRATION OR IS IN SHOCK, DO NOT TRY TO GIVE HIM LIQUIDS OR ORAL MEDICATION. GET PROFESSIONAL HELP IMMEDIATELY.**

▶ **CALL THE DOCTOR FOR ADVICE IF A CHILD (ESPECIALLY AN IN-FANT OR TODDLER) HAS PERSISTENT SYMPTOMS THAT WOULD PUT HER AT RISK FOR DEHYDRATION:**

- Vomiting and/or diarrhea that is not slowing or stopping with home treatment measures.

- Refusal to drink at least half of her usual amount of liquid in a twenty-four-hour period, regardless of the reason (especially if there is also a fever).

353

RECOGNIZING
AND
MANAGING
SERIOUS OR
POTENTIALLY
SERIOUS
ILLNESS

- Marked reduction in the number of wet diapers or the amount of urine, or very concentrated (dark, strong) urine.

Dehydration: A Wide Spectrum

Dehydration—abnormal lack of body fluid—can result from a variety of problems. It is potentially more of a risk for younger infants and toddlers than for older children, but it can occur at any age. It can happen gradually or very suddenly, depending on the cause.

Dehydration most often develops when a small child is losing more fluid than he is drinking. The fluid loss may be due to vomiting, diarrhea, or even a large burn that is oozing body fluid. Vomiting is an especially difficult problem, not only because the youngster is losing excess fluid, but because he is also unable to take in enough liquid to replenish what has been lost. Diarrhea is a somewhat easier situation to manage— since the youngster can (at times) drink enough liquids to make up for what is lost.

Very sick or weak infants and children are especially prone to dehydration in very hot weather or when they have fevers. Usually, what happens is that they are not able to drink enough to keep ahead of their fluid losses (through urine, sweating, vomiting, and diarrhea). Since infants and nonverbal children are dependent on adults to "read" their signals that they're thirsty, they may also not be offered quite enough to drink. Also, youngsters who are breathing very fast have extra liquid requirements, as do those who sweat a great deal (for whatever reason, including vigorous exercise).

Dehydration: Signs and Symptoms

Normally, a youngster has a built-in mechanism to prevent dehydration: when his body is getting low on fluid, he gets thirsty—and drinks just the right amount to keep ahead of his losses. This system works very well for verbal children and older youngsters who can tell someone they are thirsty or get themselves something to drink. It also works well for infants and nonverbal children as long as they are offered enough liquids to drink or do not have any unusual fluid losses. However, the system works well only if the liquid used to replace losses has the right amount of salt in it, as well (for example, juices, commercial drinks such as Gatorade, carbonated beverages, and so on). If the system is altered—the results can be disastrous.

The kidneys function to keep the fluid balance in the body correct. When there is

354

ILLNESS IN
INFANTS,
CHILDREN,
AND
ADOLESCENTS

a low supply of fluid or unusual losses, the kidneys slow down their urine production, and the urine becomes concentrated (strong). When smaller amounts of urine are made and it becomes concentrated, it is very dark yellow in color. If the body is still not able to keep ahead of fluid losses, other signs and symptoms of dehydration begin to occur.

As the fluid supply dwindles, *thirst* increases, and *urine production decreases further*. Then the cells and tissues begin to show signs of dryness. The *lips*, then the lining of the *mouth and the tongue get sticky and dry*. *No tears* are formed, and the *eyes* begin to look glassy and *sunken*. With further water loss, the *skin* loses its elasticity and *wrinkles* easily when it is pinched and lifted. The youngster becomes weaker, more sleepy, and more irritable. If an infant or small child, his cry becomes weak, and he doesn't seem to care what is done to him. (For example, if you pinched the bottom of his foot, he might not even respond—when, normally, he would holler.)

As the youngster loses even more liquid, the amount of blood being circulated by the heart is reduced, and she slips into *shock*. She then breathes very fast and sometimes irregularly, with her pulse being fast, not weak. Her skin is cool and dry, and pale, gray, mottled, or bluish. If the situation is not corrected quickly (with intravenous fluids)—permanent damage to organs and tissues or even death can occur.

While water lack is the major problem in dehydration, salt imbalance (called electrolyte disturbance) also plays a role. Sometimes, the body's level of sodium (one of the body salts) becomes very high or very low. Potassium (another salt) may also become low. When dehydration occurs, the acid content of the cells and tissues usually increases. Once all of these events are added up—the result is an assault on the organs and tissues. The severity of these occurrences will influence how seriously ill the youngster will be. Electrolyte disturbances are particularly likely to occur with certain diseases (such as cystic fibrosis or chronic diarrhea) or if a youngster who has been vomiting or had diarrhea is given the wrong liquids to drink (for example, *large* quantities of plain water, boiled skim milk, or homemade salt solutions and other folk-medicine remedies that don't work).

The Treatment for Dehydration: What to Expect

Since dehydration is such a potentially serious problem—especially in young infants and toddlers—it is important that you call the doctor if you notice *any* signs of dehydration (even if the youngster is experiencing only a dry mouth and excessive thirst). The doctor will talk with you about *why* the youngster might be dehydrated and determine if you can try to treat the child at home (for a time) or if more drastic measures are warranted. The doctor will recommend liquids to give the youngster and the amount necessary to prevent further difficulty, as well as to correct the body's fluid imbalance.

355

RECOGNIZING
AND
MANAGING
SERIOUS OR
POTENTIALLY
SERIOUS
ILLNESS

Most often, you will be advised to give the youngster small servings of liquids that contain a small amount of salt, potassium, and sugar (as well as water). This might be in the form of juices, carbonated beverages, or electrolyte solutions such as Gatorade, Pedialyte, Infalyte, or Lyte-Pops. Follow the doctor's instructions about the amount and type of fluid intake, as well as when to call him or her back.

When dehydration has progressed beyond the dry-mouth stage, intravenous fluids are almost always necessary. This means the youngster will need to be hospitalized— usually for at least twenty-four hours. When hospitalized and the cause of dehydration is vomiting and/or diarrhea, the youngster will usually not be permitted to drink anything for a number of hours and will then gradually be started back on liquids after the dehydration is corrected. Most often, it takes twelve to forty-eight hours to completely replenish all fluids and electrolytes that have been lost (but this depends on the severity of dehydration).

THE DON'TS

Don't overlook the early signs of dehydration, including a decrease in urine production or concentrated urine, thirst, and dry mouth. The earlier treatment is begun, the shorter the recovery period will be—and the lower the risk is for permanent damage to various body tissues.

Don't concoct a homemade electrolyte solution or salt solution for a youngster who might become dehydrated. Older children and teenagers usually do well drinking fruit juices or carbonated beverages. Young infants and toddlers who are borderline dehydrated may need to drink a commercially available electrolyte solution. If you have questions about what would be best for your child, check with your doctor.

Don't forget that the younger the infant, the more prone he is to dehydration, and the quicker he will run out of body liquids. Be alert for signs of dryness and call the doctor if you are concerned.

Don't fail to prevent dehydration in situations that put a youngster at risk. Excessive heat, excessive exercise when the weather is very hot, fever, rapid breathing, and unusually large losses of water (due to vomiting, diarrhea, burns) are all situations where dehydration can occur. Offer additional fluids whenever the risk for dehydration increases.

PLEASE NOTE: Now that you have a grasp of how to recognize and manage dehydration, it would be extremely helpful for you to go back to the Emergency Quick Reference With the Steps in Detail and review it carefully. The more familiar you are with that material, the more useful it will be to you when you need it.

356

ILLNESS IN
INFANTS,
CHILDREN,
AND
ADOLESCENTS

EMERGENCY QUICK REFERENCE

Diabetes Mellitus

Suspect diabetes mellitus (also called juvenile diabetes or "sugar diabetes") in a child or older youngster who shows the following symptoms:

▶ **MARKED INCREASED IN THIRST AND CONSUMPTION OF LIQUIDS.**

▶ **MARKED INCREASE IN APPETITE.**

▶ **WEIGHT LOSS IN SPITE OF THE INCREASE IN LIQUID AND FOOD INTAKE.**

▶ **INCREASED URINATION, SOMETIMES OUT OF PROPORTION TO THE AMOUNT OF LIQUIDS THE YOUNGSTER IS DRINKING.**

▶ **PROGRESSIVE WEAKNESS AND LACK OF ACTIVITY.**

▶ **ABDOMINAL PAIN, VOMITING, AND PROGRESSIVE SLEEP-INESS ALONG WITH OR FOLLOWING THE ABOVE SYMPTOMS.**

Call your doctor for advice and an appointment if you recognize the above-stated symptoms. If you do not have a doctor, go to an emergency room, especially if the youngster seems weak or very sick along with increased thirst and urination.

Diabetes Mellitus: What You Should Know

Diabetes mellitus (often called "sugar diabetes") is a serious chronic disease that can suddenly appear at any age. If the disease is detected before the age of eighteen and the youngster is insulin-dependent, then it is commonly referred to as "juvenile diabetes."

Most often, the cause of diabetes in children is unknown. However, in some children, there is a link between diabetes and previous infections with certain viruses that appear to damage the insulin-producing cells of the pancreas (an organ located in the middle of the abdomen). There also appears to be a genetic link—in that there is a tendency

357

RECOGNIZING
AND
MANAGING
SERIOUS OR
POTENTIALLY
SERIOUS
ILLNESS

for diabetes to occur in children who have family members with the type of diabetes that requires insulin.

Insulin is a hormone needed by the body to convert the blood sugar, glucose, into energy. Normally, the glucose produced in the body from foods eaten is processed by insulin. Once processed, the glucose can be very efficiently used by the cells as energy.

With diabetes mellitus, this entire process goes crazy, causing serious problems. It can best be described as a chronic disease that produces a domino effect in the body. The basic problem is that the pancreas is not able to produce enough insulin. (This is different from the common type of diabetes in older adults, in which the insulin is not as effective as previously.)

When there isn't enough insulin, the body is unable to break down and therefore use the blood glucose (also called blood sugar) for energy. Instead, glucose continues to build up in the blood. Once it reaches very high levels, it escapes from the body in the urine, taking extra body water with it (the reason someone with uncontrolled diabetes is so excessively thirsty). The liver tries to make up for the cells' "lack" of glucose by converting stored body fats into glucose. This process is inefficient and results in the buildup of fat-breakdown products called ketones—a condition known as ketosis.

Meanwhile, the domino effect continues. The cells are literally "starving," in spite of the excessive amount of glucose in the bloodstream. In response, they produce excessive acids, which build up in the body and act like poisons. When this occurs, the problem is called acidosis.

When you add ketosis to acidosis, you get a very serious problem called ketoacidosis. Essentially, the body is poisoning itself. Initially, this entire process can take days or weeks to occur, because the pancreas continues to produce some insulin. As the insulin supply gets lower, ketoacidosis worsens—and can lead to diabetic coma and even death if not diagnosed and treated promptly.

Diabetes Mellitus: Signs and Symptoms

The symptoms of diabetes in children can start slowly, with *increased thirst and appetite* for days or weeks before more serious signs of this disease appear. Often, parents remember the first signs only after the youngster has gotten quite ill, because the first signs are so subtle. At first, the youngster drinks excessive liquids and eats voraciously only during the daytime. Later, he or she might even wake at night to eat and drink, as well as urinate. Sometimes, bed-wetting after years of being dry at night is a clue to this disease.

In spite of the amount of food the youngster consumes, he begins to *lose weight* and seem listless and out of sorts. His school performance and play activity worsen, and he seems weak. If the disease is not recognized at this point, more serious symptoms begin to appear.

358

ILLNESS IN
INFANTS,
CHILDREN,
AND
ADOLESCENTS

Easily recognized symptoms of diabetes often show up when a youngster develops an infection. With fever and illness, the cells are further stressed, and *weakness*, as well as *dehydration*, occur—in spite of the voluminous liquids the youngster is drinking. She shows signs of dehydration (dry mouth, sunken eyes, and so on) but continues to urinate in large amounts. She may complain of abdominal pain and become progressively less alert, even slipping into coma (unconsciousness) if the problem is not treated.

Diabetes Mellitus: What to Expect

If diabetes is suspected, your doctor will most likely perform a simple urine analysis to look for glucose (sugar) and acetone, which are present in the urine in children with diabetes. (This is different from most adults with diabetes, who might not have sugar in the urine at all times.) A simple blood test for blood sugar will usually confirm the diagnosis, but additional tests will probably be ordered, to help the doctor with planning treatment.

If diabetes is diagnosed, the youngster will need to be admitted to a hospital, even if he is in the early stages of the disease. In addition to confirming the diagnosis, the doctor and a team of other professionals (dieticians, nurses, physical therapists, and others) will begin treating the youngster. Treatment includes daily injections of insulin, along with a special diet, and involves carefully monitoring his blood glucose (sugar) and urine. It often takes several days or even weeks to "regulate" the youngster's diabetes—that is, balance his diet, exercise, and insulin as much as possible.

A youngster who has more advanced diabetes, with dehydration and ketoacidosis (the condition in which excess acids and ketones are present in the body) might need to be in an intensive-care unit for several days and receive intravenous treatment. After her condition is stabilized, her insulin needs will be regulated and a special diet prescribed.

One of the most important parts of diabetes treatment is teaching children and their parents about the disease and how to manage it at home. This process of education is usually carried out by a team headed by your youngster's doctor or a specialist in childhood diabetes. Once the youngster is regulated and all teaching is completed, he will be sent home. You, your child, and his doctor then remain a team in caring for the youngster for the rest of his life. The goal of treatment: to provide the most normal life possible for the youngster—with the best possible control of the diabetes—in order to reduce the complications of the disease.

THE DON'TS

Don't overlook the symptoms of diabetes in a child or older youngster: increased thirst, increased urination, and increased appetite, along with weight loss. The earlier

359

RECOGNIZING
AND
MANAGING
SERIOUS OR
POTENTIALLY
SERIOUS
ILLNESS

you and your youngster's doctor are aware of this chronic disease, the faster the youngster can be treated and continue his or her normal life.

Don't be fooled by the symptoms if they occur in a thin youngster. While adult-type diabetes most often strikes people who are overweight, juvenile diabetes appears in thin, normal, and overweight youngsters and most often actually causes weight loss.

Don't hesitate to talk to your youngster's doctor and have the youngster examined if you suspect diabetes. The tests that detect diabetes in children are very simple and are very accurate in determining whether a youngster has this chronic disease.

Don't despair if your child has developed diabetes. While this is a serious disease that will require daily treatment and painstaking medical care, there are advances each year that make controlling the disease easier and preventing long-term complications more possible.

PLEASE NOTE: Now that you have a grasp of how to recognize and manage diabetes mellitus, it would be extremely helpful for you to go back to the Emergency Quick Reference and review it carefully. The more familiar you are with that material, the more useful it will be to you when you need it.

360

ILLNESS IN
INFANTS,
CHILDREN,
AND
ADOLESCENTS

EMERGENCY QUICK REFERENCE

With the Steps in Detail

Meningitis

▶ **SUSPECT MENINGITIS IN A YOUNG INFANT, CHILD, OR TEENAGER WHO:**

- Has a tense, bulging soft spot (infant or young toddler only).

- Has a stiff neck (can't touch her chin to her chest).

- Has fever, irritability, headache, and/or lethargy, along with a stiff neck.

- Has had a convulsion with fever (although meningitis is rarely a cause of febrile seizure).

▶ **GET IMMEDIATE MEDICAL ATTENTION FOR YOUR CHILD IF YOU SUSPECT MENINGITIS. CALL YOUR DOCTOR RIGHT AWAY TO DETERMINE WHETHER THE CHILD SHOULD BE SEEN IN HIS OR HER OFFICE OR WHETHER THE DOCTOR WANTS TO MEET YOU AT THE EMERGENCY ROOM OR WANTS YOU TO TAKE THE YOUNGSTER TO THE EMERGENCY ROOM FOR EVALUATION BY THE EMERGENCY-ROOM PHYSICIAN. FOLLOW THE INSTRUCTIONS WITHOUT DELAY.**

Meningitis: Life-Threatening Infection

Meningitis is an inflammation and infection of the membranes that cover the surface of the brain and spinal cord. Infection of these membranes, especially by bacteria, is potentially life-threatening. For those youngsters who survive bacterial meningitis, there is a significant risk for permanent brain damage or disability. If lifelong disabilities are to be prevented or their severity reduced—early recognition and prompt treatment are imperative!

361

RECOGNIZING
AND
MANAGING
SERIOUS OR
POTENTIALLY
SERIOUS
ILLNESS

The most deadly form of meningitis—*bacterial meningitis*—is caused by one of several bacteria. These germs, which usually travel to the area around the brain by means of the respiratory tract, usually make the youngster quite ill very quickly. One minute, she's healthy, and the next, she's critically ill. While bacterial meningitis is still potentially devastating, progress is being made each year. The combination of high doses of antibiotics, sophisticated monitoring, and prompt recognition and treatment of complications has led to much better results. Treatment requires several weeks of hospitalization. Many infants and children recover without any residual complications, while others are left with such problems as muscle weakness, hearing loss, partial paralysis, seizures, and delay in development.

Viral meningitis, on the other hand, is generally a much milder disease. It affects older children more often than bacterial meningitis does, can follow a number of flulike illnesses, and is more common in the warmer months of the year. While there is no specific treatment to cure viral meningitis, it usually resolves itself on its own in five to seven days and leaves no residual damage. There are exceptions to this. For example, the meningitis that can complicate measles is a much more serious disease.

Meningitis: Signs and Symptoms

In young infants and toddlers (who are more prone to certain forms of bacterial meningitis than older children), the earliest signs of meningitis are sometimes subtle. Meningitis may complicate a respiratory illness or ear infection. If the child gets sicker than you would expect with one of these illnesses, that may be a signal that meningitis or another serious complication could be involved.

Almost all youngsters with meningitis have a *fever*, usually above 102 or 103 degrees. Most become progressively *lethargic* and intensely *irritable*. As the inflammation of the brain progresses, pressure builds up inside the head, and the *soft spot bulges* (in infants and young children whose soft spot is still present). Most infants with meningitis *will not eat or drink* and have an *unusual, high-pitched cry*. Some will have *seizures*, as well. As the meningitis advances, the little ones become less and less arousable and more limp—but stiffen when you try to bend their necks. They may show signs of *shock* and develop a *rash* (which is caused by bleeding under the skin).

In older children who no longer have soft spots (fontanels), you will not be able to use this as an indicator of a problem. Instead, the verbal child or older youngster will complain of a *severe headache* and *stiff neck* early in the disease. Along with these two symptoms, the child will have a *fever* and be *lethargic* and *irritable*. He may also complain that light bothers his eyes and that moving his eyes to look around hurts.

In a child who cannot talk, suspect a headache and stiff neck if she really fusses or

362

ILLNESS IN
INFANTS,
CHILDREN,
AND
ADOLESCENTS

cries with any movement or when you pick her up. (Most infants and children who are ill enjoy being picked up and cuddled. Those with headache, stiff neck, or other severe pain object to being picked up or cuddled because the *movement* causes them intense pain.)

The signs of *viral meningitis* are similar to those of bacterial meningitis but are usually less severe and appear more gradually. Older children with this problem will complain of *severe headache, stiff neck, sensitivity to light, nausea*, and generally *feeling bad*. They will usually sleep more than is normal for them but will act more like themselves when awakened than the child with bacterial meningitis.

Meningitis: What to Expect

While it is sometimes possible to make an educated guess that meningitis is either bacterial or viral, it is imperative that infants, children, and adolescents with symptoms that suggest meningitis be seen and evaluated medically as soon as possible. The evaluation will include a careful medical history and physical examination, as well as a spinal tap (also known as a lumbar puncture).

A spinal tap is done by inserting a needle through the space between the vertebrae in the lower back—into the spinal canal at the base of the spinal cord. A small amount of fluid (which normally surrounds the brain and spinal cord) is removed and analyzed (for infection) in the laboratory. If the doctor feels the fluid looks suspicious (it is cloudy and has pus in it), he or she will usually immediately give antibiotic(s) intravenously while waiting for the laboratory results. In this way, treatment is not delayed if it does turn out to be bacterial meningitis.

With bacterial meningitis, antibiotic treatment is almost always given intravenously for about two weeks (with the timing dependent on how the youngster progresses). Most hospitals institute precautions to prevent the spread of the infection to others. Therefore, parents who visit their youngsters may be required to wear gowns and masks while in the room. Infants and children with this disease are carefully observed for any signs of complications. At least one and sometimes more spinal taps are performed to follow the progress of treatment and to determine if additional modes of treatment (or longer antibiotic therapy) are necessary.

With viral meningitis, the situation is somewhat different. If the spinal tap results overwhelmingly suggest viral infection, *no antibiotics will be given* (because they are totally ineffective), and the youngster would be observed for one to three days in the hospital. Some children feel markedly improved after the spinal tap (because removing a small amount of the fluid relieves some of the pressure on the brain) and are ready to go home almost immediately. Treatment for these youngsters is to relieve symptoms—pain relievers for the headache and discomfort, as well as fluids (sometimes intravenously if vomiting is severe).

How Contagious Is Meningitis?

363

RECOGNIZING
AND
MANAGING
SERIOUS OR
POTENTIALLY
SERIOUS
ILLNESS

Hearing that someone has meningitis strikes terror in many people and causes others to become very nervous and scared—both for the person who has it and for others who may have had some contact (even remote contact) with the person. Most people believe that meningitis is very deadly *and* very contagious!

Most people have heard about meningitis epidemics. The fear is universal: "Will my family or I be at risk?" Certainly, there are types of meningitis that are contagious enough to start epidemics. The meningococcus bacteria is the bacteria that most commonly causes epidemic meningitis, because it spreads easily in crowded conditions. It has caused the worst problems among young military recruits but occurs in other situations, as well.

Another type of meningitis, which in the past had been thought not to be particularly contagious, is now known to pass from one child to another quite easily. This is the most common type of bacterial meningitis found in infants and young children. The bacteria, called Hemophilus influenzae ("H. flu" or "Hib," for short), affects infants and children under six years of age, in particular. Besides meningitis, this bacteria can cause other serious infections (epiglottitis, a serious infection around the eye called periorbital cellulitis, and pneumonia, for example). (If you would like further information, Chapter 3 presents more detailed discussions about Hemophilus influenzae infections and the protection of older toddlers and preschoolers through immunization.)

Because of the particularly contagious nature of meningitis caused by the meningococcus or Hemophilus influenzae bacteria, those with very close contacts with a youngster (or adult) with one of these types of meningitis are treated with a drug (usually Rifampin) for several days to prevent their contracting the disease. This kind of preventive treatment is restricted to family-type contacts, particularly when there are children under six years old in the home, as well as day-care–center contacts (where the disease can also spread). Other less close contacts are not particularly susceptible and are therefore not routinely treated.

The viruses that cause viral meningitis—although quite contagious—don't always produce meningitis in those who are infected. Some youngsters with the virus will get meningitis, while others will get only mild "flu" symptoms. It is always prudent to avoid contact with youngsters who have viral meningitis (for one or two days after they are without fever and are feeling well). However, there is no reason to panic if you hear a youngster has viral meningitis. We often forget that exposure of others has usually already taken place before the youngster knew he or she was ill (for the day or two before symptoms started). The disease can develop anywhere from five to ten days after the initial exposure. Again, viral meningitis is not generally a deadly disease in a normally healthy youngster (or adult), and contact often produces only a mild "flu."

The important thing to remember when it comes to exposure to meningitis is to *ask*

364

ILLNESS IN
INFANTS,
CHILDREN,
AND
ADOLESCENTS

what kind of meningitis a youngster has. Once you know this, it is important to call your doctor for advice. He or she will ask how close contact has been and when it occurred. If others should be treated to prevent the spread of the disease, hospital and public health personnel will pass on this information to the family of the sick youngster. Otherwise, watch your youngster for signs of illness, and call your doctor if you have any concerns. One last thing. There is a great public service you can perform when it comes to meningitis: be the one to *stop* the rumors of epidemic and panic—rather than spread them. If concerned, keep in contact with your doctor and public health department. They will not hesitate to take measures if they feel others are in particular danger of contracting meningitis caused by either meningococcus or Hemophilus influenzae bacteria.

THE DON'TS

Don't delay in getting medical care if a youngster has signs of meningitis. The sooner the diagnosis is made and antibiotic treatment started (if there is bacterial infection), the better are the chances that the youngster will have a good recovery.

Don't panic when you hear that another youngster has meningitis. First find out the kind of meningitis the youngster has. Then call your doctor for advice, especially if the contact was as close as a family contact or in a day-care center and your child is under six years old.

PLEASE NOTE: Now that you have a grasp of how to recognize and manage meningitis, it would be extremely helpful for you to go back to the Emergency Quick Reference With the Steps in Detail and review it carefully. The more familiar you are with that material, the more useful it will be to you when you need it.

365

RECOGNIZING
AND
MANAGING
SERIOUS OR
POTENTIALLY
SERIOUS
ILLNESS

EMERGENCY QUICK REFERENCE

With the Steps in Detail

Overwhelming Infection (Sepsis)

▶ **WITH OVERWHELMING INFECTION, AN INFANT, CHILD, OR ADOLESCENT WILL LOOK VERY SICK:**

- He or she is usually lethargic, irritable, and inactive and does not eat or drink normally.

- There is generally fever and weakness, as well.

- The youngster is usually pale and may have signs of shock.

- There may be a rash caused by broken blood vessels (this signals a *life-threatening emergency*).

- You will not have difficulty knowing there is something seriously wrong.

▶ **WHEN A YOUNGSTER LOOKS SERIOUSLY SICK, IT IS IMPORTANT THAT HE OR SHE BE EVALUATED BY A DOCTOR AS SOON AS POSSIBLE. CALL YOUR DOCTOR FOR AN URGENT APPOINTMENT OR GO TO AN EMERGENCY ROOM.**

- When possible, talk with the doctor before you rush to an emergency room, so he or she can meet you there or tell you things to do before you go.

- Obviously, skip this step and call the paramedics if there are signs of shock or breathing difficulty.

366

ILLNESS IN
INFANTS,
CHILDREN,
AND
ADOLESCENTS

Overwhelming Infection: What Is It?

Often called "blood poisoning" in the past, overwhelming bacterial infection, or sepsis, is a serious, life-threatening infection. It can be associated with other serious infections—such as meningitis, pneumonia, and deep-organ infections seen in infants and children—or it can stand alone, without another body site that is obviously infected.

This infection occurs when bacteria (germs) get into the bloodstream and are carried throughout the body in the blood. The bacteria multiply rapidly and can potentially infect every organ and other tissue. Bacteria can invade the bloodstream from an already infected part of the body or can enter from the outside. Sometimes, the origin of the bacteria is never found. The nose and respiratory tract, the skin, open wounds, and the urinary system are places that we usually suspect when an overwhelming infection occurs. The traveling bacteria can be deposited in other, new sites and cause their damage there or lead to shock because of poisons they make while in the body.

Although anyone can be at risk for sepsis, specific situations make it more likely to occur. Certain infants and children are more susceptible than others. Very young infants—those under one or two months of age—are at risk for sepsis due to bacteria that usually live in the intestine. Older infants and toddlers are at risk for overwhelming infection due to Hemophilus influenzae (the bacteria that also cause meningitis and other deep-organ infections) and pneumococcus (a type of bacteria that causes one form of pneumonia, as well as ear infections). Older, active children and teenagers are at some risk for infections due to staphylococcus bacteria if they have an infected wound.

Infants and children who are weak (for a countless number of reasons) and those who have a chronic illness or severe disability are somewhat more susceptible than otherwise healthy children. Youngsters with sickle-cell disease and those who have no spleen are at particular risk for pneumococcus infection (which can lead to sepsis). Children with some types of heart defects can be at risk for infections from skin and mouth germs (for example, during dental work). Because these infections can turn into sepsis, these youngsters are routinely given penicillin before dental work is started. Youngsters whose immune systems are not normal—such as those taking strong drugs for cancer and some other chronic diseases—are also at risk for sepsis and may not have the same symptoms and signs as other basically healthy children. But remember, sepsis *can* affect the very healthy, as well.

Overwhelming Infection: Signs and Symptoms

Infants and children with overwhelming infection *look sick*. They usually have fevers, are most often very lethargic and irritable, and refuse to eat or drink. They tend to get progressively sicker *despite* what you do. Some may go into shock, and others may

367

RECOGNIZING
AND
MANAGING
SERIOUS OR
POTENTIALLY
SERIOUS
ILLNESS

have a spreading rash caused by broken blood vessels under the skin. This rash—which looks like red dots that don't disappear when you push on them or extensive bruising—signals a potentially life-threatening situation. The youngster may have signs of another type of infection, as well (for example, an ear infection; an infected cut; a swollen joint; a very red, swollen eye). However, the youngster with sepsis will look sicker than what you would expect with one of these localized infections (which is another signal that the problem may not simply be an eye infection, infected cut, or whatever).

A few infants and young children get sepsis without an associated infection anywhere in the body—and for no apparent reason. These youngsters *appear very ill*, and their *fever* may be the only gauge you have to guide you. Most often, fevers are over 103 degrees and cannot be reduced, or the child does not look or feel any better even if you get the fever down. A careful examination by the doctor may not turn up a source for the infection. However, blood tests may point to a bacterial infection.

Overwhelming Infection: What to Do and What to Expect

Early recognition and prompt treatment are the keys to turning the odds in favor of halting the often devastating effects of sepsis. Hospitalization and administration of intravenous antibiotics (which fight the "culprit") must occur immediately once sepsis is identified or highly suspected. Your job, then, is to recognize the signs and symptoms that point to possible sepsis and call the doctor or take the youngster to an emergency room.

Again, here are the symptoms that point to possible overwhelming infection (sepsis). While most high fevers mean a mild to moderate illness, you should not hesitate to call the doctor if: the child looks sicker than you would expect; you can't reduce the fever; or the youngster doesn't look or feel any better even if you can reduce the fever. If the youngster has a known infection (ear infection, infected cut, and so on) that is being treated by the doctor and you recognize that the youngster is *not improving* or appears to be *getting worse*—then suspect sepsis (or another complication) and call the doctor.

When the doctor sees the youngster, he or she may suspect sepsis based on the youngster's signs and symptoms and wish to begin treatment immediately *after* doing certain laboratory tests. Several blood tests are ordered, including a blood culture (a special test that encourages the offending bacteria to grow in a bottle so they can be identified).

Because it takes twenty-four to seventy-two hours for the bacteria to grow in the laboratory, the doctor will probably hospitalize the youngster and start intravenous antibiotic therapy immediately if he or she suspects sepsis. The antibiotic(s) chosen

368

ILLNESS IN
INFANTS,
CHILDREN,
AND
ADOLESCENTS

will be based on experience and a knowledge of the bacteria most likely to be responsible for the overwhelming infection. Once the test results are back and the bacteria responsible are identified, the antibiotic(s) may need to be changed (since certain bacteria are sensitive to specific antibiotics, while others are not).

Besides the blood tests, a spinal tap is usually performed, as well as a chest X ray and a urine culture. These tests often verify the diagnosis but, more important, may point to or find a hidden source of the infection.

Infants and children with sepsis must be treated in a hospital with intravenous antibiotics for a week or more, depending on the type of infection and the child's other problems. You should expect gradual improvement in his or her symptoms over time. Part of the youngster's care is for hospital personnel to diligently watch for possible complications—especially localized infection in an area or organ of the body.

One note: In most cases, when overwhelming infection (sepsis) is recognized and treated promptly, infants, children, and teenagers recover—even though they may have been critically ill. There are times, however, when the best and most sophisticated medical care cannot reverse this type of rampant, overwhelming infection, and the child is not able to survive.

THE DON'TS

Don't hesitate to get an infant or child evaluated by a doctor if the youngster seems seriously ill. The only way overwhelming infection can be discovered early is to know the warning signs and to recognize that it might have occurred. But don't overreact to minor illnesses. Remember, the child with sepsis will look and feel really sick.

Don't be surprised if your doctor says your child with suspected sepsis must be hospitalized and needs to receive antibiotics intravenously. This is the only predictable way to get the antibiotic drug in the bloodstream—where the infection is—and to control the problem quickly.

PLEASE NOTE: Now that you have a grasp of how to recognize and manage overwhelming infection, it would be extremely helpful for you to go back to the Emergency Quick Reference With the Steps in Detail and review it carefully. The more familiar you are with that material, the more useful it will be to you when you need it.

369

RECOGNIZING
AND
MANAGING
SERIOUS OR
POTENTIALLY
SERIOUS
ILLNESS

EMERGENCY QUICK REFERENCE

With the Steps in Detail

Pneumonia

▶ **CALL YOUR DOCTOR FOR ADVICE OR MAKE ARRANGEMENTS TO HAVE THE YOUNGSTER EXAMINED IN THE DOCTOR'S OFFICE OR EMERGENCY ROOM WITHIN A FEW HOURS IF A CHILD DEVELOPS SYMPTOMS THAT MIGHT SUGGEST PNEUMONIA:**

- The child has rapid breathing, chest retractions, and fever.

- The child looks much more ill than you would expect with a simple cold.

- There may or may not be unusual noises with breathing.

Pneumonia: Not as Frightening as Before

Years ago, even the word *pneumonia* struck fear and terror in many parents—and for good reason! Before the advent of antibiotics, pneumonia (infection in the lungs) often led to death. Youngsters who did not die were very sick for days or weeks. All that could be done then was to watch and wait—and try to keep the fever under control. It was a greatly feared disease, much like polio, rheumatic fever, and a handful of other deadly diseases that can now be prevented or treated.

Today the situation is very different. Since the discovery of antibiotics in the 1940s and the addition of many new, sophisticated antibiotics to those already available to fight bacterial infection, most pneumonias are now successfully treated. Pneumonia can be caused by many types of germs. Pneumonia caused by bacteria (bacterial pneumonia) is usually the most serious—but also the most treatable. It can be cured by antibiotics. That makes it a much less difficult problem, because nearly all the bacteria that cause pneumonia are susceptible to one or more of the available drugs.

Pneumonia caused by viruses (viral pneumonia) is much more common and generally much more mild. It is not helped at all by antibiotics, but the disease usually improves with time.

While we usually think of pneumonia as an infection, inflammation of the lung (and

370

ILLNESS IN
INFANTS,
CHILDREN,
AND
ADOLESCENTS

therefore pneumonia) can occur as the result of other causes. Such events as choking and inhaling (aspirating) material from the stomach, inhaling irritating materials (for example, water), and certain chronic diseases can cause pneumonia. These forms of pneumonia are quite unusual in otherwise healthy children and therefore won't be discussed here.

Pneumonia: Signs and Symptoms

The symptoms and signs of pneumonia depend on how much of the lung is inflamed and what germ is to blame. Viral pneumonia, by far the most common type, is usually quite a mild disease but involves large areas of the lungs. Bacterial pneumonia, on the other hand, usually affects only one lobe or segment of a lung but causes enough inflammation that the youngster is very sick.

When a youngster has bacterial pneumonia, he *looks very sick*. While the disease may seem like a bad cold at first (with congestion, cough, and fever), the symptoms get worse quickly. As the lung inflammation increases, the youngster develops a higher fever (often 102 to 105 degrees) and is obviously feeling lousy. You will notice that he has increasing trouble breathing and breathes rather rapidly (usually over forty times a minute and sometimes even faster). Retractions (abnormal movements of the chest) often occur, and the youngster becomes increasingly lethargic and irritable. The cough of early pneumonia is tight and gets worse over a six- to twenty-four-hour period. Older youngsters may complain of pain in an area of the chest (which is caused by irritation from the inflammation).

An infant's color may be poor (pale or even somewhat bluish). In fact, these little ones are so sick they often cannot or will not eat. You may or may not hear or feel unusual noises in the chest. With all these symptoms occurring, you needn't worry about not recognizing that your little one is very ill. You'll notice!

With viral pneumonia, on the other hand, symptoms are not nearly so obvious. In fact, you may think the youngster has a severe cold—at worst. The most common symptoms she will have are fast breathing, along with a cough and moderate fever. Here you look to see if the cold symptoms seem more severe than usual or if the fever seems higher or lasts longer. You might see chest retractions in more severe cases, the youngster's appetite may be less than usual, and her activity level may decrease.

While it frightens many people to think that viral pneumonia is not as obvious in some youngsters—it really shouldn't. In fact, it is reassuring to know that the disease is most often not very serious in normally healthy children. One note: It's important to remember that there is no medication presently known today that will kill viruses and cure this type of pneumonia. Therefore, the most important thing for you to be aware of, when it comes to pneumonia, is to be able to recognize the signs and symptoms that signal trouble: very rapid breathing, poor color, lethargy, refusal to drink, or being generally sicker than you would expect with a cold.

How Pneumonia Is Treated

371

RECOGNIZING
AND
MANAGING
SERIOUS OR
POTENTIALLY
SERIOUS
ILLNESS

If you suspect that your youngster might have pneumonia, call his doctor to discuss if (and when) the youngster should be seen in the doctor's office *or* in an emergency room. As noted earlier, with bacterial pneumonia, the youngster will obviously be very ill, and while you may not be sure what is wrong, you will be certain there is a serious problem requiring immediate attention. With viral pneumonia, on the other hand, the situation is rarely as serious, and a few hours can very safely elapse before the youngster is evaluated.

The only way to tell if a youngster has pneumonia is for a doctor to examine her. The doctor will carefully look at the youngster and listen to her lungs. The doctor may hear unusual noises in the lungs that signify possible infection. He or she will more than likely want to have a chest X ray taken to confirm the suspicion. The X ray gives the doctor information about the pneumonia, as well as clues to the type and severity of the problem.

As previously noted, bacterial pneumonia requires antibiotic treatment. Most often, the child is sick enough to be hospitalized and given the antibiotic by injection or intravenously (by "IV"). She may also need oxygen and special breathing treatments, as well as other medications to make her more comfortable and manage the effects of the pneumonia until the antibiotics destroy the disease. Some older children with certain types of bacterial pneumonia can be treated at home with antibiotics and checked by the doctor often.

Viral pneumonia, on the other hand, can usually be treated at home. However, most doctors would prefer to hospitalize young infants with this disease (for a day or two) so they can observe them carefully to see whether the disease worsens or complications occur. Young infants tire out easily if breathing is very rapid. For some youngsters with viral pneumonia, antibiotics (administered by mouth or injection) are prescribed, especially if the doctor is concerned that what looks like viral pneumonia might be the early stages of bacterial pneumonia. If you don't understand the prescribed treatment, ask your doctor about it. Medications for congestion and cough might be recommended, as well. With most youngsters, you can expect the worst of the illness to pass in three or four days. However, the child will usually not get "well" for as long as two or three weeks—the time it takes for the virus to run its course.

THE DON'TS

Don't assume that a child has pneumonia merely because he or she is severely congested. As with many other illnesses, how the youngster looks and the combination and severity of symptoms (and lab tests) determine what disease is causing the problems. Remember, there are many things that can cause congestion that are not pneumonia.

372

ILLNESS IN
INFANTS,
CHILDREN,
AND
ADOLESCENTS

Don't rush an infant, toddler, small child, or teenager to the doctor or emergency room if he or she is congested—because you are afraid of pneumonia. You will recognize the serious forms of pneumonia because the youngster will look very sick. If a youngster is congested and you are concerned, call your doctor for advice.

Don't panic if the doctor says your child has pneumonia. Ask what kind of pneumonia he or she has and what treatment the doctor prescribes. Remember, the vast majority of pneumonias can be successfully treated today.

PLEASE NOTE: Now that you have a grasp of how to recognize and manage pneumonia, it would be extremely helpful for you to go back to the Emergency Quick Reference With the Steps in Detail and review it carefully. The more familiar you are with that material, the more useful it will be to you when you need it.

EMERGENCY QUICK REFERENCE

With the Steps in Detail

Reye Syndrome

▶ **SUSPECT REYE SYNDROME IF A YOUNGSTER WHO HAS OR IS RECOVERING FROM CHICKENPOX OR INFLUENZA SHOWS THE FOLLOWING SYMPTOMS:**

- Severe or persistent vomiting.

- Intense, violent headaches.

- Unusual behavior, such as severe sleepiness or lethargy, irritability, restlessness, disorientation, combativeness, or delirium.

▶ **IF YOU RECOGNIZE THESE SYMPTOMS IN YOUR YOUNGSTER, CONTACT YOUR DOCTOR OR TAKE YOUR CHILD TO AN EMERGENCY ROOM IMMEDIATELY. DO NOT WAIT FOR THE SYMPTOMS TO PASS, AND DO NOT TRY TO TREAT THE YOUNGSTER AT HOME.**

Reye Syndrome: What Is It?

373

RECOGNIZING
AND
MANAGING
SERIOUS OR
POTENTIALLY
SERIOUS
ILLNESS

Reye syndrome is a condition that can result as a complication of certain viral infections in children—most commonly chickenpox and influenza (true "flu"). Reye syndrome is a serious, life-threatening emergency that requires quick, intensive medical treatment.

Most people do not realize that Reye syndrome is *not* a new disease or "syndrome" (combination of signs and symptoms). Originally, it was thought to be a form of meningitis (inflammation of the tissues covering the brain) or encephalitis (inflammation of the brain itself). In the early 1960s, this serious problem was finally recognized for what it really is—swelling of the brain, coupled with malfunction of the liver and other body organ systems.

The cause of Reye syndrome is not known. We do know that it complicates the quite common diseases of chickenpox and influenza (and occasionally other viral infections) in only a very small number of children who get these childhood diseases. The problem is, when Reye syndrome occurs, it is life-threatening and can affect children from infancy through late adolescence.

While no one has yet identified the specific cause of this devastating problem, it is now recognized that there is a *possible* relationship between Reye syndrome and the use of aspirin when a youngster has influenza or chickenpox. In the past, other medications have been suspected, as well. Currently, studies are being done to determine the possible relationship between Reye syndrome and aspirin.

While aspirin and other medications *are not known to cause* Reye syndrome, it is best that youngsters with chickenpox, influenza, or other unidentified viral infections *not be treated with aspirin*. In fact, when at all possible, avoid the use of any medication for the treatment of mild symptoms of flus, colds, and so on. You might want to check with your doctor (at one of your child's visits) about what his or her recommendations are if your youngster experiences mild symptoms of a viral illness.

Reye Syndrome: Signs and Symptoms

The symptoms of Reye syndrome most often appear when a child or youngster seems to be *in the recovery stages* of chickenpox, influenza, or another mild viral illness. The youngster starts to *vomit* uncontrollably, has severe *headaches*, and exhibits *unusual behavior* (for example, he or she may be *very sleepy* or *lethargic* at first but, within a few hours, becomes *disoriented, combative, and delirious*). These symptoms can progress very quickly in some youngsters. If the problem continues without treatment, the youngster may slip into *unconsciousness*.

374

ILLNESS IN
INFANTS,
CHILDREN,
AND
ADOLESCENTS

Reye Syndrome: What to Do and What to Expect

Reye syndrome is a life-threatening emergency. Call your child's doctor or take him or her to a hospital emergency room without delay. Do *not* attempt to treat the symptoms at home.

When Reye syndrome is suspected, the doctor will immediately perform several tests. Certain blood tests will help make the diagnosis, and the youngster may need to have a lumbar puncture (spinal tap)—if there is any question whether the problem might be meningitis.

If Reye syndrome is confirmed or seriously suspected, the child will be immediately hospitalized (usually in an intensive-care unit). He or she will be watched and monitored for signs that the disease is worsening (especially increased pressure in the brain) and treated aggressively if these signs occur. A special instrument (an intracranial pressure monitor) is normally used, therefore, to monitor pressure inside the skull (and on the brain). As part of the treatment, the sick youngster may need a respirator (a machine that can breathe for the youngster or assist his or her breathing) and other life-sustaining treatments. Nutritional support is also very important and is given intravenously.

With Reye syndrome, the goal of treatment is to *prevent* the advancement of the increased pressure on the brain and failure of other organ systems. To do this, early diagnosis and treatment are necessary. Most often, the youngster requires hospital treatment for three days to as long as two weeks. As the youngster starts to improve, his or her breathing, brain function, and body chemistry will begin to stabilize. A youngster is usually considered "out of danger" when he or she is stable or showing improvement for at least forty-eight hours.

The most serious problem with Reye syndrome is an uncontrollable increase in pressure on the brain—due to brain swelling. This is such a serious and difficult problem to treat that sometimes even the earliest, most aggressive treatment is unsuccessful in controlling this pressure, and permanent brain damage or even death can result. When a youngster survives severe Reye syndrome, the recovery and rehabilitation period can be long and difficult.

THE DON'TS

Don't delay in calling your doctor or going to an emergency room if a child shows signs of Reye syndrome. Youngsters with severe vomiting, headache, or changes in behavior after seemingly mild viral illnesses require prompt medical evaluation and treatment.

Don't treat youngsters under the age of sixteen with aspirin if they have chickenpox, influenza, or another mild viral illness. While aspirin and other medications have not been shown to cause Reye syndrome, their use is associated with the development of this devastating problem. Since research is ongoing and relatively little is presently known about Reye syndrome, it is important to watch for new information and recommendations regarding this serious illness. If you are unsure about anything you hear, read, or are told—make sure you ask your doctor, so you get the most up-to-date information about this problem and are not misinformed because of hearsay or incorrect interpretations.

PLEASE NOTE: Now that you have a grasp of how to recognize and manage Reye syndrome, it would be extremely helpful for you to go back to the Emergency Quick Reference With the Steps in Detail and review it carefully. The more familiar you are with that material, the more useful it will be to you when you need it.

Recognizing and Managing Common Symptoms and Illnesses

Included in this chapter is information on how to recognize and manage the common symptoms and illnesses listed below. The page numbers in parentheses indicate where the Quick Reference for each condition can be found.

377

RECOGNIZING
AND
MANAGING
COMMON
SYMPTOMS
AND ILLNESSES

QUICK REFERENCE

With the Steps in Detail

Abdominal Pain

▶ **EVALUATE THE YOUNGSTER TO DETERMINE WHAT KIND OF AB-DOMINAL PAIN HE OR SHE IS EXPERIENCING, AS WELL AS THE SEVERITY OF THE PAIN.**

- Is this a first-time occurrence, or does the youngster have this pain off and on?

- Try to find out exactly where the pain is located and how severe it is. Is the pain constant, or does it come and go?

- What other symptoms are also present? (Pay attention to the youngster's appetite, activity level, and the presence or absence of fever, nausea, vomiting, and change in bowel pattern.)

▶ **CALL THE DOCTOR FOR ADVICE OR GO TO AN EMERGENCY ROOM IF:**

- The pain is severe and has persisted for longer than two to three hours.

- The pain is associated with other symptoms that suggest serious illness.

378

ILLNESS IN
INFANTS,
CHILDREN,
AND
ADOLESCENTS

- The pain follows an injury to the abdomen.

▶ **MAKE AN APPOINTMENT FOR AN EVALUATION BY THE DOCTOR WITHIN A DAY IF:**

- The pain is not severe, but there has been no improvement after one to two days and the youngster seems uncomfortable.

- There have been no other symptoms that indicate the source of the problem.

▶ **MAKE AN APPOINTMENT FOR A MEDICAL EVALUATION IF THE CHILD SEEMS TO HAVE FREQUENT COMPLAINTS OF ABDOMINAL PAIN.**

Abdominal Pain: A Common Occurrence in Childhood

Abdominal pain (the infamous ''stomachache'') is one of the most common complaints in childhood and causes a great deal of concern—sometimes unnecessarily—for both parents and children. It can signal a serious problem but most often does not. Making the distinction between a simple stomachache and a more serious problem is based (as in other illnesses) on looking not only at the youngster's complaint of pain but at the ''set'' of symptoms also associated with the discomfort.

The list of possible causes of abdominal pain in children is very long. Again, it's important to remember that most of the time abdominal discomfort, while bothersome, does not signal serious illness. In very young infants and toddlers, your challenge is great—even in being sure that what *looks* like a stomachache really is a stomachache. In older children, your challenge is different—to determine how severe is ''severe'' and what this, as well as their entire set of symptoms (if there are others), might mean.

Abdominal pain can result from such mild, inconsequential problems as eating too much or eating something that did not ''agree'' with a youngster, having a cold or the flu, being mildly constipated, or even having overused the muscles on the outside of the abdomen. Mild abdominal pain, especially if it is associated with rectal itching and restless sleep, often points to pinworms in preschoolers and even older children. You do, however, need to evaluate abdominal pain carefully, since it may be a symptom that points to more severe or serious problems—such as appendicitis, intestinal infection, urinary infection, the presence of a tumor, and even pneumonia. Making this kind of distinction often causes parents—and sometimes doctors—much concern.

The Acute Bellyache: Being a Detective

379

RECOGNIZING
AND
MANAGING
COMMON
SYMPTOMS
AND ILLNESSES

Abdominal pain—whether high up in the area of the stomach or lower down in the belly—should be looked at carefully. Do your best to determine:

- What kind of pain the youngster is having.

- How severe it is.

- What makes it better or worse.

- How the pain affects him. (Does the pain interfere with his activity and appetite—or not?)

You need to ask about the pain and also watch the youngster's behavior. Try to distinguish between true pain in the abdomen and the discomfort of nausea or the feeling that the youngster has right before she vomits. Being able to describe "the feeling" may be very difficult for a young child, but you can often get a clue as to what is actually going on when she seems much better after belching or vomiting. These are sensations that a youngster only learns to identify after a bout or two with the "flu" or having had a few simple upset stomachs. You might try asking if the young person feels "butterflies" in her stomach, since that tends to be nausea and not "true" abdominal "pain."

Most often, children will say their pain or discomfort is in the middle of their abdomen—around the belly button (umbilicus). Have your youngster point with one finger to the place that hurts the most. Ask if the hurting is all the time or comes and goes. Try to determine whether it makes a difference if she is lying still or moving around. Is it better, worse, or the same if she stands up, walks, or jumps?

Check to see whether or not the youngster has a fever and whether he has been eating or is hungry. Has he eaten anything unusual (for him)? Has there been vomiting or diarrhea? Has he had a bowel movement in the last twenty-four hours? Does it hurt to urinate or have a bowel movement? Has he been hit or kicked in the abdomen or fallen (for example, onto the handlebars of his bike)? Are there any symptoms of other illness—headache, sore throat, congestion, earache, leg or body aches?

Next, look at the young person's abdomen. Does it appear swollen compared to usual? Does he or she seem to have a lot of gas? Is there any bruising or discoloration of the skin?

Now have the youngster lie down and try to relax, so you can feel her abdomen. First push gently all around the abdomen. Does it feel hard? Is there a spot that is especially sore to the touch? Now push a bit harder. Is the sore spot really tender or just a little tender? Push inward firmly, then quickly release your pressure. Does she cringe or cry out, as if letting go hurts more than pushing in? Do you feel any unusual lumps in the abdomen? Is the pain more on the surface or deeper in the abdomen? Is the pain located more in the front than in the back? All of this information is helpful,

380

ILLNESS IN
INFANTS,
CHILDREN,
AND
ADOLESCENTS

not only to you but to the doctor if you have to talk to the doctor by telephone or the youngster needs to be seen.

All of this may seem fine if the child can talk and describe these things, you may be thinking, but what if he is too little to talk or is just an infant? Actually, parents or someone close to a little child can often get more information about whether a toddler really has tenderness in the abdomen than a doctor can! As you know, your toddler is often afraid of strangers and may cry loudly when his doctor approaches. But your child is used to you touching and being close. So don't hesitate to try these things with a little one. You may not be as sure of yourself as a doctor would be, but don't let that feeling get in your way. You *can* usually get enough information to help you determine whether you need to contact the doctor or can wait a little while to see if the symptoms subside, stay the same, or further symptoms occur.

The Acute Bellyache: When to Be Concerned

Most people think first of and fear the presence of *appendicitis* (inflammation and infection of the appendix) when a youngster has abdominal pain. While many youngsters don't "read the book" about what symptoms they should or shouldn't have, there are certain things that *do* indicate a cause for concern and others that *don't*.

The appendix is a small, fingerlike outpouching of the small intestine and is usually found in the lower right part of the abdomen. It has a very narrow opening into the intestine, which sometimes gets blocked or swollen. When this happens, inflammation and infection can result—much as you would see with a boil on the skin. This is called appendicitis. As pus is formed, the appendix swells, and the inflamed appendix rubs and irritates the lining of the abdomen (called the peritoneum). If the pus continues to form, the pressure can cause the appendix to burst, spilling the pus into the abdominal cavity—called a ruptured appendix. This results in a more serious problem, called *peritonitis* (inflammation and infection of the abdominal lining).

At the beginning, true appendicitis starts gradually and most often cannot be distinguished from the other causes of mild to moderate abdominal pain. But the *symptoms do not disappear over several hours*, and the youngster continues to complain about pain or discomfort. He also shows *other signs* of a problem more serious than a simple bellyache. He has little or no appetite and may have some nausea. If he has a fever, however, it is usually mild. Most people do not realize that the *initial pain* is generalized in the abdomen and not usually focused in the right side only (or at all).

At this point (with continued generalized discomfort or pain, tenderness to the touch, and little or no appetite), it's time to call the doctor for consultation. The doctor may want to see the youngster right away or may want you to watch for further symptoms.

The next set of symptoms you will notice are as follows. As the inflammation progresses, the pain gets more and more severe and becomes localized to one spot—

381

RECOGNIZING
AND
MANAGING
COMMON
SYMPTOMS
AND ILLNESSES

most often in the lower right side of the abdomen. The youngster experiences tenderness when you push on the abdomen and hurts more when he moves or walks. You'll notice that he prefers to lie quietly—often curled up. This is because the inflamed appendix rubs on the internal lining of the abdomen and irritates it in that spot. Lying curled up helps relieve some of the discomfort. Vomiting may begin, but diarrhea is rare. The abdomen is somewhat swollen and hard, and he has pain both when you push on his abdomen and when you let go. The youngster will often walk stooped over or limp. With these additional symptoms, he appears more and more sick.

At this point, the youngster really *must* be evaluated. You want the young person evaluated and treated *before* the appendix ruptures, if at all possible. If you cannot reach your doctor and these symptoms have occurred, then take the youngster to the nearest emergency room and have your doctor contacted by the ER professionals as the young person is being evaluated. If appendicitis is suspected, the youngster will be admitted to the hospital, and the appendix will be removed surgically.

If the appendix ruptures, the youngster may seem improved for a short time (no more than a few hours) but then becomes very sick. She develops high fever and has a very swollen, hard, and tender abdomen. She moves hardly at all and will usually cry or complain if you force her to move. The youngster, at this point, often vomits and may develop diarrhea. There is no doubt that she is seriously ill.

Most children over the age of four or five years have their appendicitis detected *before* the inflamed appendix bursts. However, a few can "fool" the most vigilant parent and the most attentive doctor. Likewise, a certain number of youngsters have the appendix removed, only to find that they did not have appendicitis after all. This can occur because other problems can mimic this disease. Interestingly, very young children's appendicitis almost always goes undetected until there is rupture—because their symptoms seem so mild or confusing.

While appendicitis is by far the most common cause of what doctors call an *"acute abdomen,"* there are others. With many of these, the symptoms that occur along with the abdominal pain are often the tipoff.

Bowel obstruction—blockage of the intestine—is heralded by persistent vomiting, with vomiting of bile (green, bitter liquid) and increasing swelling and hardness of the abdomen. This can result from a twisting of the intestines (called volvulus), telescoping of a part of the intestine into itself (called intussusception), a hernia that has been "stuck," or even blockage of the intestine by a tumor. The pain of bowel obstruction usually starts as cramping pain that comes and goes, then progresses to be a steady, unrelenting pain.

Severe, unrelenting abdominal pain can also mean such diverse problems as *pancreatitis* (inflammation of the pancreas, located in the upper abdomen), *cholecystitis* (gallbladder inflammation, relatively rare in children), *sickle-cell crisis* (severe pain caused by blocking of blood vessels in youngsters, usually black, who have sickle-cell anemia), *kidney stone* (again, not common in children, but possible), *urinary infection*, and occasionally *peptic ulcer*. With each of these, the youngster is in moderate

382

ILLNESS IN
INFANTS,
CHILDREN,
AND
ADOLESCENTS

to severe pain and has other symptoms such as vomiting and fever. In girls, especially teenagers, abdominal pain can result from problems of the *ovary, infections of the Fallopian tubes and uterus*, and *complications of an unknown pregnancy*.

In all cases of abdominal pain where the pain is persistent (constant for a few hours, or off and on for several hours or days) and there are other symptoms, as well, the doctor should be called for consultation or the youngster taken to the nearest emergency room for evaluation.

Injuries to the abdomen can also cause pain and may herald potentially serious internal injury. *Bleeding around the spleen* may follow a fall (for example, onto the handlebars of a bicycle) or a kick in the belly. Likewise, *bleeding in the liver* or *damage to the pancreas* is possible. (Abdominal injuries are discussed in detail in Chapter 16.)

Cramping abdominal pain usually originates in the intestines. If a youngster can talk, he or she can usually tell you that the pain starts slowly, then builds up but gradually disappears—only to start again. It often precedes a loose or watery bowel movement or the passage of gas. If a child has crampy pain, he or she tends to writhe around rather than lie still, and there is usually not much if any tenderness when you push on the belly.

The bottom line on abdominal pain is to recognize the combination of pain with *other symptoms*. This helps determine what is the likely cause of the pain. As a review, call the doctor for advice or go to an emergency room if:

- The youngster's abdominal pain is severe and has persisted for longer than two to three hours.

- The pain is associated with other symptoms that suggest serious illness—vomiting, especially of bile or blood; high fever; bloated, hard, and tender abdomen; severe diarrhea, especially if it contains blood or mucus; or if the youngster seems unusually "sick."

- The pain follows an injury to the abdomen.

Abdominal pain that does not seem unusually severe and has no other or few other symptoms associated with it does not require an immediate call to your doctor. Instead, watch the youngster closely and have her rest and drink or eat what she wants for a while. Most temporary problems (such as flu, gas, or eating something that does not agree with the youngster) will disappear within hours to a few days. You will want to contact your child's doctor for advice or an appointment if:

- There has been no improvement after one to two days, and the youngster still seems uncomfortable.

- There have been no other symptoms that indicate the source of the problem, but the discomfort or pain persists.

Acute Abdominal Pain: What to Expect

383

RECOGNIZING
AND
MANAGING
COMMON
SYMPTOMS
AND ILLNESSES

When your child's doctor is contacted about a problem of acute abdominal pain, he or she will want to ask you (and your youngster, if possible) questions about the pain. The doctor will also want to perform a careful examination—not just of the young person's abdomen but also of his or her entire body. A rectal examination (an uncomfortable procedure, at best) may be necessary, and the doctor will have to press hard enough on the youngster's abdomen (to feel for enlargement of organs or the presence of a tumor, for example) that it hurts. Blood and urine tests are frequently ordered, and certain X rays may be needed, as well.

If your doctor is concerned about the possibility of appendicitis or another cause of an "acute abdomen," he or she may ask that a surgeon also evaluate your child. Often, the youngster is admitted to the hospital for observation—even if an operation is not immediately planned. The youngster may not be allowed to eat or drink until it is clear what the problem is and will receive IV (intravenous) fluids and/or medications. Sometimes, surgery is the only sure way to determine what is wrong and is often the only way to correct the problem.

Recurrent Abdominal Pain: Often a Puzzle

Many youngsters, especially those of grammar-school age, repeatedly complain of abdominal pain. In these youngsters, discovering the cause of their pain may be difficult, if not impossible. Some children miss a great deal of school because of unexplained, recurrent abdominal pain. There are many possible explanations for the pain. Sometimes, children are subjected to a variety of medical tests—sometimes to no avail.

The scenario may go something like this. The youngster complains of pain in the morning—often before school. She (girls are bothered somewhat more often than boys) seems listless and may look pale. She might have dark circles under her eyes and look "as if she is coming down with something." She plays with breakfast rather than eats. She just doesn't feel well. As the morning wears on, she feels better and better and often is free of pain by afternoon. This may happen for several days in a row or may occur occasionally. The pattern is the same—whether she goes to school or not. There is usually no fever and rarely vomiting or diarrhea. This pattern may repeat itself for several months or even years, then simply disappear.

With the first few episodes, parents often think of all the "bad" conditions this pain may signal and call or visit the doctor often. The doctor may say there is nothing wrong, with or without doing any "tests." There may be implications that the pain is "in the youngster's head"—while the parents know it is "real." This most often leads to dissatisfaction and mistrust of the doctor and demands to find out what is wrong.

384

ILLNESS IN
INFANTS,
CHILDREN,
AND
ADOLESCENTS

What is really needed is a careful evaluation of the child and his problem. You, as a parent, can start the process by looking carefully at the pattern of your child's pain. When does it happen? Keep a record of the days and times of day when it occurs. Ask your child about his bowel habits. Most parents find they know little about them, because school-aged youngsters are rather self-sufficient when it comes to their bladder and bowel habits. All too often, you find that the youngster is irregular—because he does not take the time to empty his bowels when he has the urge. In this case, the recurrent pain the youngster experiences may be the body's signal for the need of a bowel movement. Likewise, a youngster may not tell you that he has loose bowels or discomfort upon urination.

If your youngster tends to have allergies, consider the possibility that certain foods may be bothering her. Likewise, eating in a rush or too many "junk foods" might be a problem in today's busy household.

But don't stop with these possibilities. Notice whether the pain happens after a bad day or week at school or after the youngster has been in trouble for something. *Is* there something going on at home that could be worrying your child? Children *do* react to stress and worry. Often, this is expressed through a bellyache or upset stomach (just as is the case with many adults). While certain illnesses or physical problems can be the cause of this kind of pain in some children, stress, worry, depression, and/ or anxiety are also likely culprits.

But don't stop here either. Now that you are armed with concrete information, make an appointment with the youngster's doctor for a thorough evaluation. Careful questioning might lead the doctor to suspect a reason for the pain. The doctor will want to do a thorough examination and maybe even some laboratory tests, depending on what you have said and what is found during the physical examination. Sometimes, a blood count, urine tests, and stool (bowel movement) examinations are important. Occasionally, X rays might be needed, as well.

Only after these steps have been taken can all of you work together to try to solve the problem. The result may be the detection of a hopefully minor but bothersome problem and a means of treating it. (Fortunately, truly serious physical problems are usually uncommon as a cause for this kind of abdominal pain.) The solution may even be as easy as having your child spend a little more time in the bathroom (on the toilet) in the morning. At times, the solution may include helping your child deal with stresses he or she is facing—either by resolving them or by getting professional counseling for the youngster. Your doctor's and your goal is the same—helping your youngster be as happy and as free of pain as possible.

THE DON'TS

Don't assume that every bellyache means appendicitis. While this is a relatively common problem in children, there are other causes of abdominal pain. Look for other symptoms associated with the pain, and contact your doctor promptly if you are worried or concerned.

Don't overlook the situations where abdominal pain signals a potentially serious illness. Persistent vomiting, fever, and a bloated, tender abdomen should lead you to act promptly. Call your doctor or take the youngster to the nearest emergency room.

Don't despair if your child has a problem with frequent abdominal pain. Be sure to have him or her carefully evaluated by a doctor, and work with the doctor to help solve the problem.

PLEASE NOTE: Now that you have a grasp of how to recognize and manage abdominal pain, it would be extremely helpful for you to go back to the Quick Reference With the Steps in Detail and review it carefully. The more familiar you are with that material, the more useful it will be to you when you need it.

385

RECOGNIZING
AND
MANAGING
COMMON
SYMPTOMS
AND ILLNESSES

QUICK REFERENCE

With the Steps in Detail

Colds, Coughs, and Congestion

▶ **USE SIMPLE, COMMONSENSE HOME TREATMENT TO HELP YOUR CHILD WITH A COLD FEEL MORE COMFORTABLE.**

- Offer plenty of liquids to drink, and don't worry if the youngster is not interested in solid food.

- Use a humidifier in the bedroom, if you can.

- Use acetaminophen (aspirin substitute) in the correct dosage for fever and general discomfort.

- Suction your infant's nose with a bulb syringe to clear it of mucus, especially before he tries to nurse or drink his bottle.

- Try a decongestant medication (in the recommended dose) suggested by your child's doctor or a pharmacist. Do not give these medicines to infants under six months of age except upon your doctor's recommendation.

386

ILLNESS IN
INFANTS,
CHILDREN,
AND
ADOLESCENTS

- Give cough-suppressant medications at bedtime if the cough keeps your child awake at night. Again, do not use these medications for infants under six months old unless recommended by your doctor.

▶ **CONTACT YOUR CHILD'S DOCTOR (OR GO TO AN EMERGENCY ROOM IF YOU DON'T HAVE A DOCTOR OR CAN'T REACH YOUR DOCTOR) IF YOUR INFANT OR CHILD HAS ANY OF THE FOLLOWING:**

- Rapid or difficult breathing, wheezing, or stridor (a crowing sound when breathing in).

- Fever over 103 degrees with cold symptoms.

- Fever over 101 degrees lasting for more than three days or developing after the youngster seems to be getting well.

- Thick, dark yellow or green mucus in the nose or brought up when coughing.

- Earache (or ear rubbing in an infant or nonverbal child) during or after a cold.

▶ **CONTACT YOUR DOCTOR FOR ADVICE AND/OR AN APPOINTMENT IF YOUR INFANT OR CHILD HAS CONSTANT OR FREQUENT CONGESTION OR COUGH FOR NO APPARENT REASON.**

The Common Cold: What You Should Know

Colds, with their congestion and coughs, are the most common illnesses children have. Called "URIs" (*upper respiratory infections*) by health professionals, these bothersome afflictions account for more "sick days" for infants and children than any other problems. There never has been a cure, and we are all left to suffer with them, trying to feel better by using a variety of home remedies and medications—none of which work really well!

A cold is a viral infection and can be caused by any one of the hundreds of tiny viruses around. The offending virus infects the mucosal linings of the upper respiratory system—the nose, the throat, the larynx (voice box), the trachea (windpipe), the Eustacian tubes (small openings between the back of the nose and the middle ear), the sinuses, and the eyes. It causes inflammation, mucous production, and swelling of all these membranes. As you well know, the common cold is highly contagious, not only during the early phases when a person knows he has it, but for a day or two *before* he even feels bad. The sneezing and coughing that herald its arrival serve to spread the virus particles to others.

Colds are most common during the winter months—for a variety of reasons. For one, this is a season when children (and adults) spend more time indoors, where one sneezing, coughing person can infect a large number of people. Children are also in school and in contact (in an enclosed area) with many other children who might be sick. School-aged children often bring the viruses home to younger brothers and sisters and to parents. Crowded public places—especially enclosed areas like shopping malls, stores, and theaters—also contribute to the "epidemic."

Colds are *not* caused by getting wet or cold or going outside without a jacket or hat. They *are* caused by being exposed to a respiratory virus to which you are not immune (in other words, it's a "new" virus to you). They *do* seem to strike at times of stress—but the exposure to the virus is the key.

Many parents worry because their young children have so many colds. Youngsters who are exposed to many colds *get* many colds. They may have as many as eight to twelve a year and still be quite normal. This simply depends on their exposure. Infants and toddlers in group baby-sitting arrangements of day-care settings spend much of the first year ill, then tend to get fewer illnesses each year. If a youngster's first exposure to other children is in kindergarten, then that will be the "bad" year. Babies usually get colds from older brothers or sisters who are in preschool or school. This is always very upsetting but very normal.

Colds: Signs and Symptoms

The signs and symptoms of a cold are well known to most people:

- Watery eyes and nose, sneezing, and a scratchy throat.

- Stuffy nose, a dry, hacking cough, along with slight hoarseness and "plugged-up" ears follow, usually within twelve to twenty-four hours.

- There may be a slight fever for one to three days, and the cough worsens. The first three or four days are usually the most miserable, but these symptoms can last for as long as a week.

- Coughing and some congestion can last for as long as two or three weeks, but each day seems a bit better.

Infants and toddlers with colds often have a fever as high as 102 degrees for the first few days. They are understandably cranky and have little appetite for food, although

387

RECOGNIZING
AND
MANAGING
COMMON
SYMPTOMS
AND ILLNESSES

388

ILLNESS IN
INFANTS,
CHILDREN,
AND
ADOLESCENTS

they'll usually drink juices and other liquids. Because of their nose congestion, they have trouble sucking or eating (it's hard to suck or eat and breathe through their mouths at the same time). They are listless and generally like to be cuddled more than usual.

At first, the nasal mucus is clear and watery, but after a few days, it becomes thicker and more gray or milky. The cough that started as dry and hacking often becomes more "wet," and you may be able to hear or feel a "rattle" in the chest. This rattling comes from thicker mucus in the back of the throat and the upper windpipe and not usually from the chest itself. It normally disappears or improves after coughing or sneezing.

Small children with colds often have noisy breathing, especially at night. You can almost always tell that it comes from the nose and upper airways and not the lungs if you watch closely. Coughing may also seem worse at night—but it usually does not keep the youngster awake after the first few days. The cough that started as a "tickle" becomes one that clears mucus out of the upper airway and throat.

Colds and Congestion: The Complications

Most colds run their course without complications. However, in certain infants and children, the common cold leads to other difficulties. All of these complications require prompt medical evaluation and treatment.

Middle-ear infection (called otitis media) is one of the most common aftermaths of colds and nose congestion, especially for infants and toddlers. The problem usually appears after several days of congestion. Suspect an ear infection if your youngster develops fever, along with extreme fussiness (especially during the night), or rubs his or her ears repeatedly and cries. Older youngsters, of course, can usually tell you their ears hurt.

A large amount of thick green or deep yellow mucus in the nose can signal *bacterial infection* in the nose or *sinusitis* (especially in older children). There may be a higher or more prolonged fever than you would expect or a headache, as well. *Eye infection* can also occur, since the tear ducts drain into the nose. Suspect this if there is a lot of yellow drainage in your youngster's eye(s).

Lower respiratory infection (such as tracheobronchitis, bronchitis, pneumonia) can also complicate the common cold. Most often, the youngster will have persistent fever, difficult or rapid breathing, and a severe cough. He or she will usually appear much sicker than you would expect with a cold.

Although quite rare, *meningitis* (infection of the coverings of the brain) or *sepsis* (overwhelming infection) follow what appears to be a normal cold. With either of these serious infections, the youngster appears very seriously ill and leaves no doubt in your mind that something is definitely wrong. Seek medical attention immediately if you suspect either of these life-threatening infections. (See Chapter 13 for a review.)

389

RECOGNIZING
AND
MANAGING
COMMON
SYMPTOMS
AND ILLNESSES

When Is It Not a Cold?

Parents often worry when their tiny infant sneezes, fearing a cold. When there are no other signs of sickness, this means the little one is merely clearing his nose in the only way he can. Occasional coughing should not worry you either.

Constant nasal congestion, even in young infants, deserves a bit of attention. This may be a response to dryness of the air, especially in the winter. Try a humidifier or put out a pan of water to evaporate. (Be sure you clean the pan or humidifier often so you don't develop a mold problem.) If this does not solve the problem, discuss the situation with the baby's doctor. Early morning stuffiness may be related to the stuffed animals in the crib. Remove them and see if the baby is better.

In older youngsters, constant or frequent nose congestion with watery mucus most often means allergy. *Allergic rhinitis* (so-called hay fever) is common and might explain your child's problem. This is especially likely if there are other members of your family with allergies, hay fever, "sinus problems," asthma, or food allergy.

Another cause of frequent runny nose is *frequent crying!* Remember, the tear ducts drain into the nose. This may be part of the reason so many mothers say their infant's nose runs because of *teething*.

One-sided nose drainage in a toddler or small child often signals a *foreign body* stuck in the nose. With this problem, the drainage can be bloody or purulent (containing pus) and often smells terrible. Look yourself or take the youngster to the doctor. If you find something, don't try to remove it yourself, since damage may occur if removal is not performed properly.

Whooping cough (pertussis) is a serious, preventable disease that starts just like a cold. After about a week, a progressively worse cough develops. The little one has coughing spells so severe that she turns blue and cannot catch her breath. Another infection, *chlamydia pneumonia*, can produce a similar illness in very young infants. A baby (or older child) who has severe coughing spells should be seen by his doctor as soon as possible.

Chronic cough, with or without congestion, also deserves investigation by your child's doctor. It may signal *allergy, asthma*, or another *chronic lung condition*.

THE DON'TS

Don't treat a cold with leftover antibiotics or expect your youngster's doctor to prescribe them for a cold. Antibiotics do not help cure viral infections, nor do they prevent complications of the common cold.

Don't use decongestant cold medications in infants under six months old without your doctor's recommendation. Use them in older children if symptoms are severe, but don't exceed the recommended dosage.

390

ILLNESS IN
INFANTS,
CHILDREN,
AND
ADOLESCENTS

Don't hesitate to have your youngster evaluated by his doctor if you suspect a complication—middle-ear infection, bacterial nasal infection, lower respiratory infection, sinusitis, and so on.

Don't forget to ask your doctor about your youngster if she seems chronically congested or has a chronic cough.

PLEASE NOTE: Now that you have a grasp of how to recognize and manage colds, cough, and congestion, it would be extremely helpful for you to go back to the Quick Reference With the Steps in Detail and review it carefully. The more familiar you are with that material, the more useful it will be to you when you need it.

QUICK REFERENCE

With the Steps in Detail

"Colic"

▶ **SUSPECT COLIC IF YOUR YOUNG INFANT HAS REPEATED EPISODES OF UNCONSOLABLE CRYING AT A CERTAIN TIME OF THE DAY.**

▶ **THINK CAREFULLY ABOUT WHETHER THE LITTLE ONE IS CRYING FOR A REASON OTHER THAN COLIC.**

  • Is he hungry, thirsty, wet, uncomfortable, sick?

  • If you are breast-feeding, have you had anything unusual in your diet in the last twelve to twenty-four hours?

  • Does she show any signs of being ill—vomiting, refusing feedings, diarrhea, fever?

▶ **TRY TO CONSOLE THE INFANT BY ROCKING, WALKING, OR MOVING IN SOME WAY** (SUCH AS A DRIVE IN THE CAR OR PLACING THE BABY IN A SPECIAL INFANT SWING). **DO NOT OVERFEED HER!**

▶ **IF THE BABY HAS NOT STOPPED CRYING AFTER TWO HOURS, CALL YOUR DOCTOR FOR ADVICE AND SUPPORT.**

391

RECOGNIZING
AND
MANAGING
COMMON
SYMPTOMS
AND ILLNESSES

▶ **IF YOUR BABY'S CRYING SEEMS REALLY EXCESSIVE, OR YOU
ARE HAVING TROUBLE COPING WITH HIM, MAKE AN APPOINT-
MENT WITH YOUR DOCTOR FOR CONSULTATION.**

Colic: What Is It?

When people think about colic, they usually think of abdominal pain in babies—pain
that leads to a lot of crying. Experienced parents or grandparents often groan at the
thought of having a colicky baby, and for good reason—because the little one is so
miserable, and so are his or her parents!

It's easier to describe how a colicky baby acts than to define exactly what colic is.
Typically, colic starts at two to three weeks of age in a baby who was previously not
especially fussy. Suddenly one evening, the baby begins to cry. At first, the crying
does not appear to be particularly different, but in a short time, the baby seems
hysterical. He screams and screams, and nothing his parents do to comfort the infant
lasts very long. He might calm down for just a minute when being fed, rocked, or
walked—but then starts crying hysterically again. Pretty soon, his little tummy seems
bloated, and he draws up his legs as if his tummy really hurts. He might burp a great
deal and pass a lot of gas. After what seems like an eternity (but is usually less than
two hours), he may settle down and go to sleep. Everything seems fine until the next
night—when the cycle starts all over again.

Considering this set of symptoms, it's easy to see why people have thought (for a
long time) that colic is caused by gas. Babies who have colic do have a lot of gas, to
be sure, and they certainly scream as if they hurt. But *all* babies have gas, and *not
all* cry hysterically about it. So what makes the difference?

Nearly all babies have occasional "fussy periods" where nothing much that you do
for them is quite right. Many also have an occasional screaming episode. These episodes
usually start when the baby is about two to three weeks old and decrease or disappear
when the baby gets to be around three to four months old. Most parents can handle
an occasional screaming bout but begin to lose their confidence *and* patience if these
occur too often.

A baby who has what we call "colic" is, in general, a bit more "difficult" than
the average baby. She is a bit more demanding when hungry and tends to gulp her
feedings rather greedily. In doing that, she swallows quite a bit of air—from around
the nipple (whether breast- or bottle-fed). She tends to be a little more difficult to
"schedule"—that is, her eating and sleeping schedule is very unpredictable. She often
likes to suck on things more than the average baby. If she can't get her fingers or
thumb into her mouth, then she gropes for a pacifier if it is offered. And she seems

392

ILLNESS IN
INFANTS,
CHILDREN,
AND
ADOLESCENTS

to sleep fewer hours in the day than her noncolicky friends (as much as two hours less!). The little one may not always be fussy, but she spends a lot of time just looking around and moving. In a sense, then, she is more "sensitive" and "active" and reacts to many things by crying. And cry she does!

To make matters worse, all babies swallow a great deal of air when they cry. If the air is not released from the stomach with a burp, it passes quickly down into the intestine, causing bloating and probably crampy pain. So crying leads to air swallowing, air swallowing leads to pain, and pain leads to more crying—a vicious cycle.

Most colicky crying occurs in the evening hours. The reason is not really known, but there are several theories. For one, mothers who nurse their babies tend to have a little less milk in the evening, so some of the crying may be from hunger. However, that does not explain colic in formula-fed babies who eat the same formula (and the same amounts) throughout the day and evening. Some think colic means a baby is not tolerating his milk—whether breast milk or formula. This doesn't make sense either, since he drinks the same thing twenty-four hours a day but only cries unconsolably during one short part of the day. Other people say the crying happens because the baby's mother (and father, too) are upset and tired—and the baby can sense their frustration. But there is no proof of this hypothesis. Boredom? Fatigue? Who knows? But the fact remains—most colicky crying happens at the same, predictable time each night.

It's true that colic is more often a problem with first-time parents than with those who are more experienced with babies, but colic can and does occur in later children (much to the surprise and dismay of their parents). While babies do seem to sense whether a person is comfortable and calm, a colicky baby is a colicky baby, no matter who handles him or her!

The good news about colic is that it does go away in time. The bad news is that it lasts until the baby is three or four months old. It seems to decrease as the baby is more able to concentrate on her surroundings—mobiles, people, and her fists, which she can usually get into her mouth by around three months of age. While some of the "personality traits" or temperament characteristics of the "colicky baby" persist— the tendency to be more sensitive to change, more difficult to schedule, less likely to sleep, and more aware of the surrounding world—the crying spells decrease and then stop.

Colic: How Can I Be Sure It's Nothing Serious?

The first time a baby cries unconsolably, it is very difficult to be sure the reason is "colic." But usually, just as you're really getting concerned about what is wrong, the baby stops crying and goes to sleep, then acts perfectly normal. By the second and third time, the truth is more obvious, and what's left is confirming your suspicions with your doctor.

393

RECOGNIZING
AND
MANAGING
COMMON
SYMPTOMS
AND ILLNESSES

Occasionally, though, a baby doesn't stop crying for several hours. If this happens, think carefully about how the baby acted *before* the crying started, and call your doctor to discuss the problem. If the problem does not seem particularly obvious, the doctor may want to see and evaluate the baby. Once in a while, an ear infection, eyelash or scratch in the eye, urinary tract infection, bowel obstruction, or sepsis (overwhelming infection) might look like colic, so it's best to call your doctor to make sure the problem actually is colic.

What Can I Do for My Colicky Baby?

While nothing magical is available to stop a colicky baby from feeling so bad or crying, there are some things you can try that work better than others.

- Before assuming your baby is crying because of colic, be sure he is not hungry or otherwise uncomfortable. If he hasn't eaten in two hours, try feeding him. Try rocking, burping, and changing his diaper.

- Try swaddling the baby in a light blanket. Some like the feeling of "containment."

- Many babies will settle down somewhat if they are kept in motion. Try rocking in a rocking chair, walking her, swaying back and forth while you hold her (either standing or sitting), placing her in an infant swing, or taking a ride in the family car (with the infant in an approved car restraint, of course).

Each baby is a little different, so what works for one might not work for another. If everything fails and you find yourself getting very frustrated—then put the baby in his bed, turn on some soothing music, close the door, and leave the room. He will stop crying eventually and *will not be harmed* by the crying. If you have really tried everything you know and it did not work, then there is no sense in getting more and more upset and frustrated by trying and trying and trying and feeling like a failure—when you're not!

If your baby is particularly difficult, be sure to see or call his or her pediatrician or your family physician. The doctor will make sure there is really nothing other than colic wrong with your baby and may have some additional suggestions for you. Some babies are so miserable that their doctors will prescribe a mild sedative to help them over the difficult times.

Staying Sane with a Colicky Baby

Colicky babies stress the coping skills of their parents. The crying happens at a time when parents are very tired and often feel insecure about whether they can or will be good parents. The crying is frustrating, and many mothers and fathers feel as if they

394

ILLNESS IN
INFANTS,
CHILDREN,
AND
ADOLESCENTS

might lose control and hurt their baby if the crying continues. The best of parents can find themselves feeling this way. But sometimes, the feeling unfortunately turns into destructive action. Parents find themselves handling the baby roughly and feeling angry that the baby will not stop crying. Some even lose control and shake or hit the baby.

It's especially important for you to find relief for yourself if your baby has colic. Arrange to give each other a break, or get someone you trust to watch the baby for a few hours so you can get out of the house for a while. Find someone you trust to talk to when you are frustrated. Above all, *call for help*—even if you must call a child-abuse hot line—if you feel as if you are losing control. Gently put the baby in his bed and shut the door rather than continue to try to comfort him if you feel close to shaking or hitting him. It's normal to feel this frustrated, but it would be devastating to lose control and hurt your little one.

You should also know that most parents with colicky babies feel like failures at some point. This is far from the truth. If you realize you can only do so much and that this problem will end in a few months, then you will not blame yourself or the baby. Instead, you will do what you can to comfort the baby and find some relief for yourself, too (as previously discussed).

THE DON'TS

Don't stop breast feeding, severely limit your diet if you're nursing, or change the baby's formula without talking with your baby's doctor. Colic is rarely caused by milk intolerance unless the crying is continuous, day and night, and associated with vomiting, diarrhea, or both.

Don't overfeed your colicky baby. Overfilling an already gassy, uncomfortable stomach is likely to make the situation worse.

Don't try sedatives or medications recommended by well-meaning friends or relatives without consulting your baby's doctor. If your baby needs something to calm him, his doctor will prescribe or recommend a medication that is safe.

Don't hesitate to call the doctor if you are not sure whether the baby is colicky or has another problem. Better yet, make an appointment to see her doctor for an examination and advice.

Don't hesitate to call someone for help—to talk to someone you trust—if you feel as if you will lose control and hurt your crying baby. Frustration is the rule rather than the exception, and talking about the problem and arranging to get a break can do wonders.

PLEASE NOTE: Now that you have a grasp of how to recognize and manage colic, it would be extremely helpful for you to go back to the Quick Reference With the Steps in Detail and review it carefully. The more familiar you are with that material, the more useful it will be to you when you need it.

395

RECOGNIZING
AND
MANAGING
COMMON
SYMPTOMS
AND ILLNESSES

QUICK REFERENCE

Constipation

▶ **CONSTIPATION MEANS HAVING LESS FREQUENT THAN USUAL, HARD, DRY, AND PAINFUL BOWEL MOVEMENTS.**

▶ **IF AN INFANT, TODDLER, OR OLDER YOUNGSTER HAS AN OCCASIONAL PROBLEM WITH CONSTIPATION, TRY CHANGING HIS DIET BEFORE YOU CONSIDER USING LAXATIVES.**

▶ **DO NOT GIVE AN INFANT OR SMALL CHILD AN ENEMA WITHOUT CONSULTING YOUR DOCTOR.**

▶ **IF YOU THINK YOUR YOUNGSTER HAS A PROBLEM WITH CHRONIC CONSTIPATION, MAKE AN APPOINTMENT FOR HER WITH HER DOCTOR.**

What Is Constipation?

Each of us has our own "normal" pattern of bowel movements. While many people believe that everyone should have at least one bowel movement (stool) each day, the fact is, it can be perfectly normal to have a bowel movement as often as three or four times a day or as infrequently as once every three to four days. The key is being sure that the stool is normal. The normal stool is neither runny or without form nor hard, dry, and pelletlike.

Few people would argue that a very dry, hard stool that was difficult to eliminate signaled constipation, especially if it caused tearing and bleeding around the anus (the opening of the rectum to the outside of the body). But what about a perfectly soft, formed bowel movement that was passed every three days? The point is, it can be just as normal for one child to have a bowel movement every third day as it is for another to have three a day.

Straining to have a bowel movement, however, and what it means in infants and children, leads to concern among parents. It is very common for young infants and toddlers to grunt, turn red, and make all sorts of noises, then have a perfectly normal,

396

ILLNESS IN
INFANTS,
CHILDREN,
AND
ADOLESCENTS

soft stool. This is *not* constipation but rather the only way the little one (who is often lying flat) can get enough pressure behind the stool to push it out. It is also a reflex in response to having stool in the rectum. Next time you see your young infant or toddler doing this, try pushing against the child's feet and see if you notice a difference. Unless this characteristic behavior is marked by excessive fussing or crying, or the bowel movement is very dry or streaked with blood, it shouldn't worry you. If you are concerned, ask the doctor about it.

Diet and Constipation

What and how much a youngster eats pretty well determine what his or her bowel movements are like. Young infants who are breast-fed, for example, tend to have watery stools with very little solid material in them. Their bowel movements can be very ''explosive,'' and happen as often as every feeding or as infrequently as every three to five days. There is very little solid waste in breast milk, so the material left for elimination is mostly liquid. Formula-fed infants, on the other hand, tend to have more solid material in their stools, but they, too, can have frequent to infrequent bowel movements (like the breast-fed baby).

As an infant begins to eat solid foods (and a more varied diet), his or her stools also change. They first tend to get somewhat pasty, then become more formed. Many of the foods little children eat are ''constipating''—that is, they have very little fiber or bulk. Therefore, some youngsters will have more and more dry stools. Even older youngsters who are rather irregular eaters will have a problem with occasional constipation—dry, hard stools—when they have eaten relatively little.

Certain foods that children like to eat are by their very nature constipating. Cow's milk, especially in large quantities, cheese, and certain starches (for example, rice) are constipating. Likewise, some of the most popular fruits for infants and toddlers— bananas and apples—are the natural sources for kaolin and pectin, which are substances often recommended for diarrhea because of their tendency to produce firmer stools. Also, most youngsters do not eat large amounts of foods containing fiber (leftover material that fills the intestines with bulk), and some do not drink enough liquid to keep their stools soft.

Constipation: When to Be Concerned

True constipation, especially in a young infant, can at times be a signal of an underlying problem. A young infant who cannot or does not have a bowel movement more often than every four or five days, or who only empties her bowel after she is given a suppository, might have a congenital problem called *Hirshsprung's disease*. In this condition, certain areas of the bowel do not contain the normal intestinal muscle, so

397

RECOGNIZING
AND
MANAGING
COMMON
SYMPTOMS
AND ILLNESSES

intestinal action is abnormal. Consult your doctor if you notice an ongoing problem with your young infant. If the doctor suspects this problem, he or she will recommend X rays and probably a biopsy of the rectal lining.

Another unusual cause of severe constipation in early infancy is *infantile botulism.* The symptoms of infantile botulism—increasing weakness that can progress to the point of paralysis, poor cry, and inability to feed, along with severe constipation—are caused by the toxins (poisons) produced by botulism bacteria, which can be detected in the sick baby's stool. The disease has been linked with honey fed to some young infants who have had infantile botulism. Avoid giving honey to infants under one year of age to reduce the risk of this potentially deadly disease.

Hypothyroidism (underactive thyroid gland function) in infancy is also associated with constipation. Screening of newborn infants for hypothyroidism is routinely carried out now, but occasionally, this problem surfaces after the first month of life or so. Other symptoms of this very serious problem include general sluggishness, a hoarse cry, umbilical hernia, a large tongue, and poor growth. Because hypothyroidism is such a serious condition, your doctor may want to retest your baby if he or she has any suspicion that it might be present.

Excessive straining with bowel movements is often blamed on a baby's having a very tight rectal muscle. While this is possible in a very small number of infants, it is probably overrated as a cause of constipation.

In older infants and toddlers, firm, dry stools (constipation) can lead to a vicious cycle of further constipation. Because firm stools cause pain, the child, who now has some control over her bowels, simply refuses to go. The longer she waits, the harder the stool becomes. Finally, she cannot control herself any longer, but the large stool tears her anal opening, producing a *fissure* (a "crack" in the skin), which causes further pain and bleeding. Afterward, each time she feels the urge to empty her bowel, she remembers the pain and again withholds the stool. The cycle goes on and on. All this happens most often during a critical time—the time of toilet training. The risk is for the child to refuse to use the toilet and to continue her cycle of chronic constipation.

Older youngsters who have mild to severe chronic constipation (often because they just don't pay attention to their natural urge to have a bowel movement) may complain of *recurrent abdominal pain*. They may also fall prey to *chronic laxative use* and dependence. A serious physical and psychological problem called *encopresis* (stool withholding, coupled with soiling) is also associated with chronic constipation. You will need professional help in dealing with these long-standing problems.

What Can I Do to Help My Child?

As a first step in helping your constipated child, look carefully at what he does and doesn't eat. Encourage him to *drink more liquids*—especially fruit juices. Prune or apple juice, as you probably know, can be particularly helpful in regulating bowel

398

ILLNESS IN
INFANTS,
CHILDREN,
AND
ADOLESCENTS

patterns. Go easy at first, though, or you may overdo it! If your baby is only a few months old and is having constipation problems, offer extra water or dilute apple juice. Do not use honey for babies under one year old, and avoid corn syrup unless your doctor recommends it. If the baby is formula-fed, talk with your doctor about possibly trying a different formula.

Encourage the child or young person to eat vegetables, especially raw vegetables, which contain a large amount of *fiber*. Discourage excessive milk drinking (of regular cow's milk, that is) and too much reliance on cheeses. Use whole-grain breads and cereals, instead of highly processed ones. Also, increase the amount of raw fruit he or she eats. Substitute these ''healthy'' foods for more highly processed foods—both at meals and for snacks. You'll not only help with the constipation problem but will also begin training your youngster to have a lifetime of good health habits.

If your child is having discomfort and is unable to have a bowel movement, but does *not* otherwise seem sick, you can help by using a *glycerin rectal suppository*. Insert the suppository (which dissolves and lubricates the hard stool) well into the rectum by pushing it in with your finger or by using your thermometer. Put it in far enough so your finger or the thermometer is inserted about one inch. There is also a liquid glycerin preparation you can buy if it seems easier for you. You can also have the youngster spend more time in the bathroom in the morning, so she has a chance to empty her bowels without rushing. You may need to use commercial products that increase stool bulk—such as Maltsupex or Metamucil—or mineral oil (but never use force, or the child may choke) to soften the stool. Check with your doctor about the use of these products. Your doctor might have further suggestions for you, as well.

Never use laxatives of any kind without consulting your youngster's doctor. Especially avoid them if a youngster is having abdominal pain or seems sick. Many of them are especially strong for children and will cause a great deal of cramping. You don't want to start a bad habit of dependence on laxatives either.

Also, *never administer enemas* to an infant or child without consulting your doctor first. When giving an enema to an infant or child, it is easy to use too much force and cause serious damage to the intestine. In addition, you can cause a serious imbalance of the youngster's body water and electrolytes, especially with repeated, large enemas. On a psychological level, enemas are uncomfortable and embarrassing—something all of us would like to avoid, if at all possible.

You should also be aware of the fact that serious conflicts between you and your child can result from forcing him to move his bowels. Therefore, regardless of what you do to help your child, do it with as little emphasis on the constipation as you can. This is especially important when you are dealing with a young toddler or preschooler.

THE DON'TS

Don't assume that an infant or child is constipated if he doesn't have a bowel movement every day. Each youngster has his own normal pattern.

399

RECOGNIZING
AND
MANAGING
COMMON
SYMPTOMS
AND ILLNESSES

Don't forget that diet has a lot to do with how hard or soft a bowel movement is and how often it is passed. Make changes in her diet as a first step in controlling occasional constipation problems.

Don't treat chronic constipation yourself without consulting your child's doctor. While uncommon, certain potentially serious problems can have constipation as a symptom.

Don't use or rely on stimulant laxatives or enemas to control your youngster's bowels. You can cause serious physical as well as psychological problems.

PLEASE NOTE: Now that you have a grasp of how to recognize and manage constipation, it would be extremely helpful for you to go back to the Quick Reference and review it carefully. The more familiar you are with that material, the more useful it will be to you when you need it.

QUICK REFERENCE

With the Steps in Detail

Diarrhea

▶ **YOU CAN TRY HOME TREATMENT FOR DIARRHEA IF IT IS MILD AND YOUR YOUNGSTER SHOWS NO SIGNS OF DEHYDRATION:**

- For the first six to twelve hours, offer small amounts of diluted juices (except apple), carbonated beverages, or a prepared solution such as Gatorade, Pedialyte, or Infalyte. Eliminate cow's milk or formula during this time.

- Introduce the so-called "BRATT" diet for older infants and toddlers— fresh, ripe *b*ananas, *r*ice or rice cereal, *a*pplesauce, *t*oast (dry or with jelly), and weak *t*ea, in addition to the liquids. Gradually resume the normal foods over a few days as the youngster tolerates them and is hungry.

- Restrict older youngsters to bland foods—cereals, soups, gelatins, and crackers or bread along with the juices are best.

- After twelve to twenty-four hours, introduce milk or formula in small amounts. Gradually increase the amount over a day or so.

400

ILLNESS IN
INFANTS,
CHILDREN,
AND
ADOLESCENTS

- If you are breast-feeding, continue to offer the breast, even through the first few hours of diarrhea. Breast-fed infants rarely need to be taken off breast milk because of diarrhea.

- Be sure you offer some foods or beverages that contain calories and protein after the first twenty-four hours.

- Do not give medications to stop the diarrhea unless you have checked with your doctor.

▶ **CONTACT YOUR CHILD'S DOCTOR (OR GO TO AN EMERGENCY ROOM IF YOU DON'T HAVE A DOCTOR OR CAN'T REACH YOUR DOCTOR) IF ANY OF THE FOLLOWING OCCUR:**

- Your young infant or toddler has bowel movements that are large in volume and watery (more than six to eight per day), and you see no improvement in twenty-four to forty-eight hours by restricting her diet.

- The diarrhea contains blood or large amounts of mucus.

- The youngster shows signs of dehydration—little or no urine in eight to twelve hours, dry mouth, severe listlessness, excessive thirst, sunken eyes, doughy skin.

- There is a lot of abdominal pain or high fever with the diarrhea.

- The youngster is vomiting (more than once or twice) along with severe diarrhea.

- You see no improvement after two or three days, even by limiting his diet.

Diarrhea: What You Should Know

Diarrhea is the frequent passage of much looser than usual or liquid bowel movements. It can be nothing more than a bothersome result of dietary indiscretion or can signal a potentially serious condition. However, the diarrhea most infants and young children suffer is of the mild variety and lasts only a few days.

The bowel movements (stools) become looser than usual or watery because food products pass very quickly through the intestine. Diarrhea stools can be of many colors (from yellow to brown to green to clear and watery), depending on the cause of the problem and how fast the food moves through the digestive system. This "rapid-transit" bowel movement may also contain *small* amounts of intestinal mucus, as well.

When an infant or child has diarrhea, he or she loses more water than usual in the bowel movement. This water most often comes from fluid intake but may also include ''extra'' water stored or used by the body (found in tissues, organs, and the bloodstream). This water is released from areas of the body and is secreted into the intestines if the intestines are inflamed. This process leads to dehydration (excessive loss of body fluids). If true diarrhea with intestinal inflammation persists for more than several days, the delicate lining of the intestine can be temporarily damaged, and the youngster is not able to normally absorb foods (especially fats, as well as some proteins and sugars). This problem can be further complicated by not feeding a youngster for a long time. For these reasons, prolonged diarrhea is a signal for medical attention.

Before you can be sure whether your youngster has serious diarrhea, you need to compare what is happening to *his or her* normal pattern. Are the stools just a little looser and more frequent than normal, or are they large in volume, liquid, and watery? Are they a normal color, or green or clear? Green bowel movements that are not much looser than normal often are the result of a change in the child's diet—or a change in the nursing mother's diet, for breast-fed infants. They also occur when normal bile from the gallbladder does not have enough time (because of ''rapid transit'') to be changed in color. Is there blood or large amounts of mucus? Is there a lot of pain or gas associated with the diarrhea? Are the stools passed explosively? These questions can help you decide how serious the problem is or isn't.

Diarrhea: The Causes

The most common cause of diarrhea is probably *dietary indiscretion*, especially in anyone other than exclusively breast-fed or formula-fed infants. And even in babies who are nursing, a change in the mother's diet can lead to ''rapid transit.'' This kind of diarrhea lasts only a short time—hours or a day or so.

Intestinal virus infections (so-called *gastroenteritis*) are the next most common culprit that causes diarrhea. Here again, the problem usually lasts only a few days and may have vomiting associated with it. There may be mild fever and some cramping. Resting the inflamed intestine by having the child eat *very small amounts* of very bland food and encouraging the intake of *plenty of liquids* are the cornerstones of treatment. These intestinal viruses are contagious within the family or in baby-sitting situations, especially if the infant or child is in diapers (it's changing the diaper that heightens the risk for transmitting the virus).

Bacterial diarrhea is a more serious problem in which a youngster seems quite sick (with fever and usually abdominal pain) in addition to having diarrhea. The stools may have blood or quite a bit of mucus in them. The bacteria that cause these problems are also very contagious. They can be transmitted from person to person or caught through contaminated water or food. Certain *intestinal parasites* can also lead to this kind of illness. If these culprits are suspected, the doctor's help is needed, and he or

401

RECOGNIZING
AND
MANAGING
COMMON
SYMPTOMS
AND ILLNESSES

402

ILLNESS IN
INFANTS,
CHILDREN,
AND
ADOLESCENTS

she will usually want to have the stool studied (called a stool culture) to identify the cause.

Infants and children often have mild diarrhea when they have other infections—such as *colds* and *ear infections*. Some infants and toddlers have ''rapid transit'' when they are *teething*, as well. Certain *medications* can also be the culprits—especially antibiotics, which eliminate some of the ''normal'' intestinal bacteria and allow other bacteria and yeasts to overgrow. With these problems, the diarrhea is temporary and goes away when the medicine is stopped or the problem causing it has disappeared.

Chronic diarrhea requires medical evaluation. It can be caused by a low-grade parasite infection, food allergy, and chronic inflammatory diseases of the intestine. Check with your child's doctor if you think your youngster has too many episodes of loose bowels. While it can be his or her ''normal'' reaction to illness or stress, there may be an underlying problem that treatment can remedy.

Diarrhea: The Complications

The most common complication of severe diarrhea—especially in infants and young children—is *dehydration*. This risk is especially great if the youngster is also vomiting. It's important to watch for signs of dehydration: low urine production, extreme thirst, dry mouth, sunken eyes and abdomen, and doughy skin. Whenever you recognize these symptoms, seek medical help.

Undernutrition can be a problem if diarrhea is prolonged, especially if a youngster is kept on a liquid or very limited diet for longer than a few days. So-called *starvation stools* can be misinterpreted as persistent diarrhea, leading to continued restriction of the diet. (Starvation leads to the passage of very small but frequent greenish, loose stools with mucus.) Contact your doctor if diarrhea continues for longer than a few days and you are not making progress in feeding the child.

Prolonged or particularly severe diarrhea can result in temporary damage to the lining of the intestine, leading to intolerance of certain foods. Most commonly, fats are not well absorbed by the intestine, and the youngster may not tolerate certain sugars or proteins either. For example, cow's milk may not be tolerated. You need your doctor's help in deciding what substitutes have to be made and for how long these substitutes must be continued.

THE DON'TS

Don't overreact if your youngster has mild diarrhea. Try a bland diet and plenty of liquids for a day or two, then call your doctor if you are not seeing the problem resolve.

403

RECOGNIZING
AND
MANAGING
COMMON
SYMPTOMS
AND ILLNESSES

Don't misinterpret the loose, watery yellow stools of the breast-fed infant as diarrhea. This is normal, even if the baby has six to ten bowel movements a day. Formula-fed babies also have less-formed stools than older youngsters and adults (who are eating a variety of foods).

Don't treat mild or moderate diarrhea with liquids only for longer than two or three days. Contact your child's doctor for advice.

Don't hesitate to call your doctor if the diarrhea is very severe, the youngster is also vomiting, there is blood or mucus in the stool, or there are any signs of dehydration. Your youngster probably needs medical evaluation and even hospitalization to treat the problem.

Don't give antidiarrhea medicines to your child without your doctor's approval. While mixtures of kaolin and pectin are safe and may be helpful, stronger medicines can be dangerous and cover up a more serious problem.

PLEASE NOTE: Now that you have a grasp of how to recognize and manage diarrhea, it would be extremely helpful for you to go back to the Quick Reference With the Steps in Detail and review it carefully. The more familiar you are with that material, the more useful it will be to you when you need it.

404

ILLNESS IN
INFANTS,
CHILDREN,
AND
ADOLESCENTS

QUICK REFERENCE

With the Steps in Detail

Earaches, Ear Infections

▶ **MIDDLE-EAR INFECTION (OTITIS MEDIA) IS A COMMON COMPLI-CATION OF A COLD OR NOSE CONGESTION. SUSPECT THIS PROB-LEM IF:**

- Your infant or toddler seems cranky, cries unconsolably (especially during the night), or pulls or rubs his ears during or after a cold (with or without much fever).

- Your older child tells you her ear(s) hurt.

- You see pus draining from a youngster's ear(s).

▶ **IF YOU SUSPECT MIDDLE-EAR INFECTION:**

- Give the youngster the correct dose of aspirin substitute to help with the pain.

- Sometimes, lying down makes the pain of ear infection worse, because it increases the pressure inside the ear. Pick up a small child and hold him, or have an older youngster try to sleep with his head slightly elevated.

- If there is *no drainage* from her ear, you may want to put a few drops of warm oil (olive oil, vegetable oil, baby oil, ear oil from a previous earache) in her ear. Do *not* do this if you see any liquid in the ear.

- You do not need to see the doctor right away if it's in the evening. Instead, call your doctor in the morning for an appointment (or take the youngster to an emergency room, if you don't have a doctor or can't reach your doctor), even if the pain has gone away. If you suspect the problem and it's daytime, call the doctor right away for an appointment. The point is, the child should be seen by a doctor *within* twenty-four hours from the time you recognize the symptoms. (If the youngster appears to be in extreme pain, call the doctor immediately for advice.)

405

RECOGNIZING
AND
MANAGING
COMMON
SYMPTOMS
AND ILLNESSES

▶ **SUSPECT "SWIMMER'S EAR" (OTITIS EXTERNA) IN AN OLDER YOUNGSTER WHO HAS BEEN SWIMMING IF:**

- He complains of an earache, *and* it is painful if you touch or gently pull the outer ear.

- You see swelling of the ear canal, there is a drainage from the ear, and the ear is tender or painful.

▶ **IF YOU SUSPECT "SWIMMER'S EAR":**

- Treat the youngster's pain with aspirin substitute (in the correct dosage).

- Place warm compresses or a heating pad (set on low) over the ear(s) to help ease the discomfort. (Do not allow a youngster to go to bed with a heating pad!)

- Make an appointment with the doctor for an examination to be sure the problem is not a middle-ear infection.

Middle-Ear Infection: *What You Should Know*

A middle-ear infection (otitis media) is probably the most common complication of colds and respiratory infections. While some youngsters never seem to get middle-ear infections, others are literally plagued by them nearly each and every time they have a cold.

The middle ear is a cavity closed from the outside by a thin membrane called the eardrum. It is lined by the same kind of mucous lining found in the nose and is connected *inside* the head to the nasal cavity by a very narrow opening called the Eustacian tube. The middle ear normally contains air and the tiny bones that vibrate to transmit sound. The Eustacian tube opens and closes to allow air into the middle ear and keeps the pressure inside the ear the same as that outside the ear. This opening and closing is what causes your ears to "pop."

When the lining of the nose is inflamed or swollen—as it is during a cold or with allergies—the Eustacian tube often becomes blocked. It can also be blocked by large adenoids (tonsillike structures in the back of the nose). This blockage leads to a buildup of fluid in the middle ear. Infection of the fluid occurs from viruses and bacteria that were in the nose. As pus forms and the pressure builds up, an earache results. If the pressure is great, the eardrum might even rupture (develop a hole), allowing the pus to drain through the eardrum into the ear canal (and that is why you can see the

406

ILLNESS IN
INFANTS,
CHILDREN,
AND
ADOLESCENTS

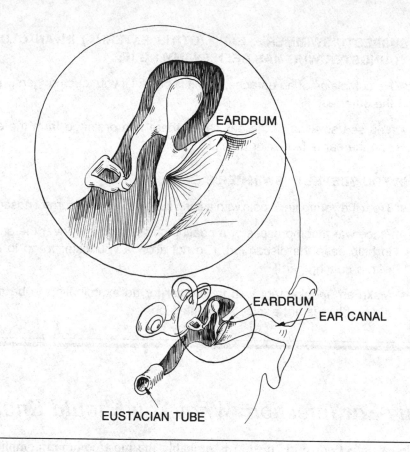

EARDRUM

EARDRUM

EAR CANAL

EUSTACIAN TUBE

Most ear infections involve the middle ear—the cavity behind the eardrum—and are caused by problems with the Eustacian tube.

drainage). If the eardrum bursts, the pain usually improves or disappears, but the infection remains unless it is treated. Most perforations (holes) in the eardrum heal quickly when the infection is treated.

As previously noted, certain youngsters are more prone to getting ear infections than others. Infants and young children have narrow Eustacian tubes and relatively large adenoids. In some, the tubes just don't function as well as they might. These youngsters tend to get ear infections often (with or without a cold as the initiator). Youngsters with allergies or chronically congested noses are at risk for ear infections. Certain problems such as cleft palate and Down's syndrome also predispose a child to ear infections.

Children who get frequent ear infections tend to have most of them in infancy, then get fewer and fewer of them each year after that. In some babies, the culprit seems to be (at least in part) drinking or nursing while lying down. It's worth the effort to hold an infant more upright during feeding or to try the type of bottle with disposable bags in bottle-fed babies (because the baby can sit straight up and still drink if she is

407

RECOGNIZING
AND
MANAGING
COMMON
SYMPTOMS
AND ILLNESSES

old enough to hold her own bottles). Your doctor may also suggest that you treat your little one with a decongestant at the first sign of nose congestion—in the hope of preventing another ear infection.

Otitis Media: Signs and Symptoms

The most important symptom of a middle-ear infection is pain in the ear. If your youngster is old enough to tell you about it, you are ahead of the game and can make an appointment for his doctor to examine him.

Young infants and toddlers who don't talk are a little more difficult, but there are signs that should make you suspect an ear infection. Consider the possibility of an earache if your baby or toddler wakes up at night crying as if she hurts, especially if she also has nose congestion and/or a cold. She might rub her ears or head, or poke her fingers into her ears. A fever may also develop, although ear infection can be present without fever. Some youngsters with ear infection vomit or have loose bowel movements, as well. *Always* suspect middle-ear infection if you see drainage of pus from the ear, even if the baby, toddler, or older child seems to have no pain. Children who have repeated ear infections tend to show the same symptoms each time, so you will soon recognize the pattern.

Interestingly, earache most frequently strikes at night (or during a nap, if you're lucky). Babies and nonverbal toddlers usually wake up crying and continue to cry for a time. They may go back to sleep only to wake up again and do the same thing. Don't be confused when these children seem better in the morning, then do the same thing the next night. The crying probably happens during naps and at night because the youngster is lying down, and the pressure inside the ear is likely to cause more pain at that time.

While most infants and children who have a middle ear infection seem to experience pain with their infections, some do not. As many as one in five infants and nearly that many older children with an ear infection do not show obvious signs of ear pain. Their infections are usually found when the doctor examines them because of problems which might seem unrelated—diarrhea or vomiting, for example—or even during well-checks. Even older children who usually can communicate well may not complain about earache when they have a middle ear infection. So don't be overly surprised when the doctor tells you that your youngster has a middle ear infection—when you thought the problem was teething, the flu, or strep throat!

Otitis Media: The Complications

Before antibiotics were available to treat ear infections effectively, *chronic ear infection, mastoiditis, and hearing loss* were the most common complications. These complications still occur, although much less frequently. However, it's still important that

408

ILLNESS IN
INFANTS,
CHILDREN,
AND
ADOLESCENTS

a youngster's ear infection be treated quickly and completely in order to prevent these serious complications.

Persistent otitis media and *serous otitis media* (fluid behind the eardrum—middle ear effusion) are the most common complications of middle-ear infection now that antibiotics are available. Your child's doctor will want to recheck his or her ears after the antibiotic treatment is completed (to make sure no fluid or infection remains in the middle ear cavity). If there are still signs of infection (persistent otitis media), the youngster will need further antibiotic treatment. Sometimes, the infection clears, but fluid remains within the middle-ear cavity. This is called serous otitis media or middle ear effusion, and can lead to *repeated infections* and *hearing loss*. If fluid does remain, then the doctor will want to continue treating and monitoring this problem.

Some youngsters' ears just cannot be kept clear of fluid, and treating each new infection by medication alone does not remedy the problem. For some of them, giving a low dose of an antibiotic every day for several weeks or even months will reduce the number of new infections they experience, or even prevent new infections completely. Other children with repeated infections, or those who experience new infections in spite of long-term antibiotic treatment, will benefit from the insertion of ventilation tubes (so-called PE—polyethylene—tubes) surgically placed through the eardrum. For them, this is a better alternative (because it drains the fluid continuously) than the repeated infections and fluid accumulation.

Occasionally, ear infection can lead to more serious complications like *meningitis* (infection of the coverings of the brain) or *sepsis* (overwhelming infection)—even after antibiotic treatment has been started. If your youngster seems to get worse with an ear infection and is suddenly very sick—even if he or she is taking an antibiotic—contact your doctor immediately or go to an emergency room (if you don't have a doctor or can't reach your doctor). (For information about these very serious problems, you can review Chapter 13.)

"Swimmer's Ear": What You Should Know

The ear canal—the part of the ear outside the eardrum—is lined by skin. It contains small glands that make cerumen (so-called earwax). This skin of the ear canal can become inflamed if it is irritated, then infected by bacteria or fungi. Irritation can occur from scraping the canal during improper (and unnecessary) cleaning or, most commonly, because the ear canal is constantly wet. The skin infection can be mild and bothersome, or quite dramatic.

This skin infection is called *otitis externa*, or more commonly, "swimmer's ear." The ear canal swells and becomes reddened, and debris and pus form. The outside of the ear can even become swollen, and the little lymph nodes below, in front of, and behind the ear can swell and become painful or tender.

409

RECOGNIZING
AND
MANAGING
COMMON
SYMPTOMS
AND ILLNESSES

Because the ear is draining, it is important for a youngster to be evaluated by his or her doctor, to make sure there is no middle-ear infection, as well.

"Swimmer's Ear": Signs and Symptoms

As with middle-ear infection, the most common complaint you'll hear is "my ear hurts." If you look at the ear, you may see the pus and irritation of the ear canal and even the skin at the outside. There is usually no fever. "Swimmer's ear" is a more common problem of the older youngster who spends a great deal of time in the water.

Since this infection is in the ear canal and not behind the eardrum, the outside of the ear is sore to touch. When you try to tell the difference, touch the outer ear first. Pull on it gently, and push on the little "knob" in front of the ear canal. If the youngster complains bitterly, you can be pretty certain "swimmer's ear" is the problem.

Some youngsters seem to get "swimmer's ear" frequently. If your child has this problem, you may be able to prevent it in the future. Have him shake the water out of his ears right after swimming. Then place two to four drops of an alcohol/vinegar solution into each ear. (Make the alcohol/vinegar solution by mixing together equal parts of rubbing alcohol and distilled vinegar.) If these steps are not effective, ask your doctor for additional suggestions.

THE DON'TS

Don't overlook the signs and symptoms of middle-ear infection in a youngster who has nasal congestion, earache, ear pulling or rubbing, night crying, unusual fussiness, and/or ear drainage (with or without fever). Make an appointment for your youngster to see the doctor, even if she seems better in the morning.

Don't put ear drops or oil in a draining ear unless the doctor recommends it. The drainage usually means there is a hole in the eardrum, and you will be putting drops into the sensitive middle-ear cavity. The only way to know ear drainage is caused by "swimmer's ear" is for the doctor to look inside with an otoscope (a special instrument that allows him or her to see the eardrum).

Don't stop giving antibiotics for middle-ear infection just because the youngster is feeling better. The symptoms disappear long before the infection is eliminated, so it's important for the child to complete his prescription.

Don't restart antibiotics for your ear infection–prone child without talking with or seeing her doctor first.

Don't overlook the importance of having the doctor recheck your youngster after treatment for middle-ear infection is completed. The infection might not be completely gone, or there may be leftover fluid, even though the youngster now seems

410

ILLNESS IN
INFANTS,
CHILDREN,
AND
ADOLESCENTS

fine. This recheck is an important part of preventing or detecting the complications of middle-ear infection (serous otitis media, repeated infection, and hearing loss).

Don't overlook the signs of serious complications of ear infection (meningitis, sepsis, and mastoiditis) even if your child is receiving antibiotics. These serious problems occasionally occur even if the youngster is being treated.

PLEASE NOTE: Now that you have a grasp of how to recognize and manage earaches and ear infections, it would be extremely helpful for you to go back to the Quick Reference With the Steps in Detail and review it carefully. The more familiar you are with that material, the more useful it will be to you when you need it.

QUICK REFERENCE

With the Steps in Detail

Eye Infections

▶ **MILD EYE INFECTIONS (THOSE WITH SOME REDNESS, ITCHING, OR BURNING, AND SMALL AMOUNTS OF MUCOUS OR PUS FORMATION) CAN OFTEN BE TREATED EASILY AT HOME.**

- Gently wipe away mucus or pus with a cotton ball or soft cloth moistened with warm water.

- Try placing a cool, wet cloth over the eyes for a short time.

- Treat styes (small pimples of the eyelids) with frequent warm, wet soaks.

- If your child seems to have a problem with only one eye (especially if he or she is reluctant to open it), look in the eye carefully to see whether there is something there—a bit of sand, an eyelash. If you find something, gently flush the eye with warm water. (Do not try to remove it in any other way.)

- Do not use eye drops or ointment—prescription or over-the-counter—without checking with your doctor first.

- Call your child's doctor for advice (and/or an appointment) if there is a

411

RECOGNIZING
AND
MANAGING
COMMON
SYMPTOMS
AND ILLNESSES

great deal of pus formation, redness, or swelling or if the problem is limited to one eye only.

▶ **CALL TO SEE THE DOCTOR (OR GO TO AN EMERGENCY ROOM IF YOU DON'T HAVE A DOCTOR OR CAN'T REACH YOUR DOCTOR) IF THE YOUNGSTER SHOWS SIGNS OF SERIOUS EYE INFECTION OR INFLAMMATION:**

- Deep red or purplish discoloration of the eyelid, along with severe swelling.

- Red eye(s) and pain in the eye(s).

- Marked swelling of the eyelids, lots of pus formation, or severe redness of the conjunctiva (the white part of the eye).

▶ **MAKE AN APPOINTMENT TO SEE YOUR YOUNGSTER'S DOCTOR OR CALL TO SEE IF HE OR SHE RECOMMENDS THAT YOU SEE AN OPHTHALMOLOGIST** (A MEDICAL DOCTOR WITH SPECIAL TRAINING IN THE EVALUATION AND TREATMENT OF EYE PROBLEMS) **IF YOUR YOUNGSTER HAS REPEATED EYE PROBLEMS, SUCH AS:**

- Frequent discharges from the eye, styes, chronic or periodic eye irritation, or excessive rubbing.

Eye Infections: An Overview of What You Should Know

Fortunately, most eye infections and inflammations infants and children get are mild and easily treated. A few, however, are serious and require prompt and careful treatment.

The insides of the eyelids and the eyeball itself are covered with a thin, clear mucous lining called the conjunctiva. Inflammation of this membrane is called *conjunctivitis* (commonly known as "pink eye"). Most often, conjunctivitis involves *both eyes*.

Inflammation that involves only *one eye* should make you suspicious about the probability that the problem is something other than conjunctivitis. Among the most simple causes of soreness, redness, and increased tears is a foreign object in the eye— an eyelash, a speck of dust, or something else. Serious infections can also be the cause of inflammation of one eye and need to be recognized and treated quickly.

412

ILLNESS IN
INFANTS,
CHILDREN,
AND
ADOLESCENTS

Sometimes, it's hard to distinguish between infection and irritation. Irritated eyes look red because of dilatation (widening) of the small blood vessels in the conjunctiva. This accounts for the redness you see after crying, eye rubbing, and when a person is tired. This dilatation of blood vessels also accounts for the eye redness seen in older youngsters and teens who use marijuana.

Because the eyes are so sensitive and inflammation and infection so potentially serious, it is important that you contact your doctor if you are not sure about your youngster's eyes. Do not treat what appears to be an infection with eye medications without your doctor's agreement. It's better to be safe and have the youngster evaluated than to overlook a serious problem or, because of self-treatment, cause damage to the eye(s) by using an incorrect medicine.

Eye Infections in Young Infants

Because newborn infants are susceptible to eye infections caused by bacteria they are exposed to during the birth process—by law, their eyes are treated at birth. Drops or ointment (antibiotics like erythromycin or tetracycline, or the older silver nitrate) are put into the newborn's eyes to prevent such diseases as gonorrhea, chlamydia, and other possible infections. These drops, particularly silver nitrate, can cause temporary eye inflammation, which accounts for some of the eyelid swelling in tiny newborns.

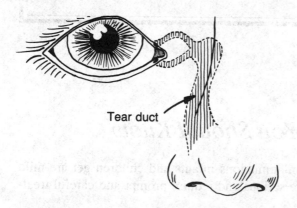

Tear duct

A blocked tear duct does not allow tears to drain into the nose.

In the first few weeks of life, many infants have problems with mucous or pus formation, especially in the inside corners of their eyes. This is usually the result of a partially *blocked tear duct* on one or both sides. Tears cannot drain into the nose, and the little pocket of tears is infected by the normal bacteria of the nose and the outside environment. Suspect a blocked tear duct if you see:

• Accumulation of white or yellowish discharge in the corner of the eye (one or both eyes).

413

RECOGNIZING
AND
MANAGING
COMMON
SYMPTOMS
AND ILLNESSES

- *No* redness of the conjunctiva.

- Increased tearing on the side of the eye with the mucus (because tears cannot drain into the nose through the blocked duct).

- Redness and swelling (although this is rare) along the side of the nose. (This suggests more serious infection if it is present.)

Most of the time, the problem of a blocked tear duct clears up in the first six months of life. If it seems to be a continuing problem or the white discharge occurs off and on, call the baby's doctor or mention it at your next visit. The doctor may want you to use antibacterial eye drops and massage the tear duct for a period of time. Occasionally, the tear duct might need to be widened (this is a simple procedure) if it doesn't open by itself by the time the baby is six to twelve months of age.

Gonococcal infection in young infants is unusual because of the use of preventive drops. However, when it occurs, it produces a serious infection that can lead to blindness if not treated vigorously and promptly. The infection produces a great deal of swelling and redness of the eyelid and copious amounts of purulent (pus-containing) discharge.

Chlamydial eye infection affects infants under two or three months old and can be associated with pneumonia. Chlamydia bacteria are acquired in the birth canal but do not cause infections until weeks later. The eye infection is rather mild, with pus forming in the eye, mild eyelid swelling, and redness. Although chlamydia infections usually do not cause permanent damage to the eyes, they should be treated with oral antibiotics and/or antibacterial drops. An infant with chlamydia pneumonia may not appear very ill but coughs in a characteristic way—in prolonged spells of high-pitched coughs, which can interfere with feeding and sleeping. This potentially serious infection should be treated by the doctor.

Conjunctivitis ("Pink Eye")

The insides of the eyelids and the eyeball itself (as previously noted) are covered with a thin mucous lining called the conjunctiva. This lining extends down into the top of the nasal cavity through the tear duct, which is located at the inside corner of the eye. Most eye inflammation and infection involves this sensitive membrane, which turns red when irritated and will even secrete mucus and pus. Inflammation of this membrane is called *conjunctivitis* (commonly known as "pink eye").

Mild conjunctivitis is often associated with colds. This makes sense, since the viruses and bacteria in the nose are in direct communication with the eye sac through the tear duct. In addition, most youngsters with respiratory infections rub their eyes and can transfer germs from the nose discharge directly into the eye.

Viruses probably cause most conjunctivitis, although bacteria can invade the already

414

ILLNESS IN
INFANTS,
CHILDREN,
AND
ADOLESCENTS

inflamed eye linings and lead to further inflammation and pus formation. This is why your doctor might have you treat conjunctivitis with antibacterial drops or ointment. Suspect conjunctivitis if your child has this group of signs and symptoms:

- Redness of the conjunctiva in *both eyes*, along with the formation of pus.

- Itching or burning and excessive tearing.

- Mild eyelid swelling.

- Mild cold symptoms or sore throat.

Sometimes, there is a great deal of pus formation with conjunctivitis. The secretions may be heavy enough to stick the eyelids shut by morning after sleeping all night. With some forms of conjunctivitis, the inflammation is so severe that there is actual bleeding in the conjunctiva.

You should try to remember that conjunctivitis is very contagious and is spread by coming into contact with the drainage from the eye. Contact with nasal mucus is probably another way to contract conjunctivitis, as well. Take care to wash your hands before and after touching your youngster's eyes and face (be careful to do this each and every time). Also, make sure you have the youngster use separate washcloths and towels from the rest of the family (to avoid possible spread of infection). If your youngster is in preschool or school, he or she should not go to school until the infection is totally cleared up.

Sty: A Pimple on the Eyelid

A sty is essentially a pimple on the eyelid (usually right at the edge of the lid), in one of the little eyelash follicles. It starts as a painful lump, then "comes to a head" and drains pus. It is caused by a bacterial infection, usually the staphylococcus ("staph") germ, and is contagious to other people.

Most of the time, a youngster has only one sty, but a few children are prone to getting them often. When this happens, your doctor might want to look for a source of the infection—in the youngster's nose or in the noses of family members. Staph germs are common on the skin and in the nose but don't cause problems for everyone.

You can treat a sty at home most of the time, unless your child has many styes or seems to get them all the time. Simply use warm, wet compresses on the eye several times a day until the pimple either opens and drains, or just fades away. Be careful to wash your hands well with soap and warm water each time you touch the child's eye or face or apply compresses, and have the youngster use separate washcloths and towels. Also, try to keep your child from rubbing or playing with the infected eye. Rubbing may lead to greater problems or result in infecting the other eye.

Sometimes, styes become more seriously infected and lead to much swelling and redness around the eye. They might also be associated with impetigo—a skin infection around the eyes and face. If either of these problems occurs, you will need your doctor's help.

415

RECOGNIZING
AND
MANAGING
COMMON
SYMPTOMS
AND ILLNESSES

Periorbital Cellulitis: A Very Serious Infection

Periorbital cellulitis is an inflammation and infection of the tissues around the orbit of the eye—the eyelids, the adjacent face, and even the supporting tissues of the eyeball itself. It is a potentially life-threatening infection and needs immediate antibiotic treatment (usually in the hospital). Youngsters with this infection often have sepsis (generalized, overwhelming infection), as well.

Suspect periorbital cellulitis in an infant or child who develops:

- Severe swelling of one eye with red or purplish discoloration.

- High fever and other signs of serious illness (listlessness, irritability, vomiting, and/or loss of appetite).

If you think your child might have a serious eye infection, contact your doctor immediately or go to an emergency room if you don't have a doctor or can't reach your doctor. This infection can worsen rapidly, so do not try to treat it at home. Instead, seek medical assistance as soon as possible.

Unusual Eye Infections

Herpes simplex virus can cause a serious eye infection that affects the cornea (the clear membrane right in front of the pupil through which you see). The virus (the same one that causes "cold sores" or "fever blisters") invades the cornea and causes an ulcer (crater or hole) to form on the cornea. This can lead to scarring of the cornea and loss of vision, because the scar often occurs right over the pupil.

The symptoms of herpes simplex infection of the eye are redness, pain, and light sensitivity in one eye, as well as blurry vision. Be especially suspicious of this infection if your child also has a fever blister or has been in close contact with someone who has one. Get the youngster to his or her doctor or an ophthalmologist (an eye specialist) as soon as possible, since it is imperative that the child receive prompt evaluation and that proper treatment be started immediately.

Children with *chickenpox* can also get little pox ulcers in and around the eye during the disease. Fortunately, these ulcers are rarely serious and should not cause undue worry—unless the youngster complains of trouble seeing or has a pox ulcer right over the cornea. However, *herpes zoster (shingles)*, which is caused by the same virus as

416

ILLNESS IN
INFANTS,
CHILDREN,
AND
ADOLESCENTS

chickenpox, can occur on the face around the eye and can be more serious. Shingles causes blisters that crust over in a very limited area on the face or another part of the body. See your doctor if there is any question of herpes zoster near the eye.

Noninfectious Causes of Eye Irritation and Inflammation

One of the most common causes of eye irritation and inflammation is *allergy*. The eyes are irritated and inflamed because of sensitivity to one or more things in the environment (such as pollen, dust, smoke, animal dander, or pollutants). Usually, the young person has other signs and symptoms of having an allergy, as well, such as allergic rhinitis (hay fever), hives, or asthma. You might suspect allergic eye irritation when a youngster has the following signs and symptoms:

- Mild pinkness of the conjunctiva, along with a lot of tearing.

- Itching and burning of the eyes.

- "Sandy" feeling in the eyes.

- Dark circles under the eyes and mild swelling of the eyelids.

- Frequent sneezing and runny nose, with clear mucus.

- Redness and irritation of the edges of the eyelids.

One of the more frightening things that can happen with eye allergy is marked swelling of the conjunctiva itself. The mucous membranes swell enough to stick out of the eyelids, which are often swollen, as well. The grayish, puffy membranes leave only the iris (colored part) of the eye visible, so the eye looks "buried." This is a temporary condition and will go away if the allergy is treated (without leaving any damage to the eye itself).

Another common cause of a swollen eye is an *insect bite* on the eyelid. The eyelid suddenly appears swollen (usually in the morning) and slightly pink, but the youngster does not seem to have any discomfort at all. You might be able to see the tiny bite if you look closely. The conjunctiva is not red, and there is no eye drainage. The swelling improves after a day or so. While no treatment is necessary, you can try putting cold compresses on the swollen area, particularly if the youngster is concerned or is experiencing some minor discomfort.

You are probably all too familiar with the problem of a *foreign body* (for example, an eyelash, a speck of dirt) in the eye. If your child complains of pain in the eye, has a red eye that is tearing a lot, and has trouble opening it, then look for something in the eye. If you see something there, flush the eye with plain lukewarm water. (See

417

RECOGNIZING
AND
MANAGING
COMMON
SYMPTOMS
AND ILLNESSES

Chapter 16 for details.) If he or she feels better and the symptoms disappear, you need do nothing more. If the problem persists, see your doctor.

A *corneal abrasion* (scratch on the eye) can also cause a young person to have a red, painful eye and experience sensitivity to light, as well as blurry vision. The pain can be very intense! Have the youngster keep his or her eye shut (it's best to patch both eyes). Be sure to contact the doctor immediately if you think your child might have a scratch on the eye. The doctor will want to examine the youngster and will recommend treatment to prevent infection and reduce the pain. Fortunately, almost all corneal abrasions heal well in one to two days and without complications.

If your older youngster or teenager has frequent red eyes (without tearing or other symptoms), be sure to consider *marijuana* use as a possible cause. Here the problem is not inflammation but rather dilatation (widening) of the small blood vessels in the conjunctiva. This same blood-vessel dilatation is the cause of red eyes after *crying* or when a youngster is *very tired*. No medical treatment for the eyes is necessary.

THE DON'TS

Don't put drops or ointment—whether over-the-counter or previously prescribed—into your youngster's eyes without your doctor's approval. Certain types of drops and ointments can cause more harm than good.

Don't hesitate to call your doctor if you think your child has an eye infection. Be especially concerned if the youngster has a great deal of eye swelling and discoloration or a lot of purulent eye discharge.

Don't hesitate to call your doctor immediately if you think the youngster has a corneal abrasion. Anytime a youngster experiences severe pain and can't open his or her eye easily or without severe pain, you should immediately call the doctor for advice.

Don't assume that all red eyes are infected. Look for other possible causes, especially if the problem occurs over and over again.

PLEASE NOTE: Now that you have a grasp of how to recognize and manage eye infections, it would be extremely helpful for you to go back to the Quick Reference With the Steps in Detail and review it carefully. The more familiar you are with that material, the more useful it will be to you when you need it.

418

ILLNESS IN
INFANTS,
CHILDREN,
AND
ADOLESCENTS

QUICK REFERENCE

With the Steps in Detail

Hives

▶ **IF YOU SUSPECT HIVES AND YOUR YOUNGSTER ALSO HAS MOUTH OR TONGUE SWELLING, TAKE HER TO AN EMERGENCY ROOM IMMEDIATELY. IF SHE IS ALSO EXPERIENCING DIFFICULTY BREATHING, HAVE SOMEONE ELSE CALL THE PARAMEDICS WHILE YOU TREAT THE CHILD. IF NO ONE IS WITH YOU, CONTINUE TREATING THE CHILD WHILE YOU PERIODICALLY SHOUT FOR HELP. WHEN HELP ARRIVES, HAVE THAT PERSON CALL THE PARAMEDICS.** (If you are unable to remember the details of managing this problem, turn to the Emergency Quick Reference on page 324, entitled "Anaphylaxis," for a review.)

▶ **IF YOU SUSPECT HIVES AND YOUR CHILD IS OTHERWISE FINE, YOU CAN TRY HOME TREATMENT:**

- Remove heavy clothing, especially wool or other rough clothing, and keep him as cool as possible.

- Have your child soak in a tub of *cool* water for as long as he will stay there.

- If you have an antihistamine medicine in the house, give him one dose (be sure you give the recommended dose if it is an over-the-counter drug, or check with your doctor if you are uncertain about a prescribed medication).

- If your treatment is successful but the hives come back, repeat the treatment.

▶ **CONTACT YOUR CHILD'S DOCTOR FOR ADVICE OR AN APPOINTMENT IF:**

- Your treatment is not successful after a few hours in making the youngster feel more comfortable or in controlling the hives.

- The rash you thought was hives becomes deep red or purple in color.

419

RECOGNIZING
AND
MANAGING
COMMON
SYMPTOMS
AND ILLNESSES

- Your child has repeated bouts of hives.

- You think the hives were caused by a medication prescribed for your child, especially if it was prescribed for an infection or seizure control. Call the doctor to see if you can discontinue the medication until the child can be seen.

Hives: What You Should Know

Hives, or *urticaria* (the medical name for hives), are caused by allergy. Foods, medicines, and materials that touch the skin are the most common culprits. Finding the exact cause for an outbreak of hives can be very frustrating. In many youngsters, the cause is never really identified.

A mild case of hives lasts only a few hours, but often the rash comes and goes for days. This may mean that your child is still coming into contact with whatever it is that is causing the rash, but sometimes the rash comes and goes even without further contact. Some children have only one attack of hives, while others are plagued with repeated bouts. In many of these youngsters, you will have other indications that they are inherently allergic—for example, they might have eczema (a chronic skin condition), allergic rhinitis (so-called hay fever), or asthma.

In some youngsters (or adults), hives can occur as a response to cold, heat, or even stress. In general, these youngsters do not have a serious problem and don't require any special treatment. However, if your child seems to have the typical skin rash of hives often, check with your doctor about whether he or she suggests any testing or treatment.

Hives: Signs and Symptoms

Typically, hives start as unusually shaped, flat, red areas. The youngster will look blotchy (red spots of varying sizes). If you look carefully, some of the blotches will have raised, white areas in the center. The problem with hives is that they itch like crazy, and the size of the welt often increases if the young person scratches it. At first, you might think the spots are mosquito bites, since they look much like a scratched bite. The rash usually fades a little—only to reappear on other areas of the body. The good news is that hives disappear completely, leaving no marks or scars on the skin.

Since heat tends to make hives worse, expect to see more rash if your child is warm (for example, after a warm bath, when he or she wakes up in the morning, after running

420

ILLNESS IN
INFANTS,
CHILDREN,
AND
ADOLESCENTS

or playing hard). In some young people, you might see the hives in warm areas only (for example, on the abdomen and back, in the body creases, or under a diaper or other clothing). It is common to see hives in all different stages at once, so don't be alarmed if some are blotchy, some are small welts, and some are large and irregular (almost maplike).

"Hives" That Are Not Hives

While most youngsters with hives have only a mild (but bothersome) problem, others will experience more serious symptoms. *Anaphylaxis* (overwhelming allergic reaction) should be suspected if your child has lip, mouth, or tongue swelling; hoarseness; any trouble breathing; eye swelling; or general body swelling. *This is a medical emergency. Go to an emergency room immediately, or call the paramedics if there is breathing trouble.* (Review Chapter 13 for more information about anaphylaxis.)

Allergic reactions to some medications look like hives at first, but then the welts become discolored. The welts may at first look white, then become deep purple in color or even look like bruises. When these "hives" fade away, they leave (temporarily) a purple or brownish discoloration on the skin. These welts usually do not itch very much—unlike true hives. The youngster might also have sores in his mouth, burning upon urination, or bleeding (usually minor) in his intestines (which, of course, you can't see). He may have a fever and *look* more sick than he would with hives. This problem is called *erythema multiforme*. It can follow infections, such as strep throat and some viral infections.

Call your doctor, explain the symptoms, and arrange for an appointment. In the meantime, eliminate any nonprescription medications the youngster is taking, and check with the doctor about whether he or she wants you to eliminate prescribed medicines, as well, until the youngster can be evaluated. (Don't stop giving prescription medications, especially antibiotics or medications for seizure control or asthma, without contacting the doctor first.)

Henoch-Schönlein purpura is an unusual disease with a rash that looks at first like hives. The rash is most often concentrated on the legs and buttocks and looks as if there were bruises in the hives. The youngster often has painful joints—ankles, knees, elbows—and may have swelling of these painful joints. Your doctor should see the youngster, because kidney inflammation and sometimes bowel bleeding can complicate this disease.

THE DON'TS

Don't panic if your youngster shows signs of hives unless he also has mouth, face, or eye swelling or trouble breathing. If it's only hives, then cool him down in a tub of water and reevaluate the situation.

421

RECOGNIZING
AND
MANAGING
COMMON
SYMPTOMS
AND ILLNESSES

Don't hesitate to call your doctor if your child has hives and you are not able to keep her comfortable. Antihistamine medications can be very useful and might need to be given for several days or weeks if the hives come back.

Don't hesitate to call the doctor if what looked like hives now looks discolored or if there are other signs that worry you. You might be dealing with another problem, such as erythema multiforme or Henoch-Schönlein purpura.

Don't forget to call your doctor if you think the hives were caused by a prescribed medication. The doctor may want you to substitute another medication and will want to record this possible reaction in your child's record.

Don't give a youngster foods or medications that you thought caused hives again. If he or she is allergic, the same reaction is likely to occur and may be worse the second time around.

PLEASE NOTE: Now that you have a grasp of how to recognize and manage hives, it would be extremely helpful for you to go back to the Quick Reference With the Steps in Detail and review it carefully. The more familiar you are with that material, the more useful it will be to you when you need it.

422

ILLNESS IN
INFANTS,
CHILDREN,
AND
ADOLESCENTS

QUICK REFERENCE

With the Steps in Detail

Mouth Sores, Mouth Infections

▶ **MOST MINOR MOUTH SORES ARE CAUSED BY VIRUSES OR MOUTH IRRITATION AND CAN BE TREATED AT HOME:**

● If the sore is in the front part of the mouth, try applying a pain-relieving substance, such as Orajel or Glyoxide, to the sore (using a cotton swab) to relieve some of the pain. (Check the product label to make sure the youngster is not allergic to any of the ingredients.)

● An older child or teenager can swish the mouth with 3 percent hydrogen peroxide or a pain-relieving mouthwash, such as Chloraseptic, if there is more than one sore or a sore is located near the back of the mouth. (Again, check the product label to make sure the youngster is not allergic to any of the ingredients.)

● Have the youngster avoid salty or rough foods, as well as acidic or carbonated drinks. These have a tendency to cause pain.

● A young infant with mouth sores often does not want to suck from a bottle. Give nonirritating liquids by cup or with a teaspoon or plastic syringe.

▶ **YOU WILL NEED TO CONTACT YOUR DOCTOR IF:**

● Your young infant or toddler has many sores inside the mouth, has a fever, and will not drink liquids.

● There is redness, swelling, and pain around your youngster's teeth.

● Your young infant has more than very mild "thrush" (described below).

Mouth Sores and Infections: What You Should Know

423

RECOGNIZING
AND
MANAGING
COMMON
SYMPTOMS
AND ILLNESSES

The inside of the mouth is wet, warm, and filled with bacteria. You might think this would make mouth infections very common. However, it also contains enzymes (chemicals to keep the acidity correct), which help fight infections from "bad" bacteria and some viruses. The lining of the mouth (cells and tissues) is also replaced often, so most mouth sores heal themselves quickly, without drastic treatment. For this same reason, most simple mouth injuries—such as minor cuts of the lining or the tongue—heal so quickly and well that they don't need sutures (stitches) or special care.

Because of this ideal situation, many mouth sores are caused not by infection but rather by injury to the lining of the mouth or by allergy or because of a sensitivity to certain things that are eaten or chewed. Infections that do occur happen because the normal bacteria found in the mouth are reduced—for example, by antibiotic use—or because of an infection caused by certain viruses.

Canker Sores

A canker sore (technically called an *aphthous ulcer*) is a small sore that usually develops on the inside of the cheek or in the groove between the cheek lining and the gums. No one knows what causes a canker sore, but irritation seems to be the culprit in some youngsters (and adults)—for example, a scratch by harsh food or by a tiny particle of food that gets trapped in the groove between the teeth and the cheek—or sensitivity or allergy to certain foods. Many children (and adults) suffer from occasional canker sores, and they are usually nothing to worry about.

A canker sore starts as a red spot on the mouth lining. A tiny blister forms, then the blister breaks and leaves a gray ulcer (crater) with a small area of redness around it. You will often miss the blister stage because it breaks so quickly. The ulcer is most painful in the first day or two after it appears, then becomes less sore as it heals. Canker sores can last as long as a week.

Canker sores heal themselves, but the pain can be moderate to severe. Have your child avoid irritating foods—salty or spicy foods, acidic juices, and carbonated beverages—particularly while the pain is most intense. You can try to dab a small amount of anesthetic mouth medication on the sore before meals or have the youngster swish a small amount of hydrogen peroxide in the mouth several times a day. (Read the product label of any mouth preparations to make sure the youngster is not sensitive or allergic to any of the ingredients.)

Don't be confused if the sore that you see looks rough and has a little bleeding. Some youngsters bite or chew on the inside of their mouths—often as a habit or just because there is a sore there. These "chew marks" usually look slightly swollen and

424

ILLNESS IN
INFANTS,
CHILDREN,
AND
ADOLESCENTS

rough and are located on the cheek lining in the *area between the teeth*—where the youngster *can* chew. While these sores are painful and bothersome, they heal quickly if the youngster just stops chewing on the sore spot.

Herpes Simplex Infections

Herpes simplex virus causes two types of infections in and around the mouth. This very contagious virus invades the cells around the mouth and causes painful sores. Although the sores heal, the virus lies dormant in the area for an indefinite period of time, only to flare up again in the future. No one knows why some people are more prone to having this infection than others, nor why this virus has the capacity to lie dormant and recur over and over again.

A child's first infection with this virus is usually quite severe. Suspect *herpes gingivostomatitis* (infection of the mouth and gums with herpes simplex virus) if your toddler, preschooler, or older child has:

- Severe enough mouth pain that he or she refuses to eat or drink.

- Redness and swelling inside the mouth—with sores and ulcers scattered over the tongue, the gums, and the cheek linings.

- A fever (sometimes as high as 104 degrees) for three or four days.

- Sores in the mouth along with one or more sores on the lip margins.

- A blisterlike sore on a thumb or fingers of an infant or toddler who sucks the thumb or fingers, in addition to mouth sores.

The major problem with this mouth infection is that it is so painful that some infants and children refuse to eat or drink. This puts them at serious risk for dehydration. The fever they experience adds to the need for more, rather than less, liquids. Some even refuse to swallow their saliva, so you'll notice a great deal of drooling. Youngsters with this infection appear very ill. Sores, pain, and fever occur over the first few days, but the sores do not disappear for a week to ten days.

Your hardest job is to be sure the little one is getting enough liquid. If an infant refuses a bottle or the breast, try giving cold, nonacidic liquids from a spoon, dropper, or syringe. Keep track of how much you are able to get in, and call your doctor if the infant or toddler refuses to take at least sixteen to twenty-four ounces of liquid a day or shows signs of dehydration (little urine output, lethargy, or doughy skin). You won't be able to use the "dry mouth" sign of dehydration because of the oozing and drooling from his or her inflamed mouth.

Liquid acetaminophen (Tylenol, Datril, Tempra, and so on) will help with fever and pain control in youngsters with herpes gingivostomatitis. Most young infants and children cannot or will not cooperate if you try to spray or paint the mouth with a local pain reliever, so this is usually futile. Ice, popsicles, slushed drinks, and cold liquids are usually more successful. Interestingly, many youngsters with this infection refuse even very cold milk or ice cream!

425

RECOGNIZING
AND
MANAGING
COMMON
SYMPTOMS
AND ILLNESSES

Recurring herpes simplex virus infections usually appear as the typical *"cold sore"* or *"fever blister."* You can be pretty sure your child has this infection if he or she has:

- One or more blisters on the lip (with some swelling, itching, or burning pain).

- Yellow crusting of the blisters after a day or two.

- Similar blister(s) on the "sucking fingers" of a little one who sucks a thumb or finger.

- A cold, fever, exposure to the sun, or some other "stress" that might lead to a flare-up of this viral infection.

Herpes simplex lip infections occur at the *margin* of the lip (where it meets the skin). You might confuse the yellow crusting of a cold sore with impetigo unless you notice that the worst of the sore is on the lip margin rather than on the skin. Antibiotics, whether given by mouth or put on the sore, do not help the herpes sore to heal.

Try to keep the youngster from picking or rubbing the cold sore, and try to keep it moist with a lip cream or petroleum jelly. A pain-relieving ointment or cream, such as Blistex or Camphophenique, might be helpful. Try to avoid exposing others to this infection by using separate eating and drinking utensils, as well as towels, and by avoiding kissing and contact with the youngster's saliva. If *you* have an active cold sore, try to avoid passing the infection to others, including your children.

An additional note: Herpes infections of the lips and mouth are almost always caused by herpes simplex virus, type 1. This is very different from the herpes simplex virus, type 2, that causes genital herpes. Because there is a great deal of confusion about the two different herpes viruses, parents sometimes panic when a child gets cold sores, fever blisters, or mouth sores and hear that the youngster has "herpes."

Herpes simplex, type 1, is contagious and can be spread to other people and to other areas of the youngster's body (usually above the waist, however). Therefore, excellent handwashing and other commonsense precautions are always wise when caring for a child who has active gingivostomatitis or a cold sore.

Genital herpes—herpes simplex virus, type 2—is transmitted from one person to another through sexual contact nearly all of the time. (One exception is that a newborn infant can acquire a very deadly form of this infection during or shortly after birth if his mother has active genital herpes.) In children, however, sexual contact (usually sexual abuse) is most often the cause of genital herpes. If a youngster has suspicious blisters on the genitals, the doctor can take a culture to determine whether herpes simplex virus, type 2, is the cause.

426

ILLNESS IN
INFANTS,
CHILDREN,
AND
ADOLESCENTS

Gingivitis: A Gum Infection

Inflammation and infection of the gums around the teeth is a serious problem. It usually results from poor tooth care and needs to be evaluated and treated by your dentist. Suspect this problem, often called "trench mouth," if your older youngster has:

- Pain, swelling, and redness on the gums around the teeth.

- Pus formation around the tooth margins.

- Loose teeth that are painful if he or she chews.

- Tender, swollen lymph nodes under the chin.

- *No* sores or swelling on the tongue or the cheek lining.

Gingivitis is inflammation and often bacterial infection of the sockets of the teeth and the gums right around the teeth. It is usually caused by accumulation of food particles and debris around the base of the teeth and poor dental hygiene (inadequate tooth brushing and flossing and not rinsing the mouth after meals or snacks). It is the leading cause of early tooth loss and can occur *without* tooth decay.

If you suspect this potentially serious problem, take your youngster to a dentist for care and enforce good tooth brushing, flossing, and other measures the dentist will suggest. The youngster may need to be treated with an antibiotic for this problem if it is severe.

Thrush: Yeast Infection in the Mouth

Thrush is caused by a yeast called Candida albicans, a tiny organism that is usually present in the mouth and intestines. It causes inflammation in certain situations where the normal bacterial population is disrupted.

Thrush is most common in very young infants. Suspect it if your little one has:

- White patches that look like curdled milk stuck on the tongue or the insides of the cheeks.

- Mild pain or discomfort during nursing.

- A fiery red diaper rash with small bumps and blisters, along with white patches in the mouth.

Often, this infection appears in the weeks or few months following birth. It is sometimes contracted during delivery, because the yeast that causes it is frequently found in the vagina during pregnancy. Mothers with this infection might know they

427

RECOGNIZING
AND
MANAGING
COMMON
SYMPTOMS
AND ILLNESSES

have a yeast infection or may not have any symptoms at all. Sometimes, nursing mothers have soreness of the nipples when their infants have this infection because of a mild skin infection of the nipple with the same yeast. Contact your infant's doctor if you suspect this problem, since a prescribed medication is often needed to cure it.

Older infants, children, and even adults can get yeast infection, as well. It usually occurs after taking certain antibiotics that destroy some of the normal bacteria in the mouth and intestine. It can also occur after taking cortisonelike drugs, especially if they are taken by inhaler—for example, for asthma. Once in a while, yeast infections become bothersome or recurrent in children and adults who have diabetes.

In older youngsters with mild thrush of the mouth, eating plain yogurt will often control the infection. Yogurt contains some of the "normal" bacteria usually found in the mouth and intestines (therefore, it helps "rebalance" the tissue chemistry). However, it is still best to contact your doctor for advice if you suspect your youngster (whatever his or her age) has thrush.

Hand-Foot-Mouth Disease

Hand-foot-mouth disease is a mild viral infection that usually appears in the springtime and bothers toddlers and children who are in school settings. It tends to occur in sporadic outbreaks, because it is quite contagious. The infection goes away without treatment and should not cause you serious worry. Suspect this infection if your child complains of a sore mouth or throat and has:

- Two to ten small, ulcerlike sores in the back of the mouth—often on the soft palate (roof of the mouth)—and on the cheek lining near the tonsils.

- One or more blisterlike sores on the hands (often the palms), feet (check the soles), or buttocks.

- Little or no fever.

There is no treatment for this disease, which lasts about a week. Because it is contagious, use separate eating and drinking utensils and towels for the youngster. Have the youngster avoid irritating foods, and encourage him or her to drink plenty of liquids. You can try using pain-relieving mouthwash or spray if the youngster can cooperate.

Problems with the Tongue

Many parents worry unnecessarily about changes they see in their child's tongue—especially when the youngster is sick.

Most of the time, *"coated tongue"* means nothing more than lack of eating or

428

ILLNESS IN
INFANTS,
CHILDREN,
AND
ADOLESCENTS

drinking, because the little papillae (normal tongue bumps) are not irritated and worn off as they are after eating. Don't worry about it if the youngster is not bothered by it and does not seem uncomfortable. A heavy white coating may be a sign of thrush (yeast infection), especially if there are white patches inside the cheeks.

Discoloration of the tongue can have a variety of causes. You are very familiar with the colors caused by eating colored foods or drinks, or the yellow or brown coating seen in smokers. Certain medications can also cause tongue discoloration. Some antibiotics change the bacteria in the mouth and lead to yellowing or even blackening of the tongue. Other medications can cause blackening, too—for example, the bismuth in Pepto-Bismol can cause this and is nothing to worry about. The discoloration goes away when the offending medication is stopped. Brushing the tongue with a toothbrush will remove the colored coating without damaging the tongue.

Sore, red tongue can be a signal of irritation from "irritating" foods. It can also be the first sign of thrush infection of the mouth, especially in older youngsters who are taking antibiotics or who have certain vitamin deficiencies. Check with your doctor if the cause is not obvious to you. Very red tongue that is not especially sore is seen in scarlet fever (a strep infection with a rash), which is discussed later in this chapter.

Geographic tongue is a interesting phenomenon. In this common disorder (not a disease), the normal papillae (tongue bumps) disappear in patches, leaving pink spots of different shapes scattered among the white coating of the tongue. If you look at your youngster at different times, the patterns look different and may seem maplike. While this is seen in some allergic children, it has no real significance and causes no problems.

THE DON'TS

Don't worry if your youngster has occasional problems with mouth sores. Most mouth sores are caused by irritation or viral infection and don't require treatment.

Don't worry if your child won't eat solid foods if he has sores in the mouth. Encourage nonirritating liquids while his mouth is sore.

Don't hesitate to contact your doctor if your infant or toddler has mouth sores and refuses to drink liquids or shows any signs of dehydration.

Don't fail to take your youngster with a gum infection to a dentist for care. Gingivitis is a serious cause of early tooth loss but can be successfully treated.

PLEASE NOTE: Now that you have a grasp of how to recognize and manage mouth sores and mouth infections, it would be extremely helpful for you to go back to the Quick Reference With the Steps in Detail and review it carefully. The more familiar you are with that material, the more useful it will be to you when you need it.

429

RECOGNIZING
AND
MANAGING
COMMON
SYMPTOMS
AND ILLNESSES

QUICK REFERENCE

With the Steps in Detail

Nosebleeds

▶ **TREAT SIMPLE NOSEBLEEDS AT HOME TO STOP THE BLEED-ING:**

- Have your youngster sit down quietly.

- Press the nostrils together firmly for ten minutes without releasing the pressure during that time.

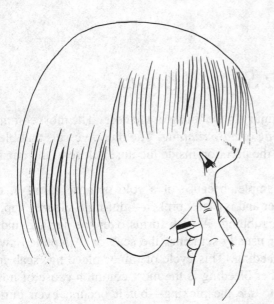

To stop a nosebleed: Press the nostrils together firmly and steadily.

- If the nose is still bleeding after this time, again apply steady pressure for ten minutes.

- When the bleeding stops, make sure the youngster does not blow (or pick) the nose for an hour or two, or the bleeding is likely to start again.

430

ILLNESS IN
INFANTS,
CHILDREN,
AND
ADOLESCENTS

▶ **CONTACT YOUR DOCTOR FOR ADVICE OR AN APPOINTMENT IF:**

- You are not able to control the bleeding (by applying pressure) after an hour.

- The bleeding is really heavy and you are unsuccessful in stopping it, or it starts again after numerous attempts at controlling it.

- The bleeding follows an injury to the nose, and the youngster's nose looks crooked.

- The bleeding follows a head injury *without* a direct injury to the nose.

- Your youngster seems to have frequent nosebleeds.

- Your youngster has other bleeding problems, as well.

- You see some bleeding, along with a smelly, purulent (pussy) drainage.

Nosebleeds: What You Should Know

Most nosebleeds are caused by minor injury to the lining of the nose. The most common cause, by far, in children is *nose picking* or *nose rubbing*. The blood vessels that bleed most often are located on the septum (the partition inside the nose) close to the outside and are very near the surface.

When the nose is irritated (for example, because of a cold or nose allergy), the lining over these blood vessels is tender and is easily broken—during a sneeze, wiping of the nose, or because of picking or rubbing. A scab forms over the surface and is irritating or itches; then the youngster usually scratches the scab or it is pulled away by sneezing, leading to more nose bleeding. This cycle of minor bleeding, scab formation, picking or sneezing, and further bleeding is the most common cause of nosebleeds in children. You don't need to *see* the picking—but it occurs, even during sleep.

Most nosebleeding in children is minor and involves very little blood loss—often just a few drops. The amount may look greater than it is—because there is usually some nasal mucus with the blood. Young children can swallow some blood during a nosebleed, especially if they lie down while you try to stop it. If they happen to vomit, you will see blood in what they vomit. If it is a small amount, this should not worry you, as long as you know there was a nosebleed.

431

RECOGNIZING
AND
MANAGING
COMMON
SYMPTOMS
AND ILLNESSES

More Serious Causes of Nosebleeds

Injury to the nose—from a fall, being hit—can cause a nosebleed. Here, your concern should be whether the nose is broken or not. If the nose looks crooked or swells a great deal, then contact your child's doctor. He or she will make sure the inner portions of the nose, as well as the outer bones, are in their normal position (or if they're out of alignment, the doctor will recommend evaluation by an ENT—ear, nose, and throat—specialist).

If your youngster has nose bleeding after a *head injury*, check to see whether there is any indication that his or her nose was also injured (swelling, crooked nose, a cut inside the nose, and so on). If not, contact your doctor. Nose bleeding can follow certain types of *skull fracture*, and the youngster needs medical attention.

Youngsters who have frequent nosebleeds *without* nose irritation or nose picking, or for no apparent cause, occasionally have more serious problems. *Hypertension* (high blood pressure) is not a common cause of nosebleeds in children and teenagers but can occur. *Severe* nosebleeding can be a signal of a *bleeding disorder* (for example, a disorder of the platelets—clotting particles—or even leukemia, a form of childhood cancer) in some children. Think of this possibility if your child bruises easily, has had problems with bleeding a lot with other injuries, or seems otherwise ill. Some bleeding disorders are hereditary and are detected early in infancy, while others can appear unexpectedly later in childhood or adolescence.

Keep in mind, too, that a *foreign object in the nose* can cause enough inflammation and swelling to lead to a nosebleed. Usually, you will see other characteristic signs of this problem: one-sided nose congestion; a persistent, one-sided nose drainage with pus and blood; and a very pungent, foul odor. Most often, you cannot get the object out and should not try. Call the doctor for an appointment.

THE DON'TS

Don't rely on cold packs on the nose (or neck) to stop simple nosebleeds. Apply direct pressure by squeezing the nostrils together for ten minutes.

Don't forget that the most common cause of frequent nosebleeds in children is irritation and nose picking. All children rub or pick their noses, whether you are aware of it or not.

Don't hesitate to contact your doctor if you think your child's nosebleed(s) may mean a more serious problem. A medical evaluation will help to determine if your youngster does have a more serious problem and requires treatment.

Don't attempt to remove a foreign object from your child's nose. You will often be unsuccessful and can cause further damage to the delicate nasal structures.

432

ILLNESS IN
INFANTS,
CHILDREN,
AND
ADOLESCENTS

PLEASE NOTE: Now that you have a grasp of how to recognize and manage nosebleeds, it would be extremely helpful for you to go back to the Quick Reference With the Steps in Detail and review it carefully. The more familiar you are with that material, the more useful it will be to you when you need it.

QUICK REFERENCE

With the Steps in Detail

Rashes and Skin Infections

▶ **THE MOST COMMON CAUSE OF SKIN RASH IN INFANTS AND CHILDREN IS IRRITATION AND INJURY TO THE SKIN.**

▶ **"MEASLES" IS AN UNUSUAL CAUSE OF SKIN RASH IN CHILDREN, ESPECIALLY THOSE WHO HAVE RECEIVED IMMUNIZATION AGAINST IT.**

▶ **MANY MINOR SKIN RASHES REQUIRE NO TREATMENT AT ALL AND GET WORSE IF YOU DO TOO MUCH:**

- Avoid overwashing irritated skin. Soap and water dry the skin and lead to more irritation.

- Keep baths cool and short, and pat the skin dry rather than rub it.

- Apply a mild moisturizing cream or lotion to dry, irritated skin.

- Avoid rough, harsh clothing on itchy, rashy skin. This leads to more itching and scratching.

- Avoid oils or ointments unless they are recommended by your child's doctor.

▶ **LEARN TO RECOGNIZE THE SKIN RASHES THAT CAN MEAN SERIOUS ILLNESS AND CONTACT YOUR CHILD'S DOCTOR IF YOU SUSPECT THEM:**

- A rash that looks as if there were bleeding in the skin, or bruising within a rash.

Fresh-Savert

1-800-508-1991

Valentines to
Grandma - Heart
Timmy
Eric
Mary

From Grandma to:
Timmy
Eric
Mary
Jenny
Rob
Bob
Arnold/Cindy

433

RECOGNIZING
AND
MANAGING
COMMON
SYMPTOMS
AND ILLNESSES

- Blisters on the skin in a young infant.

- Bright red, swollen skin, with or without peeling.

- Any rash that occurs along with other signs and symptoms of a serious illness—high fever, lethargy, breathing problems, shock, joint swelling, abdominal pain, convulsion.

▶ **CONTACT YOUR DOCTOR IF YOU THINK YOUR CHILD HAS A SKIN INFECTION OR AN INFECTION UNDER THE SKIN:**

- More than one infected insect bite or sore (for example, reddened, swollen skin around sores, pus in the skin, yellow crusting on sores).

- Warm, tender swelling on a body part or area, even if you see no pus.

Skin Rashes and Infections: What You Should Know

The skin is the largest organ of the body. Human skin is composed of four layers of cells and lies over the top of a layer called subcutaneous tissue (which protects the muscle tissue beneath it). Each of us loses many skin cells every day—they simply dry out and flake or rub off.

Skin injury—such as scrapes, rubbing, burning, or infection—normally causes this process to happen more rapidly than usual. You're very familiar with the peeling of a sunburn and the flakiness of some skin rashes.

The skin and the subcutaneous tissue underneath have a rich blood supply that helps in the repair process. When the skin is injured, blood flows to the injured area through dilated blood vessels, and the skin becomes quite red. Certain cells in the blood gather to seal off any open areas and to fight off infection. This results in a scab or crust beginning to form. The healing process goes on underneath this protective crust, which falls off when it is no longer needed. If there is long-standing irritation, the healing process continues, and the skin becomes thickened and rough. Sometimes, its color changes, as well.

Skin rashes can occur if just the very top layers of skin are damaged, or they can result from infections or conditions inside the body. Skin rashes may be found only in the top layers of skin, or they can affect thicker layers of the skin and subcutaneous tissue. What you see on the outside is determined by both the *cause* of the problem and the *depth* of the skin injury or infection.

The layers of skin contain tiny sweat glands, hair follicles, and sebaceous (oil-

434

ILLNESS IN
INFANTS,
CHILDREN,
AND
ADOLESCENTS

secreting) glands. These tiny but important structures can also be part of the problem with rashes and skin infections.

Body Rashes in Small Infants

The skin of a normal newborn baby is very soft and downy—and very sensitive. In general, the less you do to it or for it, the less likely it is that the baby will have skin rashes. However, there are certain "normal" rashes that occur.

Many full-term newborn infants, especially those who were even a little bit overdue, have skin *peeling* that is normal. The top layer of skin, which was protected from rubbing off before birth by the amniotic fluid, peels or flakes off for several weeks after birth. This is *not* dry skin. Sometimes, there will be a few areas of oozing or bleeding, especially in creases, during this process. You don't need to put lotions or oils on the baby's skin, since the skin underneath is perfectly healthy. Wash the baby no more often than every other day and only with a mild soap and warm water. Limit washing the baby between these times to a refreshing wipe with a washcloth and warm water.

A day or two after the baby is born, you might notice a blotchy rash scattered over his or her body, and some of the blotches might have a little welt in the middle. This rash will disappear after several hours, only for new spots to appear. This can continue for a few days to a few weeks. This rash is called *erythema toxicum*, or more descriptively, "flea-bite rash"—because it looks as if the baby has been bitten by fleas. Consider it a signal that your little one is healthy. Don't try to treat it with oils or lotions.

Beginning around the third or fourth week of life, your baby might have red bumps on his forehead and cheeks. If you look closely, the little one's skin appears more oily than before, and his hair might also seem to get oily more quickly than it once did.

This is *"baby acne"* and is a response to a temporary change in hormones after birth. Wash her face with water (use mild soap and a rough washcloth if severe) several times a day, and shampoo her hair every day. Don't put creams or oil on the rash, since this might make the problem worse. Baby acne will disappear by the time she's about two or three months old.

White spots on the bridge of the nose and scattered over the cheeks and forehead are also normal. These little spots are called *milia* and are clogged sebaceous glands. They disappear gradually after a few weeks or months without treatment.

Diaper Rash: A Common Problem

The warm wetness of the genital area in a baby or toddler who wears diapers is a perfect environment for breeding diaper rash. Minor skin irritation caused by urine or

435

RECOGNIZING
AND
MANAGING
COMMON
SYMPTOMS
AND ILLNESSES

stool is made worse by the constant wetness and action of the skin and stool bacteria on the skin. The result? A diaper rash.

Some babies seem to always have diaper rash, while others seem curiously free of the problem, especially early in infancy. Blond, light-complected babies are more likely to have problems than darker-skinned infants. Most babies, however, have a diaper rash at some time before they are toilet-trained.

Most *ordinary diaper rash* looks red and dry. It may start right around the anus or seem to appear "overnight" and affect the whole area that was covered. It may seem most pronounced right under the plastic edges of disposable diapers or the elastic of plastic pants and is less obvious in creases than on the flat surfaces of the skin.

Diaper rash is sometimes easier to prevent than to clear up. Avoid using soap as much as possible (use water, and only as necessary), because it can cause diaper rash by drying out normal skin. Avoid using commercial diaper wipes as much as possible, because they contain scents and sometimes alcohol, which can dry and irritate sensitive skin. Besides, alcohol *burns* if you put it on irritated skin, as you well know. These products are fine when you are away from home, but stay with plain water when you can.

If your baby develops diaper rash, try to think about what might have caused it. Consider new foods in his or her diet, irritation by the plastic edges of disposable diapers or the elastic of plastic pants, the new detergent you used to wash cloth diapers, or the scent in the new brand of disposable diapers you bought. Some infants have mild diarrhea and diaper rash each time they cut a tooth. Others react to certain soaps or creams you might put on their skin. Sometimes, there is just no good explanation!

The treatment for mild diaper rash is simple:

- Change the baby's diaper more often than usual.

- Wash the baby's bottom with water (avoid soap as much as possible) and pat it dry, then apply petroleum jelly or a soothing cream, lotion, or ointment in a thin layer when you change the diaper.

- Avoid plastic pants as much as possible.

- Change brands of disposable diapers if you think this might be the problem. Look for diapers that are unscented.

- If you wash your own cloth diapers, use a low-suds detergent and use less of it, then rinse the diapers well (you can put diapers through two rinse cycles) and avoid fabric softeners.

- Expose the baby's bottom to air for fifteen or twenty minutes several times a day, but don't forget to protect your furniture!

- Check with your doctor before you use cortisone-containing or medicated creams or ointments. Overuse of these products can damage the skin over a period of time.

436

ILLNESS IN
INFANTS,
CHILDREN,
AND
ADOLESCENTS

Older babies and toddlers are susceptible to diaper rash caused by *ammonia*. Ammonia is essentially made in the diaper by bacteria from the skin and bowel that act on the urine. When ammonia stays on the skin, it causes a burnlike rash. Sometimes, an ammonia burn can even cause blisters and open sores. Suspect this problem if an *older* infant or toddler wakes up after a long night with a very red, sore bottom and smells "strong" like ammonia. Chronic ammonia rash looks dry, red, and scaly, and the little one is likely to cry when he urinates, because it hurts when the urine hits the skin.

You can usually prevent ammonia diaper rash in an older infant by applying a layer of petroleum jelly to her clean, dry bottom before the last diaper change at night. Ammonia diaper rash, once it has appeared, is treated the same way as ordinary diaper rash. If it is particularly severe and you are not successful in controlling the problem, contact your doctor for additional suggestions.

Monilial diaper rash is caused by the yeast Candida albicans (also called monilia). It is often seen along with thrush infection in the mouth but can be present without visible thrush patches. It is most common in very young infants and in infants and toddlers who have taken certain antibiotics, especially ampicillin and its relatives.

The first patches of a monilial diaper rash look red and bumpy. Tiny blisters (pinhead-sized and smaller) form, then break, leaving raw skin underneath. The rash spreads outward (often starting in the creases and spreading from there), with a few "satellite" blisters at the edges. The rash looks wet and sore.

Diaper rash caused by yeast almost always needs to be treated with a prescription cream or ointment in order to kill the yeast. Before you call the doctor, look into your child's mouth to see if you can find spots that look like curdled milk on his or her tongue or cheeks. This will help the doctor know whether the little one will need oral medication (taken by mouth), as well as cream or ointment for the rash. Feeding an older infant small amounts of plain yogurt is frequently helpful in replacing some of the normal bacteria that prevent yeast infection, but medication is often necessary, as well.

Heat Rash

Infants and young children are more susceptible to heat rash because they are often too warmly dressed and are sensitive to heat. Remember, these nonverbal infants and toddlers don't have any way of telling their parents they are too warm!

You can recognize heat rash easily. Red, raised bumps appear in the warm places of the body—around the neck, in the armpits, and in the groin. A heat rash is itchy and irritating, and if the little one can scratch, he or she will. Sometimes, there will be tiny blisters on some of the bumps, and some infants will have raw, wet areas in the "hot spots," as well.

437

RECOGNIZING
AND
MANAGING
COMMON
SYMPTOMS
AND ILLNESSES

Older youngsters, especially those who perspire a lot, can also be plagued with this kind of rash. You might see it in the armpits, around the neck, in the groin, at the waist, and under the breasts of well-developed girls. In these older youngsters, the combination of warmth, sweat, and rubbing leads to red bumps and raw, wet areas of rash.

The treatment of heat rash is simple:

- Use cool water to rinse the rashy areas, and pat the area dry. Do not rub.

- Use a talcum powder or medicated powder to keep the area dry.

- Dress the youngster in lighter, more absorbent clothing! Avoid scratchy fabrics like wool and synthetic clothing that does not absorb moisture well (cotton is best).

- Avoid tight-fitting clothing or anything that rubs on the area.

If you are not successful in treating or controlling heat rash, contact your doctor. Older youngsters sometimes get a fungal infection on top of the heat rash.

Scaly Rashes

Eczema (atopic dermatitis) is the most common scaly rash found in infants and children and is usually a chronic, bothersome problem. In some children, it is caused by allergy—usually to foods. In others, it seems to be a problem of dry skin and constant itching and scratching.

In infants, eczema usually starts on the cheeks as a red, chafed rash. The little one tries to scratch by rubbing his or her face on sheets and blankets and is often very irritable. The rash may spread to the back, neck, arms, and legs. Severe eczema looks dry and raw and may have some oozing of clear or yellow fluid from the open areas. Being too warm, wearing scratchy clothing, and perspiring tend to make the rash worse.

Older youngsters with eczema usually have the worst of the rash in the folds of the body—the insides of the elbows, backs of the knees, the neck, and ankles. They may have other scattered areas of eczema, as well. With this problem, older youngsters usually have dry, scaly, and thickened skin and may have open areas from scratching. The inflamed skin itches a great deal, and it may be almost impossible to keep the youngster from scratching.

You will need your doctor's help in treating and controlling all but the most mild eczema. Your main goals are to control itching and scratching, eliminate any known foods or fabrics that seem to make it worse, keep the skin moist, and reduce skin inflammation and damage. Your doctor might recommend:

438

ILLNESS IN
INFANTS,
CHILDREN,
AND
ADOLESCENTS

- Few or no baths and no soap.

- Moisturizing cream or lotion for the skin.

- Light, soft cotton clothing.

- Elimination of certain foods if they seem to make the skin worse.

- Use of steroid (cortisonelike) cream or ointment in the worst places (for a short period of time).

- Medication to control itching, especially at night.

Some youngsters have scattered patches of dry, scaly skin that come and go. This is often mild eczema and is worse in winter or dry seasons. Try having your child take fewer baths and apply a lubricating skin lotion or cream right after baths. Have him or her wear loose, soft clothing to reduce the amount of itching. If the problem is more than very mild, your doctor might suggest that you use a cortisonelike cream or ointment occasionally when the spots are at their worst.

Seborrheic dermatitis is easy to confuse with eczema, especially in young infants. This rash is caused by oily rather than dry skin and appears on different parts of the body—the scalp, the eyebrows, around and under the ears, in the armpits, and in the genital area. You can easily remember these locations if you think of this as a problem of hair-bearing skin.

The rash of seborrheic dermatitis is red and oily looking, with yellowish, greasy scales. Scaling of the scalp—called "cradle cap" in infants and "dandruff" in older youngsters (and adults)—is usually present, as well. It is less itchy than eczema and is more likely to be "picked at" than scratched.

Most of the time, you can recognize and control seborrhea without your doctor's help. The most important part of controlling this condition is keeping the scalp free of oil and scales and keeping the skin as free of oil as possible:

- If the scales on the scalp are really thick, apply oil to the scalp for thirty to sixty minutes before shampooing.

- Shampoo the hair often, daily at first, and try to remove the scales by brushing them gently with a soft toothbrush or hairbrush. In infants, you don't usually have to use an antidandruff shampoo, but older youngsters might need this.

- Shampoo often enough to keep the hair and scalp from looking oily and to prevent reaccumulation of the scaling.

- Bathe the youngster, using a mild soap, as often as necessary to keep her from being "oily." Don't use soap on her face, even if she has seborrheic rash there, unless your doctor recommends it. Try not to rub the skin very much.

- Avoid using creams, lotions, and oils on the skin and on the hair or scalp. This often promotes more oil production and traps the oil on the skin.

439

RECOGNIZING
AND
MANAGING
COMMON
SYMPTOMS
AND ILLNESSES

If you have a problem with controlling seborrhea or your youngster's rash seems unusually extensive, contact your doctor for his or her recommendations.

Psoriasis is a chronic skin condition that can start during childhood or adolescence. This problem tends to run in families and can be very mild to quite severe. The most severe cases require the help of a dermatologist (a medical doctor with special training in the diagnosis and treatment of conditions of the skin).

Patches of psoriasis can be large or small and have varying shapes. They usually have a rather thick white or silver scale on top of a very red, shiny patch of skin. While they can appear on any part of the body, they often are most obvious on the elbows or knees. Suspect psoriasis if your youngster has a problem with "dandruff," but the scalp underneath the scales is very red and shiny. You will need your doctor's help to treat psoriasis.

Fungus Infections of the Skin

Most parents think of "ringworm" when they see a round sore on their youngster's skin, but many times, what they are seeing is not ringworm at all.

True *"ringworm"* is a fungus infection of the skin. It starts as a tiny red patch that grows in size over days to weeks. As it grows, the center becomes pale and scaly, while the growing border stays red and slightly raised. It is mildly contagious and can be caught from animals as well as people. Ringworm is easily treated with antifungal creams if it is recognized early, although the treatment takes weeks or months. Check with your doctor if you think your child might have this kind of fungus infection.

People often confuse a very common skin condition called *pityriasis alba* with ringworm. Children with this condition have a few pale patches with very fine, almost powdery scales on their skin. This condition is most common in darker-skinned children, especially those who are mildly allergic. Although this skin problem doesn't need any treatment, if your youngster has more than a few of these pale patches, ask your doctor about them, so you can be sure they are not a skin fungus called *tinea versicolor*.

Fungus infections of the *scalp* are quite common in school-aged children. These are contagious and can be transmitted from other children or animals. They are usually not found in very young children and adolescents. It is important that this kind of fungus infection, called *tinea capitis* (scalp ringworm), be diagnosed correctly and treated appropriately. A youngster with this infection has an enlarging bald spot, in which the hair is broken off rather than just missing. Make an appointment with the doctor if you think your youngster might have scalp ringworm. It is treated with oral medicine that kills the fungus. Other causes of bald spots in children include hair pulling and a condition called alopecia areata, in which the hair falls out in patches for no apparent reason.

"Athlete's foot" is a contagious fungus infection that causes blistering, peeling, and

440

ILLNESS IN
INFANTS,
CHILDREN,
AND
ADOLESCENTS

painful cracking *between* the toes. This infection usually starts in late childhood or adolescence and is difficult to completely cure. It tends to remain an off-and-on problem through adulthood for those youngsters who get it during childhood. Athlete's foot can be spread in locker rooms and by wearing the shoes of someone who has it. You can treat the problem at home by:

- Having the youngster wash his feet carefully and pat the sore areas dry. (Use separate towels to prevent spreading the fungus infection to others in the family.)

- Have her apply antifungal cream or powder between the toes twice a day for two or three weeks. You can ask your pharmacist what product to use.

- Be sure the child or youngster wears cotton socks, preferably white, rather than nylon or synthetic socks, and changes shoes often, in order to keep his feet as dry as possible.

People often confuse *contact dermatitis* of the feet with athlete's foot. A youngster who has contact dermatitis—because of sensitivity to parts (materials) of the shoes—has a red, peeling rash on the tops, sides, or bottoms of the feet rather than between the toes. If you look closely at the youngster's feet, you can compare the shape of the rash to the shoe lining. Here, the treatment is first to eliminate contact with the offending shoe and then to treat the rash by keeping it dry and applying a soothing lotion or cream. Sometimes, a mild hydrocortisone cream applied for a few days will hurry the healing process.

Impetigo

Impetigo is a skin infection caused by bacteria. The most common type of impetigo is caused by streptococci bacteria (the group of bacteria that cause so-called strep throat). At times, the youngster gets a "mixed" infection—streptococci combined with staphylococci bacteria (the bacteria that cause boils).

Most often, impetigo appears after the skin is irritated or inflamed for another reason—for example, the upper lip or face is a bit raw because of a cold, or an insect bite or other sore becomes infected because of scratching. The sore then becomes red and crusted with honey-colored material. If the crust is removed, the sore oozes and crusts over again. It spreads quite rapidly to infect other areas nearby and can even infect areas far from where it started. Impetigo is also contagious to other youngsters, so care should be taken not to expose them. Do not allow them to share towels, dinnerware, or cups or to touch the sores.

Your best weapon against impetigo is *soap and water*. Wash the infected skin well, dry it, and keep it covered if the youngster is prone to scratching or picking at it. You

441

RECOGNIZING
AND
MANAGING
COMMON
SYMPTOMS
AND ILLNESSES

might apply an antibiotic ointment, although this may not be as helpful as you might think. Skin antiseptics are *not* as effective as plain soap and water.

If there is more than one small spot of impetigo, your youngster will need to take an antibiotic by mouth for ten days. This will eliminate the bacteria that cause it and sometimes prevents complications of strep infection. Since the strep bacteria that cause impetigo sometimes cause inflammation of the kidneys, and less often rheumatic fever, it's important to contact your doctor if your child has more than one spot of impetigo.

Bullous impetigo is a form of skin infection that results in pus-containing blisters. This kind of infection is caused by staph bacteria and most often affects newborn infants. In them, the blisters, which vary from one-sixteenth to one-half inch in size, often start in the diaper area or near the umbilical cord. The blisters form quickly, then break, leaving a red, raw base with peely edges. If you think your tiny infant might have bullous impetigo, contact your doctor immediately, since the baby is at some risk for developing overwhelming infection (scpsis). Older children who get bullous impetigo usually have the blisters start on their buttocks, but they can start in other areas of the body, as well. In addition to thorough washing, this form of impetigo always requires treatment with oral antibiotics.

Cellulitis: Infection of the Subcutaneous Tissues

Cellulitis is inflammation and infection of the tissues under the skin. It is caused by bacterial infection and often spreads quickly. It may start under an obvious sore or appear without any warning "out of the blue." Untreated cellulitis can result in serious, overwhelming infection (sepsis), especially in young infants and children and in youngsters with poor immunity. If you suspect it, contact your doctor promptly or take your youngster to an emergency room if you don't have a doctor or can't reach your doctor.

Suspect cellulitis if your youngster has a warm, deep red, painful swelling under the skin. The swelling usually increases rapidly, and you might see red streaks leading away from the swollen area. The child might also have a fever and seem sick—listless, cranky, and without an appetite.

Certain types of cellulitis are especially dangerous because of the complications that can arise. *Periorbital cellulitis* refers to inflammation and infection in the tissues around the eye. The youngster's eyelid and even cheek are deep red or even purple, massively swollen, and tender. This infection can easily lead to sepsis (overwhelming infection) and possibly meningitis.

Facial or buccal (cheek) cellulitis, usually a problem in infants and toddlers, is equally serious. With this problem, the little one develops a red "spot" on the cheek. Within hours, the cheek is deep red or purple, hot, hard, and tender. He or she usually has a fever and appears quite ill. This, too, is often associated with sepsis and needs prompt antibiotic treatment (usually intravenously) in a hospital. So-called popsicle

442

ILLNESS IN
INFANTS,
CHILDREN,
AND
ADOLESCENTS

panniculitis also causes a red, hard swelling, usually of the cheek. This inflammation of the fatty tissues is caused by sucking on ice or popsicles long enough that the cold actually injures the tissue. Usually seen in infants and young children, it looks very much like facial cellulitis. If you suspect this problem, contact the doctor.

Cellulitis of the *hand* or *foot* is a serious problem but for a different reason. Cellulitis in these areas can lead to serious damage to the tendons and nerves because of pressure from massive swelling and inflammation. Youngsters with deep infections of the hand or foot might need surgery to relieve the pressure—in addition to antibiotic treatment.

Abscesses in the Skin

An infection with a collection of pus is called an abscess. A small abscess under the skin is commonly called a *boil*. A boil starts as a small, hard, painful bump under the skin. As it develops, the area around it becomes very red, swollen, and tender. As pus forms, the center becomes whitish or yellowish and softer than the surrounding bump. As it heals, it may just "melt away" or rupture and drain the pus.

Boils are caused by infection with staphylococcus bacteria. Most often, a youngster has only one boil, but occasionally, he or she is bothered by several boils at a time, frequent boils, or a collection of boils clustered together (called a *carbuncle*). You can treat a single boil at home:

- Apply warm, wet compresses to the boil for fifteen to thirty minutes three or four times a day.

- If the boil "pops" on its own, *pull* the edges apart gently to allow the pus to drain out.

- Do not squeeze a boil or open it yourself with a needle. You can cause a more serious infection this way.

Make an appointment with your doctor if your youngster seems unusually sick or uncomfortable with a boil, has a boil in the area around the rectum, has more than one at a time, or seems to get boils frequently. He or she may need antibiotics, or the doctor may want to open (incise) the boils.

Contact Dermatitis

Contact dermatitis is inflammation of the skin caused by allergy or sensitivity to something that touched the skin. The rash is red and itchy or painful and may have blisters form on it after hours or days. The rash and skin irritation will continue or

443

RECOGNIZING
AND
MANAGING
COMMON
SYMPTOMS
AND ILLNESSES

worsen as long as the offending material stays in contact with the skin and will reappear later if the child comes into contact with the substance again.

Often, the location or shape of the rash will give you a clue about what is causing it. Common causes of contact dermatitis are: poisonous plants (poison ivy, poison oak, poison sumac); metals, especially nickel (inexpensive ''gold'' jewelry—earrings, rings, chains); perfumes; dyes (shoe-leather dyes, toilet tissue); soaps; cosmetics; adhesive tape; and laundry products (detergents, rinses).

Obviously, the most important thing you can do to treat contact dermatitis is to *identify its cause* and *eliminate contact* of it with your child. Wash the rash with water and try to prevent the youngster from rubbing or scratching it. Sometimes, a mild astringent, such as witch hazel or Burow's solution (see your pharmacist), will help with the itching and oozing. If the rash is in a very small area (but not on the face), try using a mild hydrocortisone cream. However, if the rash is widespread or is not improving after a few days, be sure to call your doctor.

Scabies: Skin Mites

Scabies is a very common skin infection caused by a tiny mite (insect) called Sarcoptes scabei. It is very contagious and can be transmitted through contact with a person or animal who has the infection (this is the disease called ''mange'' in dogs). Scabies is common in school-aged children, who then bring it home to the rest of the family.

Days or weeks after contact with an infected person, the typical skin bumps of scabies appear. Most often, the problem starts with intensely itchy tiny bumps between the fingers. Soon rows of bumps appear on the arms, then the trunk (especially around the beltline) and legs. If you look closely at scabies bumps, you might see a tiny dark spot in the center, but you cannot see the mite without a microscope. Soon the youngster is scratching incessantly, and some of the bumps begin to bleed or ooze. By this time, other members of the family might also be itching! Young infants with scabies usually have most of their bumps on their abdomen, buttocks, and genitals, because that is where they are touched by others (in diaper changing and picking the baby up).

If you suspect scabies, have your doctor see your youngster. If you are correct, he or she will recommend treatment for both *your child and the rest of the family*. Treatment of scabies involves applying one of several prescription medications on the skin. Since these drugs are potent pesticides, be sure to follow the doctor's directions carefully, do not overuse the medication, and keep it locked up after every use (if you have small children in the home or visiting frequently). The medication(s) will kill any active mites, but the rash may continue for several weeks (because some of the dead mites are trapped under the skin). If your youngster is itching a lot, the doctor might also recommend a soothing lotion and an oral medication to help ease the itching, especially at night.

444

ILLNESS IN
INFANTS,
CHILDREN,
AND
ADOLESCENTS

Acne

As you probably know, acne can be an unpleasant, chronic skin condition that usually starts during adolescence. It is a disorder of the sebaceous (oil) glands of the skin and is most often related to changes in the body hormones, especially to an overbalance of the male hormones (androgens). Acne is actually more common in boys than in girls. The problem can be very mild or very severe.

Most often, a teenager will have acne on the forehead and over the nose (and its folds), but it can also appear on the back and chest. The first sign of acne is oily skin. The overactive sebaceous glands produce excessive amounts of sebum (oil), a whitish material that clogs the glands. These "whiteheads" become "blackheads" when the sebum is exposed to the air. (Blackheads do not mean the youngster is dirty.) "Pimples" are a result of the sebum's leaking into the skin, causing inflammation; then the bacteria on the skin cause tiny areas of infection (pimples here or there). However, the more infection there is, the worse the acne becomes. Chronic skin inflammation and infection can lead to permanent scarring.

In contrast to what you might think, acne is influenced very little by what your youngster eats. Greasy foods, chocolate, and cola drinks do not really make the problem worse for most youngsters. There is no reason to limit your teenager's diet because of acne, unless he or she and you can pinpoint certain foods that do seem to make a difference.

Your teenager can treat mild acne without medical help:

- Encourage him to wash his face (and back or chest if they are involved) twice a day with a soft washcloth, warm water, and a mildly abrasive soap. (Do not encourage vigorous scrubbing, since this can cause skin inflammation and worsen the problem.)

- Mild skin-peeling agents, such as benzoyl peroxide lotion or gel, can be rubbed or dabbed on once or twice a day. If the skin becomes red, dry, or sore, reduce the number of times she uses it.

- Discourage the use of hair oils or pomades and makeup.

- Emphasize the importance of not picking or squeezing pimples or blackheads.

Get help from your youngster's doctor or a dermatologist if the teenager has many pimples or pustules or if the amount of acne is severe. The doctor may suggest treatments such as antibiotic lotions, oral antibiotics, stronger peeling agents, and the use of retinoic acid. Sometimes, abscesses and large cysts will need to be carefully opened, as well. Medical knowledge about acne is improving each year, and in most youngsters, this condition can be controlled quite well. Everyone's goal is to reduce the discomfort and embarrassment of acne during the teenage years, as well as prevent permanent scarring.

445

RECOGNIZING
AND
MANAGING
COMMON
SYMPTOMS
AND ILLNESSES

It's particularly important for you to be sensitive about this problem. Teenagers are experiencing so many physical changes and times of confusion that, for some, having even a few pimples is a catastrophe, and serious acne is enough to make them embarrassed even to be seen. It is essential to seek professional care if even the smallest amount of acne causes your youngster to become overly self-conscious about it. Being sympathetic and supportive also helps. We often forget what a difficult experience acne was for us or our friends when we were teenagers. To hear "Don't be ridiculous. It will go away someday" can be devastating. "Someday" isn't very comforting when you feel the whole world is staring at your face. Saying you know that it's not a pleasant experience, explaining the reason acne occurs (physical changes/hormonal changes at that time in his or her life), and indicating that you are certainly willing to see if a doctor can help at least let the teenager know you do understand, are sympathetic, and are willing to help if you can.

Pityriasis Rosea: An Unusual Disease

Pityriasis rosea is a strange skin disease that usually affects older children and teenagers. No one knows the cause, but it behaves a little like a viral infection (because it tends to occur in outbreaks). It is a mild disease with no known complications.

The rash of pityriasis is faint pink or salmon colored and appears on the trunk—the back and chest—and sometimes on the upper arms. The rash is slightly raised and dry and may itch. The individual bumps of the rash tend to be oval and fall into the skin lines (so if you look at the youngster from a distance, his or her back has a rash in "lines" that look like the branches of an evergreen tree).

If you think back, you might remember that a week or two ago, your child had a dry, scaly sore somewhere on the body (there may still be some of it left) that appeared but caused little concern. You may have thought it looked a little like impetigo or ringworm, but it didn't worry you because it began to improve. This was the first sign of pityriasis rosea.

There is no treatment for pityriasis rosea, which lasts as long as six weeks. If itching is a serious problem, your doctor can prescribe an antihistamine for the youngster to use, especially at night. As with most itchy skin rashes, keeping the youngster cool will cut down on the itching.

Chickenpox

Chickenpox (varicella) is the most contagious of the childhood rashes. Caused by a virus, it is one of the few "childhood diseases" for which there is not yet an effective vaccine, although vaccines are being developed and tested.

446

ILLNESS IN
INFANTS,
CHILDREN,
AND
ADOLESCENTS

Chickenpox is first contagious (spread) during the twenty-four to forty-eight hours *before* there are any signs of skin rash. The virus is spread by nose and mouth secretions, as well as by contact with the skin rash and secretions *until* all the little blisters are crusted over. A youngster can develop chickenpox from one to three weeks after initial contact, and the disease tends to work its way systematically through school classrooms, day-care centers, and families until all of the youngsters who have not had it get it. This virus is most commonly seen in late winter and spring.

The rash of chickenpox develops very rapidly after it first appears. Initially, you might notice a few tiny red bumps on your child's skin (often, parents think they might be insect bites). Within a few hours, these tiny bumps form a little blister (one-sixteenth to one-eighth inch in size) on top. After another few hours, the blisters look "dented." Crusts begin to form on the bumps, usually within a day. Don't think anything is wrong if each time you look at your child you see new bumps. This, in fact, goes on for three to seven days—with new crops of pox appearing one or more times a day.

Most youngsters with chickenpox seem only mildly ill and run little if any fever. The *do* itch a lot, however, and may complain bitterly about how miserable they feel. Most children manage to play and stay active in spite of the itching and scratching. There's no reason to keep children more quiet or less active than usual, and it's fine to allow them to play outdoors (but out of direct sun), as long as you keep them away from other children who have not had chickenpox already. Children are no longer contagious after the last of the pox are *firmly crusted over*. Once this has occurred, children can return to school. (You will probably welcome their departure, since they do not feel very sick with this disease, even though they may be irritable because of the itching!)

While there is nothing you can do to cure your youngster or shorten the time he has the chickenpox, you can try to make him more comfortable:

- Keep him lightly dressed. Being too warm always makes the itching worse.

- Give her frequent, cool baths. You don't need to add anything to the water, but a little baking soda won't hurt.

- Give the youngster the appropriate dose of acetaminophen (aspirin substitute) as he needs it for fever and discomfort. Do *not* use aspirin.

- Soothing lotions, such as calamine, may help, although a cold, wet washcloth applied to especially itchy pox can be just as effective and less messy.

- Call your doctor if the itching is very intense. He or she may recommend or prescribe a medication (usually an antihistamine) to help control the itching.

Fortunately, complications of chickenpox are very unusual in healthy children. Varicella pneumonia usually affects adults and children who have suppressed immunity (for example, because of cancer treatment or hereditary immune deficiency).

Two complications of chickenpox, although rare, can occur during the recovery

447

RECOGNIZING
AND
MANAGING
COMMON
SYMPTOMS
AND ILLNESSES

phase of the disease—varicella encephalitis (brain inflammation) and Reye syndrome. (Further information on Reye syndrome can be found in Chapter 13.) Contact your doctor *immediately* or go to an emergency room if your youngster recovering from chickenpox experiences:

- Unusual sleepiness or lethargy.

- Confusion, restlessness, irrational behavior, or delirium.

- Persistent vomiting.

You will probably not be able to prevent chickenpox in your other youngsters if one brings home the disease, but you might be able to prevent them from getting a severe case if you keep them as far away from the sick youngster as possible. If you have a youngster who has poor immunity and he or she has been exposed to chickenpox or develops signs of chickenpox, contact your doctor immediately for advice.

Is It Measles, Doctor?

Chances are, the first thing you (and most parents) think about when you see a red or pink, blotchy or bumpy rash on your youngster is measles. The fact is, very few rashes children get *are* measles, especially when so many youngsters are immunized against this serious childhood disease. Rashes do present a problem, in that it can be difficult to figure out just what a rash is or what it might mean.

Many viral diseases cause a "measly" rash—one that is at first flat and red or pink, then becomes bumpy or rough after a day or two. The "spots" may stay discrete and dotlike or run together to make a large area of rash. Most viral rashes start on the neck or chest and spread to cover the back and abdomen, then the face, arms, and legs. Many of the diseases that cause them also cause some fever, as well as some swelling of the lymph nodes. Most of these viral diseases occur in the spring and summer months and are caused by a group of viruses called enteroviruses.

How can you tell the difference between true measles and a "measly" rash caused by another viral disease? True *measles* (called rubeola) is a relatively uncommon disease—and could be *completely prevented if all children received measles immunization*. (Outbreaks of true measles have occurred in teenagers and young adults who received measles vaccine before one year of age, especially if the vaccine was given with gamma globulin, as was the practice when the vaccine was first developed. These youngsters need repeat vaccination.)

If you know the symptoms of this very serious disease, listed below, you will not confuse it with other causes of rash in children:

- A coldlike illness, with a runny nose, red eyes, and a cough for two to three days.

448

ILLNESS IN
INFANTS,
CHILDREN,
AND
ADOLESCENTS

- High fever that lasts for two to three days before the rash appears and a week or so afterward.

- A deep, "brassy" cough during most of the illness.

- The typical measles rash: red, flat blotches that start around the neck and behind the ears, then rapidly spread over a few days to cover the entire body. After a few days, the rash feels a little rough to the touch, and there may be mild skin peeling toward the end of the disease.

- If you look carefully, you might see Koplik's spots on the day before and the first day of the rash: tiny white dots that look like little grains of sand attached to the mouth lining, usually near the back teeth, and in the conjunctivae (mucous linings) of the eyes.

In a word, children with measles look *sick*. They are susceptible to complications, such as pneumonia, ear infection, encephalitis, and even appendicitis. A few actually die from the disease.

About one-third of youngsters who receive *measles immunization* develop a mild measleslike illness five to fourteen days after they are immunized. The symptoms are mild, but the rash may look like the real disease. This happens because the vaccine is a live-virus vaccine that essentially gives the little one a mild case of measles, protecting him or her from the full-blown disease. Many parents forget about this possibility, even if they have been warned that it can occur, because it happens so long after the shot was given. No treatment is needed, the youngster is not contagious, and you don't have to report this reaction to your doctor unless it seems unusually severe.

Rubella (German measles) is a much more mild disease and can be confused with the many other causes of "measly" rashes. In fact, even doctors can be sure only by doing special blood tests—unless, of course, there is an epidemic of rubella. Suspect rubella in an *unimmunized* youngster who has:

- Mild cold symptoms and a mild fever for one to three days.

- A pink, dotlike rash starting on the neck, chest, and back and spreading to the rest of the body over another day or two. The rash tends to run together and feels rough after the first day.

- Slightly enlarged, tender lymph nodes in the back of the neck, just under the base of the skull.

One of the complications of rubella infection is joint pain and swelling. If the youngster is experiencing a mild illness and also has joint pain and/or swelling, it helps raise the suspicion that the problem is rubella. This complication, however, is more common in older teenagers and adults who get the disease.

The major problem with rubella infection is the risk of infecting women who are

449

RECOGNIZING
AND
MANAGING
COMMON
SYMPTOMS
AND ILLNESSES

pregnant and thereby their unborn babies. Although a mild disease for the pregnant woman, rubella can cause devastating birth defects in the unborn baby (particularly if the unborn baby is infected with the disease during the first three months of the pregnancy). If a child with a "measly" rash comes into contact with a woman who is pregnant, it is vital to determine: (1) whether the pregnant woman is immune to rubella (has already had rubella or has been immunized against it) and, if she is *not* immune, (2) whether the child with the rash has rubella or some other viral illness that mimics it. Therefore, if you think your child has rubella or are not sure if he or she has it and might have exposed a pregnant woman, contact your doctor for advice, and immediately explain your concerns to the pregnant woman. Have her contact her doctor to find out if she is immune (there is a simple blood test that can determine if the woman is immune or not).

Roseola, commonly called "baby measles," usually affects infants under two years old. It has a very characteristic pattern:

- The infant has three days of high fever (sometimes over 104 degrees) but appears quite healthy and comfortable in spite of the fever. Some infants will have a convulsion because of the high fever that is part of this disease.

- On the third day, the fever breaks suddenly, and a fine pink or red rash appears, usually on the neck and chest. The rash may last only a few hours or for a day or so, and the little one seems completely healthy.

No one knows the cause of roseola, although most doctors suspect an as yet unidentified virus. The disease is mildly contagious to young infants who are not immune. It has no known complications, other than the febrile seizures that occur in certain infants. These can often be avoided by prompt attention to reducing the fever and keeping it down. This is done by using an aspirin substitute (acetaminophen) and by cooling the baby down with frequent sponge baths with lukewarm water.

Fifth disease (more properly called exanthem subitum) is a strange disease that also behaves like a viral infection because it is so contagious. This is a problem of preschool and school-aged children and frankly should not even be considered a disease—because youngsters who have it are not sick at all. However, you should be aware of the signs of fifth disease so you don't worry if the youngster gets it. This problem is easy to identify if you know what to look for:

- The youngster has bright red cheeks (almost as if they had been slapped) for several days, without having a fever or other problem that could cause this.

- He or she develops a lacy-looking red or pink rash that appears mostly on the outer surfaces of the arms and the upper legs. The rash does not itch, and the youngster may not even be aware of it until you notice it.

- The rash comes and goes for several weeks, often appearing after a warm bath or whenever the youngster is warm.

450

ILLNESS IN
INFANTS,
CHILDREN,
AND
ADOLESCENTS

Scarlet Fever: Strep with a Rash

Before the discovery of penicillin, scarlet fever was a dreaded disease. Caused by the streptococcus bacteria, it is now easily treated with antibiotics.

It is important to recognize scarlet fever because this rash tells us a strep infection is somewhere in the body (usually in the throat, but sometimes in the skin or another body system). The rash is caused by a toxin (a chemical "poison" made by the strep bacteria).

The signs and symptoms of scarlet fever are:

- Fever and symptoms of a strep infection (for example, severe sore throat); cellulitis (inflammation and infection of the soft tissues under the skin); an infection in a sore or wound.

- A rough, sandpapery pink rash that starts in the armpits, the groin, and the neck, then rapidly covers the body. If you look closely, you can see tiny, raised dots that seem to run together to produce the rash.

- Pale areas around the mouth and in some of the skin creases, especially around the inside of the elbows.

- So-called strawberry tongue—a shiny, bright red, sore-looking tongue.

- Fine peeling of the skin and even the palms of the hands and the soles of the feet (after about a week).

Always contact your doctor for an appointment (or go to an emergency room if you don't have a doctor or can't reach your doctor) if you suspect that your child might have scarlet fever. This infection must be treated with an antibiotic for ten days.

The most common complication of scarlet fever—*glomerulonephritis* (an inflammation of the kidney)—appears one to three weeks after the infection, whether or not the youngster was treated with antibiotics. Glomerulonephritis is caused by an antigen-antibody reaction between the strep bacteria and the cells of the kidney—a sort of immunity problem. You should look for the signs of this potentially serious problem if your youngster has scarlet fever:

- Brown, smoke-colored, or red urine and reduced urine production.
- Puffiness or swelling around the eyes and sometimes generalized body swelling, caused by accumulation of body water.

With glomerulonephritis, the structures of the kidneys' filtering system become inflamed. This inflammation results in the kidneys' failing to work as well as before. When this happens, it often leads to reduced urine production and bleeding of the kidneys (that is why you may see blood in the youngster's urine). Hypertension (high blood pressure) can result from this inflammation, as well. While acute glomerulonephritis usually heals, some youngsters can suffer mild to severe permanent kidney damage. If you suspect this problem, contact your doctor, who will want to examine your child and do certain laboratory studies.

451

RECOGNIZING
AND
MANAGING
COMMON
SYMPTOMS
AND ILLNESSES

THE DON'TS

Don't overtreat skin rashes. Use as little soap on dry rashes and as little ointment, cream, or lotion on the skin as possible. Let the normal skin oils do their job.

Don't assume that all skin rashes are measles. Measles is fortunately unusual, and many viral infections cause "measly" rashes. However, if you know or suspect that your child has German measles (rubella) and has come into contact with a pregnant woman, be sure to talk to your child's doctor (to see if the youngster really has this virus) and the pregnant woman, so she can consult her doctor to be sure she is immune to rubella.

Don't hesitate to contact your doctor if you are not sure what your child's skin rash is or how to treat it. Rashes are sometimes difficult to recognize, unless you have seen many of them.

PLEASE NOTE: Now that you have a grasp of how to recognize and manage rashes and skin infections, it would be extremely helpful for you to go back to the Quick Reference With the Steps in Detail and review it carefully. The more familiar you are with that material, the more useful it will be to you when you need it.

452

ILLNESS IN
INFANTS,
CHILDREN,
AND
ADOLESCENTS

QUICK REFERENCE

With the Steps in Detail

Sore Throat

▶ **INITIALLY, CHILDREN WITH MILD SORE THROAT OR SCRATCHY THROAT AND LITTLE OR NO FEVER CAN BE TREATED AT HOME:**

- Have the young person drink plenty of liquids—especially nonacidic, noncarbonated drinks—and eat bland foods.

- Give aspirin substitute in the correct dosage to help with pain or discomfort.

- Have the youngster gargle with a saltwater solution or hydrogen peroxide several times a day, *if* he can or will.

- Offer hard candies or pain-relieving throat lozenges for her to suck on (if the youngster is over three years old).

▶ **CALL YOUR DOCTOR FOR AN APPOINTMENT (OR GO TO AN EMERGENCY ROOM IF YOU DON'T HAVE A DOCTOR OR CAN'T REACH YOUR DOCTOR) IF YOUR CHILD HAS:**

- A very sore throat with moderate or high fever.

- Swollen, tender lymph nodes in the neck along with the sore throat.

- Very red, swollen tonsils or throat (with or without pus on the tonsils).

- A sore throat with a rough, red rash.

- A mild sore throat that lasts longer than three days.

Tonsils and Adenoids: What You Should Know

453

RECOGNIZING
AND
MANAGING
COMMON
SYMPTOMS
AND ILLNESSES

The tonsils are round, firm lumps of tissue found on both sides of the throat at the back of the tongue. The adenoids are similar structures located above the roof of the mouth at the back of the nose. Tonsils and adenoids are formed by lymph tissue, the same tissue that makes up the lymph nodes in the neck and other parts of the body. Lymph tissue (part of the body's immune system) acts to protect the youngster (or adult) from infection, by "filtering" germs. This tissue also contains special cells that form antibodies (immunity) to combat invading germs. Smaller patches of lymphoid tissue (they look like little bumps on the back of the throat) have the same function.

The tonsils and adenoids (and other lymph nodes) of children are normally larger than those of young infants and adults. This probably happens because preschool and school-aged children are exposed to many germs—viruses and bacteria—that could

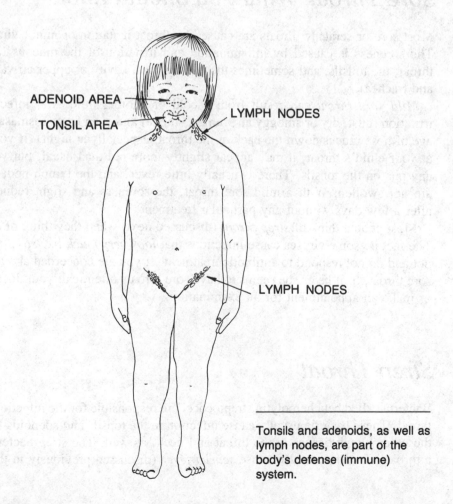

ADENOID AREA

TONSIL AREA

LYMPH NODES

LYMPH NODES

Tonsils and adenoids, as well as lymph nodes, are part of the body's defense (immune) system.

454

ILLNESS IN
INFANTS,
CHILDREN,
AND
ADOLESCENTS

or do cause infections. The tonsils and adenoids normally shrink during adolescence and adulthood to a very small size.

Having large tonsils and adenoids does not necessarily mean the youngster has an infection, nor does it necessarily mean the tonsils and adenoids need to be removed. In fact, the feeling over the last few years is to avoid removing the tonsils unless there is no other choice. Likewise, frequent sore throats do not necessarily mean a youngster's tonsils need to come out. However, chronically infected, huge tonsils that block the airway or interfere with breathing, or adenoids that block the Eustacian tube(s) or interfere with breathing, often need to be removed. If you are concerned about your youngster's tonsils or adenoids, talk with your doctor about whether he or she would recommend removing them.

Sore Throat: What You Should Know

Most sore or scratchy throats are caused by throat irritation or minor viral infections. The soreness is caused by inflammation and irritation of the mucous linings of the throat, the tonsils, and sometimes the nearby nasal cavity or upper airway (the larynx and trachea).

Mild sore throat can result from a cold or another mild viral infection or from irritation (dust, dry or smoggy air, fumes, smoke) and even from postnasal drip (drainage of nose mucus down the back of the throat, especially at night). If you take a look at your child's throat, it may appear slightly more red than usual, but you won't see any pus on the tonsils. There is usually little fever, and the lymph nodes in the neck are not swollen. With a mild sore throat, the soreness and slight redness disappear after a few days without any particular treatment.

Most people think of *strep throat* (discussed next) when they think of a sore throat. The fact is, some viruses cause infections that *look very much like strep throat* but are not and do not respond to antibiotic treatment. If you are concerned about your child's sore throat, or if he or she seems to have sore throats often, call your doctor for advice or make an appointment for an examination.

Strep Throat

Bacteria called beta hemolytic streptococci are responsible for the infection called strep throat. These bacteria usually cause infection in the tonsils and adenoids but can affect the other lymph tissues in the throat and neck, as well. The strep bacteria that cause a throat infection can also cause *scarlet fever* (discussed previously in this chapter).

455

RECOGNIZING
AND
MANAGING
COMMON
SYMPTOMS
AND ILLNESSES

Suspect strep throat infection in a youngster who has:

- Severe throat pain with swallowing and sometimes achiness in the throat at other times.

- High fever and achiness, as well as sore, swollen, tender lymph nodes in the neck (found under the angle of the jaw).

- Swollen, very red tonsils, with or without pus on the surfaces.

- *Very sore throat* with the red, rough rash of scarlet fever.

It is very difficult to be sure that strep bacteria are the cause of a severe throat infection without doing a throat culture (in order to grow the offending bacteria in the laboratory) or performing a faster test to identify the strep bacteria. To do a culture, the youngster's throat is swabbed with a cotton applicator, which is then taken to the laboratory. If strep bacteria are the culprits, they will grow enough to be recognized in twelve to twenty-four hours. Newer tests to identify strep can give this information within a few hours. Many doctors will want to do a culture *before* treating a child with antibiotics, while others will *start* antibiotics while waiting for the results of the culture.

Although a potentially serious infection, strep can be treated effectively with antibiotics. The primary reasons for treating strep throat with antibiotics are to shorten or lessen the discomfort of the sore throat—and *to prevent serious complications* of strep infection, especially rheumatic fever. If you suspect that your youngster might have a strep infection, call the doctor for an appointment, so he or she can examine the youngster and decide whether his throat needs to be cultured and he needs to be treated with antibiotics.

Penicillin is very effective in curing strep infection and can be given by mouth (orally) for ten days or by a single, long-lasting injection. Another antibiotic, erythromycin, is also effective and is usually used for children who are allergic to penicillin. If oral antibiotics are prescribed for strep throat, *be sure to give them for ten days or until they are gone*. Do not stop the oral medication just because your child is feeling better, because the infection requires ten days of antibiotic therapy to be completely eliminated.

Some youngsters suffer repeated strep throats and tonsillitis. Some of these children get strep from a member of the family who is not sick but is a "carrier" of the strep germ. Others are carriers of the strep germ themselves and periodically get reinfected. In still others, the strep infection is traced to the family dog! Talk with your doctor if your child or teenager gets frequent strep infections. The doctor may want to investigate the possible reasons for this or just have you watch him or her carefully to identify recurrent strep infection early. Occasionally, the doctor will recommend tonsillectomy for youngsters with recurring strep infections.

456

ILLNESS IN
INFANTS,
CHILDREN,
AND
ADOLESCENTS

Infectious Mononucleosis: A Cause of Severe Sore Throat

Infectious mononucleosis is an infection caused by what is called the Ebstein-Barr virus. It produces a *severe* throat infection, as well as a variety of other complaints and problems. The severe tonsillitis of "mono" is almost impossible to distinguish from strep throat just by looking at the throat.

While "mono" is most often a disease of teenagers and young adults, it can and does occur in younger children. It is moderately contagious and is spread through contact with saliva and nose secretions. However, the so-called kissing disease can be spread by sneezing and coughing, as well as kissing. "Mono" starts much like a severe cold or strep sore throat, then gets worse over a period of a week or two. Its signs and symptoms can last for six to eight weeks.

The problem with infectious mononucleosis is that it affects many organ systems of the body. It usually causes a severe throat infection, with enough pus formation on the tonsils that the pus looks like a white or yellowish membrane over the tonsils. Sinus infection, bronchitis, and even pneumonia are common in a youngster with mononucleosis. Enlargement and inflammation of the lymph nodes and the spleen are also common, and the young person can have mild hepatitis (liver inflammation) or aseptic meningitis (viral infection of the coverings of the brain and spinal cord), as well.

You should suspect that your child has "mono" if he or she shows the following signs and symptoms:

- A severe sore throat, with tonsil swelling and pus on the tonsils (particularly if these do not get better after five to seven days—even with antibiotic treatment).

- Tender, swollen lymph nodes in the neck, the armpits, and the groin (or elsewhere in the body).

- A fever plus severe fatigue or lethargy, lasting for longer than five days.

- Lack of appetite with nausea and/or vomiting. Pain and/or tenderness in the upper abdomen.

- Nose and sinus congestion and cough (along with the other symptoms of mono, as mentioned).

- A blotchy, red skin rash on the face, chest, back, arms, and legs.

Your doctor is likely to further suspect this viral disease if he or she finds that the young person's spleen is enlarged and tender and that she did not improve when her "strep throat" was treated with antibiotics. Certain blood tests can help confirm the suspicion of "mono," especially after the first week of the illness. The doctor will probably suggest having these blood tests and may also want to do another blood test

457

RECOGNIZING
AND
MANAGING
COMMON
SYMPTOMS
AND ILLNESSES

to find out if there is inflammation of the liver, as well. These blood tests are especially helpful in older children and teenagers, but not so helpful in young children.

Because "mono" is so uncomfortable and lasts for such a long time, you might be wondering whether or not an antibiotic would help. In some situations—where there is also a bacterial infection—it can. However, certain antibiotics, most notably ampicillin, not only provide no help but may also lead to a severe skin rash in almost all youngsters with the disease.

Some youngsters with "mono" are sick enough to need hospitalization and intravenous fluid treatment. A few others have serious enough swelling of the tonsils and adenoids that they need treatment with cortisonelike drugs.

The recovery phase of "mono" can be quite long and discouraging, especially for an active child or teenager. Be supportive and encouraging. Let him know that he *will* get better. It's important, too, that he and you understand how easy it is for him to become tired and that he does need extra rest and sleep. The doctor will want the youngster to avoid vigorous activities, especially contact games and sports, particularly while his spleen is enlarged. The doctor will check the youngster with mono regularly until signs of the disease have disappeared.

The best treatment, in many children, appears to be plenty of rest and sleep (to allow the body to heal itself), eating properly (to keep up their strength), and following any instructions from the doctor. Most children get into trouble because they don't listen to their body's need for rest and become active too fast. When this happens, they may become very sick again. This can turn into a vicious cycle, and you may need to step in and simply insist that the child or teenager rest properly and stay relatively inactive until the doctor feels the disease has passed. Remember, there is no treatment to cure "mono," but the doctor may be able to suggest ways to make your youngster more comfortable.

Peritonsillar Abscess

Sometimes, one tonsil can become so infected with bacteria that an abscess (collection of pus) forms inside it. This causes marked swelling of the tonsil, and the young person cannot or will not swallow at all. This serious infection *must* be treated by a doctor, as soon as possible, to prevent serious complications.

Quinsy, as peritonsillar abscess may be called, should be suspected in a youngster with severe sore throat and:

- Inability or unwillingness to swallow even sips of water or his or her own saliva.

- High fever.

- A muffled voice and pain when talking.

- One enlarged, red tonsil that is swollen enough to extend past the middle of the

458

ILLNESS IN
INFANTS,
CHILDREN,
AND
ADOLESCENTS

throat or that seems to push the uvula (the small piece of tissue that hangs down from the roof of the mouth) over to the other side.

- Difficulty breathing, along with severe sore throat and fever, in an older youngster or teenager.

If you suspect that a young person has a peritonsillar abscess, arrange for him or her to see the doctor promptly, or take the youngster to an emergency room (if you don't have a doctor or can't reach your doctor). Usually, the pus needs to be drained from the tonsil in the hospital, and antibiotics must be given intravenously to control infection. The doctor will often recommend that a tonsillectomy be performed several months after the infection has been treated successfully.

THE DON'TS

Don't assume that every sore throat is strep throat. Many viral infections cause sore throat, and certain irritants can cause a sore or scratchy throat.

Don't expect that every sore throat needs to be treated with an antibiotic. Viral infections do not respond to antibiotics.

Don't assume that your youngster needs to have her tonsils and adenoids removed just because they are large or because she gets occasional throat infections. Children's tonsils are normally quite large, and they function as part of the body's immune system.

Don't hesitate to call your doctor if you are worried about your youngster's sore throat. The doctor may wish to examine the young person or may have some suggestions to help her feel more comfortable.

PLEASE NOTE: Now that you have a grasp of how to recognize and manage sore throats, it would be extremely helpful for you to go back to the Quick Reference With the Steps in Detail and review it carefully. The more familiar you are with that material, the more useful it will be to you when you need it.

459

RECOGNIZING
AND
MANAGING
COMMON
SYMPTOMS
AND ILLNESSES

QUICK REFERENCE

"Swollen Glands"

Do not worry unnecessarily about swollen glands in the neck in a youngster who has a cold or other symptoms of a mild infection, as long as:

▶ **THERE ARE SEVERAL SMALL TO MEDIUM-SIZED "LUMPS" SCATTERED IN THE NECK, ARMPITS, OR GROIN.**

▶ **THE SIZE OF THE LUMPS SEEMS TO GO UP AND DOWN WITH ANY MILD INFECTION OR ILLNESS.**

▶ **THE LUMPS DO NOT SEEM TO BE MATTED TOGETHER, UNUSUALLY TENDER, RED, OR ROCK-HARD.**

Learn to distinguish between the swelling of mumps and the swelling of lymph nodes in the neck:

▶ **MUMPS AFFECTS THE PAROTID GLANDS, LOCATED IN FRONT OF AND JUST BELOW THE EARS.** This makes the youngster look "like a chipmunk."

▶ **LYMPH NODES ARE LOCATED UNDER THE JAWBONE.**

Treat the discomfort of neck lymph-node enlargement or infection by:

▶ **APPLYING HEAT,** either as warm, wet towels or with a heating pad (supervise the youngster while the heating pad is on, and don't allow him or her to go to bed with a heating pad).

▶ **GIVING THE CORRECT DOSE OF ASPIRIN SUBSTITUTE** to help with the discomfort.

Contact your doctor for an appointment if the youngster shows signs of a more serious problem:

▶ **ONE LARGE LYMPH NODE THAT IS WARM, RED, AND TENDER TO THE TOUCH.**

460

ILLNESS IN
INFANTS,
CHILDREN,
AND
ADOLESCENTS

▶ **ENLARGEMENT OF SEVERAL LYMPH NODES, ALONG WITH OTHER SIGNS OF MORE SERIOUS ILLNESS** (frequent or high fever, unusual paleness, easy bruising or bleeding, weight loss).

▶ **NECK SWELLING IS DOWN LOW IN THE NECK** (in the area of the "Adam's apple"), **OR THE YOUNGSTER'S NECK SEEMS TO BE BIG-GER AROUND WHERE HIS OR HER COLLAR RESTS.**

Lymph Nodes: What You Should Know

Most of the time, when you hear people talking about "swollen glands," they are really talking about enlarged lymph nodes in the neck. The lymph nodes are tiny collections of tissue scattered throughout the body (both deeper inside the body and just under the surface of the skin). They are an important part of the body's defense (immune) system and help ward off infections.

When a "foreign invader"—bacteria, virus, or fungus—enters the body, the lymph nodes and the rest of the body's immune system go to work. They "filter" the blood near where the invader entered and trap the germ. Their cells have the ability to make antibodies to fight against these germs—and hopefully prevent serious infection. Lymph nodes are strategically located throughout the body, so that all areas and organs are protected. During the process of fighting an infection—whether viral, bacterial, or fungal—the lymph nodes enlarge and may become hard and somewhat sore to the touch. After their job is done, they shrink down again to normal size.

The tonsils (located at the entrance to the throat, at either side of the tongue) and adenoids (collections of lymph tissue found in the back of the nose above the roof of the mouth) are part of the same lymphatic system. They, too, swell when a virus, bacteria, or fungus invades the body through the mouth or nose.

As previously noted, tonsils, adenoids, and lymph nodes are, in general, larger in children than they are in teenagers and adults. In fact, during the early school years, children can have as much as twice the amount of lymph tissue that they will have as adults. Therefore, it is *normal* for their tonsils and lymph nodes to seem large and "lumpy." This may be due, at least in part, to their constant exposure to viruses and bacteria—and their bodies' constant efforts to fight infection. As they approach their teenage years, the size of the lymph nodes (whether those in the neck, the tonsils, adenoids, or others in the body) gradually decreases, as the youngsters tend to have fewer colds and other infections.

Many parents worry when their child's swollen lymph nodes last longer than the infection or disease that probably caused the enlargement. It is common for the lymph nodes to stay swollen for several weeks after a youngster seems fully recovered.

461

RECOGNIZING
AND
MANAGING
COMMON
SYMPTOMS
AND ILLNESSES

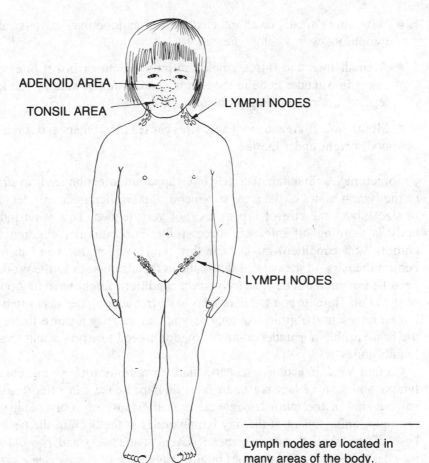

ADENOID AREA

TONSIL AREA

LYMPH NODES

LYMPH NODES

Lymph nodes are located in
many areas of the body.

Common Causes of Lymph-Node Swelling

As mentioned earlier, infection (viral, bacterial, or fungal) is the most common cause
of lymph-node swelling. The *location* of the swollen lymph node(s) often gives you
a clue as to the site of the infection. For example:

- Colds and other minor respiratory infections often lead to swelling and mild
  tenderness of one or more lymph nodes in the neck—usually under the jawbone
  and in the sides of the neck.

- The lymph nodes just under the angle of the jaw swell with tonsillitis (infection
  of the tonsils) and other throat infections.

462

ILLNESS IN
INFANTS,
CHILDREN,
AND
ADOLESCENTS

- "Swimmer's ear" or an infected pierced earlobe may cause swelling of the tiny lymph nodes just below the earlobe.

- A small infection (for example, an infected cut or insect bite) on the arm may result in a tender node in the armpit, and a similar sore on the knee or leg may lead to a corresponding problem in the groin.

- Mouth infections and tooth abscesses cause enlargement and soreness of the lymph nodes right under the jaw.

Sometimes, skin inflammation *without* apparent infection leads to slight enlargement of the lymph nodes of the area. In general, the swollen nodes are less than a half inch in size (about the size of a pea) and not very tender. This is an indication that the body is warding off infection successfully. For example, children with eczema (a chronic skin condition) might have tiny lymph nodes that you can feel in the neck, behind the ears, at the base of the skull, in the armpits, or in the groin. Children with head lice or severe seborrhea (oily scalp condition) might have tiny bumps at the base of the skull. Infants and toddlers who have frequent diaper rash often have "lumpy" lymph nodes in the groin. As long as you can identify a cause like those above, and the basic problem is under control, you don't need to worry about these tiny enlarged lymph nodes.

Certain viral infections are particularly notorious for causing enlargement of the lymph nodes in certain areas. In fact, their presence can often lead your doctor to suspect one of the following infections as the cause of your youngster's illness. For example, enlargement of the tiny lymph nodes at the back of the neck right under the base of the skull occurs in *rubella* (German measles) and *roseola* (so-called baby measles). Your doctor (and you) might suspect one of these diseases if your youngster had other signs and symptoms of these childhood rash diseases, even before the rash appeared.

More Serious Causes of Generalized Lymph-Node Swelling

Infectious mononucleosis is a viral infection that causes enlargement of the lymph tissues of the body. As discussed previously, this disease is caused by a virus and lasts for six to eight weeks. While there is no specific treatment for it, you and your doctor will want to know whether your youngster has it. The lymph nodes of the neck are usually the most enlarged and painful, but "mono" also involves the lymph nodes of the armpits and groin, the tonsils and adenoids, the lymph tissue in the back of the throat, and the lymph tissue in the spleen and liver. As a reminder, contact your doctor

463

RECOGNIZING
AND
MANAGING
COMMON
SYMPTOMS
AND ILLNESSES

if your youngster shows any of the following signs and symptoms of infectious mono-nucleosis:

- A severe sore throat, with tonsil swelling and pus on the tonsils (particularly if these do not get better after five to seven days—even with antibiotic treatment).

- Tender, swollen lymph nodes in the neck, the armpits, and the groin (or elsewhere in the body).

- A fever plus fatigue or lethargy, lasting for longer than five days.

- Lack of appetite with nausea and/or vomiting. Pain and/or tenderness in the upper abdomen.

- Nose and sinus congestion and cough (along with the other symptoms of "mono," as mentioned).

- A blotchy, red skin rash on the face, chest, back, arms, and legs.

To learn more about the signs, symptoms, and treatment of infectious mononucleosis, review pages 456–457 in this chapter.

Certain *chronic inflammatory diseases* of childhood can cause generalized enlarge-ment of the lymph nodes. These long-term conditions cause *other* symptoms that lead you to suspect a serious problem. For example, *juvenile rheumatoid arthritis* may start with a fever, rash, and generalized lymph-node swelling. Joint swelling or pain usually follows days, weeks, or months later. However, the prolonged or recurring fever of this disease is more likely to cause you worry than the enlarged lymph nodes. Make sure you call the doctor if your child experiences the above symptoms followed by joint pain and swelling days, weeks, or months later.

Childhood cancer is another cause of unexplained enlargement of the lymph nodes. *Lymphoma* (cancer of the lymph nodes) causes enlargement of one or a group of lymph nodes, which become firm or rubbery in texture and matted together in a cluster. *Leukemia* (cancer of the blood-forming tissues) can also cause enlargement of the lymph nodes. Youngsters with these serious problems will have other symptoms and signs that would also concern you, such as:

- Unexplained paleness.

- Unexplained fevers.

- Fatigue, poor appetite, weight loss.

- Problems with unusual bleeding or bruising.

- Pain in the bones or joints.

The bottom line with swollen lymph nodes, with or without other serious symptoms, is that you should make an appointment with your child's doctor if you are concerned.

464

ILLNESS IN
INFANTS,
CHILDREN,
AND
ADOLESCENTS

Arrange for an examination, and tell the doctor about your fears. He or she will recommend laboratory tests if they will help to clarify the situation, or recommend a "watch and wait" period.

Causes of a Single Swollen Lymph Node

Sometimes, a lymph node itself will become infected during the course of the "filtering" process. This infection, called *lymphadenitis,* may become so severe that an *abscess* (collection of pus) will form in the lymph node. Suspect lymphadenitis if you notice that one lymph node is enlarging a great deal and:

- The lymph node is over one-half inch in size.

- The skin over the lymph node is red or purple in color.

- The swollen area is painful and hard to the touch.

- The center of the lymph node is softer than the edges or looks whitish or yellow (as if there were pus inside).

- The youngster has a fever and other signs of a serious illness or infection (listlessness, poor appetite, weight loss, and so on).

If you suspect that your child has lymphadenitis, contact your doctor. He or she will want to examine the youngster and prescribe treatment. Most often, lymphadenitis is caused by bacteria and needs to be treated with an antibiotic. Sometimes, the treatment must be carried out in a hospital if the infection is severe or the doctor suspects more serious generalized infection. This treatment will often control the infection before pus forms in the lymph node.

If the infection is advanced enough that pus has formed in the lymph node (an *abscess* has formed), the pus will need to be drained. This involves minor surgery (a cut is made in the abscess) and packing of the abscess so all the pus drains to the outside. Antibiotics are also used, and the infected lymph node usually heals after several weeks. Occasionally, the infected lymph node will need to be removed completely.

Tuberculosis occasionally causes infection in a lymph node (usually in the neck). If the doctor suspects this possibility, he or she will want to test your child for tuberculosis with a TB (tuberculosis) skin test. Don't be surprised (or panic-stricken) if this possibility is raised. If tuberculosis is found, the treatment may include removal of the infected lymph node by a surgeon, as well as special medication for several months. Lymph-node tuberculosis is often caused by different tuberculosis bacteria than cause lung TB and is not usually as contagious as lung tuberculosis.

An unusual cause of lymphadenitis can be a cat scratch. Suspect so-called *cat-*

465

RECOGNIZING
AND
MANAGING
COMMON
SYMPTOMS
AND ILLNESSES

scratch fever if your youngster has a large, tender lymph node in the area where he or she was scratched by a cat. The scratch would look infected and would be taking a long time (usually more than a week) to heal. Until recently, the exact cause of this infection was not known, and testing for it can be difficult. It is usually treated with antibiotics.

Mumps: Less Common Than You Think

Mumps is the first thing that comes to many people's minds when a youngster has "swollen glands." Fortunately, this usually mild infection is far less common today than it was in the past, because it can be prevented by immunizing children against it. (Mumps immunization is usually given to youngsters over one year old, most often in combination with measles and rubella vaccine.)

Mumps (or epidemic parotitis, as it is more correctly called) is a viral infection that causes swelling and inflammation of the parotid gland(s). The parotid glands are located in front of the ears and extend just below the ears. The parotid glands and glands in the floor of the mouth (which can also become inflamed with mumps) secrete saliva. Suspect mumps in an unimmunized youngster who has:

- Painful swelling of the face *in front of the ear(s)* and just under the ear(s). The swollen cheeks make the child look a bit like a chipmunk with its mouth full!

- Mild fever and listlessness.

- Severe pain when he or she eats or drinks something sour—for example, a pickle or citrus juice.

The mumps virus can also cause inflammation and swelling of certain other gland tissues in the body—the pancreas (a gland located in the abdomen that secretes digestive enzymes), the testicles, and occasionally the ovaries. *Pancreatitis* (inflammation of the pancreas) may cause severe abdominal pain and vomiting. Occasionally, a youngster with this complication of mumps infection must be hospitalized to prevent or treat dehydration. Mumps *meningoencephalitis* (inflammation of the brain coverings and even the brain itself) cannot be treated and must run its course, but it rarely causes any long-term difficulty. Mumps *orchitis* (inflammation of the testicle) is not very common but is more common in teenage boys and adult men who are not immune to mumps. Although it is extremely painful, mumps orchitis is usually a temporary problem and is not (as frequently thought) a common cause of sterility. It must run its course, and the only thing you can do is to help your youngster feel more comfortable, by encouraging him to rest, take an aspirin substitute, and apply either heat or cold (whichever feels better).

The reason mumps immunization is so important is that one of the long-term com-

466

ILLNESS IN
INFANTS,
CHILDREN,
AND
ADOLESCENTS

plications of mumps is permanent hearing loss or deafness, due to damage to the auditory (hearing) nerve.

While most complications of mumps infection are usually mild, you should contact your doctor if your *unimmunized youngster* shows the signs and symptoms of mumps, along with:

- Headache and stiff neck.
- Severe abdominal pain.
- Severe vomiting.
- Swelling and pain in the testicle(s).

You have probably heard that a youngster (or you, as an adult) who has had mumps is not immune unless the disease affected "both sides" (both parotid glands). This is not correct. Immunity against the disease is formed regardless of where the virus showed its signs and symptoms. In fact, many adults (who were exposed to the disease before mumps vaccine was available) developed immunity to the virus without ever having had mumps illness.

The fact is, mumps is a preventable disease. Mumps vaccine can and should be given to all youngsters and can be given to adults who may not be immune. (There are no known serious side effects of this vaccine.) Be sure your youngsters are immune to this disease and that you are, too!

What about the youngster who supposedly "had mumps more than once"? Most often, one (or more) of the illnesses were not mumps but rather swollen lymph nodes in the neck (below the angle of the jaw). Repeated swelling of the parotid gland can occur, sometimes because of blockage of the tiny opening from the gland into the mouth or by bacterial infection of the gland. Youngsters who play wind instruments (for example, the trumpet, trombone, or tuba) or those who blow up balloons with gusto can force air into the parotid gland and cause swelling and pain. Check with your doctor if you think your *immunized* child has mumps or if he or she seems to have had it more than once, since it is another problem and may require evaluation and treatment.

Other Causes of Neck Swelling

Swelling in the neck, other than obviously mild swelling of the lymph nodes, should lead you to call the doctor for advice. There are many causes for neck swelling, and an examination is usually warranted.

The thyroid gland is located in the lower part of the front and sides of the neck. It produces vital hormones that control many of the body's functions. If the thyroid gland is swollen (called a *goiter*), you will notice this swelling in the lower part of the neck

467

RECOGNIZING
AND
MANAGING
COMMON
SYMPTOMS
AND ILLNESSES

near where a youngster's collar would be. The swelling is usually soft and painless and is often noticed only when clothing seems too tight around the neck. Goiters can occur at any time from infancy through adulthood and always need medical evaluation. A youngster with a goiter might have no other symptoms or could show signs of either underactive or overactive thyroid gland (changes in weight, appetite, energy level, and growth). Any sign of a possible thyroid problem should result in a call to the doctor to have the youngster evaluated.

Several kinds of *cysts* (collections of fluid) can occur in the neck of infants and children, causing neck swelling. Some cysts are present at birth or are seen shortly afterward, while others appear later. Cysts can be large or small and may be located right in the front or on either side of the neck. The swelling caused by a cyst is soft and not painful to the youngster. Cysts in the neck often must be removed by surgery.

Certain *hemangiomas* (swellings caused by enlargement and malformation of blood vessels) and *lymphangiomas* (swellings due to malformation of the lymph tissues) can also occur in the neck. These problems are almost always present from birth. Your doctor will want to watch a youngster with a hemangioma or lymphangioma in the neck closely, in order to detect any problems that might lead to blockage of the airway. Treatment of large neck hemangiomas and lymphangiomas is difficult and often requires very specialized care.

THE DON'TS

Don't assume that swelling in a youngster's neck means he or she has mumps. Mumps swelling is found in the cheek, just in front of and below the ear(s).

Don't be overly concerned if your young child always seems to have swollen lymph nodes without other symptoms of a serious problem. Enlarged lymph nodes are common in children and usually point to mild infection or inflammation. If you are unsure about whether or not the youngster has something really wrong, call the doctor for an appointment to have the youngster evaluated.

Don't hesitate to contact your doctor for advice or an appointment if you are concerned about swollen lymph nodes in your child. A physical examination is often all that is needed to make sure that your child is healthy.

Don't hesitate to call your doctor immediately if your youngster shows signs of serious illness, along with swollen lymph nodes.

PLEASE NOTE: Now that you have a grasp of how to recognize and manage "swollen glands," it would be extremely helpful for you to go back to the Quick Reference and review it carefully. The more familiar you are with that material, the more useful it will be to you when you need it.

468

ILLNESS IN
INFANTS,
CHILDREN,
AND
ADOLESCENTS

QUICK REFERENCE

With the Steps in Detail

Swollen Joints, Limping

▶ **IF JOINT SWELLING OR LIMPING FOLLOWS AN OBVIOUS INJURY, HAVE THE YOUNGSTER SIT DOWN OR LIE DOWN, TO AVOID FURTHER INJURY.**

- Elevate the injured arm or leg.

- Apply ice packs.

- Contact your doctor or take the youngster to an emergency room if there is a great deal of swelling, pain, or limitation of movement.

- See Chapter 16 for more information on bone and joint injuries.

▶ **CALL THE DOCTOR IF A YOUNGSTER HAS JOINT SWELLING, WITH OR WITHOUT HAVING EXPERIENCED AN INJURY TO THE JOINT.**

▶ **CALL THE DOCTOR FOR AN APPOINTMENT IF A CHILD OR OLDER YOUNGSTER LIMPS FOR LONGER THAN ONE OR TWO DAYS, EVEN IF THERE ARE NO OTHER SYMPTOMS.**

▶ **MAKE AN APPOINTMENT WITH YOUR DOCTOR IF AN INFANT OR YOUNG CHILD REFUSES TO WALK OR USE AN ARM OR LEG, ESPECIALLY IF HE OR SHE ALSO HAS A FEVER OR OTHER SIGNS OF ILLNESS.**

▶ **CALL THE DOCTOR FOR AN APPOINTMENT IF YOUR YOUNGSTER HAS FREQUENT SORE JOINTS OR EXPERIENCES PAIN IN THE BONES.**

The Child Who Limps

469

RECOGNIZING
AND
MANAGING
COMMON
SYMPTOMS
AND ILLNESSES

Limping—walking in a way that protects a leg from hurting—is always a cause for concern. It can mean the youngster is hurting because of something as minor as a nail in his or her shoe or as major as a serious illness or injury to a part of the leg or back. Telling the difference often requires some detective work on your part and that of your doctor.

Most often, limping results from pain due to a minor injury—to the foot, the ankle, the knee, the hip, or the back. All youngsters fall or twist a leg at some time during childhood. Most of these injuries are minor, and the resulting pain and damage are not a cause for worry. The pain stops, and the child walks or runs normally after a few minutes, hours, or days. You may never find out what happened, but whatever it was, it went away. (See Chapter 16 for more information on bone and joint injuries.)

Persistent limping—lasting for longer than a day or two—should raise your suspicions that the youngster might have a more serious problem. In general, you will need to make an appointment with the doctor, but before you do, collect as much information about your youngster's condition as you can:

- Ask your older child or youngster if he hurt himself in the last day or two.

- Watch her walk. Which leg seems to be the problem?

- Watch him walk in his shoes, then barefoot. Determine if the limping is the same.

- If he limps more in shoes, look at his shoes. Are there any nails or rough areas that could irritate his feet, or are the shoes too small?

- If the limp doesn't change whether he is wearing shoes or not, check his feet and legs. Is there any swelling or bruising? Are there any scrapes, blisters, or obvious sore spots on his feet?

- Feel all the way up and down his legs and feet. Do you find any obvious sore spots?

- Have the youngster move all the joints in his feet and legs—feet, ankles, knees, and hips. Is there any joint that hurts or that he will not or cannot move? Do both legs or hips move the same way?

- Check her back. Are there any tender spots? Does she stand as straight as usual? Can she bend in all directions?

- Think about whether he has had a fever or other signs of illness—rather than an injury.

When you take your youngster to the doctor, he or she will perform a careful examination. The cause of the limping might become obvious during the examination, or the doctor might suggest waiting for a few days to see if anything else develops.

470

ILLNESS IN
INFANTS,
CHILDREN,
AND
ADOLESCENTS

If the doctor suspects a potentially serious problem, he or she might recommend X rays of the child's legs, hips, and back and may want the youngster to have certain blood tests, as well, depending on his or her suspicions. You might wonder why, for example, the doctor would be concerned about the child's hips—even if the pain seemed to be in the knee or ankle. The reason is that pain in the hip or back can be "referred" to another area of the leg (because of the way the nerves that "feel" pain work). In other words, pain that comes from the hip may be felt in the knee, or even the heel, but may not be felt in the hip itself.

Treatment will depend on what the doctor finds, both during the examination and from any tests that are taken.

Some Common Causes of "Unexplained" Limping

While most "unexplained" limping in a child or older youngster is caused by a minor injury that you did not know about, it can signal a more serious problem. A youngster's age will determine, to some extent, what his or her risks are for certain problems.

Babies who are just learning to walk and older toddlers present a special problem—because they cannot tell you exactly what bothers them. They may limp but continue to walk, even without crying, or they may refuse to walk altogether. Shoes that hurt or don't fit may be the culprit, so look at that possibility first. If a small child limps for a day or two after receiving an injection in the leg or hip, then remember that soreness in the muscle is the explanation. Beyond those possibilities, you will need the doctor to help you determine what the problem is.

Regardless of a child's age, your first concern (and that of the doctor) will be an *unknown injury*. Usually, a careful examination and X rays, if they seem warranted, will solve this problem. Injuries can range from a pulled muscle to a fracture (broken bone) or sprain (injury to a ligament).

Very active young children may limp for a few days or complain of hip pain due to so-called *traumatic synovitis* (inflammation of the joint lining). A similar condition, called *toxic synovitis*, occasionally follows a mild viral infection. This condition causes only mild pain and limping for a few days and may be due to accumulation of a small amount of fluid in the joint (not enough to detect on examination). Your youngster's doctor may want to rule out an infection in the joint before making this diagnosis.

Legg-Calve-Perthes disease is a very serious problem that affects children, most commonly boys, between four and ten years old. In youngsters with this disease, disruption of the blood supply to the epiphysis (growing area) of the ball-like head of the femur (upper leg bone) causes the bone to become flattened and deformed. If this hip disease is not recognized and treated promptly, permanent deformity of the hip joint will occur. Its exact cause is not known, and it can involve one or both hips. At

471

RECOGNIZING
AND
MANAGING
COMMON
SYMPTOMS
AND ILLNESSES

first, the youngster limps but experiences no pain—sometimes for weeks. As he continues to walk on his leg, he feels pain and the constant stress of walking causes more and more deformity. The doctor can make this diagnosis by taking X rays of the hips. Treatment takes months or years and involves avoiding putting any weight on the hip. The youngster might need to stay in bed, be in a large cast, use crutches, or wear a special brace during the treatment.

In older youngsters, especially preteenage boys who are overweight, limping can be caused by *slipped capital femoral epiphysis*. In young people with this problem, the growing portion (epiphysis) of the hip gradually slips out of place, causing first a limp, then pain in the hip. Without treatment, the youngster will usually develop permanent damage and deformity of the hip joint. This serious problem can be detected through hip X rays. Treatment takes months or years to complete and will involve several measures to avoid putting pressure on the hip joint while it heals. The earlier the problem is recognized, the better the chances are that permanent damage can be prevented.

Occasionally, limping results from a *back problem*, even in young children. Most often, the youngster will also complain of pain in the back and will not be able to bend or twist the back as completely as usual. Problems with the intervertebral discs (the soft structures that are found between the bones of the back and cushion them), slippage of the vertebrae, or damage to the blood supply of one or more of the bones of the back can cause this kind of difficulty. Detection of these unusual problems requires a careful physical examination and X rays of the back. Treatment depends on the problem and may involve bed rest, bracing, or surgery.

Osteomyelitis: Infection in the Bone

When a youngster who is limping (or refusing to use a body part or joint) also has fever, the first possibility you and your doctor will consider is that of infection. This infection can be in the bone itself (called *osteomyelitis*) or in a joint (called *septic arthritis*).

Osteomyelitis is a very serious infection of a bone and can involve any bone in the body. Most often, bacteria invade the growing portion of the bone, causing inflammation and pus formation. This leads to pain in the bone, often with swelling over the infected bone, and soreness to the touch. If the infected area is close to a joint, the infection may reach the joint itself and cause swelling in it. If the infection is not recognized and treated, the bone will gradually become seriously damaged.

In young infants and children, bone infection can follow a generalized body infection (sepsis) or occur without any known illness or injury. The bacteria that cause osteomyelitis in young children are somewhat different from those that affect older, active youngsters. Be suspicious if your little child has fever and limps or refuses to use an

472

ILLNESS IN
INFANTS,
CHILDREN,
AND
ADOLESCENTS

arm or leg. (For example, a *toddler* might prefer to crawl and cry if you try to get him to stand and walk, or he might hold his arm still and cry if you move it. An *infant* might cry when you move his leg to change his diapers.)

In older, active youngsters, a bone infection often follows an injury. The injury can be as little as a bruise or can be an infected scrape or cut. For some reason, bacteria from the skin get into the bone and set up an infection, leading to pain, swelling, and fever. Check with your doctor if a youngster seems to have more pain or trouble with an arm or leg after an injury than you would expect, especially if she also has fever.

If the doctor suspects a bone infection, he or she will want to do blood tests and may want to have the child go to the hospital for treatment. X rays of the suspicious bone or a special test called a bone scan can confirm the diagnosis. The doctor will try to find out exactly which germ is causing the infection, either by aspirating the bone (inserting a needle into the bone and withdrawing pus) or by opening the bone in surgery to relieve pressure and identify the cause of the infection. Treatment for osteomyelitis is long and involves high doses of antibiotics, first given intravenously (by vein) and later by mouth (orally). The youngster may need to stay in the hospital for as long as four to six weeks.

Joint Swelling: What You Should Know

Swelling in or around a joint in a child almost always signals a potentially serious problem. If your youngster seems to have joint swelling, with or without a known injury, call your doctor promptly for advice and an appointment. Early identification of the problem and prompt treatment are very important when it comes to those things that can cause joint swelling.

Much of the time, swelling in or around a joint is caused by an *injury* to one of its structures. Damage to the bone or its growth plate (the area of the bone where growth takes place), the joint surface itself, ligaments, or tendons causes accumulation of fluid or blood in and around the joint. This leads to pain and restriction of the joint's motion. If you suspect a joint injury, have the youngster rest and apply ice packs for several hours. Contact your doctor for advice or go to an emergency room for evaluation. (See Chapter 16 for more information about joint injury.)

Arthritis (inflammation of a joint) is one of the most serious reasons for joint swelling and can have several possible causes. With arthritis, the lining of a joint (called the synovium) becomes swollen and irritated. Fluid builds up inside the joint space and leads to swelling, soreness, and restricted motion of the joint. If the fluid inside the joint contains blood or pus, the joint surfaces can be further irritated and scarred. If the amount of fluid buildup is great, pressure inside the joint can cause still more damage to the delicate lining structures.

Septic arthritis (infection in a joint) is a very serious cause of joint swelling. When

473

RECOGNIZING
AND
MANAGING
COMMON
SYMPTOMS
AND ILLNESSES

a joint becomes infected with bacteria, pus is produced. The joint becomes swollen, hot, and sore, and the youngster usually develops a fever. Septic arthritis is a common complication of bone infection (osteomyelitis) of the bone right next to the joint. In order to diagnose this very serious infection, the doctor will aspirate the joint (take some of the fluid out with a needle) and have the laboratory try to identify the cause of the infection, so the correct antibiotic treatment can be started. He or she will also look for infection in the nearby bone—and elsewhere in the body. A youngster with septic arthritis is usually hospitalized and treated with intravenous antibiotics. Care will be taken to keep the joint as free of pus and fluid as possible (by frequent removal of the pus and fluid with a needle or through surgery) and to prevent permanent damage to the joint.

Swelling of one or more joints can be a complication of *rubella (German measles) infection*, especially in teenagers and adults. It can also be a complication of *rubella immunization*, showing up sometimes as late as one or two months afterward. Think of this possibility when a youngster has the signs and symptoms of rubella infection (mild fever, listlessness, swollen lymph nodes in the back of the neck under the skull, and a red rash), along with or followed by joint pain and swelling (even if it's a few weeks to a couple of months after the rubella immunization).

Juvenile rheumatoid arthritis, although uncommon, is a chronic disease that leads to pain, swelling, and redness of one or more joints. The youngster usually has a fever and other signs of illness, and the symptoms may come and go over months to years. There are several forms of juvenile rheumatoid arthritis, and in each form, it can be very difficult for the doctor to reach what is called a definitive diagnosis (an absolute diagnosis). However, as each episode of joint swelling occurs, the diagnosis becomes more and more apparent. This disease can go on for weeks, months, or years and may disappear completely, without any residual problems, or can lead to permanent joint deformity. Treatment of juvenile rheumatoid arthritis is complicated and depends on the form of the disease the youngster has and how severe the joint inflammation is.

Serum sickness (a form of allergy or sensitivity to a medication) and *Henoch-Schönlein purpura* (an unusual immune disease that was discussed under "Managing Hives") also cause joint swelling. With both of these problems, the youngster will also have other symptoms and signs, including skin rash or swelling. Call the doctor if your youngster has joint swelling along with a skin rash, and stop any medications you might be giving the youngster.

Pain in the Bones

Many youngsters complain of leg pain at some time during childhood. Usually, this pain comes from muscle strains or cramping due to vigorous activity. You will notice that the complaints occur at night and that the youngster seems otherwise healthy.

474

ILLNESS IN
INFANTS,
CHILDREN,
AND
ADOLESCENTS

These are commonly called *"growing pains."* You may be concerned about these pains and have trouble distinguishing them from the pain of *shin splints* (discussed in Chapter 17).

True bone pain is a different matter. Youngsters who complain of pain inside the bone(s) should be evaluated by a doctor. *Leukemia* and other forms of *childhood cancer* can cause bone pain—because of a tumor inside the bone. Youngsters with these conditions may also have unusual paleness, weight loss, bruising or bleeding problems, and fever. *Bone cysts* (collections of fluid or nonbone tissue) and *bone tumors*—both cancerous (called malignant) and noncancerous (called benign)—can also cause bone pain or limping with pain. If your child has frequent pain in a bone or is limping and experiences pain in a bone, make an appointment with the doctor for a thorough examination. Make sure you explain the youngster's symptoms and your fears.

THE DON'TS

Don't overlook a limp as "not important" just because a youngster does not complain about pain. Certain potentially serious problems of the hip or back may not cause pain in their earliest stages.

Don't overlook the signs of bone or joint infection in your child: limping or refusing to use an arm or leg; fever; and pain, redness, and swelling of a joint. Contact your doctor promptly, or go to an emergency room for an evaluation.

Don't hesitate to see the doctor if your youngster has frequent problems with bone or joint pain, even if you cannot pinpoint an illness or injury associated with it. Most often, the youngster will be perfectly healthy, but occasionally, these pains will be a signal of more serious illness or injury.

PLEASE NOTE: Now that you have a grasp of how to recognize and manage swollen joints and limping, it would be extremely helpful for you to go back to the Quick Reference With the Steps in Detail and review it carefully. The more familiar you are with that material, the more useful it will be to you when you need it.

475

RECOGNIZING
AND
MANAGING
COMMON
SYMPTOMS
AND ILLNESSES

QUICK REFERENCE

With the Steps in Detail

Teething and Toothaches

It's important to distinguish between the symptoms of teething and those of a mild or more serious infection:

▶ **TEETHING MAY CAUSE:**

- Irritability and crankiness.

- Soreness of the gums.

- Increased chewing activity.

- Increased drooling.

- Mild chin and face rash.

- Runny nose, with clear mucus.

- Slightly looser than usual bowel movements.

▶ **TEETHING DOES NOT CAUSE:**

- High fever.

- Severe vomiting or diarrhea.

- Continuous nighttime (or daytime) crying.

- Other signs of infection or another serious illness.

You can help your teething baby to feel more comfortable by:

▶ **LETTING HER CHEW ON COLD, FIRM TEETHING OBJECTS.**

▶ **GIVING HIM ASPIRIN SUBSTITUTE IN THE CORRECT DOSAGE.**

▶ **RUBBING HER GUMS WITH YOUR FINGERS AND PERHAPS WITH A PAIN-RELIEVING TEETHING MEDICINE.**

476

ILLNESS IN
INFANTS,
CHILDREN,
AND
ADOLESCENTS

Be on the lookout for signs of tooth decay or gum disease in your child, and take him to the dentist if you think or know he has a problem. Delaying will only allow the problem to get worse.

▶ **TOOTHACHE THAT LASTS FOR LONGER THAN A FEW HOURS, OR OCCURS REPEATEDLY, MEANS TOOTH DECAY OR ABSCESS UNTIL PROVEN OTHERWISE. THE YOUNGSTER SHOULD PROMPTLY SEE A DENTIST.**

▶ **A YOUNGSTER WHO HAS SIGNS OF TOOTH INFECTION OR ABSCESS—TOOTHACHE, JAW OR FACE SWELLING, AND FEVER— NEEDS PROMPT DENTAL OR MEDICAL ATTENTION.**

- Contact your dentist or doctor immediately, so antibiotic treatment can begin and dental work can be done as soon as possible, in order to save or repair the infected tooth.

Tooth Eruption: What You Should Know

The formation of deciduous teeth (so-called baby teeth) begins before a baby is born and continues for a year or so after birth. The formed teeth stay protected under the gums for a varying period of time after birth, then slowly start moving until they break through the gums and into the mouth. A few infants are born with visible teeth, but most babies' teeth begin appearing when they are between four and nine months of age. The twenty baby teeth (ten on the top and ten on the bottom) are usually visible by the time the little one is two and a half years old. These deciduous teeth are pushed out by the developing permanent teeth, beginning when a child is about five to six years old, and the last ones are lost just before adolescence (around twelve years of age).

The formation of healthy teeth depends on good, balanced nutrition and health. Protein, calcium, and other minerals are important to the formation of healthy teeth, and fluoride in the diet adds further protection from decay (called dental caries). Good mouth care—tooth brushing; avoiding constant exposure of the erupted teeth to sugars, starches, and acidic foods; and regular dental care—prevents many common dental problems in children (and adults). However, none of these preventive measures has much to do with *when* teeth appear in the mouth.

The time that teeth appear is different for each baby and depends on her own makeup and heredity. If your teeth were "late," chances are your baby's teeth will appear

477

RECOGNIZING
AND
MANAGING
COMMON
SYMPTOMS
AND ILLNESSES

later than you might expect. Likewise, the time a youngster loses "the first tooth" depends on her own personal makeup. The timing is less important than most people think. Many parents worry unnecessarily about when a baby's teeth will appear and when the permanent teeth will start coming in.

Actually, premature loss of the baby teeth is more of a problem than late appearance of the baby teeth. While baby teeth are obviously important for chewing and eating, they also serve a vital function in the development of the child's face and mouth. If baby teeth are lost and not replaced by the permanent teeth (because of severe decay or trauma), the remaining teeth may "drift" in the mouth and lead to crooked or overlapping teeth. Some people are not particularly concerned about decay or loss of their children's baby teeth because they know they will fall out and be replaced later. They forget, though, that some of the baby teeth must last for approximately eight to ten years *before* they are replaced. During this time, the permanent teeth (below the gums) can be affected by decay or abscess of the baby teeth, and gum disease can also result in damage to the permanent teeth. It is therefore quite important to preserve and protect the baby teeth until the permanent teeth are ready to erupt (come in).

To be sure, there *are* serious health problems that lead to late eruption of both baby and permanent teeth. These include some inherited problems of the skin and hair, some inherited bone problems, and disorders of the thyroid gland. However, all of these potentially serious problems have *other* symptoms and signs besides delayed tooth appearance that would alert you and your doctor that there is a more serious problem.

"Teething": What Is It?

Parents and others tend to blame "teething"—the eruption of the teeth—for many of the common symptoms babies and children have. Some of the problems parents see may well be due to the discomfort associated with tooth eruption, while others are not really caused by teething.

Most parents begin to wonder if their baby is teething when they see him begin to drool and chew on his fists. However, babies begin to drool a great deal around three to five months of age—and at the same time begin to chew on *everything* in sight and reach. This chewing is a normal part of development and is not necessarily related to the teething. At this young age, babies begin to have better control of their hands and can more easily put things into their mouths (in a more coordinated way). At this point, babies are also beginning to learn how to move their mouths in a chewing motion—probably in preparation for eating solid foods rather than sucking on the breast or bottle.

If you think your child is teething, look carefully at his or her gums. (Check the lower front area first, since most infants get the lower teeth before the upper ones.) You may see some swelling right at the surface and may also see the outline of the teeth underneath, as they rise closer to the surface. Feel for any hard, sharp points. If

478

ILLNESS IN
INFANTS,
CHILDREN,
AND
ADOLESCENTS

you see these things, your guess might be correct. But when in doubt, wait until you actually see the teeth appear through the gums! It can take days or weeks for the teeth to actually push through the swollen gums.

Teething causes *minor* discomfort and symptoms in babies:

- Crankiness and irritability.

- Swollen gums, sometimes with slight redness.

- Increased drooling.

- Minor rashes (you might think of them as "spit rashes") on the chin and face.

- Runny nose with clear mucus (probably because the baby is crying more than usual, and his tears drain out through his nose!).

- Minor changes in appetite.

- Increased chewing, sucking, and mouthing of everything in reach.

- Slightly looser than usual bowel movements (but not real diarrhea) and minor diaper rashes.

Teething does *not* produce high fever. It does *not* cause vomiting or real diarrhea, or other signs and symptoms of more serious disease. Teething is rarely painful enough to cause repeated nighttime crying either (but a few babies are the exception to the rule).

The problem is, teething occurs at the same time (during most of the first two and a half years of a baby's life) when he or she is also getting minor (and sometimes more serious) infections. To further confuse the issue, some of the symptoms of teething are similar to the early symptoms of other illnesses in babies. If you check the baby's temperature, you might find that it's 100 degrees or so and think, "A-haa, this is a fever," when it's actually the baby's normal temperature in the afternoon or evening. (Everyone's temperature is higher in the late afternoon and evening than it is in the morning.) This might lead you to believe that teething caused a "fever." Consider, too, that a baby with an earache (ear infection) may also be teething, but it's the earache that keeps him or her crying at night and causes a fever. Another example is a toddler who has vomiting and diarrhea due to a minor intestinal infection and who might also be teething—and the diarrhea and vomiting are blamed on teething.

So, you see, because children who are teething are at an age where two things are happening (exposure to many infections and teething), the myth about teething goes on. Therefore, be sure to consider these other possibilities that may cause serious symptoms, and call your doctor if your baby has symptoms that can't be attributed to "sore gums" (teething). If your child is checked by the doctor and he or she absolutely cannot find another reason for the symptoms, then your child may indeed be one of the exceptions to the rule.

You can help ease your little one's teething discomfort in some simple ways:

479

RECOGNIZING
AND
MANAGING
COMMON
SYMPTOMS
AND ILLNESSES

- Give her something cold and "chewable" to gnaw on. Refrigerate teething rings, and get one or more flexible (but *safe*) toys she can put into her mouth.

- Rub her gums with your fingers. If you wish and your doctor agrees, try one of the commercially available teething gels or lotions.

- Give her *aspirin substitute* (in the correct dosage) for discomfort.

- Offer her extra liquids to drink, and don't be concerned if she is less interested in solid foods than in liquids.

If you are not successful in helping the baby feel better, reevaluate the situation to be sure you are really dealing with teething. If you're not sure, contact your doctor for further advice. Above all, do not assume that every symptom your child has is due to teething— since you may then overlook problems that require medical treatment!

Tooth Decay (Dental Caries) and Its Prevention

Teeth are covered by a hard protective coating called enamel. A break in this coating leads to tooth decay (dental caries), or "cavities." Buildup of debris (called plaque) between the teeth and along the gum margins provides a perfect environment for bacteria to accumulate and begin their destructive work. Acidic foods and drinks and those with sugar in them make the decay process easier, and eventually the enamel is dissolved. The decay works its way farther and farther into the tooth, and if it reaches the nerve endings deep inside the tooth, a toothache develops. Further invasion can lead to infection deep inside the tooth, and an abscess (collection of pus) can form.

The formation of healthy teeth that are resistant to dental caries depends on a large number of factors. A mother's nutrition during pregnancy, certain hereditary factors, a youngster's nutrition, and proper preventive measures all play a role. You should also be aware of the fact that certain illnesses weaken tooth enamel (for example, hypothyroidism—underactive thyroid gland). Fluoride can do a great deal to strengthen teeth while they are forming, if taken by an infant or child during the time of tooth development. (While fluoride use continues to be controversial, its benefits in preventing tooth decay are great.)

After the teeth have formed, other measures can help in preventing or controlling the development of tooth decay. Fluoride applied to the surface of the teeth can assist in making them more resistant to decay. Good mouth hygiene—rinsing, brushing, flossing, and avoiding poor dietary habits—can also do much toward preventing or controlling tooth decay. All of these factors play a role in a youngster's (and an adult's) having healthy teeth.

480

ILLNESS IN
INFANTS,
CHILDREN,
AND
ADOLESCENTS

There is a great deal you can do to help your infant, child, or older youngster to have healthy teeth that stay free of dental caries. Start early in infancy:

- Be sure your infant has a well-balanced diet, with an adequate fluoride supply. Check whether there is fluoride in your water supply, and ask your doctor whether he or she recommends giving your baby fluoride supplements.

- If your doctor or dentist recommends fluoride supplementation, be sure to continue it (in the dosage prescribed by your doctor or recommended by your dentist) until all the youngster's permanent teeth have formed (until ten to twelve years of age).

- Do not allow a baby or toddler to take a bottle to bed or suck on a bottle constantly during the day. (Constant sucking on a bottle "bathes" the teeth with sugar, increasing the risk of decay.)

- Begin a program of mouth care as soon as teeth appear.

- Have your infant or child drink water after eating or rinse his or her mouth after eating or drinking.

- Wipe your baby's teeth with a wet washcloth after meals—right from the start.

- Begin tooth brushing (you don't need toothpaste) when your baby is twelve to eighteen months old, and make it a habit.

- Begin to use a toothpaste that contains fluoride as soon as the little one can be trusted *not to swallow the paste* during toothbrushing.

- Teach older youngsters how to floss their teeth, and encourage daily flossing.

- Begin regular dental checkups by the time the child is three years old, and follow your dentist's recommendations about routine care and fluoride applications.

- Ask your dentist about newer techniques, such as tooth sealing (a process in which a plastic material is sealed onto the tooth surfaces, to halt or prevent further tooth decay), to provide additional protection for your youngster's teeth.

- Learn to recognize the signs and symptoms of dental caries, and get the youngster to a dentist when you recognize the indications of possible decay.

By taking these measures, you can prevent many of the problems of severe tooth decay and mouth disease that threaten your child early on and later as an adult. Remember that some serious dental problems take years to develop and may not be apparent until adulthood. Prevention starts with good oral hygiene and dental care at an early age—not after a problem exists. Therefore, you would be doing your children a great service by helping them develop excellent habits now, which would prevent serious problems later in life.

481

RECOGNIZING
AND
MANAGING
COMMON
SYMPTOMS
AND ILLNESSES

Dental Caries: Signs and Symptoms

Dental caries can develop in the teeth of infants and very young children if conditions in the mouth are just right. Toddlers and young children who constantly suck on a bottle, especially throughout the night, are at high risk for *nursing-bottle mouth* (also called nursing-bottle syndrome). This is a totally preventable problem that can lead to severe tooth decay, early tooth loss, and later problems with crooked teeth (if the baby teeth are lost long before permanent teeth are ready to appear).

This kind of tooth decay occurs because the teeth are constantly bathed with sugar-containing liquids—day and night. Although sucking on a bottle of milk all night or day is damaging, fruit juices given this way can cause even worse damage because of their sugary and acidic content. The upper front teeth are likely to show the first signs of decay, but all of the teeth are gradually attacked. At its worst, this preventable disease causes the teeth to literally rot away. Look carefully at your young child's teeth for signs of this serious problem:

- Yellow, brown, or gray discoloration of the upper front teeth.

- Brown, black, or yellow discoloration of the sides of the front teeth—in the spaces where the teeth meet.

- Worn biting edges of the teeth, areas that look chipped or worn away, or outright rotting of the front teeth.

- Beginning or advanced decay (black spots and holes) in the lower and back teeth.

If you suspect nursing-bottle caries, make an appointment with a children's dentist as soon as possible. The damage can usually be repaired and further decay halted with early treatment. Above all, completely stop allowing the youngster to drink from a bottle, or limit bottle use to water only, as a temporary alternative while you get him or her used to the idea of not having a bottle. Closely follow the dentist's recommendations for further treatment.

In older children, tooth decay continues to be a potential problem, especially in youngsters who eat unusual amounts of sweets and who do not brush and floss their teeth well. Regular dental checkups can detect dental caries before you can see the cavities developing. However, check your youngster's mouth periodically for visible signs of decay—black or brown spots in the tiny pits of the teeth, along the gum margins, and on the edges of the teeth, where they meet each other. If you see any spots that concern you, make an appointment with the dentist, so the damage can be repaired *before* decay advances to the point of causing pain and infection. "Sensitive" teeth—teeth that are painful when a youngster eats or drinks hot, cold, or sweet things—usually mean that decay is beginning. Don't overlook this early sign of tooth decay, and make an appointment with the dentist for an evaluation.

482

ILLNESS IN
INFANTS,
CHILDREN,
AND
ADOLESCENTS

If your youngster complains of a *toothache*, you can be pretty well assured that he has an area of decay. Look at the tooth that seems painful, to see whether you can see a hole or area of decay. Make an appointment with the dentist as soon as possible. While you are waiting for the appointment, you can help the youngster feel more comfortable by:

- Having her floss between the teeth right around the painful spot. (You might be able to dislodge food that is causing pressure and inflammation around the gums.)

- Giving her *aspirin substitute* as needed (use the correct dosage) for the pain.

- Soaking a piece of cotton or a small piece of cloth in oil of cloves (see your pharmacist) or a commercially available medicine for toothache and having her bite down on it for fifteen to thirty minutes.

- Trying warm or cold compresses (each person prefers a different thing) on the outside of the jaw.

- Having her rest or sleep with her head elevated slightly, to prevent throbbing in the gum/tooth.

Suspect *tooth infection* or *tooth abscess* if your child complains of toothache and has one or more of the following:

- A fever.

- Swelling of the jaw or cheek on the side of the face with the toothache.

- Swelling of the gums around the painful tooth or pus that is visible around a tooth. Sometimes, you can see a red, swollen area with a yellow center along the margin of the gums—called a "gum boil."

- Swollen, tender lymph nodes under the jaw.

- A foul taste in the mouth (because of pus drainage).

If you think your child might have a tooth abscess, call the dentist promptly, or call your doctor if you cannot reach your dentist (or do not have one). Tooth abscesses are infections that must be treated with antibiotics, which can be started before the dentist treats the tooth itself. (Some dentists prefer that antibiotic treatment be completed before working on the tooth.) You can make your child more comfortable by applying warm packs to his jaw and giving aspirin substitute. The dentist will do all he or she can to save your youngster's tooth, but occasionally, the infected tooth must be removed.

A word about *periodontal disease* (inflammation and infection of the gums and supporting structures of the teeth): Gum disease is the leading cause of early loss of teeth in older youngsters and adults. The sad thing is that perfectly healthy teeth can be lost because of infection and inflammation of the gums surrounding them. This can be completely prevented by following a routine of good mouth hygiene (correct tooth brushing, regular flossing between the teeth, and routine dental evaluations that include cleaning the teeth).

Check your youngster's mouth on a regular basis for early signs of periodontal disease. You should be suspicious if your youngster has:

- Swollen, pink, or red gums right at the edges of the teeth.

- Puffiness and redness of the tiny parts of the gums that stick up between the teeth.

- Painful gums that bleed easily with eating or tooth brushing.

- Spaces (gaps) between the gums and the teeth, with or without pus in the spaces.

- Persistent bad breath, along with any of the other signs of gum disease.

- Loose, painful teeth, especially the permanent teeth.

You will need your dentist's help in treating all but the most minor gum inflammation. He or she will carefully clean off all the plaque (debris that accumulates on the teeth) and begin treating the inflamed gums. The dentist will also teach you and the young person how to keep the teeth and gums clean and healthy in the future.

THE DON'TS

Don't assume that teething is the cause of a fever in an infant or toddler. Teething certainly causes mouth discomfort and irritability, but most people assume it causes more problems than it really does.

Don't worry about when your baby or toddler will get his or her teeth. The time teeth appear in the mouth depends on a child's own makeup, and delayed tooth eruption rarely means a serious problem of growth or development.

Don't neglect your child's baby teeth. They are important for chewing, as well as for maintaining proper spacing inside the mouth. Besides, some of them must last for as long as ten years!

Don't ever allow a baby or toddler to take a bottle to bed or suck constantly on a bottle of milk or sugar-containing liquid. Constant ''bathing'' of the teeth with milk or sugar-containing liquids leads to rampant dental decay and tooth destruction.

Don't forget to start mouth care and tooth brushing as soon as a baby gets teeth. You will be protecting your child's teeth from decay right from the start and begin a lifetime habit of good dental care.

Don't overlook fluoride as a major help in preventing tooth decay. While fluoride supplementation is somewhat controversial in the view of some people, it is very effective in promoting the formation of strong teeth. And fluoride applied to the surfaces of the teeth can be helpful in reducing dental caries, even in teenagers and adults.

484

ILLNESS IN
INFANTS,
CHILDREN,
AND
ADOLESCENTS

Don't delay in taking your child to the dentist if he or she complains of sensitive teeth or toothache. These symptoms almost always signal tooth decay.

Don't hesitate to contact your dentist or doctor immediately if your youngster shows signs of tooth abscess or infection (toothache, pain and swelling of the jaw, and fever). The youngster needs prompt antibiotic treatment, as well as care for the damaged tooth itself.

Don't forget about periodontal disease—gum inflammation and infection—as a serious problem in children and teenagers. It is a leading cause of early loss of teeth.

PLEASE NOTE: Now that you have a grasp of how to recognize and manage teething and toothaches, it would be extremely helpful for you to go back to the Quick Reference With the Steps in Detail and review it carefully. The more familiar you are with that material, the more useful it will be to you when you need it.

QUICK REFERENCE

Urinary Tract Infections

Suspect urinary tract infection (bladder or kidney infection) if an infant or toddler shows one or more of the following symptoms:

▶ **UNEXPLAINED HIGH FEVERS,** with or without vomiting and/or diarrhea.

▶ **CRYING WHEN HE URINATES.**

▶ **FOUL-SMELLING URINE.**

▶ **BLOOD ON HER WET DIAPER.**

▶ **UNEXPLAINED WEIGHT LOSS OR POOR WEIGHT GAIN.**

▶ **UNEXPLAINED REPEATED DAYTIME AND NIGHTTIME CRYING.**

Suspect urinary tract infection in preschool and older children, as well as adolescents, who have one or more of the following symptoms:

▶ **PAIN OR BURNING WITH URINATION.**

485

RECOGNIZING
AND
MANAGING
COMMON
SYMPTOMS
AND ILLNESSES

URINATING MORE OFTEN THAN USUAL, ESPECIALLY OF SMALL AMOUNTS OF URINE.

LOWER ABDOMINAL PAIN, SIDE OR BACK PAIN.

DAYTIME AND NIGHTTIME WETTING "ACCIDENTS" AFTER BEING COMPLETELY TOILET-TRAINED.

BLOOD IN THE URINE.

CLOUDY, FOUL-SMELLING URINE.

REFUSING TO URINATE OR BEING UNABLE TO START TO URINATE, EVEN WITH A FULL BLADDER.

FEVER WITH ANY OF THE ABOVE SYMPTOMS.

If you suspect your youngster might have a urinary tract infection, call the doctor for an appointment within the next day or two.
You can help your child feel more comfortable while you wait for the appointment by:

ENCOURAGING THE YOUNGSTER TO DRINK MORE LIQUIDS THAN USUAL.

HAVING THE YOUNGSTER SIT IN A TUB OF PLEASANTLY WARM WATER AND HAVING HER URINATE IN THE TUB—IF HER PAIN IS SEVERE OR QUITE UNPLEASANT.

Urinary Tract Infection: What You Should Know

Urinary tract infection—infection of the bladder and/or kidneys—is more common in infants and children than most people believe. It is also more difficult to recognize in infants and very young children than it is in older children and adolescents. Urinary tract infection, however, is a potentially serious problem—if left unrecognized and untreated—since a youngster can suffer serious kidney damage. Because of this, it is imperative that a youngster with possible urinary infection be seen by his or her doctor.

486

ILLNESS IN
INFANTS,
CHILDREN,
AND
ADOLESCENTS

Girls are more likely to have urinary infections than boys (at any age), and many girls have repeated infections during childhood. Others have their first infections in adolescence or adulthood, especially after they become sexually active. Most urinary infections in girls occur because of their anatomy—the urethra (the opening from the bladder to the outside of the body) is short and straight, allowing bacteria from the genitals to easily enter the bladder.

Urinary tract infection is detected using a laboratory test called a urine analysis (the urine is studied in the laboratory with several chemical tests, and a drop is looked at under the microscope for signs of infection) *and* with a urine culture (a few drops of urine are mixed with a solution or gel, then kept warm for a day or two to see whether bacteria grow in the laboratory). If only a urine analysis is used, some children will be incorrectly diagnosed as having infection, while real infection in some others will go undetected. For this reason, it is important that a youngster who is suspected of having urinary infection have a urine culture.

Urinary Tract Infection: Signs and Symptoms

When an infant or child has an urinary tract infection, inflammation of the bladder and urethra usually leads to pain or discomfort when urinating. The youngster usually urinates more often than usual, and may cry or complain before, during, or after emptying his or her bladder. With young infants, you may not recognize these symptoms, since they wear diapers (so you don't see them urinate), but they cry or fuss a great deal more than usual. You might instead be concerned about the fever, vomiting, or diarrhea that often accompanies the infection. Some young infants with a urinary infection—which goes undetected—eat poorly, and/or do not gain weight as expected.

An older child can usually tell you that it hurts when she goes to the bathroom. In fact, her discomfort might be so severe that she even refuses to urinate—when you know she has a full bladder! You might notice strong, cloudy, or even blood-tinged urine, and the youngster might have a fever, and complain of pain in the lower part of the abdomen.

Although most infants and children with a urinary tract infection have some symptoms with a first time or new infection, some who have recurring infection show little or no outward sign of the problem. Their urine usually contains bacteria (causing the infection), but few if any pus cells (which signal the inflammation that usually leads to the symptoms of infection). For this reason, it is important that youngsters who have had one or more urinary tract infections in the past be closely monitored by you and the doctor for repeated infection that could go unnoticed (and lead to serious kidney damage over months or years).

487

RECOGNIZING
AND
MANAGING
COMMON
SYMPTOMS
AND ILLNESSES

Other Possible Causes of Genital and Bladder Irritation

Although a urinary tract infection is a very common problem, other problems can cause similar symptoms—especially in girls. *Vulvovaginitis*—inflammation and irritation of the external genitals (the vulva) and vagina—is a very common cause of pain or discomfort. With this problem, the genitals look very red and irritated, and are tender if you touch them. You might also notice a yellow vaginal discharge or stains in the child's underwear. The most common cause of vulvovaginitis is poor hygiene— a nearly universal problem in young girls who use the bathroom without your help. Wetness and/or contamination of the delicate tissues of the vulva lead to irritation— which then leads to scratching and further irritation. Nylon or other nonabsorbent panties and chafing from clothing that is too tight add to the problem. In older girls, sensitivity to scented or colored toilet tissue, genital deodorants, or sanitary napkins can also cause problems.

Pinworm, a common parasite in young children, can also cause vulvovaginitis, and even a true urinary tract infection, because the female worm carries bacteria from the bowel onto the genitals when she lays her eggs. Check the genitals of a youngster who seems to have pain or discomfort with urination. If she looks red and irritated, have her sit in a tub of lukewarm water (without anything else in the water), and help her gently clean the outer genitals—rubbing very little. You can use petroleum jelly or an ointment like A & D on her irritated genitals to help prevent further inflammation. If her symptoms do not seem to improve in a day or two, be sure to have her examined by her doctor.

So-called *bubble bath urethritis* is another common cause of genital irritation and urinary discomfort. While it is most often a problem for girls, because of their delicate genital tissues, it can also occur in young boys. The culprit is bubble bath—or similar additives, including shampoo in some cases—in the bath water. These chemicals irritate the genital tissues and urethra, leading to pain or burning with urination. The treatment is simple—avoidance of *all* additives in a youngster's bath water, or substituting showers for baths.

Urinary Tract Infection: What to Expect

Although urinary tract infection is quite common in children, especially girls, other problems have signs and symptoms that can be similar. Because of this, your doctor will examine your youngster's genitals and abdomen carefully. Then the doctor will want to perform a urine analysis if he or she suspects an infection and also culture the

488

ILLNESS IN
INFANTS,
CHILDREN,
AND
ADOLESCENTS

urine to see whether bacteria will grow in the laboratory. If infection is found, the youngster will be treated with an antibiotic for ten to fourteen days, then another urine sample will be cultured to make sure the infection was successfully treated.

After the infection has been successfully treated, the doctor will usually want to culture the youngster's urine every few months, even if there are no further symptoms, to be sure an unrecognized infection has not appeared.

Girls who have their first urinary infection before the age of one year and boys at any age who experience a urinary tract infection sometimes have abnormalities of the urinary tract (urethra, bladder, ureters, and kidneys). For this reason, the doctor will want to rule out possible urinary tract abnormalities if your child fits the above criteria *or* if he or she has recurrent urinary tract infections. This usually will include either an ultrasound examination or X ray of the kidneys and a special X-ray examination of the bladder after the infection is treated. (The X rays of the kidneys involve the injection of a special "dye"—contrast material—into a vein, and those of the bladder require that the "dye" be put into the bladder using a small plastic catheter and that a series of X-ray pictures then be taken.) Be sure you ask the doctor about these tests in detail if they are recommended for your youngster.

THE DONT'S

Don't overlook the signs and symptoms of possible urinary tract infection in your infant or toddler, child, or teenager. Urinary tract infection is a potentially serious problem that must be carefully treated if kidney damage is to be prevented in the future.

Don't underestimate the importance of finishing any medication prescribed by your doctor to treat urinary infection or fail to return for repeat examination and urine testing. Children often feel much better after a day or two of medication, but their infections can continue to smolder for much longer. You will want to do all you can to prevent long-term kidney damage as a result of unrecognized urinary tract infection.

PLEASE NOTE: Now that you have a grasp of how to recognize and manage urinary tract infections, it would be extremely helpful for you to go back to the Quick Reference and review it carefully. The more familiar you are with that material, the more useful it will be to you when you need it.

489

RECOGNIZING
AND
MANAGING
COMMON
SYMPTOMS
AND ILLNESSES

QUICK REFERENCE

Vomiting

The treatment for vomiting is based on resting your youngster's stomach:

▶ **GIVE HIM *NOTHING* TO EAT OR DRINK FOR ONE TO TWO HOURS AFTER HE VOMITS.** You can allow an older child to rinse his mouth with water, but tell him not to swallow it.

▶ **AT FIRST, OFFER HER SIPS (A TEASPOON OR TWO) OF PLAIN WATER, GATORADE, "FLAT" SODA, OR FRUIT JUICE EVERY TEN TO FIFTEEN MINUTES FOR AN HOUR OR SO, OR ALLOW AN OLDER CHILD TO SUCK ON ICE CHIPS.**

▶ **IF HE DOESN'T VOMIT AGAIN, GRADUALLY INCREASE THE AMOUNT OF BLAND LIQUID HE DRINKS EACH TIME.**

▶ **AFTER SEVERAL HOURS, LET HER TRY BLAND SOLID FOOD,** such as crackers, toast, rice, mashed potato, banana, soup, or gelatin.

▶ **AVOID MILK AND MILK PRODUCTS, FATTY OR GREASY FOODS, SPICES, AND "HEAVY" FOODS FOR AT LEAST TWELVE TO TWENTY-FOUR HOURS AFTER THE VOMITING HAS STOPPED OR UNTIL HIS APPETITE HAS RETURNED TO NORMAL.**

▶ **CHOOSE OR SUGGEST FOODS THAT WOULD SOUND APPEALING TO YOU IF YOU HAD AN UPSET STOMACH,** and don't worry if your child eats small amounts of food for several days.

If your small infant spits up frequently but seems otherwise healthy, minor changes in how you feed and handle her may solve the problem:

▶ **TRY TO FEED HIM MORE SLOWLY AND BURP HIM MORE OFTEN THAN BEFORE.**

▶ **DO NOT ALLOW HER TO OVEREAT,** and don't encourage her to take "the last swallow" or "the last bite" if she doesn't want it. Feed her smaller amounts more frequently.

490

ILLNESS IN
INFANTS,
CHILDREN,
AND
ADOLESCENTS

▶ **HANDLE HIM GENTLY FOR THE FIRST HOUR AFTER FEEDINGS.** Don't jostle or bounce the little one around or play roughly with him.

▶ **AVOID FOODS OR DRINKS THAT SEEM TO MAKE THE PROBLEM WORSE.** Juices and acidic foods often make "spitty" babies spit up more.

▶ **TRY POSITIONING HER ON HER ABDOMEN AFTER FEEDING, OR PROP HER SO HER RIGHT SIDE IS DOWN FOR AN HOUR OR SO AFTER SHE EATS.** Avoid placing her on her back, so she doesn't aspirate (inhale) stomach contents if she spits up. While a few babies do better when they are propped up in an infant seat, others spit up more in this position.

Call the doctor or take the youngster to an emergency room for evaluation if there are signs of potentially serious illness or injury:

▶ **THE VOMITUS CONTAINS BLOOD OR DARK MATERIAL THAT LOOKS LIKE COFFEE GROUNDS OR IS YELLOW OR GREEN.**

▶ **SEVERE ABDOMINAL PAIN.**

▶ **SWOLLEN, HARD ABDOMEN THAT IS SORE TO THE TOUCH.**

▶ **SEVERE DIARRHEA, ALONG WITH VOMITING.**

▶ **SIGNS OF DEHYDRATION:** decreased urine production, severe thirst, lethargy or irritability, dry mouth, sunken eyes, or doughy skin.

▶ **REPEATED VOMITING WITH CHANGES IN BEHAVIOR IN A YOUNGSTER WHO IS RECOVERING FROM CHICKENPOX OR A "FLU"-LIKE ILLNESS.**

▶ **PERSISTENT VOMITING IN A VERY YOUNG INFANT.**

▶ **VOMITING MORE THAN ONCE AFTER A HEAD INJURY.**

▶ **VOMITING FOLLOWING AN INJURY TO THE ABDOMEN.**

Contact the doctor for advice and/or an appointment if:

▶ **A VERY YOUNG INFANT HAS REPEATED VOMITING OF MOST OR ALL OF HIS FEEDINGS FOR ONE DAY.**

491

RECOGNIZING
AND
MANAGING
COMMON
SYMPTOMS
AND ILLNESSES

▶ **AN OLDER INFANT, CHILD, OR YOUNGSTER HAS PERSIS-TENT VOMITING,** in spite of attempts to rest his stomach, then feed small amounts of liquids or solids.

▶ **A YOUNGSTER WHO IS VOMITING APPEARS TO BE LOSING WEIGHT.**

▶ **A BABY SPITS UP (REGURGITATES) MORE THAN ONCE OR TWICE A DAY FOR MORE THAN A WEEK,** and changes in handling or positioning don't seem to help.

▶ **A YOUNGSTER HAS REPEATED EPISODES OF VOMITING,** and you cannot identify the reason.

Vomiting: What You Should Know

Vomiting is the forceful throwing up of the stomach contents. It is caused by a reflex that makes the stomach contract (get smaller), then empty itself through the mouth. Vomiting can be a sign of minor illness or dietary indiscretion, or the hallmark of a more serious illness or injury. Some children are prone to vomit with almost any upset, while others seem to have very few experiences with vomiting during childhood.

Young infants tend to vomit more readily than older children. This probably results from immaturity of the stomach and the nervous system, which also plays a role in the reflex that leads to vomiting. For example, almost all infants vomit occasionally without being sick. In most infants, this tendency disappears after the first year or so, although some older youngsters react to many stresses—from eating too much to being frightened—by vomiting. As long as this type of vomiting does not occur frequently (more often than once or twice a week in young infants, or repeatedly in older children), and the youngster seems generally healthy, active, and energetic, you need not worry.

Nausea is the feeling you get right before vomiting—an unpleasant sensation, at best. Infants and young children usually cannot tell you when they are nauseated, because they can't talk or don't know how to describe the feeling. You can, however, often suspect nausea by their behavior. They might become quiet and prefer to lie still, may look pale and drool, swallow a great deal, or retch. They will often refuse to eat anything and sometimes prefer not to drink anything either. In some situations, you might not notice anything unusual before the vomiting occurs, especially in very young infants. (Also, these little ones might seem perfectly normal and hungry right after vomiting.) Older children can tell you they feel "funny" or sick or that they have an upset stomach. In all but a few situations, nausea precedes vomiting by at

492

ILLNESS IN
INFANTS,
CHILDREN,
AND
ADOLESCENTS

least a few minutes. (One note: Nausea does not always end in vomiting and can simply go away.)

Your first concern when your infant or child vomits will be to try to determine what caused the vomiting. Think back about what and how much the youngster ate in the last few hours. Then look for other symptoms that might give you additional clues. Remember that young children often react with their whole bodies to minor illnesses and upsets. In general, you don't need to worry a great deal, unless the vomiting is persistent or the youngster looks very ill, as well.

If vomiting is persistent, it can lead to serious dehydration and abnormalities of the body salts. With pending or present dehydration, the young person is losing not only the liquids that he or she drank, but also vital stomach juices and acid. Because of this, your goal in treatment is to stop the vomiting. After the vomiting has stopped, you can then worry about getting small amounts of liquids and foods into the youngster. At first, then, it is important to offer the youngster only liquids or foods that are easy to digest and do not continue to irritate the stomach.

Let the little one's stomach calm down before you give her something to drink. Then, go slowly, and limit the amounts that a youngster drinks and eats for the first few hours after she vomits. Gradually increase the amount of food you offer the youngster as soon as it seems the youngster is better and no longer vomiting. Your judgment will be excellent if you think about what would taste good and stay down if you put yourself in the youngster's place and remember how *you* feel when you have an upset stomach.

It is important to distinguish between true vomiting and *"spitting up,"* which is regurgitation of small amounts of the stomach contents. Spitting up is very common in young infants, who spend much of their time lying down. Occasional spitting up during the first four to six months of life in a baby who is otherwise normal should not cause you undue worry. If, however, the baby looks sick and begins spitting up, consider it one of the symptoms of an illness. If her other symptoms suggest serious illness, contact your doctor.

Common Causes of Vomiting

Dietary indiscretion is probably the most common cause of vomiting, regardless of a youngster's age. Infants may occasionally drink too much (of breast milk, formula, or fruit juice), and children and older youngsters often eat too much (of favorite foods, new foods, or "junk" foods)—especially when their routines are different from the usual. This may lead to only an "upset stomach," but some youngsters will vomit once or twice in order to rid the stomach of the upsetting foods. Certain children are sensitive to some foods, and vomiting is the body's own way of preventing further illness. For example, a nine-month-old who is allergic to cow's milk might vomit or spit up cow's milk if it is given to him or her. An older youngster who cannot digest

493

RECOGNIZING
AND
MANAGING
COMMON
SYMPTOMS
AND ILLNESSES

strawberries might complain of a stomachache after eating strawberries and vomit a short time later. Usually, the young person feels much better after vomiting and is ready to eat and drink again in a matter of hours.

Mild to moderate viral intestinal infections can also cause vomiting—with or without diarrhea, as well. With so-called stomach flu, the child feels queasy and nauseated and usually vomits several times. He or she has little or no appetite. You might notice a mild to moderate fever and some diarrhea, depending on where in the digestive tract the virus is most active. Many viral intestinal infections can also cause mild muscle aching, mild abdominal pain, and even rashes. These viral infections usually run their course in one to three days, without any particular treatment—other than letting the digestive system rest and preventing dehydration. Intestinal viruses are potentially more serious in young infants and toddlers than in older youngsters—because the risk of dehydration is greater with smaller children.

Other infections can also lead to vomiting, especially in infants and young children. For example, *middle-ear infection* (otitis media) is a notorious culprit in causing vomiting in some children. Here vomiting might result from dizziness or upset equilibrium due to the increased pressure inside the middle ear, or from the pain of the earache. Youngsters with *respiratory infections* (such as a cold or croup) often vomit after coughing or because mucus that they swallow irritates the stomach. Some children with *urinary tract infections* have fever and vomiting as their only symptoms.

Motion sickness is quite common in preschoolers and older children. Vomiting might be your first clue that the youngster is bothered by riding in the car. Most youngsters who suffer from motion sickness feel better if they can see outside the car and learn to look at things far in the distance. If your youngster has frequent and severe trouble with motion sickness, contact your doctor for advice about medications that can be used to help with this problem.

Poisoning is probably the cause of more vomiting in toddlers, children, and teenagers than people recognize. So-called *food poisoning* can result from eating or drinking food that is clearly spoiled or poorly handled and stored. Be suspicious if vomiting follows a large party where food was not refrigerated for a long period of time before it was served or if several people became ill at the same time. Most food poisoning is caused by a toxic material produced in spoiled food rather than an actual infection. Severe vomiting, diarrhea, and abdominal cramping that last for several hours are common. Food poisoning resulting from actual bacterial infection usually causes more diarrhea than vomiting and lasts for several days.

Toddlers and young children frequently "taste" or eat nonfood objects, some of which are poisonous. Even those things that are not serious poisons often cause stomach upset and vomiting. Household materials and plants commonly cause vomiting, which might be your first clue that the little one ate something he or she shouldn't have. If you suspect poisoning as a cause of vomiting, contact your local poison control center, your doctor, or an emergency room for advice. If you find an empty or partially empty container, always take it with you to the emergency room. (For more information on poisoning, review Chapter 10.)

494

ILLNESS IN
INFANTS,
CHILDREN,
AND
ADOLESCENTS

Certain medications cause vomiting in some youngsters. Aspirin and aspirin substitutes, drugs used to treat asthma, and certain antibiotics can be the offenders in some youngsters. If you suspect a medication as the cause of a child's vomiting, avoid using that medicine if you can. However, contact your doctor immediately for advice before stopping prescribed medication, so substitution can be made.

Vomiting as a Sign of Serious Illness

Youngsters with *intestinal obstruction* (blockage of the intestine) vomit because nothing can pass the blocked area. The intestines, which normally contract to push digesting material through the digestive tract, stop working, and food, liquid, and bile back up into the stomach. Suspect intestinal obstruction in a child who vomits yellow or green liquid; has a painful, distended abdomen; and seems generally sick. Contact your doctor or take the youngster to an emergency room if you suspect this problem.

Meningitis (infection of the coverings of the brain and spinal cord) and *encephalitis* (infection and inflammation of the brain itself) often have vomiting as one of their symptoms. Here vomiting results from irritation of the center in the brain that controls or initiates vomiting. This irritation occurs because of increased pressure or inflammation in that area of the brain. Contact your doctor immediately or go to an emergency room if your child has signs and symptoms of meningitis or encephalitis: fever, headache, stiff neck, lethargy or extreme irritability, shock, or bulging fontanel (soft spot) in a young infant. (Review Chapter 13 for more information about these very serious infections.)

Children with *sepsis* (overwhelming infection) often vomit several times. Young infants with sepsis may also spit up rather than vomit forcefully. Suspect sepsis in a child who is vomiting if he or she is also lethargic, has a high fever, seems dazed or "out of it," and has very poor color. Young infants with sepsis frequently do not have a fever but show other signs of being seriously sick and refuse feedings. Contact your doctor immediately, or go to an emergency room if you suspect overwhelming infection. (Review Chapter 13 for more information about sepsis.)

Hepatitis is inflammation and infection of the liver (usually caused by a virus) and has as one of its symptoms prolonged vomiting. At first, the youngster looks as if he has "intestinal flu," but the vomiting and lack of appetite persist for longer than two or three days. He is tired, has little or no appetite, and may complain of vague abdominal pain, especially high in the right side of the abdomen. The urine looks dark brown, and the youngster may develop jaundice (yellow color of the skin and of the white part of the eyes). His bowel movements may be lighter in color than usual or even almost white. Although there is no specific treatment for this very contagious infection (except rest, not taking any medications that can further inflame the liver, and maintaining good nutrition), it is important that it be recognized, so other people can be protected from getting it.

495

RECOGNIZING
AND
MANAGING
COMMON
SYMPTOMS
AND ILLNESSES

Reye syndrome is a life-threatening condition in which swelling of the brain, along with damage to the liver and sometimes the kidneys, occurs—during the recovery stages of certain viral illnesses. Suspect this problem in a youngster who develops severe vomiting during the recovery stages of chickenpox or influenza and shows increasing sleepiness or lethargy, irritability, and behavior changes. Contact your doctor *immediately* or go to an emergency room if these symptoms develop.

Vomiting of blood most often signals a serious problem. Bleeding in the stomach can result from irritation and inflammation due to a viral infection, medication use (aspirin is a common culprit), or an ulcer. Always contact your doctor if you notice more than a few flecks of blood in vomited material. (The exception here is if a youngster vomits blood after having a nosebleed. He or she may have swallowed blood, then vomited it.) Vomited material that looks like *"coffee grounds"* usually contains blood that was in the stomach long enough for the stomach acid to chemically change it. Contact your doctor or go to an emergency room if a youngster vomits what looks like "coffee grounds" material and has not had a nosebleed.

Vomiting and Injury

Youngsters who have suffered a serious *head injury* often vomit as a result of it. While one episode of vomiting right after the injury in a child *who did not lose consciousness* does not signify serious injury, repeated vomiting usually indicates at least mild to moderate brain injury. If the youngster *vomits more than once*, contact your doctor for advice, or go to an emergency room. (For more information on head injury, see Chapter 16.)

Vomiting after an *injury to the abdomen* can also signal serious internal injury. Here again, a single episode of vomiting immediately after the injury may mean nothing more than that the youngster was hit in the stomach. However, repeated vomiting can indicate a deeper, more serious injury to one or more of the abdominal organs. Have the youngster evaluated by your doctor or in an emergency room *without delay*. (See Chapter 16 for more information about abdominal injury.)

Pyloric Stenosis: A Problem of Early Infancy

Congenital hypertrophic pyloric stenosis is the formidable name for a rather common problem of early infancy, which causes increasingly severe vomiting in the first few weeks or months of life. In this condition, the muscle that surrounds the outlet of the stomach (the pylorus) progressively enlarges (hypertrophies), causing blockage of the stomach outlet. In other words, as the muscle enlarges, the narrowing (stenosis) of the stomach outlet gets worse. Thereby, less and less milk can empty from the stomach,

496

ILLNESS IN
INFANTS,
CHILDREN,
AND
ADOLESCENTS

and the infant vomits. This condition is thought to be present at birth (is congenital) and worsens over the next few weeks or months after birth.

Pyloric stenosis is slightly more common in boys than in girls and tends to run in families. It is more common in firstborn children but can certainly affect later children. Most often, the baby seems perfectly fine for several weeks after birth, then begins to vomit occasionally. Over the next few days or weeks, vomiting becomes more frequent and more severe. Vomiting occurs shortly after feedings, or even during feedings, and shoots like a projectile (the vomited milk forcefully shoots a distance in the air). The baby digests less and less milk and may not gain weight or may even lose weight. Throughout all of this, the little one *seems perfectly healthy* and is ravenously hungry right after vomiting. You may notice that the baby has very few bowel movements (because there is little food to digest). If the vomiting continues without the baby's being treated, he will become malnourished and dehydrated (both very serious problems and potentially life-threatening).

Contact your doctor if your baby has increasing problems with vomiting in the first few weeks or months of life. The doctor will want to examine the infant and feel her abdomen carefully to detect a small, "olivelike" mass, which is the overgrown pyloric muscle. If he or she suspects this problem but cannot feel the lump, your baby may need an X ray of the stomach (an upper GI [gastrointestinal] series, in which the radiologist will have the baby drink barium to outline the stomach and pylorus).

If your baby has pyloric stenosis, he will need a simple operation to correct the problem. If he is dehydrated or has a disturbance of his body acids and salts because of the vomiting, the doctor will want to give him fluids intravenously (through a vein) in the hospital before the surgery is performed. Although there are risks associated with every surgical procedure, even the simplest one, almost all babies do well with this surgery and recover very quickly. They usually leave the hospital within one to two days after the surgery and have few if any further problems with vomiting. Recovery from their malnutrition occurs quickly.

The Baby Who Spits Up: Gastroesophageal Reflux

Occasional spitting up is common and normal in early infancy and probably results from overfilling of the baby's immature stomach. The "extra" mouthful of breast milk or formula comes up gently with a burp or when the baby moves around. The baby seems perfectly happy and grows well but is messy! She outgrows this problem after the first twelve months of life—as she matures.

In some infants, the muscle at the top of the stomach (called the gastroesophageal sphincter) is more relaxed than normal. These babies spit up often and may lose significant amounts of the breast milk or formula they drink. This problem is called *gastroesophageal reflux* (regurgitation through the gastroesophageal sphincter). The

497

RECOGNIZING
AND
MANAGING
COMMON
SYMPTOMS
AND ILLNESSES

spitting up lasts until the baby is around a year old—when he begins to spend most of his time in an upright position. Almost all babies outgrow this problem, but a few need special medical attention. If you think your baby is spitting up excessively, contact your doctor for an evaluation and advice.

In some babies, spitting up seems to be related, at least in part, to what they drink. Formula-fed babies who spit up are often tried on different formulas to see if they do a bit better. Mothers of breast-fed babies can sometimes control the spitting up by adjusting their own diets somewhat. Parents often notice that their babies spit up more when they are in certain positions or if they are unusually active right after eating. In some babies, thickening feedings with rice cereal helps, and these little ones do better when they begin to eat more solid foods. In some infants with gastroesophageal reflux, medications that increase the movement of food from the stomach into the intestines are very helpful.

While most babies with so-called GE reflux do very well, a few suffer complications of the problem. These can include poor weight gain and growth; aspiration pneumonia (lung inflammation due to inhaling the regurgitated stomach contents); wheezing because of inhaling the stomach material; irritation and inflammation of the lower end of the esophagus; and even infant apnea (breathing stoppage because of inhaling the stomach contents). In these babies, the doctor will want to do special studies to find out how severe the reflux is and will recommend steps for you to take to lessen the problem. In a few infants, stomach surgery is needed to correct the problem.

Bulimia: A Special Consideration in Teenagers

With today's emphasis on thinness equaling attractiveness, vomiting to control weight gain (called *bulimia*) has emerged as a serious health problem in certain teenagers (and adults). Bulimia is thought to be one aspect of the spectrum of eating disorders and may be associated with *anorexia nervosa* (a condition in which a young person voluntarily starves to control his or her weight).

Anorexia nervosa is a complicated eating disorder that can lead to death or permanent physical damage if it is not recognized and treated by professionals who are experienced with this problem. It usually appears in teenagers, most often girls, who feel they are not quite thin enough. It may follow an episode of dieting that is carried to extremes— even to the point where the young person is literally starving to death. Suspect this problem if your youngster continues to diet and lose weight, even after he or she is very thin and literally emaciated. Girls with anorexia nervosa stop having menstrual periods, lose their hair, feel cold all the time, and become more and more listless and weak. They also try to hide the problem from parents, peers, and professionals. If you suspect anorexia nervosa, get medical help *immediately*. Do not try to treat it yourself without professional assistance. It often requires a period of hospitalization and forced feeding to literally save the youngster's life, along with psychiatric therapy.

498

ILLNESS IN
INFANTS,
CHILDREN,
AND
ADOLESCENTS

Bulimia (voluntary vomiting) has become a dangerous way for some girls with eating disorders to control their weight. Girls with this problem are usually older, sometimes in their late teens or early adulthood, and are generally compulsive overeaters. They "binge" on food, then—in order to control their weight—vomit and/or use laxatives to purge themselves of the food. As they learn that this is a successful way to stay thin—it becomes a life-threatening habit. Bulimia is especially common in college students, as well as in athletes who must control their weight in order to compete.

If a young person seems to lose an undue amount of weight, even if you see him or her eating what seems to be a normal or excessive amount of foods, and otherwise has no symptoms of another serious illness (such as fever, excessive urination, tremors, or excessive sweating), suspect bulimia or laxative abuse. Most often, the vomiting is not apparent to anyone else, and the youngster will deny it or claim to be ill if you detect an episode of vomiting. Like the starvation form of anorexia nervosa, bulimia requires prompt medical and psychiatric treatment. As bulimia, anorexia nervosa, and other eating disorders have become more and more known to professionals and the public, eating-disorders programs have been developed across the country to help youngsters with these problems. If there is no program in your area, ask your local hospital information service or local medical society about doctor(s) or psychiatrist(s) in the area who have special interest and expertise in eating disorders.

Important: Unexplained weight loss can also be a sign of potentially serious diseases (hyperthyroidism, diabetes, cancer, or others). Whether you suspect a serious eating disorder or a potentially serious illness, call the doctor to schedule the earliest possible appointment for the young person to have a complete physical examination. The sooner any of these problems is recognized, the better the odds are that the youngster can be successfully treated.

THE DON'TS

Don't continue to feed a youngster who is vomiting because you are afraid he will starve or become dehydrated. Wait for a few hours after he has vomited, then offer him small amounts of liquids.

Don't overreact if a baby vomits occasionally or spits up once in a while. All babies vomit or spit up occasionally, because their stomachs are immature or they overeat.

Don't hesitate to contact your doctor if your youngster has persistent vomiting—in spite of your attempts to stop it.

Don't delay in getting medical help (call the doctor or go to the emergency room) if your vomiting youngster shows signs of dehydration: dry mouth, excessive thirst, decreased urine production, doughy skin, sunken eyes, or weakness and sleepiness. Dehydration requires prompt medical treatment, usually in a hospital.

Don't delay in calling your doctor or taking a baby or child who is vomiting to an emergency room if he or she shows signs of serious illness. Blood in the vomited material, yellow or green vomit, high fever, lethargy, headache, changes in behavior, or severe diarrhea along with the vomiting can be signs of a very serious illness and require immediate professional evaluation.

Don't overlook vomiting as a signal to get medical help in a youngster who has had a head injury or an injury to the abdomen. Vomiting more than once after a head or abdominal injury can be a sign of serious brain injury or swelling or of damage to the internal organs.

Don't hesitate to contact your doctor if your young infant seems to spit up excessively. While spitting up occasionally is normal, babies who spit up a great deal may have more serious underlying problems.

Don't try to treat your youngster with suspected anorexia nervosa, bulimia, or another eating disorder without professional assistance. These are life-threatening problems that require expert treatment.

PLEASE NOTE: Now that you have a grasp of how to recognize and manage vomiting, it would be extremely helpful for you to go back to the Quick Reference and review it carefully. The more familiar you are with that material, the more useful it will be to you when you need it.

499

RECOGNIZING
AND
MANAGING
COMMON
SYMPTOMS
AND ILLNESSES

S E C T I O N 4

Injuries in Childhood and Adolescence

Every single child learns to *play* as she grows older (unless, of course, the child has such severe physical disabilities that she can only remain immobile). Whether you have a toddler, preschool-aged child, school-aged child, or teenager—she will be involved in playing.

From swings to bicycles to organized sports—young people experience injuries. Most injuries, of course, are quite minor and can be cared for at home. Others will need medical evaluation and treatment. At times, a young person may experience a serious or potentially serious injury that would need intensive medical or surgical care.

Today in the United States more than 33 million young people aged five to thirteen are involved in sports activities. That doesn't even include those who play at recess, in unorganized sports activities after school, at parks, in backyards, or in the streets. That means that most of the children in this country are playing a sport or involved in some activity where injury can easily occur.

Section 4 (Chapters 15, 16, and 17) gives you the information you need to recognize serious or potentially serious injuries and take appropriate action, as well as how to treat more common and minor injuries at home. Again, the more you know, the better equipped you are to help the youngster and guarantee proper medical intervention when needed.

CHAPTER 15

How to Evaluate
Your Injured Child

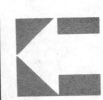

EMERGENCY QUICK REFERENCE

With a Step-by-Step Formula

Assessing Injury

If the Youngster Is Unconscious

▶ ALWAYS ASSUME A HEAD, NECK, OR BACK INJURY IS POSSIBLE AND MOVE THE YOUNGSTER ONLY IF YOU HAVE NO OTHER CHOICE; THEN DO SO WITH THE GREATEST OF CARE. REMEMBER TO SUPPORT THE HEAD AND NECK IF ANY MOVEMENT IS NECESSARY.

▶ DETERMINE WHETHER THE YOUNGSTER IS BREATHING.

- If she *is breathing*, go on to the next step, but ensure an open airway (and periodically recheck to see whether the youngster is still breathing).

503

- If she *is not breathing*, open the airway carefully (in case there is a head, neck, or back injury) and begin rescue breathing. (If you are unable to remember the details of performing rescue breathing, turn to the Emergency Quick Reference on page 113, entitled "A Review of the Six Steps of CPR.") Have someone else call the paramedics while you treat the child. If no one is with you, continue treating the child while you periodically shout for help. When help arrives, have that person call the paramedics.

▶ **CHECK FOR A PULSE (HEART FUNCTION).**

- If there *is a pulse*, continue rescue breathing. Check for a pulse periodically. If at any point the pulse stops, begin full CPR (rescue breathing with chest compressions). (If you are certified in CPR and are unable to remember the details of the procedure, turn to the Emergency Quick Reference on page 113, entitled "A Review of the Six Steps of CPR.")

- If there *is no pulse*, begin full CPR.

- If there are other people who can assist you, direct them in assessing and treating other injuries or problems. (For example, control bleeding, treat shock, treat any other injuries, such as splint or immobilize fractures or dislocations.)

If the Youngster Is Conscious but Found Lying Down (Since He Is Conscious, You Also Know He Is Breathing and His Heart Is Functioning)

▶ **TELL HIM NOT TO MOVE AT ALL UNTIL YOU CAN DETERMINE WHAT (IF ANY) INJURIES HE HAS SUSTAINED.**

▶ **ASK QUESTIONS AS YOU VISUALLY EVALUATE THE YOUNGSTER'S STATUS AND NOTE ANY INJURIES:**

- Do you remember what happened?

- Where are you?

- How do you feel?

- Do you hurt anywhere?

- Does your head, neck, or back hurt or feel different or funny?

- Is there tingling or a numb feeling in your arm(s), leg(s), or on one side of your body?

- Can you wiggle your toes for me?

- Can you move your right leg? How about your left leg?

- Can you wiggle your fingers for me?

- Can you move your right arm? How about your left arm?

- Are you nauseated (do you feel sick to your stomach), dizzy, or light-headed?

- Is your vision blurry?

- Do you have any abdominal pain? (Does your stomach ache?)

- Are you having any trouble breathing?

▶ **IF YOU OBSERVE ANY OF THE SIGNS LISTED BELOW, DO NOT MOVE THE YOUNGSTER. INSTEAD, HAVE SOMEONE ELSE CALL THE PARAMEDICS WHILE YOU TREAT THE CHILD.** IF NO ONE IS WITH YOU, CONTINUE TREATING THE CHILD WHILE YOU PERIODICALLY SHOUT FOR HELP. WHEN HELP ARRIVES, HAVE THAT PERSON CALL THE PARAMEDICS.

- There is any numbness or tingling in the leg(s), the arm(s), or on one side of the body.

- The youngster is unable to wiggle his toes or fingers or move his leg(s) or arm(s).

- She has head, neck, or back pain.

- There is any possibility of a head, neck, or back injury or you are unsure about what injuries exist.

- She has multiple injuries (fractures, possible internal bleeding, severe external bleeding, and so on).

▶ **IF THE YOUNGSTER DOES NOT HAVE A HEAD, NECK, OR BACK INJURY OR OBVIOUS MULTIPLE INJURIES, THEN TRY TO DETERMINE WHETHER THERE ARE OTHER DEEP INJURIES. IF SO, HAVE SOMEONE CALL THE PARAMEDICS.**

- Watch the youngster's chest move if there is any difficulty breathing. Does it move normally when breathing, or does it collapse in on one side or area with breathing?

- Is there any pain in the abdomen or any soreness when you touch an area of the abdomen, chest, pelvis, and so forth?

▶ **MANAGE WHAT INJURIES YOU CAN WHILE WAITING FOR THE PARAMEDICS.**

- Control any bleeding.

- Cover the youngster with a blanket or coat, but do not elevate either his head or feet if there is any possibility of a head, neck, or back injury or multiple injuries.

If There Are No Head, Back, or Neck Injuries and You Are Quite Sure There Are No Other Deep Injuries, Then Examine the Youngster Carefully to See What Injuries Do Exist

▶ **START WITH THE HEAD AND WORK TOWARD THE TOES—LOOKING CAREFULLY FOR SIGNS OF INJURY.**

▶ **IN SOME SITUATIONS, YOU'LL NEED TO "FEEL" AS WELL AS LOOK FOR INJURIES. BE A DETECTIVE.**

▶ **LOOK FOR BRUISES, SCRAPES, CUTS, AND SWELLING. CHECK FOR ANY DEFORMITY OR ABNORMAL POSITION (OF AN ARM, FOR EXAMPLE). ASK THE YOUNGSTER WHETHER SHE FEELS PAIN (IF SHE CAN TALK) AS YOU FEEL DIFFERENT AREAS AND PARTS OF HER BODY, OR WATCH THE REACTIONS OF A YOUNG, NONVERBAL CHILD AS YOU TOUCH OR MOVE PARTS OF THE BODY.**

▶ **THE FOLLOWING LIST INCLUDES SOME OF THE LESS OBVIOUS PROBLEMS TO LOOK FOR. CALL YOUR DOCTOR FOR ADVICE IF YOU FIND ANY OF THESE:**

- Unequal pupils of the eyes or eyes that don't move together as a unit in *all* directions.

- Clear, watery, or bloody drainage from the ear(s) or nose.

- Mouth or tooth injury; jaw injury.

- Chest or rib injury. (Squeezing the chest gently or having the youngster take a deep breath might lead you to suspect this, since either would hurt.)

- Pain, bruising, or swelling of the abdomen or soreness when you push gently on the abdomen.

- Genital injury. Look at the genitals to see if there is any swelling or bruising, and also check later to see if there is any blood in the urine when this kind of injury is possible.

- Pain, swelling, or tenderness of or around a joint.

Your Role: The Vital Link

For years, it was the general feeling in medicine that *speed alone* in getting someone who was injured or seriously ill to medical care made *all the difference*. Once was the time, for example, when an injured or seriously ill person was merely swept up and swiftly placed in the back of an ambulance or car. This is often called the "scoop and run" principle, and the point was to get the injured or ill person to a hospital as quickly as possible. Little or nothing was done for the person before moving him, because transporting him was *the* main objective.

That's all changed now! As more was learned, it became clear that speed *was* important, but it became just as clear that *managing the injuries (or illness), doing everything possible to stabilize the person, and preparing him or her "at the scene" for safe transport* were also vital. This new information and advances in care led to the establishment of emergency medicine as a medical specialty area, the development of paramedic training programs, and the establishment of trauma centers across the country.

These changes in the last ten years have also included one other very important aspect. It became obvious that you, too, are a vital link in emergency care. Your knowledge, commitment, and awareness may mean the difference between life and death—between a lifelong disability and a minor injury.

Studies have shown that when someone "on the scene" administers proper emergency care and performs CPR (when indicated), not only are lives saved that otherwise would not have been, but overall results are also better.

The links in the emergency chain go like this:

- Someone (you) begins evaluation, management, and necessary treatment when the injury or serious problem occurs and calls or has someone else call the paramedics (or an ambulance if there are no paramedics in the area).

- The paramedics stabilize and treat the injured or seriously ill person and prepare him or her for transport to an emergency-care facility.

● Specially trained emergency medical care professionals begin sophisticated evaluation and treatment at the hospital's emergency room or trauma center.

In order for this system to work, each of us needs to know as much as we can about what steps to take (and what not to do) when a youngster (or adult) experiences injury or another serious medical problem. Taking a CPR certification course (and a first aid class), as well as learning the basic guidelines for evaluating, managing, and treating a youngster until professional help arrives, is the key to your role.

How important is your role? Every year, more than 100,000 children are seriously crippled by injuries, and another 2 million are temporarily incapacitated. "Accidents" in the home account for some 21 million injuries each year (involving both children and adults). And one-half of all deaths in the childhood years to age fourteen are the result of trauma (injury). Some statistics show that an injury occurs in this country every three seconds. Therefore, learning what to do and what not to do when an infant, child, or youngster (or adult) experiences an injury is vital.

Evaluating Your Injured Child: What You Should Know

Injuries in children and teenagers can range from the very minor to the potentially serious or even life-threatening. It is vital, then, that you be able to rapidly (but carefully) evaluate the extent of an injury or injuries and determine the need for and type of medical care required.

As always, the only way to properly and quickly evaluate a youngster is to stay calm and proceed in an established, *step-by-step* manner. In this way, you "train" yourself to respond in a specific way when a young person (or adult) is injured.

The most important aspect of injury *assessment* and *treatment* is this: do *not* move the youngster or allow the youngster to move (at all) until you have determined the extent and possible types of injuries that may have occurred. There are *only two exceptions* to this rule.

First of all, if you must perform CPR (the youngster is not breathing and/or has no heart function), then you have no choice but to move her. Second, if leaving the young person where he is would threaten his life or put him in continued danger (for example, he is imminently threatened by fire, water, being hit by a car, truck, train, or falling debris), then you must take the risk of moving him, knowing permanent injury may occur. The reason you do not move the youngster (unless absolutely necessary) is because there is always a possibility that the youngster has sustained a head, neck, or back injury. With some injuries, the slightest movement might mean the difference between a treatable injury and a lifelong disability (as discussed in detail in Chapter 16).

Interestingly, people are more than likely to remember not to move older children and teenagers (because of their size) but totally forget about this vital safety precaution when it comes to infants, toddlers, and small children. Because of these little ones' small size, parents and others quickly pick up an injured infant, toddler, or small child without thinking about potential head, neck, or back injuries. If a small, "portable" child is injured and you are tempted to scoop him up and rush to an emergency room, STOP! Leave him lying down, and check to see whether there might be a head, neck, or back injury. Assume this is likely if the little one fell from a high place, or is unconscious, or is not moving part(s) or area(s) of her body, or does not seem to "feel" you touching her.

If the little child is moving around wildly, or will move around when you ask her to do so, then it is probably safe to pick her up. However, do this carefully. Support the head, neck, and back, and try to keep them still during any movement.

Whenever you *must* move an injured older youngster—do so with the greatest care, as well. Always assume there could be a head, neck, or back injury, and try to protect these areas from *any* movement. The more people who can help you move the youngster, the safer the move will usually be. Try to move the youngster *as a unit*. Support the head and neck (try to keep them in the same position in which you found them), and support the legs and arms so they do not flop around. In this way, you give the young person the best chance of not furthering the extent of his or her injuries.

Injury Assessment: Why Use a Step-by-Step Formula?

Assessment of injuries should always be approached in a systematic way. It is essentially a ruling-out process. You start by looking for the most serious problems first and progressing down to the least serious ones. Again, do not move the youngster unless you have no other choice. The best and easiest way to remember the injury-assessment process is to think from "serious to minor" and from "head to toe." Here's the order of assessment and treatment:

- Is there or do you suspect a head, neck, or back injury?

- Is the youngster unconscious?

- Is the youngster breathing?

- Is the heart functioning?

- Is there any serious external bleeding?

- Are there possible internal injuries (or bleeding)?

- Is the youngster in shock?

- Are there any other obvious injuries (fractured leg(s), large gash on the head, bruise on the abdomen, and so on)?

- Are there any not-so-obvious injuries?

Whether a youngster falls down a short stairway or is hit by a car—the assessment steps remain the same. The reason for this is very logical, since the most serious or potentially life-threatening problems must be identified and treated first.

Therefore, at each step in the process, an assessment must be made and/or action taken. That's why it's important to memorize the step-by-step assessment formula, as well as what action to take if the youngster has (or does not have) that specific problem.

THE DON'TS

Don't move a youngster if you have any reason to believe there could be a head, neck, or back injury, except when you have no other choice (as discussed). This goes for infants and small children, as well as for larger children and teenagers.

Don't forget to look for serious hidden injuries (abdomen, chest, and so on). Remember, what you observe "visually" may not always tell you the whole story and the severity of the situation.

PLEASE NOTE: Now that you have a grasp of how to recognize and manage injury, it would be extremely helpful for you to go back to the Emergency Quick Reference With a Step-by-Step Formula and review it carefully. The more familiar you are with that material, the more useful it will be to you when you need it.

C H A P T E R 16

Recognizing and Managing Serious or Potentially Serious Injuries

Included in this chapter is information on how to recognize and manage the serious or potentially serious injuries listed below. The page numbers in parentheses indicate where the Emergency Quick Reference for each type of injury can be found.

513

RECOGNIZING
AND
MANAGING
SERIOUS OR
POTENTIALLY
SERIOUS
INJURIES

EMERGENCY QUICK REFERENCE

With the Steps in Detail

Abdominal Injuries

▶ **ALWAYS CONSIDER THE POSSIBILITY OF AN ABDOMINAL INJURY IF A YOUNGSTER WHO HAS MULTIPLE INJURIES BUT NO OBVIOUS SEVERE BLEEDING SHOWS SIGNS AND SYMPTOMS OF SHOCK:** EXTREME PALENESS; COOL, CLAMMY SKIN; EXTREME THIRST; A WEAK, RAPID PULSE; POOR CIRCULATION IN THE SKIN; FAINT-NESS OR UNCONSCIOUSNESS.

- Have the youngster lie down (if he is not already lying down) and try to keep him calm.

- Elevate his feet ten to twelve inches and cover him with a blanket if you can.

- Check again for any obvious bleeding and control it with direct pressure.

- While you treat the child, have someone else call the paramedics or an ambulance to transport the young person to an emergency room. If no one is with you, continue treating the child while you periodically shout for help. When help arrives, have that person call the paramedics or an ambulance.

- While you are waiting for help, watch the youngster closely. If his breathing stops, begin rescue breathing; or begin full CPR (chest compressions with rescue breathing) if his breathing and heart have both stopped. (If you are certified in CPR and are unable to remember the details of the procedure, turn to the Emergency Quick Reference on page 113, entitled "A Review of the Six Steps of CPR.") Continue your efforts until help arrives.

▶ **SUSPECT A POTENTIALLY SERIOUS INTERNAL ABDOMINAL IN-JURY IF A CHILD OR YOUNGSTER HAS SUFFERED A BLOW (FOR EXAMPLE, A FALL ONTO AN OBJECT, A HANDLEBAR INJURY, A KICK TO THE ABDOMEN) AND HAS:**

- Pain in the abdomen.

- Signs and symptoms of shock: extreme paleness; cool, clammy skin; extreme thirst; a weak, rapid pulse; poor circulation in the skin; faintness.

- Vomited more than once.

- A swollen, tender abdomen.

- Blood in the urine.

- A bruised or discolored area on the abdomen.

▶ **IF YOU SUSPECT AN ABDOMINAL INJURY, GET MEDICAL ASSISTANCE AS SOON AS YOU CAN.**

- If the young person is in shock or seems very ill, have someone call the paramedics or an ambulance, or go to a hospital emergency room as soon as possible.

- If the youngster is uncomfortable or in pain but seems stable, promptly call your doctor for advice, or go to an emergency room if you are unable to reach the doctor within thirty minutes.

- Do not give the youngster anything to eat or drink.

▶ **ALWAYS GET MEDICAL HELP IMMEDIATELY IF A YOUNGSTER HAS A PENETRATING INJURY TO THE ABDOMEN (FOR EXAMPLE, A STAB WOUND, A GUNSHOT WOUND TO THE ABDOMEN).**

- Place a clean cloth (or anything else you have available) over the wound and apply pressure to stop bleeding, if there is bleeding.

- Have someone call the paramedics or an ambulance, and get the young person to an emergency room.

Abdominal Injuries: What You Should Know

Injuries to the internal organs of the abdomen are increasingly frequent as children become more active and explore their environments. Understanding these injuries is particularly important because they can be "silent" for some time, then lead to serious problems.

So-called blunt injuries to the abdomen—those caused by a kick or falling on an object like bicycle handlebars or rocks or toys—are quite common and account for about 5 percent of all serious injuries to children and adolescents. Penetrating injuries—for example, gunshot wounds or falling on a sharp stick—are less common but do occur. With the increase in violence in our society, gunshot wounds and stab wounds have become more commonplace, even in young children.

The internal organs of infants, children, and older youngsters are particularly vulnerable to injury for several reasons. The abdominal muscles are relatively poorly developed and do not protect the internal structures as well as they do in teenagers and adults. In addition, the liver and spleen are less protected by the rib cage in smaller children than in older youngsters. In younger children, these organs lie farther down in the abdomen. Even the bladder, which usually rests deep down in the pelvis (where it is better protected), might be distended in younger children and extend upward toward the umbilicus (belly button), especially if the youngster has not emptied the bladder recently.

The potential seriousness of a penetrating injury to the abdomen is obvious. These injuries often damage the intestines, as well as the so-called solid organs—the liver, spleen, and kidneys. They are almost always recognized —because they leave a "mark" on the abdomen.

Blunt injuries, on the other hand, can be relatively subtle, because they may not be apparent for hours or even days after the injury. They most often involve damage to the spleen, the liver, the pancreas, or the kidneys. However, in very young children, blunt injuries can cause damage to the intestine or the bladder.

It is particularly important to remember that an abdominal injury may have occurred if a youngster has another serious injury. Always assume the possibility of an internal abdominal injury if a youngster who has been seriously injured is in shock and there is no obvious visible source of bleeding.

Abdominal Injuries: Understanding the Problem

The most serious consequence of abdominal injury is bleeding into the abdomen. The *spleen*, an organ that is part of the immune system and has a very rich blood supply, is the most common organ damaged when a blunt abdominal injury occurs in children. Located in the upper left side of the abdomen, it can be damaged by a blow to the abdomen or left side or can be injured when the blow strikes the rib cage (the ribs then hit the spleen and cause damage).

If the spleen is damaged (for example, by a fall onto bicycle handlebars or a kick), blood vessels are broken, and blood builds up under the capsule (the outside, protective tissue) of the spleen. As the pressure builds up, the capsule may tear (so-called rupture of the spleen), and blood will leak into the abdominal cavity. This bleeding, which can be severe enough to result in shock, will cause pain in the abdomen and irritation (not infection) of the peritoneum (the lining of the abdominal cavity). Sometimes, the bleeding will be so slow that a youngster may not show symptoms or signs of spleen injury for hours or days after the accident occurred.

Like the spleen, the *liver*, which is located in the right upper part of the abdomen and extends just past the middle of the abdomen, has a rich blood supply. It is most commonly damaged by severe trauma to the lower right side of the chest but can be damaged by blunt injury to the upper abdomen. It can bleed if injured, leading to extreme loss of blood and shock. If its capsule and structures are torn, it can also leak bile into the abdominal cavity, leading to severe inflammation of the peritoneum. For some unknown reason, the liver seems less likely to be injured than the spleen, and small tears often heal over without serious bleeding.

Being hit in the center of the abdomen can also lead to damage to the *pancreas*, an important organ located in the middle part of the abdomen. The pancreas manufactures digestive juices, as well as insulin, which is important in the body's metabolism of sugar. Bleeding in the pancreas can cause blockage of the ducts that lead into the intestine from the liver. In addition, a tear in the pancreas can cause the digestive juices to spill into the abdominal cavity, leading to severe inflammation. A late complication of pancreas injury is the formation of a tumorlike cyst of the pancreas, which may be recognized months or years after a blunt injury to the abdomen.

The *kidneys* are located in the very back of the abdomen, behind the abdominal cavity at the level between the waist and the rib cage. They are nestled in protective layers of muscle and other tissues and usually protected, at least at their top ends, by the lower part of the rib cage. A blow to the abdomen at either side of the body or near the back can cause bleeding under the capsule (outer membrane) of the kidney or even rupture of the kidney, sometimes with damage to the tiny ureters (the tubes that lead from the kidneys to the bladder). In addition to problems due to unrecognized blood loss, this kind of injury can cause permanent damage to the involved kidney.

Injuries to the so-called hollow organs—the *stomach*, the *intestines*, and the *bladder*—are most often the result of penetrating injuries. When a sharp object (like a stick) or a projectile (like a bullet) penetrates the abdomen, it may perforate one of these structures. When this occurs, the major problem is leakage of the contents of the organ(s) into the abdominal cavity. Leakage of stomach acid is irritating, as is urine leakage. Perforation of the intestine causes spillage of bacteria-containing intestinal contents. The end result? Peritonitis (inflammation of the abdominal lining) and infection. Obviously, there is damage to the perforated organ itself, as well.

While rupture or perforation of the stomach, intestine, or bladder most often results from penetrating trauma to the abdomen, blunt injury (from, for example, a hard kick in the abdomen) occasionally leads to similar problems. This is more common in smaller infants and children than in teenagers and adults. In addition, a hard blow occasionally results in bleeding within the wall of one of these organs (called an intramural hematoma). Bladder injuries often result from severe injury to the bones of the pelvis.

Abdominal Injuries: Signs and Symptoms

517

RECOGNIZING
AND
MANAGING
SERIOUS OR
POTENTIALLY
SERIOUS
INJURIES

When a youngster has suffered a penetrating injury to the abdomen, there is little question that the damage to internal organs is potentially serious. The youngster will obviously have an open wound—whether a cut, stab, or hole—in the abdomen. Your goals here are obvious: stop any bleeding by putting pressure on the wound; keep the youngster calm; and get someone to call the paramedics or an ambulance immediately.

The real problem arises when a youngster has been hit in the abdomen or has fallen on something and there are no obvious external injuries. Here you are left to decide whether there are any internal injuries.

You will easily recognize the signs and symptoms if a youngster merely has "the wind knocked out of him." He will immediately bend over or fall down and become pale. He usually writhes around in pain for a short time and may even faint. He often vomits immediately. In a matter of minutes, he feels better and is up and ready to play again, although he may be somewhat subdued for a time. He may complain of slight soreness in the abdomen, but no other symptoms develop.

Most often, the signs and symptoms of more serious internal injury are subtle and develop gradually—over hours rather than minutes. Suspect a potentially serious internal abdominal injury if the youngster has any of the following:

- Persistent or increasing paleness (because of unrecognized internal bleeding).

- Signs and symptoms of shock: extreme paleness or a gray color; cool, clammy skin; weak, rapid pulse; dizziness; confusion or delirium; poor circulation to the skin; and finally, collapse.

- Persistent or increasing pain in the abdomen, especially if he or she also complains of pain in either shoulder (pain from certain injuries can be *referred* to the shoulder—because the nerves that cause some types of abdominal pain also cause shoulder pain).

- Soreness or tenderness deep in the abdomen.

- A swollen abdomen.

- Bruising or discoloration of the abdomen.

- Vomiting more than once.

- Vomiting of blood, green or yellow liquid (bile), or material that looks like "coffee grounds."

- Blood in the urine.

- Blood in the bowel movement or black, tarry bowel movements.

If the youngster's signs and symptoms seem minor or you are not sure whether they are significant, call the doctor for advice. If the youngster's symptoms obviously point toward internal abdominal injury, then promptly get the youngster to an emergency room for evaluation. When it comes to internal abdominal injury, it is better to err on the side of safety and have the youngster evaluated by a doctor.

Abdominal Injuries: What to Expect

Whenever an abdominal injury is caused by a penetrating object, surgery is needed to explore the extent of the damage and repair it. An intravenous (IV) infusion will be started immediately, so the youngster can be given fluids, blood, and medications that are needed. If the youngster is stable, tests might be done before surgery. After the surgery, the youngster will need to stay in the hospital, often in an intensive-care unit, until he or she recovers from the surgery and the injury.

If blunt internal abdominal injury is suspected, the doctor will ask you (and your youngster) exactly how the injury occurred and will want to know in detail how the youngster is feeling and acting. He or she will do a very careful examination, looking for signs of internal injury.

If bleeding is possible or suspected, the youngster will need one or more blood tests. A urine sample will be examined for blood, and the youngster may need to have a rubber catheter (tube) inserted into the bladder. Special X rays and other tests (scans) to evaluate the spleen and liver, as well as the kidneys, might be recommended. Sometimes, a procedure called peritoneal lavage (in which a needle or plastic catheter is inserted into the abdominal cavity to determine if there is any bleeding there) is carried out.

Usually, a youngster with a suspected internal abdominal injury will need to stay in the hospital for careful observation. Repeated blood tests can help the doctor to tell if there is continued bleeding inside the abdomen. The youngster will not be allowed to eat or drink anything for a time and will be given fluids and medications by vein. Sometimes, surgery is needed to determine the location and extent of internal injury or to control severe bleeding and repair the damage.

In the past, tears or ruptures of the spleen were always treated by removing the spleen. Recently, the trend has changed, and injuries to the spleen are treated differently. If possible, no surgery is performed, and the spleen is allowed to heal itself. If surgery is needed to control bleeding, all attempts are made to repair the organ rather than remove it.

THE DON'TS

Don't delay in calling the paramedics or an ambulance if a youngster has an obvious, serious abdominal injury.

519

RECOGNIZING
AND
MANAGING
SERIOUS OR
POTENTIALLY
SERIOUS
INJURIES

Don't overlook the subtle signs and symptoms of internal abdominal injury after a youngster receives a blow to the abdomen or falls on a blunt object. Internal bleeding can develop gradually. Take the youngster to the doctor or to an emergency room if you suspect internal abdominal injury.

Don't panic if a youngster "has the wind knocked out of him or her." The dramatic reaction that follows—severe pain, paleness, sweating, and vomiting—passes in a matter of minutes. However, if the symptoms continue for more than a few minutes, get medical help promptly.

PLEASE NOTE: Now that you have a grasp of how to recognize and manage abdominal injuries, it would be extremely helpful for you to go back to the Emergency Quick Reference With the Steps in Detail and review it carefully. The more familiar you are with that material, the more useful it will be to you when you need it.

EMERGENCY QUICK REFERENCE

With the Steps in Detail

Chest (Thoracic) Injuries

▶ **SUSPECT A POTENTIALLY SERIOUS CHEST INJURY IF A YOUNG-STER HAS ANY OF THE FOLLOWING AFTER A SEVERE BLOW TO THE CHEST OR A FALL ONTO THE CHEST:**

- Difficulty breathing, especially if he is blue (cyanotic).

- Pain in the chest, particularly when taking a deep breath.

- Obvious deformity of the chest (the ribs stick out or are sunken in) that is made worse by breathing in.

- Part of the chest seems to sink in or collapse when the youngster breathes in and bulges outward when he breathes out.

- There is an open wound, and you hear air sucking in and out through it when the youngster breathes.

▶ **ALWAYS ASSUME THERE IS A SERIOUS CHEST INJURY IF A YOUNGSTER HAS HAD A CRUSH INJURY TO THE CHEST—FOR EXAMPLE, HER CHEST HAS BEEN RUN OVER BY A CAR.**

➤ **IF THERE IS AN OBVIOUS OR SUSPECTED CHEST INJURY, HAVE SOMEONE ELSE CALL THE PARAMEDICS OR AN AMBULANCE WHILE YOU TREAT THE CHILD. IF NO ONE IS WITH YOU, CONTINUE TREATING THE CHILD WHILE YOU PERIODICALLY SHOUT FOR HELP. WHEN HELP ARRIVES, HAVE THAT PERSON CALL THE PARAMEDICS OR AN AMBULANCE. DO WHAT YOU CAN FOR THE YOUNGSTER WHILE YOU ARE WAITING FOR THE PARAMEDICS OR AMBULANCE:**

- Keep the youngster lying down and try to calm him.

- Make sure the airway is open. Tilt the youngster's head back slightly so her jaw is jutted forward (the "sniffing position"). Clear her mouth of any debris.

- Check to make sure he is breathing. If not, begin rescue breathing. Start CPR (chest compressions with rescue breathing) if he is not breathing *and* there is no pulse. (If you are certified in CPR and are unable to remember the details of the procedure, turn to the Emergency Quick Reference on page 113, entitled "A Review of the Six Steps of CPR.")

- If there is an open chest wound and you can hear air sucking in and out through it, put a thick piece of cloth over the hole and apply very firm pressure over it with the palm of your hand to seal off the hole.

- If the youngster is awake but uncomfortable breathing while lying down, elevate his head and shoulders slightly to see if that will help.

Chest (Thoracic) Injuries: What You Should Know

The rib cage acts as a protective shield for the vital organs within the chest—the heart and its major blood vessels, the lungs and their supporting structures. Very severe blows to the chest or crush injuries (for example, being run over by a car) can lead to rib fractures (breaks), as well as damage to the lungs, heart, and blood vessels. When a serious chest injury occurs, the greatest problem is that the vital functions of breathing and circulation are affected.

The ribs of infants and children are very pliable and are only broken if excessive force is applied to them. Therefore, most blunt injuries (for example, blows to the chest or falls onto the rib cage) that involve the chest cause little if any damage to the ribs. As youngsters get older, the tendency to fracture (break) ribs increases. Usually, if there is no damage to the ribs, the underlying vital organs are damaged little, if at all.

If an injury is caused by a penetrating object (for example, a bullet, a knife, a sharp piece of metal or wood), the damage can be very severe or surprisingly slight. The extent of the injury is determined by what was in the way of the object: the lung(s), the heart, the blood vessels—or none of these vital structures. Sometimes, the greatest amount of damage is to the structures of the chest wall itself—the ribs and the blood vessels between them.

Trauma to the lower part of the rib cage is more often associated with abdominal injuries than with injuries to the internal organs in the chest. Bleeding in the spleen (on the left side) and liver (on the right side) often results from fractures of the ribs or penetrating injuries of the lower rib cage.

Chest Injuries: Understanding the Problem

Rib fractures (broken ribs), as we discussed earlier, are not very common in young children, except when the force of the injury is very great. In general, a single rib fracture does not cause much of a problem (unless the rib is splintered and is poked into the lung underneath it). Taking deep breaths, coughing, or laughing might cause some pain, because the ends of the broken rib move against each other. However, the fracture heals within a few weeks without any particular treatment.

When several ribs in the same area are broken, the broken ends can protrude into the chest and bruise the lung tissue underneath. The blood vessels that are found in the rib cage (between the ribs) can be torn and bleed into the space between the chest wall and the lung (called the pleural cavity). Buildup of blood in the pleural cavity—called a *hemothorax*—puts pressure on the lung and restricts its ability to expand during breathing. This causes pain and, if severe, difficulty in breathing, as well as in getting enough oxygen into the lungs. Usually, this collection of blood can be removed with a plastic tube that is inserted into the space in which the blood is trapped. The blood vessels that were broken heal over after several days.

If the broken ribs (or a sharp object) penetrate the lung tissue itself, a *pneumothorax* will result. An air leak in the lung will allow air to escape from the lung and collect in the space between the lung and the chest wall. If the collection of air is small, few if any problems develop (because the leak seals itself over, and the body eventually absorbs the trapped air after several days). Larger collections of air limit lung function and must be treated by removing the trapped air through a special tube inserted into the pleural space through the chest wall.

In certain situations, air continues to accumulate outside the lung with each breath. The trapped air will cause the lung to collapse and even push the chest structures over toward the opposite side. This so-called *tension pneumothorax* is life-threatening unless the trapped air is released. A tension pneumothorax may be caused by an open chest wound through which air is sucked into the chest from the outside with each breath but does not escape when the youngster breathes out. When the youngster breathes in, you can hear air rushing into the open chest wound. If you think this is occurring, press a bulky wad of cloth firmly over the open chest wound so no further air can be sucked into the chest. Tension pneumothorax can also result from rupture of a lung from inside because of too much pressure being used to breathe artificially for a person. It is a rare complication of rescue breathing but could occur if the breaths delivered to the nonbreathing youngster were too forceful. This is one of the reasons it is important to learn rescue breathing and CPR from professionals trained to teach these lifesaving techniques!

Lung contusion (essentially a bruised lung) may result from blunt injury of the lung itself by the rib cage. With this injury, the lung tissue is actually bruised and torn, leading to bleeding and swelling. Unless lung contusions are massive, they heal after several days or weeks without any special treatment. A person with a lung contusion usually has mild to severe difficulty breathing.

Heart damage due to blunt chest injury is usually minimal, if present. However, on occasion, a blood vessel will rupture and cause blood to collect in the pericardium (the sac around the heart). This blood collection outside the heart prevents the heart from filling completely with blood that needs to be pumped to the rest of the body. If there is a great deal of blood outside the heart and putting pressure on it, then the heart's pumping action cannot work efficiently, and the youngster's pulse becomes very faint—if detectable at all. Tears and lacerations of the heart itself and its large blood vessels most often follow a penetrating injury to the chest. In this case, it is obvious that the problem can be resolved only with emergency medical care. In this situation, apply firm pressure over the wound, while someone calls the paramedics (or an ambulance if there are no paramedics in your area).

Chest Injury: Signs and Symptoms

Most often, potentially serious chest injuries are not difficult to recognize. However, they may be overlooked if a youngster has other serious injuries, as well. The cardinal symptoms of serious chest injury are breathing difficulty and pain in the chest, especially when taking a deep breath. The youngster might be cyanotic (blue) if the damage is severe and may have a weak, thready, or nonfeelable pulse. The chest cage may move in an unusual way. One side might bulge out a great deal farther than the other (suggesting trapped air—pneumothorax), or a section of the rib cage might move in a paradoxical way—that is, that portion of the rib cage would cave in when the youngster breathes in and push out when he or she exhales.

Chest Injury: What to Expect

523

RECOGNIZING
AND
MANAGING
SERIOUS OR
POTENTIALLY
SERIOUS
INJURIES

Whenever there is a potentially serious chest injury, the emergency physician will do a complete and careful physical examination of the hurt youngster and order X rays of the chest. If there is evidence of a chest injury, the youngster will have to stay in the hospital for a matter of days or weeks and will be watched very closely. An intravenous (IV) infusion will be started and continued for one or more days.

While most chest injuries heal themselves with time, some youngsters with chest injuries must have a special tube inserted through the chest wall into the space between the rib cage and the lungs and other vital structures. This tube is used to withdraw air (pneumothorax) or blood (hemothorax), if present. Sometimes, a respirator (breathing machine) is needed to help a youngster with a serious chest injury breathe while the injuries to the lungs and other structures heal. Youngsters who have injuries to the heart or the major blood vessels need emergency surgery to repair the damage.

THE DON'TS

Don't overlook the symptoms and signs of a serious chest injury. A youngster who has difficulty breathing or pain in the chest after an injury requires immediate medical attention.

Don't hesitate to call the paramedics if there is an obvious puncture wound to the chest. Remember to put firm pressure over the wound until the paramedics take over.

PLEASE NOTE: Now that you have a grasp of how to recognize and manage chest injuries, it would be extremely helpful for you to go back to the Emergency Quick Reference With the Steps in Detail and review it carefully. The more familiar you are with that material, the more useful it will be to you when you need it.

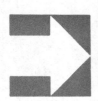

EMERGENCY QUICK REFERENCE

With the Steps in Detail

Cold Injury (Hypothermia) and Frostbite

▶ **SERIOUS LOWERING OF BODY TEMPERATURE CAN OCCUR WITHIN MINUTES IF A YOUNGSTER IS SUBMERGED IN VERY COLD WATER OR WITHIN HOURS OF BEING IN A VERY COLD ENVIRONMENT. TAKE ACTION IMMEDIATELY, EVEN IF YOU THINK IT MIGHT BE TOO LATE BECAUSE THE CHILD APPEARS DEAD.**

- Remove the youngster from the cold immediately.

- If she is unconscious, check to see whether she is breathing and has a heartbeat. If not, begin CPR (rescue breathing and chest compressions) immediately and continue until you get help or someone takes over for you. (If you are certified in CPR and are unable to remember the details of the procedure, turn to the Emergency Quick Reference on page 113, entitled "A Review of the Six Steps of CPR.")

▶ **WHETHER HE IS CONSCIOUS OR NOT, BEGIN WARMING HIM IMMEDIATELY.**

- Remove any wet clothing and dry the skin.

- Wrap the youngster in blankets.

- If you are far from medical help or you will need to wait for some time for help, place the youngster in a tub of warm (but *not* hot) water. Continue to watch carefully for signs of breathing difficulty, and check for a pulse frequently.

- If you must go for help, treat the youngster first (explained above), then get her to an emergency room for an evaluation. Make sure to keep her warm while you travel.

▶ **IF A YOUNGSTER HAS A LOW BODY TEMPERATURE AFTER BEING WET IN A VERY COLD ENVIRONMENT OR HAS PLAYED TO THE POINT OF EXHAUSTION IN THE COLD, CHECK HER TEMPERATURE. IF IT IS LESS THAN 97 DEGREES FAHRENHEIT AND SHE IS AWAKE BUT SLEEPY, BEGIN TO WARM HER.**

525

RECOGNIZING
AND
MANAGING
SERIOUS OR
POTENTIALLY
SERIOUS
INJURIES

- Remove any wet clothing.

- Place him in a tub of warm (*not* hot) water until shivering stops and he is comfortable.

- Call the doctor for advice if she does not seem perfectly normal after she is warm again.

▶ **IF A YOUNGSTER SHOWS SIGNS OF FROSTBITE (VERY COLD, WHITE, HARD, PAINLESS FINGERS, TOES, NOSE, OR EARS, FOR EXAMPLE), BEGIN WARMING IMMEDIATELY.**

- Put the frostbitten area into warm (but *not* hot) water, or wrap it with warm, wet towels. Do not rub the frostbitten part.

- Continue to rewarm the area until it is pink or red, swollen, and painful.

- Protect it from further cold.

- Call the doctor or go to an emergency room if blisters form on the frostbitten area. Keep the frostbitten area warm while traveling.

Hypothermia: What You Should Know

Infants and young children are more prone to cold injury or hypothermia (a generalized lowering of body temperature) than young adults are (for a variety of reasons). Some of these reasons include the following: young infants cannot shiver to conserve their body heat or increase their activity level enough to raise their body heat; children are more likely to ignore early signals of being cold if they are outside playing in very cold climates; and older youngsters are likely to play to the point of exhaustion, which makes them more at risk for hypothermia. Certain problems such as anorexia nervosa, alcohol use, and malnutrition add to the risk of hypothermia.

Hypothermia can result from prolonged exposure to cold if a youngster is improperly dressed or not moving. For example, an injured child who is lost will lose heat very rapidly, even in moderately cold weather. If clothing is wet and there is a wind, cooling occurs even more rapidly. Immersion or submersion in cold water can drop the body temperature dangerously in a matter of minutes.

If not recognized and treated, cold injury can lead to death quite rapidly. It is imperative that you recognize the conditions that lead to cold injury, as well as the signs and symptoms of hypothermia, and take action quickly if it occurs.

Hypothermia: Understanding the Problem

When a youngster is exposed to cold, her body responds by starting to produce extra heat. At first, she begins to move and shiver in order to produce additional heat. However, this extra activity uses up her body's stores of energy and increases her need for oxygen. Her body temperature falls in spite of the efforts to generate heat.

As the body temperature falls, blood circulation slows down, and blood is directed from the skin and surface to internal organs. The youngster becomes pale or cyanotic (blue). He becomes sleepy and listless, moving very little, and may lapse into unconsciousness. His heartbeat slows and gets very weak, and his breathing first slows down, then stops. If the child is in a freezing environment, his arms and legs will begin to freeze. If he is not resuscitated, death will shortly follow.

When hypothermia is severe, it can mimic death—or end in death. However, minimal body function can continue for relatively long periods of time when the body temperature is low, because at low temperatures, the body tissues require very little oxygen. For this reason, it is important that you not assume that a very cold infant or child is dead even if she is very, very cold and you cannot feel a pulse or see her breathing. Remarkable recoveries can occur if the youngster is vigorously but carefully resuscitated.

Hypothermia: Signs and Symptoms

The signs and symptoms of lowered body temperature develop over time and become more severe as the temperature falls. They include the following:

- A feeling of intense cold.

- Repeated shivering, with increasing stiffness of muscles between violent shivers.

- A white, blue, or mottled coloring of the skin.

- Numbness of fingers, toes, and skin, especially if the youngster is wet.

- Progressive sleepiness and sluggishness.

- Slow, shallow breathing.

- Faint, slow pulse.

- Coma.

- Respiratory and cardiac arrest (the lungs and heart stop).

527

RECOGNIZING
AND
MANAGING
SERIOUS OR
POTENTIALLY
SERIOUS
INJURIES

Since the earliest of these symptoms and signs can occur with even minimal drops in body temperature, it is important that you pay attention to such signs as a youngster's shivering and turning blue while swimming or playing outdoors. Remove the youngster from the cold environment and rewarm him or her immediately. If hypothermia has progressed to its later stages, it is imperative that you treat the youngster as you quickly get medical help.

Frostbite: Understanding the Problem

Frostbite is the actual freezing of body tissues—with ice formation. It usually affects the smallest, most exposed parts of the body—for example, fingers, toes, nose, ears, and chin. However, with prolonged exposure to extreme cold, it can involve entire arms or legs and large surfaces of the body. When the skin and underlying tissue freeze, blood circulation stops, and the tissues gradually die if the blood circulation is not restored. If the freezing is prolonged and deep, permanent damage can be extensive.

As with hypothermia, the risk of frostbite increases when a youngster is wet or improperly clothed, especially in windy weather. In addition, young children may not be aware that the numbness and pain they feel mean they are too cold. They may not be aware of steps they can take to keep themselves warm, so tissue damage gets worse.

Mild frostbite affects only the skin surface, while deep frostbite, like a burn, leads to blistering and damage to deeper layers of skin. The most severe freezing injuries result in gangrene of the frozen body part.

Frostbite: Signs and Symptoms

The earliest warning signal of impending frostbite is numbness. This early indication is followed by whiteness of the frostbitten area. As freezing deepens, first the skin and then the deeper tissues under the skin become firm and hard to the touch. There is little or no sensation or pain at this point. With very severe frostbite, blisters may form, even before the area is rewarmed.

When a frostbite injury is rewarmed, it becomes easier to tell how severe the injury really was. With superficial injuries, the child will complain of pain and burning, and you will notice that the finger or toe becomes very red, swollen, and tender. It might even look mottled with red and purple—giving it a bruised look. With deeper frostbite, blisters develop on the surface of the frozen part, and swelling is severe. A youngster who has had a serious frostbite injury should always be evaluated and treated by a doctor.

THE DON'TS

Don't assume that a youngster who is found in a very cold environment and appears to be dead is dead. Hypothermia can mimic death, so you should always begin resuscitation and continue until you get help. Death cannot be assured unless there is still no sign of life after a person has been warmed to normal body temperature.

Don't rub ice on a frostbitten area, and don't rub the area at all during rewarming. Rubbing can cause further damage to the already damaged tissues.

Don't expose a frostbitten body part to cold again after it has been rewarmed. Keep it warm to avoid further injury. Therefore, if you must transport the young person to medical care, make sure he or she is well covered and protected against the cold.

Don't hesitate to have the child or young person evaluated by a doctor if you're not sure whether the cold injury is severe or may need treatment.

PLEASE NOTE: Now that you have a grasp of how to recognize and manage cold injury (hypothermia) and frostbite, it would be extremely helpful for you to go back to the Emergency Quick Reference With the Steps in Detail and review it carefully. The more familiar you are with that material, the more useful it will be to you when you need it.

529

RECOGNIZING
AND
MANAGING
SERIOUS OR
POTENTIALLY
SERIOUS
INJURIES

EMERGENCY QUICK REFERENCE

With the Steps in Detail

Crush Injuries

▶ **ALL BUT THE MOST MINOR CRUSH INJURIES TO AN ARM, LEG, HAND, OR FOOT SHOULD BE EVALUATED BY A DOCTOR IMMEDIATELY:**

- Apply a splint (a pillow, firm cardboard, or board) in case there is a fracture or joint injury.

- Elevate the injured arm or leg as much as possible.

- Get the youngster to an emergency room for evaluation.

▶ **YOU CAN TREAT AND OBSERVE AN APPARENTLY MINOR CRUSH INJURY AT HOME:**

- Wash the injured area with soap and water. Firmly scrub scrapes or cuts (if present) to remove any dirt or debris.

- Have the youngster keep the injured area elevated as much as possible to prevent or control swelling. Prop a leg or foot up on a stool or pillows during the daytime and on pillows at night. Have him keep an injured arm or hand at or above the level of his heart. (You can use a towel or scarf as a sling, if necessary.)

- Apply cold, wet towels (not ice) for several hours, to help control swelling and bleeding.

- Treat minor pain or discomfort with the appropriate dose of aspirin substitute (*not* aspirin).

- Check the injury every hour for six to eight hours, then every few hours for a day. Look for swelling and other signs of a more serious injury (listed below).

- You may apply heat after twenty-four to forty-eight hours if there is continued discomfort but little or no swelling.

▶ **CALL THE DOCTOR OR GO TO AN EMERGENCY ROOM IF A YOUNGSTER WHO SUSTAINED WHAT LOOKED LIKE A MINOR CRUSH INJURY DEVELOPS ANY OF THE FOLLOWING:**

● White or blue fingers or toes that are cool or cold to the touch on the arm or leg that was injured.

● Severe or increasing pain.

● Increasing swelling of the injured area, especially if the swollen area becomes hard to the touch.

● Numbness, tingling, or inability to move the fingers or toes below the injury.

● Blistering or darkening of the skin over the injury.

● Signs of infection in the injured area: pus formation in an abrasion, redness and warmth of the area, or fever.

Crush Injuries: What You Should Know

Active children are at risk for crush injuries to their arms, legs, hands, and feet. Fortunately, one of the most common and serious crush injuries in the past—called wringer injury (which occurred when a child or youngster got a hand and arm caught in a washing-machine wringer)—is now uncommon. However, the same kind of injury can occur in other ways. A child or youngster can: get a foot caught in a bicycle wheel; be run over by the wheel(s) of a bicycle, motorcycle, or car; get an arm, leg, hand, or foot caught in a power gate; be injured by belts or rollers on power equipment; or have fingers or toes crushed in car doors.

The major problem with crush injuries is that most of the damage is below the skin. In fact, most of the time, the only visible effects right after the injury are bruising and abrasions (scrapes) of the skin. This might lead you to think there is little or no serious damage—in spite of the amount of force involved in the injury.

The serious effects of the injury—swelling, bleeding, and pressure on nearby blood vessels and nerves—develop over the first few hours after the injury. Therefore, it is vitally important that the youngster be evaluated by the doctor after a serious crush injury or watched carefully by you after what appears to be a less serious injury.

Crush Injuries: Understanding the Problem

531

RECOGNIZING
AND
MANAGING
SERIOUS OR
POTENTIALLY
SERIOUS
INJURIES

When a youngster suffers a crush injury, the tissues of the leg, arm, hand, or foot are subjected to severe crushing (where the injury got its name), as well as pulling, rubbing, and twisting. This leads to swelling and bleeding below the skin—in the muscles and supporting structures. Friction and pressure may also cause abrasions of the skin and even deeper layers of tissue, but true cuts that need sutures (stitches) are unusual. Occasionally, a fracture (break) of a bone might occur, as well.

The swelling that follows a serious crush injury usually develops within a few hours and can be massive. Swelling can be caused by both bleeding from broken blood vessels and oozing of tissue fluids. As swelling increases, it puts additional pressure on vital blood vessels, nerves, and muscles and leads to the more serious consequences of a crush injury—loss of circulation and nerve damage.

Lack of circulation to an area causes whiteness or blueness of the skin, coolness or hardness to the touch, and severe pain. If circulation is not restored, cells will die, and permanent damage can occur. This damage can affect the skin, which may blister or turn black. When the lack of blood supply affects muscle tissue, it can also be permanently damaged.

Nerve damage after a crush injury is caused either by direct injury to the nerve or by pressure due to severe swelling. Nerve damage causes severe pain, as well as numbness and tingling in the area beyond the injury. It also causes weakness or complete inability to move the muscles (and thereby the injured extremity) supplied by the damaged nerve. This nerve damage can be temporary or permanent.

Tissues damaged by crushing are particularly susceptible to infection because of the severe swelling and bleeding. Infecting bacteria can invade the injured tissue through broken skin or even travel from more distant parts of the body. They multiply quite easily when circulation of blood is not normal (blood cells that would normally clear the area of bacteria cannot carry away the invading microorganisms). Infection can also be caused by unusual bacteria that thrive when there is a poor supply of oxygen.

Crush Injuries: Signs and Symptoms

When you first look at an arm, leg, hand, or foot that is crushed, you might be fooled about how serious the injury is because there might be little or no visible damage. You might see abrasions (skin scrapes), slight bruising, or tiny blood spots that look more like a rash than a bruise. Swelling will develop quickly, usually in a matter of a few hours, if the problem is more serious. The youngster might complain of very little discomfort initially but then have more and more pain as swelling begins.

When a youngster has had an obviously serious crush injury, he needs to be evaluated by a doctor immediately. If, however, the injury seems mild at first, you should observe the youngster for a short time. Wash the crushed area well with soap and water, paying particular attention to any scrapes or cuts. Elevate the crushed arm or leg, apply cool, wet cloths, and watch for signs of more serious injury. You can give the youngster the appropriate dose of aspirin substitute (*not* aspirin, because it can lead to further bleeding) if he has mild pain or discomfort.

It is vitally important that you call the doctor or take the youngster to an emergency room if you notice any of the signs of more serious injury, as listed in the Emergency Quick Reference.

Crush Injuries: What to Expect

When a youngster has had a serious or potentially serious crush injury, the doctor will be most concerned about swelling and hidden damage caused by the injury and swelling. He or she will carefully examine the youngster, looking in particular for signs of poor blood supply or nerve damage. X rays might be taken to check for fractures (broken bones) or joint injury.

The doctor will want to admit the youngster to the hospital for observation and treatment if the injury is potentially serious. The crushed area will be cleaned carefully and may be wrapped tightly to help control swelling and bleeding. It will be elevated until swelling is reduced, and the youngster will be checked frequently to detect any loss of circulation, nerve injury, or infection. He or she will be allowed to go home when the danger of further swelling is gone.

If swelling is severe enough to put pressure on blood vessels or nerves, surgery is needed to relieve this pressure. If there is extensive skin or muscle damage, skin grafts and other special surgical procedures might be necessary. If infection occurs, antibiotic treatment will be started immediately.

THE DON'TS

Don't be fooled by the lack of visible damage if a youngster has had a crush injury. Severe bleeding and swelling can develop quickly, even with apparently minor injuries.

Don't overlook the signs of worsening damage due to a crush injury: severe swelling; severe or increasing pain; white, blue, or cool skin below the injury; numbness, tingling, or weakness in an injured arm, leg, hand, or foot; blistering or darkening of the skin; or signs of infection. Call the doctor or go to an emergency room if any of these problems develop.

533

RECOGNIZING
AND
MANAGING
SERIOUS OR
POTENTIALLY
SERIOUS
INJURIES

PLEASE NOTE: Now that you have a grasp of how to recognize and manage crush injuries, it would be extremely helpful for you to go back to the Emergency Quick Reference With the Steps in Detail and review it carefully. The more familiar you are with that material, the more useful it will be to you when you need it.

EMERGENCY QUICK REFERENCE

With the Steps in Detail

Electric Shock and Electrical Burns

▶ **HIGH-VOLTAGE ELECTRIC SHOCK MAY LEAD TO CARDIAC ARREST, AS WELL AS SERIOUS BURNS. TAKE ACTION IMMEDIATELY IF A YOUNGSTER IS SHOCKED BY, FOR EXAMPLE, A POWER LINE OR LIGHTNING.**

▶ **REMOVE THE CHILD FROM THE SOURCE OF ELECTRICITY AS QUICKLY AS POSSIBLE, WHILE PROTECTING YOURSELF FROM INJURY.**

- Turn off the power, if possible.

- If the wire is still "hot," use a *nonconductive material* such as a wooden pole to remove the wire. Take care to avoid standing in water while you do this.

▶ **CHECK TO SEE WHETHER THE YOUNGSTER IS BREATHING AND HAS A PULSE. IF NOT, BEGIN RESCUE BREATHING AND/OR CPR.** (If you are trained in CPR and are unable to remember the details of this procedure or how to perform rescue breathing, turn to the Emergency Quick Reference on page 113, entitled "A Review of the Six Steps of CPR.")

- Have someone else call the paramedics while you treat the child. If no one is with you, continue treating the child while you periodically shout for help. When help arrives, have that person call the paramedics. Continue your resuscitation until someone arrives who can assist or take over for you.

▶ *ALWAYS* GET THE YOUNGSTER TO AN EMERGENCY ROOM FOR AN EVALUATION, EVEN IF YOU DON'T SEE ANY OBVIOUS BURNS OR IF THE SURFACE BURNS SEEM MINOR.

▶ IF A YOUNGSTER IS SHOCKED OR BURNED BY A HOUSEHOLD SOURCE OF ELECTRICITY AND IS NOT UNCONSCIOUS, CHECK CAREFULLY FOR ANY SIGNS OF A BURN.

● Take the youngster to his or her doctor or an emergency room for evaluation. This is especially important if the burn is around the mouth.

Electric Shock and Electrical Burns: What You Should Know

Electricity can cause serious surface burns, as well as deeper burns, because electrical current, with its heat and energy, tends to travel through body tissues. This means that deep tissues of the body can be more damaged than it would appear on the surface. While some youngsters who suffer electricity-related burns have serious surface burns, the great majority have deep, destructive burns under the surface.

In addition to causing burns, electrical current can lead to instantaneous death. It can cause breathing to stop if the current passes through the respiratory center in the brain stem (the area at the base of the brain). It can cause the heart to stop pumping blood if it passes through the heart and causes ventricular fibrillation (abnormal electrical activity that makes the heart muscle quiver rather than beat effectively). If either of these unfortunate events happens, immediate CPR is the only hope for a youngster to survive.

Fortunately, less life-threatening injuries are most common. However, the initial appearance of any electrical burn is deceiving, so it's important that any youngster who is burned by electricity be evaluated by a physician.

Electrical Burns: Understanding the Problem

As we mentioned previously, electrical current tends to travel through part or all of the body, following tissues that conduct its current most easily. Nerves, blood vessels, muscle, and skin are most likely to carry electrical current. This means that nerves, blood vessels, muscle, and skin are the most likely to sustain serious burns.

Electrical burns usually look innocent enough at the start. You might see a blackened or charred area where the current entered the body. This small area is surrounded by a white or gray area. Farther out from the center, there is redness and swelling. This type of burn completely destroys all the tissue in the center and a large amount of tissue surrounding it. Any blood vessels in the path of the current are immediately clotted, so there is no blood supply for the surrounding tissues. At first, swelling and inflammation appear, then the tissues that have no blood supply gradually die and harden (so-called gangrene). At this point, it becomes obvious that the burn is serious and destructive.

Serious electrical burns are almost always treated in the hospital, because multiple operations to remove the destroyed tissue are required. Infection is a very real risk, as well. Many electrical burns leave permanent deformity or scarring, and plastic surgery is usually required.

Electrical Mouth Burns: A Special Problem for Infants and Toddlers

The most common type of electrical injury in a young child is a burn around the mouth caused by sucking on an electrical cord or chewing through its insulation. The "female" end of an extension cord is especially dangerous. Like other electrical burns, this kind of burn is deceiving, because, at first, it looks small and innocent. In fact, it is a deep, third-degree burn that extends farther into the tissues of the face than you initially think.

Most often, the burn involves the tissues of the corner of the mouth, the lips, or the tongue. At first, you see only a small area of darkening surrounded by the telltale gray or white area. Over the next few days, the tissue damage becomes more and more obvious.

Electrical mouth burns must be cared for by plastic surgeons who are familiar with this kind of burn. Initially, little or nothing is done with the burn, other than to keep it clean and watch for signs of infection and bleeding. After one to two weeks, the surgeon may need to operate on the burned area to remove any of the dead tissue. Later, he or she will attempt to correct as much of the deformity caused by the burn as possible. Most often, however, the youngster is left with permanent scarring and deformity around the mouth. Prevention is therefore the best medicine (see Chapter 2 for information regarding prevention of electrical, flame, and scald burns).

THE DON'TS

Don't delay in beginning rescue breathing or full CPR if a youngster has had an electrical burn or shock and is unconscious, is not breathing, or has no heartbeat. Respiratory or cardiac arrest following electric shock is not rare.

Don't be deceived by the surface appearance of an electrical burn. There is always deeper damage (to the tissues underneath) than meets the eye. Get medical help immediately.

Don't consider electrical mouth burns in infants and toddlers to be minor. These are serious burns that should be treated by a plastic surgeon.

PLEASE NOTE: Now that you have a grasp of how to recognize and manage electric shock and electrical burns, it would be extremely helpful for you to go back to the Emergency Quick Reference With the Steps in Detail and review it carefully. The more familiar you are with that material, the more useful it will be to you when you need it.

EMERGENCY QUICK REFERENCE

With the Steps in Detail

Eye Injuries

Objects Embedded in the Eye

▶ **IF THE EMBEDDED OBJECT IS SMALL AND *DOES NOT EXTEND BEYOND THE EYELID:***

- Do not touch or try to remove the object (splinter, glass, nail, pencil lead, piece of metal, or whatever).

- Quickly but carefully cover *both* eyes to restrict movement of the eyes. Use a gauze wrap, eye patches, a scarf, strip of clean sheet, necktie, handkerchief, sanitary napkin, dish towel, or knee sock.

- Have the youngster lie down and try to keep him or her calm.

- Call your ophthalmologist if you have one. (An ophthalmologist is a medical doctor who has special training in the evaluation and treatment of eye diseases, disorders, and injuries.) He or she may have you bring the youngster to the office, wish to meet you at the nearest emergency room, or have the emergency-room physician see and treat the youngster.

- If you do not have an opthalmologist, call the youngster's doctor for advice, or go calmly but quickly to an emergency room while keeping the youngster as calm as possible.

537

RECOGNIZING
AND
MANAGING
SERIOUS OR
POTENTIALLY
SERIOUS
INJURIES

Object Impaled in the Eye

▶ **DO NOT TRY TO REMOVE AN IMPALED OBJECT (PENCIL, STICK, TOY, AND SO ON).**

▶ **HAVE THE YOUNGSTER LIE DOWN AND STAY THERE. KEEP HIM CALM AND DO NOT ALLOW HIM TO TOUCH THE EYE.**

▶ **IMMOBILIZE THE EYES:**

- If the object is relatively small, you can immobilize the eyes by using a cup or similar object. First, patch the *uninjured* eye shut (using tape and a patch or cloth). Then place a cup over the injured eye and securely tie or tape it in place. This prevents movement of both eyes (remember, they move together).

- If the object is very large, hold it carefully *so it does not move.* Try to keep it from causing further damage.

▶ **HAVE SOMEONE ELSE CALL THE PARAMEDICS OR AN AMBU-LANCE WHILE YOU KEEP THE YOUNGSTER STILL AND CALM. IF NO ONE IS WITH YOU, CONTINUE TREATING THE YOUNGSTER WHILE YOU PERIODICALLY SHOUT FOR HELP. WHEN HELP AR-RIVES, HAVE THAT PERSON CALL THE PARAMEDICS OR AN AM-BULANCE. THE YOUNGSTER NEEDS TO BE MOVED CAREFULLY TO AN EMERGENCY ROOM WHILE LYING DOWN.**

Cut on the Eyeball

▶ **IT IS VITAL THAT YOU NOT TOUCH THE EYE, RUB IT, OR APPLY ANY PRESSURE TO CONTROL OR STOP BLEEDING.**

▶ **HAVE THE YOUNGSTER LIE DOWN AND STAY CALM.**

▶ **LOOK AT THE EYE TO TRY TO SEE WHETHER THERE IS REALLY A CUT OR TEAR OF THE EYEBALL ITSELF AND HOW DEEP OR EXTENSIVE IT IS.**

- Can you see any fluid draining from the eye or any of the contents of the inside of the eye?

- Is there damage to the front structures (the pupil, the clear cornea) of the eye?

▶ **PATCH BOTH EYES TO PREVENT MOVEMENT.**

- Gently but quickly cover the injured eye with a preferably sterile or clean gauze wrap, cloth, sanitary napkin, or patch. Cover the uninjured eye, as well.

- Tape or tie the patching material in place.

▶ **HAVE SOMEONE ELSE CALL THE PARAMEDICS OR AN AMBULANCE (SINCE THE CHILD NEEDS TO BE TRANSPORTED LYING DOWN). IF NO ONE IS WITH YOU, CONTINUE TREATING THE CHILD WHILE YOU PERIODICALLY SHOUT FOR HELP. WHEN HELP ARRIVES, HAVE THAT PERSON CALL THE PARAMEDICS OR AN AMBULANCE.**

▶ **IF THE CUT IS MORE SUPERFICIAL (SURFACE OF THE EYEBALL ONLY), IT STILL NEEDS TO BE EVALUATED.**

- Keep the youngster calm.

- Patch both eyes.

- Call your doctor or ophthalmologist, or go to an emergency room.

Blow Directly to the Eye

▶ **HAVE THE YOUNGSTER LIE DOWN IMMEDIATELY AND RESTRICT ALL MOVEMENT.**

▶ **EVALUATE THE INJURY:**

- Is the eye red?

- Does the eye hurt?

- Is the youngster experiencing blurred vision?

- Are the pupils uneven?

- Does her head hurt?

- Is she nauseated?

- With these symptoms, the youngster should not be moved until you have received instructions from a professional.

539

RECOGNIZING
AND
MANAGING
SERIOUS OR
POTENTIALLY
SERIOUS
INJURIES

▶ **TREATING THE INJURY:**

- Cover *both* eyes with gauze wrap, a scarf, towel, sanitary napkin, or other similar material. This restricts movement and rests the eyes.

- Call your ophthalmologist or your doctor for instructions.

- If you do not have a doctor or cannot reach your doctor, call the paramedics or an ambulance or go carefully but quickly to an emergency room. When there is a blow directly to the eye, bleeding inside the eye (which you can't see) can take place. The youngster needs to be moved carefully and in a lying-down (supine) position.

▶ **IF THE BLOW WAS TO THE CHEEKBONE OR EYE SOCKET BUT NOT DIRECTLY TO THE EYE:**

- Check to make sure there are no symptoms of direct eye injury (explained under "Evaluate the Injury").

- If not, have the youngster lie down and rest.

- Close both eyes and cover with gauze wrap, a towel, scarf, or other similar material—to rest the eyes.

- Place an ice pack on the injured area (cheekbone, forehead, eye socket) to reduce swelling.

- Call the doctor if the youngster begins to complain of eye pain and/or blurred vision or you're concerned about the amount of swelling.

Solvents, Poisons, and Chemicals in the Eye(s):

If you are unable to remember the details of managing this problem, turn to the Emergency Quick Reference on page 172, entitled "Managing Poisoning," for a review.

Instant-Bonding Glue (Cyanoacrylate) in or near the Eye(s):

If you are unable to remember the details of managing this problem, turn to the Emergency Quick Reference on page 172, entitled "Managing Poisoning," for a review.

Eyelash, Dust, or Dirt in the Eye

▶ **KEEP THE YOUNGSTER CALM; TELL HIM NOT TO RUB HIS EYE BUT TO CLOSE IT GENTLY—AND KEEP IT CLOSED UNTIL YOU ARE READY.**

- Wash your hands with soap and warm water.

- Now lift the upper lid of the eye with your thumb and forefinger. Gently pull the upper lid down *over* the lower lid and hold it there for a moment. Tell the youngster this is supposed to feel funny. It will make his eye water and hopefully wash out the eyelash, dust, dirt, or whatever.

- If this technique does not work, find an eyedropper, bulb syringe, or drinking glass. Fill it with lukewarm (never hot) water. Turn the youngster's head to the side and flush the water (a slow, steady stream) through the eye. Pour the water from the inside corner of the eye (next to the nose) and allow it to flush across the eye to the outside corner.

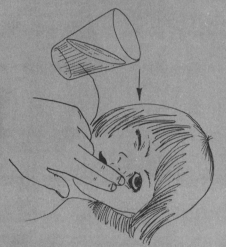

Flush the eye with water to try to remove a foreign object.

- If you cannot remove the foreign object by flushing with water, call the doctor. He or she may give you additional instructions or have you bring the youngster into the office for evaluation. Do not manipulate the eye any further unless instructed to do so.

▶ **IF YOU CANNOT SEE ANYTHING IN THE EYE, BUT THE YOUNGSTER STILL FEELS AS IF THERE IS SOMETHING THERE, SUSPECT A SCRATCH ON THE EYE (CORNEAL ABRASION).**

- The youngster will have an intense feeling of "something in his eye" and eye pain, and he will usually refuse to open his eye in the light or

541

RECOGNIZING
AND
MANAGING
SERIOUS OR
POTENTIALLY
SERIOUS
INJURIES

say he is unable to. He may have a headache and suffer nausea, as well. The white part of the eye will be red and inflamed.

- Cover both eyes with a scarf or patches. Do this gently but firmly to prevent the eyes from moving.

- Call your doctor to arrange for an evaluation, or go to an emergency room.

Eye Injuries: What You Should Know

Eye injuries are really frightening for both parents and the injured youngster. Our eyesight is so precious to us that any potential problem is considered a threat to our vision—and it could be. Although some eye injuries can be very serious—most are minor. The important aspects of treating eye injuries are to *cause no further harm*, to quickly evaluate the need for professional help, and to rapidly get that help for the young person if needed.

Most young people (and adults) panic whenever there is an injury to the eye. The first step is to calmly evaluate the problem and determine whether medical care is necessary or not. If it is not needed, then make sure you are careful *not* to cause further injury while providing first aid. If medical care is needed, your job is to act swiftly, but calmly, so the youngster doesn't panic and accidentally cause further damage to the eye. When it comes to the potentially serious or serious eye injuries, a review of the Emergency Quick Reference guide shows that all actions you should take are aimed at *preventing further damage*.

Many people wonder why patching *both eyes* is recommended when only one is injured. Patching is used to discourage the eyes from moving (looking around, and moving up and down when the lids are opened and shut). If the "good eye" was not patched, it would continue to move, and since both eyes move together, the injured one would move with it. Patches should not be put on with undue pressure but should be snug enough to prevent eyelid movement. (Most youngsters *hate* patches, so try to explain how important this is—but if the child resists, you may need to be firm with him or her until the injury has been professionally evaluated.)

As much as you would like to do more, particularly when there is an object impaled in the eye, remember not to take any action without instructions from the ophthalmologist or family doctor. Any attempt to remove an impaled object may result in more severe and permanent damage than the original injury caused. So the most important points to remember are to keep the youngster calm and reassured, protect the eyes from further damage, and call your doctor or ophthalmologist for instructions.

Alternatively, go to the nearest emergency room or call the paramedics or an ambulance, if warranted. Eye injuries are frightening, but your actions and promptness *can* make a major difference in many situations.

A few words about *corneal abrasions*—scratches on the cornea: These are common injuries and usually heal well on their own, but they do cause a lot of worry and pain. Most often, a youngster gets something stuck in her eye for a few minutes. Before it is removed, an abrasion (a scrape) of the cornea (the area covering the pupil) occurs. This causes severe pain, redness of the eye, tearing, and difficulty opening the eye. She may have a severe headache and nausea, as well, and complain that something is stuck in her eye.

Fortunately, the surface layers of the cornea (which are damaged with a corneal abrasion) heal rapidly—generally in twenty-four to forty-eight hours. This kind of injury needs to be evaluated by a doctor, who usually stains the eye with a special dye that allows the scrape to become fluorescent. In this way, he or she can actually see the abrasion and evaluate it. Treatment is simple and includes rest, patching the eye(s) to control pain and limit movement, as well as taking an aspirin substitute or another stronger, prescribed pain reliever. Some doctors also recommend eye ointment and reexamination in one to two days. The good news is that complications as a result of this injury rarely occur.

THE DON'TS

Don't ever try to remove an object impaled in the eye. Remember, this can lead to more damage.

Don't manipulate or probe in or around the eye—for any reason. Our eyes are very sensitive and can easily be injured and permanently damaged.

Don't hesitate to call your doctor or ophthalmologist if you are not sure whether a problem requires evaluation and/or treatment. As a precaution, always have the youngster lie down, restrict all movement, and patch both eyes—until you have instructions from the ophthalmologist.

PLEASE NOTE: Now that you have a grasp of how to recognize and manage eye injuries, it would be extremely helpful for you to go back to the Emergency Quick Reference With the Steps in Detail and review it carefully. The more familiar you are with that material, the more useful it will be to you when you need it.

543

RECOGNIZING
AND
MANAGING
SERIOUS OR
POTENTIALLY
SERIOUS
INJURIES

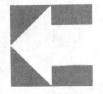

EMERGENCY QUICK REFERENCE

With the Steps in Detail

Flame and Scald Burns

▶ **IDENTIFY THE TYPE OF BURN THE YOUNGSTER HAS SUFFERED.**

▶ **MOST *SCALD* BURNS—THOSE THAT HAPPEN BECAUSE OF CONTACT WITH A HOT LIQUID—ARE FIRST- OR SECOND-DEGREE BURNS.**

- *First-degree burns* are pink or bright red and have no blisters. They are tender to the touch.

- *Second-degree burns* have areas of blistering or areas that are raw because blisters have already broken. Also, the skin is deep red, swollen, and raised. The burn is very painful and tender.

▶ ***FLAME* BURNS MAY HAVE AREAS OF SECOND-, THIRD-, AND FOURTH-DEGREE BURNS.**

- *Third-degree burns* are dry and may look white, brown, or charred. The burned area is hard and sunken compared to the surrounding skin and is not painful if you press on it.

- A *fourth-degree burn* involves deeper layers of fat, muscles, tendons, and even bones.

For Scald Burns (Those Caused by Hot Liquids)

▶ **IF THE BURNED AREA IS COVERED WITH CLOTHING, FIRST POUR COOL WATER ON THE BURN, THEN REMOVE THE CLOTHING.**

▶ **IMMEDIATELY COVER THE BURN WITH COOL, WET TOWELS. POUR COOL WATER OVER THE TOWELS AS THEY GET WARM. CONTINUE THIS FOR TEN TO FIFTEEN MINUTES.**

▶ **REMOVE THE TOWELS AND LOOK AT THE BURN TO DETERMINE WHETHER IT IS A SERIOUS OR POTENTIALLY SERIOUS SECOND-DEGREE BURN:**

- The blistered area is larger than three or four inches in size.

- There are blisters that are broken or leaking fluid.

- The burn involves the face, hands, feet, or genitals.

▶ **THE YOUNGSTER SHOULD BE TREATED BY HER DOCTOR OR IN AN EMERGENCY ROOM IF THERE IS A SERIOUS OR POTENTIALLY SERIOUS SECOND-DEGREE BURN:**

- Cover the burn with a clean, dry cloth or sheet.

- If the burn involves a large part of the youngster's body, wrap her in a blanket to keep her from getting chilled.

- Get him to the doctor (for a small second-degree burn) or to an emergency room (for a large second-degree burn).

▶ **IF THE CHILD HAS A SMALL SECOND-DEGREE BURN, AND THE BLISTERS HAVE NOT BROKEN, YOU CAN CONTINUE TO TREAT HER AT HOME:**

- Gently wash the burn with a mild soap and water and pat it dry.

- Apply a thin layer of antibiotic ointment (such as Bacitracin).

- If the burn is in an area that is likely to get dirty or be irritated, cover it with nonstick gauze and fasten it in place with tape or wrapping. Otherwise, leave it uncovered.

- Give the youngster appropriate doses of aspirin substitute if she has pain or discomfort.

- Remove the dressing (soak it off if it sticks), gently wash the burn, and reapply the ointment and dressing twice a day until the raw area of the burn is not sore when you touch it (about five to seven days), then once a day until the new skin is smooth and dry. Each time, look at the burn to see if any blisters have broken or if there are signs of infection.

▶ **CALL THE DOCTOR FOR ADVICE AND/OR AN APPOINTMENT IF YOU SEE SIGNS OF INFECTION OR POTENTIAL INFECTION IN A BURN YOU HAVE BEEN TREATING AT HOME:**

545

RECOGNIZING
AND
MANAGING
SERIOUS OR
POTENTIALLY
SERIOUS
INJURIES

- Blisters that have broken or are leaking fluid.

- Redness, swelling, or severe pain at the edges of the blistered area.

- Pus on the surface of the burn or in a blister.

- A white or gray color in the base of the burned area.

- Fever and/or chills.

▶ **MOST FIRST-DEGREE BURNS CAN BE MANAGED AT HOME:**

- Cover the burned area with cool, wet towels for another fifteen to thirty minutes. For larger first-degree burns, you might put the youngster into the bathtub in cool (but not cold) water.

- Give the youngster aspirin substitute in the appropriate dosage to control pain or discomfort.

- Aloe vera gel sometimes takes some of the sting away if you rub it onto a first-degree burn.

- Dress the youngster lightly, in soft clothing, while the burn heals. Sometimes keeping the burn lightly covered will help control pain.

▶ **CALL YOUR DOCTOR FOR ADVICE IF:**

- An infant or young child has a first-degree burn that covers more than one-fourth of his or her body.

- A youngster has severe chills, fever, nausea, or vomiting after a first-degree burn or seems more sick than you would expect.

For Flame Burns

▶ **REMOVE THE YOUNGSTER FROM THE FLAMES AND INTO FRESH AIR AND PUT OUT ANY REMAINING FIRE BY SMOTHERING IT WITH BLANKETS OR CLOTHING OR DOUSING IT WITH WATER.**

▶ **IF THE YOUNGSTER IS UNCONSCIOUS, CHECK TO BE SURE HE IS BREATHING. IF NOT, BEGIN RESCUE BREATHING OR FULL CPR, IF NECESSARY.** (If you are Certified in CPR and are unable to remember the details of this procedure or how to perform rescue breathing, turn to the Emergency Quick Reference on page 113, entitled "A Review of the Six Steps of CPR.")

▶ **IF SHE IS CONSCIOUS, COOL HER DOWN QUICKLY BY COVERING THE BURNED AREAS WITH COOL WATER IF POSSIBLE.**

▶ **REMOVE ANY WET OR SMOLDERING CLOTHING AS BEST YOU CAN.**

▶ **WRAP THE YOUNGSTER IN A CLEAN SHEET, THEN A BLANKET, TO KEEP HIM FROM LOSING BODY HEAT. HAVE SOMEONE ELSE CALL THE PARAMEDICS WHILE YOU TREAT THE CHILD. IF NO ONE IS WITH YOU, CONTINUE TREATING THE CHILD WHILE YOU PE-RIODICALLY SHOUT FOR HELP. WHEN HELP ARRIVES, HAVE THAT PERSON CALL THE PARAMEDICS. IF PARAMEDICS OR AN AM-BULANCE ARE NOT AVAILABLE, GET THE YOUNGSTER TO AN EMERGENCY ROOM AS SOON AS POSSIBLE.**

▶ **ALWAYS ASSUME THAT THERE IS A POSSIBILITY OF SMOKE IN-HALATION, INHALATION OF POISONOUS FUMES AND/OR CARBON MONOXIDE POISONING IF THE YOUNGSTER WAS INVOLVED IN A FIRE.** (For information on managing this problem, turn to the Emergency Quick Reference on page 597, entitled "Smoke Inhalation and Carbon Monoxide Poisoning," for details.)

Flame and Scald Burns: What You Should Know

Each year, more than 2,500 children die from burns, and many more suffer pain and long-term problems as a result of less serious burns. Most burns in children occur in or around the home, and many could have been prevented.

In infants and children under three years old, the greatest danger is from spilled hot liquids or foods or from burns in hot baths or showers. These scald burns can cause first- and second-degree burns of large or small areas of the body. Older youngsters are commonly victims of flame burns because of clothing that has been ignited.

While small, minor burns can be treated at home, serious or potentially serious burns must be treated carefully in a hospital whose professionals are well trained and experienced in the most up-to-date burn treatments available. The most serious burns should be managed in a regional burn center.

547

RECOGNIZING
AND
MANAGING
SERIOUS OR
POTENTIALLY
SERIOUS
INJURIES

Flame and Scald Burns: Understanding the Problem

Normally, the skin is a tough barrier that protects the tissues underneath it from losing heat and fluid and serves as a defense against infection. When a hot liquid or flame comes into contact with the skin, one or more of the skin's layers are damaged or destroyed. The resulting burn not only damages the skin itself but also leads to several other potentially serious consequences.

Burns are described as first-, second-, third-, or fourth-degree, depending on how deep the skin destruction is. A *first-degree burn* involves destruction of only the outermost, thin layer of skin called the epidermis. This layer of skin is constantly being replaced by the body, and a first-degree burn heals in seven to ten days, without leaving scars. The damage is temporary.

In a *second-degree burn*, the damage extends down into the deeper layer of the skin called the dermis. The burn causes blisters to form and break, and the open, raw surface oozes body fluid. The broken skin is an ideal ground for infection, if care is not taken to prevent or control it. With proper care, second-degree burns will heal in two to four weeks, leaving no permanent scarring. However, the burned skin may be pinker or darker than the surrounding normal skin for several months and is very sensitive to further burning or rubbing during the early healing stages.

A *third-degree burn* involves all the layers of the skin and extends down into the tissue beneath the skin, called the subcutaneous tissue. Also called a full-thickness burn, it completely destroys the skin and all its blood vessels, hair, and sweat glands. All but the smallest third-degree burns cause serious problems with body-fluid and heat loss, and most require skin grafting to heal.

So-called *fourth-degree burns* extend down to the deep tissues of the body and destroy muscle, tendons, and bone. In addition to the very serious risks for fluid and heat loss, they result in permanent deformity and disability.

When a youngster suffers a serious burn, some of the skin damage is obvious within minutes to hours after the burn. In addition, large burns—whether second-, third-, or fourth-degree—can cause a youngster to lose a great deal of fluid and body protein, because the tiny blood vessels in the dermis become damaged. The body also loses its protection against heat loss, so the youngster's body temperature can drop dangerously. The fluid loss, along with low body temperature, leads to a shocklike state, with poor circulation to the vital organs.

One of the most serious, life-threatening risks of flame burns is damage to the respiratory system. Smoke inhalation, as well as actual heat damage to the linings of the airways and lungs, leads to almost immediate problems with breathing and providing oxygen to vital organs and tissues. These very dangerous problems, along with the fluid loss and heat loss, must be recognized and treated immediately.

Infants and young children are especially at risk for losing large amounts of fluid through what look like relatively small burns. For this reason, along with the serious risk for infection, it is vital that a youngster receive excellent, up-to-date care for serious or potentially serious burns. Infants and children with all but the smallest second-degree burns are best cared for in a hospital with a burn unit—at least for the first few days after the burn.

Flame and Scald Burns: Signs and Symptoms

The signs and symptoms of scald and flame burns depend on how the burn occurred, what clothing the youngster was wearing, and for how long the hot object, flames, or liquid was in contact with the child. In addition, with scald burns, the temperature of the hot liquid is important.

- *First-degree burns* are pink at first and are quite painful. After several hours, they become bright pink or red, and the burned skin looks puffy if you compare it to the skin next to it. There are no blisters, but the burned area is sore if you touch it. If a first-degree burn covers most or all of a youngster's body, he or she may develop chills, fever, nausea, and vomiting after a few hours.

- *Second-degree burns* develop blisters within minutes to hours after the burn. If you look carefully at what appears on the surface to be a first-degree burn, you might see a very deep red or purple color to the skin before the blister forms. Blisters can be large or small, or you may see open, raw areas where blisters have already broken. The tissue under the broken blisters is usually bright red and very painful, but it may appear to be whitish or gray if the burn is deep. Unbroken blisters enlarge over the hours after the burn, and open areas ooze clear or yellow fluid in large amounts.

- *Third-degree burns* are dry and may look white, brown, or charred at first. The burned area is hard and sunken compared to the surrounding skin and is not painful if you press on it. After several days, a thick, hard crust forms over a third-degree burn, and there can be a great deal of swelling of the tissue around it.

- A *fourth-degree burn* involves deeper layers of fat, muscles, tendons, and even bones. It is obviously a serious burn and develops a thick crust after several days or weeks.

Infants and children with serious burns may show signs of dehydration and shock very quickly after the burn occurs. Paleness, sweating, extreme weakness, and excitement, followed by loss of consciousness, may signal these life-threatening problems.

If a youngster has been burned by flames, it is important that you be aware of the very great possibility of smoke inhalation and/or burns of the respiratory system. Signs

549

RECOGNIZING
AND
MANAGING
SERIOUS OR
POTENTIALLY
SERIOUS
INJURIES

and symptoms of possible respiratory burns, as discussed on page 597, should prompt you to call for help immediately and watch the youngster closely until help arrives. Get the youngster into fresh air and begin rescue breathing or CPR if breathing stops. (If you are certified in CPR and would like to review the details of the procedure, see Chapter 5.) It is vital that a youngster with known or potential airway burns be evaluated and treated in a hospital as soon as possible.

Remember that relatively small burns can lead to serious consequences in infants and children, so get medical help as soon as possible if you are in doubt.

Flame and Scald Burns: What to Expect

A baby or child with all but the most minor first- or second-degree burn must be treated by physicians who are very familiar and experienced with burn care in children. When the youngster arrives in the emergency room after a potentially serious burn, the physicians and staff will first take steps to determine whether there is or might be a respiratory burn and start treatment if there is any suspicion that the problem exists. Next, they will take steps to control or prevent shock and loss of body heat. An intravenous (IV) infusion will be started, and the youngster will be given medication for pain as soon as it is safe. He or she will not be allowed to drink any liquids or eat for several hours or even days after the burn.

The physician will then quickly but carefully examine the burns to determine how much of the youngster's body is burned and how severe the burns are. This helps him or her decide what the next steps should be and where the youngster can receive the best care.

After the youngster is stable, the doctor and staff will start to care for the burns. They will be carefully washed, and any loose skin will be removed from the burned area. Antibiotic cream will be applied, and bulky dressings may be put on. The doctor will be sure the youngster has had immunizations against tetanus and give a booster shot against tetanus, if needed. The youngster might be started on antibiotics, as well.

Youngsters with serious burns must be admitted to the hospital, ideally to a burn center or intensive-care unit, until the risk of shock, fluid loss, and infection has passed. The youngster's burns will be examined, cleaned, and treated frequently, until healing has begun. Serious burns might require cleaning and debridement (removal of dead skin and crusts) in the operating room, as well as skin grafting to cover the burned area. The burn specialist will explain these procedures to you in detail, if they become necessary.

Some burns are covered with dressings and bandages during the healing process, while others are treated "open"—without surface dressings over the antibiotic cream. If a burn is treated in this way, the youngster will be kept in as sterile an environment as possible. You will probably need to wear sterile gowns, masks, and gloves when you visit or touch your child.

If a youngster's burn is not serious enough to require hospital treatment, the doctor will give you detailed instructions about how to care for the burn at home, when the youngster needs to be examined again, and what signs would signal trouble. Pay attention to these instructions and ask questions about things you don't understand. You will want to do everything you can to prevent infection and ensure the best possible healing of the burn.

THE DON'TS

Don't rub any ointment, cream, or grease on a burn. Instead, apply cool, wet towels or a clean sheet (to a large burn) and call the doctor or go to an emergency room.

Don't allow a youngster who has had a serious burn to drink or eat right after the burn. After a burn (or any moderate or serious injury), many children develop a temporary slowdown of their intestinal activity and vomit or become bloated.

Don't try to treat a burn that is more serious than a small second-degree burn without medical help. Call your doctor for advice about even minor burns if you are not sure whether the youngster needs to be seen or if you are not sure about treatment.

Don't treat a burn of the face, genitals, hands, or feet without checking with your doctor or going to an emergency room. Burns in these areas are difficult, in that they tend to scar easily, become infected, and/or lead to potentially serious disability.

Don't delay in getting medical treatment if you see signs of infection in even minor burns. Burns are ideal places for infection to develop, and the result could be a more serious scar or deformity or even generalized infection (sepsis).

Don't overlook the steps you can take to prevent unnecessary burns in your children. Refer to Chapter 2 for suggestions about burn prevention.

PLEASE NOTE: Now that you have a grasp of how to recognize and manage flame and scald burns, it would be extremely helpful for you to go back to the Emergency Quick Reference With the Steps in Detail and review it carefully. The more familiar you are with that material, the more useful it will be to you when you need it.

551

RECOGNIZING
AND
MANAGING
SERIOUS OR
POTENTIALLY
SERIOUS
INJURIES

EMERGENCY QUICK REFERENCE

With the Steps in Detail

Fractures, Dislocations, and Growth-Plate Injuries

▶ **SUSPECT A FRACTURE, DISLOCATION, OR GROWTH-PLATE IN-JURY IF A YOUNGSTER WHO HAS BEEN (OR MAY HAVE BEEN) INJURED SHOWS ONE OR MORE OF THE FOLLOWING SYMPTOMS OR SIGNS:**

- Refusal to use an arm or put weight on a leg.

- Severe swelling and inability to move a joint.

- Obvious deformity of a bone or joint (it looks crooked, or you can feel or see part of a bone jutting out).

- Swelling and tenderness over a bone.

- Numbness, tingling, severe pain, white or blue color of the fingers or toes, if associated with an injury higher up in the arm or leg.

▶ **IF A YOUNGSTER HAS AN OBVIOUS FRACTURE OR DISLOCATION, OR YOU ARE ALMOST CERTAIN HE HAS A SERIOUS INJURY:**

- Do not allow him to put weight on the injured leg or use the injured arm.

- Immobilize the injured arm or leg. Make a splint out of a pillow, some cardboard, or other firm material and tape or tie it to the injured part, so the youngster cannot move the painful bone or joint. If the arm is injured, make a sling so the arm does not hang down or swing when he moves.

- If you can, apply an ice pack to the swollen, tender part of the bone or joint.

- Call the doctor or get the youngster to an emergency room for evaluation and treatment. If the injury involves the upper part of the leg or the hip, call an ambulance (do not call the paramedics unless there are multiple injuries or a possible head, neck, or back injury, as well) to move the youngster. If you must move her yourself, you will need several people to help you.

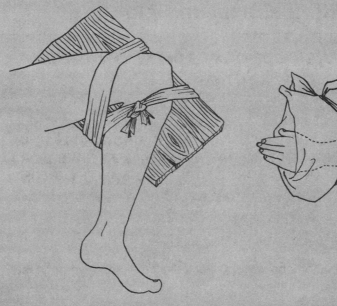

A board can be used to make a splint.

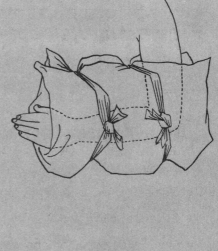

You can tie a pillow around an injured arm to "splint" it.

▶ **IF YOU THINK THE INJURY MIGHT NOT BE SERIOUS (THE YOUNG-STER CAN MOVE THE INJURED ARM OR PUT WEIGHT ON THE INJURED LEG, SWELLING AND PAIN ARE MODERATE OR MILD, AND THERE IS NO OBVIOUS DEFORMITY), TREAT THE YOUNG-STER AT HOME:**

- Have the youngster sit down or lie down and elevate the injured arm or leg on several pillows.

- Apply an ice pack over the painful area for several hours (fifteen minutes on and fifteen minutes off). Use a commercially made ice pack or make your own by putting crushed ice in a plastic bag and covering it with a towel.

- Give the youngster the appropriate dose of aspirin substitute. Repeat this every four to six hours, if needed.

- Reevaluate the injury. If there is improvement, allow the youngster to begin using the arm or leg again.

553

RECOGNIZING
AND
MANAGING
SERIOUS OR
POTENTIALLY
SERIOUS
INJURIES

- If there is little or no improvement (but no worsening of the injury), continue to apply ice packs for twenty-four hours or for as long as the youngster will tolerate it.

- After twenty-four hours, apply warm packs or a heating pad (only while you supervise the youngster), or have the child soak in a warm bath.

▶ **CALL THE DOCTOR FOR ADVICE ABOUT AN APPARENTLY MILD OR MODERATE INJURY (ESPECIALLY IF THE PROBLEM IS NEAR A JOINT) IF:**

- The youngster has increasing pain, swelling, or limitation of movement.

- Pain, limitation of movement, or swelling lasts for more than a day.

Fractures, Dislocations, and Growth-Plate Injuries: What You Should Know

The bones of infants, children, and older youngsters are particularly resilient and do not break easily. Likewise, their joints are quite resistant to dislocation, because the ligaments that hold the bones in place are firm but elastic. Because of this, falls and other injuries that would almost certainly cause fractures (broken bones) in adults often do not lead to fractures in children.

Bones are living structures—containing special cells that allow growth, repair of damaged tissue, and the laying down of calcium to make the bones hard. Bones form the supporting structures of the body. The centers of bones contain *bone marrow*—which is actually the organ that makes most of the blood cells. Bones are covered by a thick, tough membrane called the *periosteum*, which contains some of the blood vessels that nourish the bone.

Cartilage is a tough material that forms the basic structure of a bone. It contains less calcium than a fully formed bone, so it is somewhat pliable and can change shape a bit easier than bone. Young infants have more cartilage in their skeletons than bone, and as they grow and develop, this cartilage is calcified into strong bone. Cartilage also covers the joint surfaces of the bones and forms a tough cushion when bones move against each other and when an arm or leg is jarred.

In infants, children, and adolescents, each bone contains several areas that allow the bone to grow in length and width. These special areas—the *growth plates*—are found on each end of a long bone near the joint and in several other areas of certain bones, as well. Cells in the growth plate multiply, then calcium is deposited behind the growing end of the bone. The problem is that the growth plate is especially vulnerable to injury, and damage to the growth plate can lead to abnormal growth of a bone.

The bones are connected to each other at *joints*, which allow smooth movement. The bones fit together so they move in a certain way. Most joints are hinge joints—they move back and forth in one plane of the body. Other joints—such as the hip—are ball-and-socket joints, which allow some rotary motion, as well. Joint surfaces are made up of smooth cartilage, which is lubricated by joint fluid. Joints are held together by elastic structures called *ligaments*. Ligaments prevent the joints from slipping completely out of place (called a *dislocation*) or partially out of alignment (called a *subluxation*).

Serious injuries to the bones, joints, or growth plates of the arms and legs require evaluation and treatment—usually by an orthopedist (specialist in problems of the bones and joints). Your job is to determine if one of these injuries is likely or possible. To prevent further damage and pain, it's important to immobilize the injured body part and to get professional help.

(Injuries of the head, neck, spine, and chest are discussed later in this chapter. For information about injuries to the ligaments and muscles—sprains and strains—see Chapter 17.)

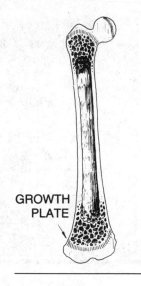

GROWTH
PLATE

Growth plates are special areas which allow bones to grow in length and width.

Fractures: Understanding the Problem

A fracture is simply a break in a bone. In general, the type of fracture a youngster has, as well as its location in the bone, will determine how serious the problem is.

There are several types of possible fractures of a long bone. The most common is a *simple* fracture, in which there is a "clean," single break through the bone. In young children, several unique kinds of simple breaks are possible because of the pliability of the bone. One of these is a so-called *greenstick* fracture, in which only the outer layer of the bone is broken. The inner portions of the bone bend without breaking, much like what you would see if you were to try to break a small branch. A *torus* fracture is another type of incomplete break, in which the outer layer of the bone "buckles" without breaking the inner part of the bone. This leaves an area on the bone that would look wrinkled on an X ray. A *compression* fracture is yet another type of incomplete break, in which the edges of the broken bone are pushed together, shortening the bone. Like a torus fracture, this can be very difficult to detect.

555

RECOGNIZING
AND
MANAGING
SERIOUS OR
POTENTIALLY
SERIOUS
INJURIES

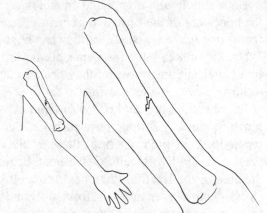

A simple fracture.

A greenstick fracture.

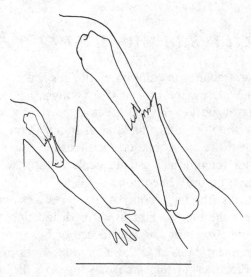

A compound fracture.

Complex fractures are often more serious than simple fractures. A *comminuted* fracture is one in which the bone is shattered, leaving several fragments of bone. A *compound* fracture is a complex fracture in which a piece of bone protrudes through the skin. This kind of break is especially serious, because the opening in the skin allows debris and dirt to enter the bone.

Both simple and compound fractures can be further complicated by movement of the bones out of their usual alignment. The edges of the broken bone can be *angulated* (bent) or *rotated* (twisted), or they can be moved so far out of place that they *overlap*. When the broken bone fragments are far out of line, they may need to be manipulated into better alignment before they heal, so healing will result in a bone that is as close to normal in shape as possible.

In general, a broken bone in a child or adolescent will heal well, without leaving much in the way of long-term damage. Because the bone is a living structure, it can repair itself in time. At first, there is bleeding and swelling around the area of the break. As the living cells of the bone begin to do their work, they first "clean up" the area of the fracture, then begin to multiply around the broken end of the bone. A *callus*—a thickened area—is formed around the broken area, and new bone is deposited to strengthen the break. (You can often feel this callus for several months after the fracture is healed.) As the youngster begins to use the arm or leg again, the broken bone is "remodeled" by the living bone cells, so it again becomes straight and strong. Because of this ability to remodel bone, a fracture with a little bit of angulation (bend) or overlap can often be allowed to heal without long-term deformity.

Common Fractures in Children and Adolescents

One of the most common fractures in children of all ages is a *clavicle* fracture (broken collarbone). This small bone can be broken if a youngster falls on his outstretched arm or on his shoulder. Suspect a clavicle break if a youngster refuses to move or cannot move his arm or shoulder after this kind of injury. You might be able to find a sore or bruised area over the collarbone or even feel the edges of the broken bone. This is a relatively minor fracture and usually heals in three to four weeks, leaving nothing more than a bump on the healed bone.

Fractures of the *humerus* (the large bone of the upper arm) can occur in the long shaft of the bone or near the elbow. Fractures (or dislocations) near the *elbow* are potentially serious, because swelling, broken pieces of bone, or poor alignment can cause temporary or permanent damage to the many blood vessels and nerves that are located at the elbow. Fractures in this area may involve the delicate growth-plate structures, as well. *Always* have a youngster with an injury around or to a joint promptly examined by the doctor.

Breaks in one or both bones of the *forearm* are especially common in youngsters and usually occur near the wrist. These bones—the radius and the ulna—are often a location for greenstick and torus fractures in children. Fractures in these bones are more common than breaks in the bones of the wrist itself, although the tiny bones of the wrist might be broken as youngsters get older.

Fractures in the *hand*, especially at or near the knuckle, are usually caused by hitting a solid object quite hard. If there is a great deal of swelling, pressure on the delicate tendons, blood vessels, and nerves can lead to serious problems. Apply ice and get medical help if swelling is severe or increasing.

Fractures of the *fingers* occur in a variety of ways. They may result from a blow to the end of the finger or when fingers are smashed—for example, in a door. Be sure to call the doctor if the skin is broken in a crush injury, since any debris left in the area of a broken bone can lead to infection. If the youngster has been hit on the end of the finger and there is swelling and soreness *between* the joints, suspect a fracture. If, on the other hand, swelling and tenderness are located over the joint, suspect a typical "jammed finger."

Fractures of the leg usually cause a youngster to be unable or unwilling to put weight on the injured leg. Breaks at the *hip* or in the shaft of the *femur* (the large bone of the upper leg) are serious fractures that can swell a great deal and may cause a significant amount of internal bleeding at the site of the fracture. In addition, the strong muscles of the upper leg may pull on the broken bone fragments enough to pull them out of alignment, causing both deformity of the leg and a great deal of pain. While they can occur with a serious fall, they more often result when a youngster is hit hard on the upper leg (for example, when struck by a car or tackled by the opposing team).

Breaks in the *tibia* (the shinbone) are relatively common in active youngsters. This strong bone of the lower leg can be fractured during a fall, especially when there is a twist involved (for example, during skiing), or by a hard blow to the lower leg. Breaks usually involve the middle or lower portion of the bone and can be compound fractures (the bone protrudes through the skin) because the bone is so close to the skin.

Fractures of the other bone of the lower leg (the *fibula*) are less serious than breaks in the tibia. The fibula is located on the outside of the lower leg and serves to strengthen the leg, but it is not the important bone in weight bearing. Therefore, a break in this bone may not cause as much pain as you might expect, and the youngster may be able to walk, although with a limp. It may be cracked when a youngster jumps down from a high place or experiences a fall. Suspect a fibula fracture when a youngster complains of pain in the outside part of the lower leg after an injury.

Simple *ankle* fractures are not very common in growing children and adolescents. Youngsters with ankle injuries are more likely to have sprains (ligament injuries) or more serious growth-plate injuries than fractures. Have the youngster elevate an injured ankle and apply ice packs for several hours, then evaluate the situation. If he or she cannot or will not put weight on the ankle, call the doctor or go to an emergency room for evaluation. Likewise, if pain, swelling, or limping persists for longer than a day or two, a medical evaluation is in order.

Fractures of the *foot bones* can occur with jumping or falling and usually lead to swelling and pain over the top or side of the foot. *Toe* fractures are common and painful but are rarely serious. In fact, there is no reason to even X-ray injured toes to be sure there is a fracture unless there is definite deformity that indicates that the toe needs to be straightened before it heals, there is numbness of the toe, or there is an open cut through which infection might enter the broken bone.

A *stress fracture* (fatigue fracture) is a type of injury in which a bone breaks because of repeated minor trauma. It is most common in young athletes who start new activities too rapidly. Usually, new stresses on a bone cause it to strengthen itself over time, so it is resistant to breaking. If, however, an activity puts unusual pressure on a bone that is not properly prepared (conditioned), a stress fracture might result. While a stress fracture can involve any bone, it is most often seen in the bones of the leg and foot.

A stress fracture can be very difficult to detect. At first, the youngster complains about a dull aching in the bone. After several days or weeks, the pain worsens, especially during the activity that caused it in the first place. If the youngster is examined at the start of the pain, there might be little you (or the doctor) can find to explain the pain. In fact, the minor hairline break might not even be visible on an X ray initially and only becomes apparent after a week or more. Think of this type of fracture if limping or pain continues for a week or so, and call the doctor for advice. He or she may wish to get another X ray or have a more specialized test called a bone scan performed to try to detect a stress fracture.

Dislocations: Understanding the Problem

Normally, the joints of the body fit together exactly. The surfaces of bone that rub together are covered by a layer of smooth cartilage and lubricated by joint fluid. Ligaments hold the joint surfaces in place and ensure that movement at the joint is allowed only in the normal direction(s). Muscles and their tendons pull across the joints to move the bones.

When a joint is subjected to excessive force in the wrong direction, the joint can be pulled or pushed out of alignment, and the bones slip out of place. When the surfaces of the joint are completely out of normal contact, the condition is called a *dislocation*. In a *subluxation,* the joint is out of alignment, but the joint surfaces are still in partial contact. Either of these injuries causes pain and can lead to stretching and damage to the ligaments, the muscles, and the joint itself.

Active youngsters often experience injuries that can result in joint dislocations or subluxations. These injuries can involve bone fractures as well as joint misalignment. A *fracture-dislocation* is a very complicated injury to a joint and involves dislocation of a broken bone. Most important, dislocations or other injuries around joints can involve damage to the sensitive growth plate(s) near the injured joint. Therefore, it is imperative that a youngster with a known or suspected dislocation be carefully evaluated by the doctor, *even if the joint slipped back into place*.

Dislocations and subluxations most often occur at the shoulder, hip, elbow, and knee. Youngsters with injuries in these areas require medical attention. Finger dislocations, while painful, are easily recognized and are less likely to cause serious long-term damage. Dislocations of the thumb tend to cause damage to the nerves and tendons of the thumb and hand—and should be viewed as serious injuries.

559

RECOGNIZING
AND
MANAGING
SERIOUS OR
POTENTIALLY
SERIOUS
INJURIES

"Pulled Elbow": A Common Problem

Toddlers and preschool children are particularly prone to "pulled elbow." This injury is often called "nursemaid's elbow" because of how it usually occurs. Most often, the little one suddenly cries and refuses to move his arm, but there has been no fall or obvious injury. What *has* happened is a sudden pull on the arm—such as might occur when he is jerked along by the hand when he doesn't want to follow. This same kind of injury can occur in an older youngster or even an adult if he tries to hold on to a very heavy object as it falls (for example, a barbell or large suitcase).

The sudden jerking of the arm pulls the radius (the bone on the thumb side of the forearm) out of place at the elbow. The radius normally is held in place by a slinglike ligament that allows the bone to rotate (twist) as well as bend. When the bone has slipped out of its sling, it can no longer rotate, and bending is painful or impossible.

A "pulled elbow" is quite easy to put back into place. In fact, sometimes the slippage is corrected before or during the doctor's examination. If the bone has been out of place for only a short time, the child will use the arm immediately afterward, without much if any pain. If there is any swelling or residual pain, the doctor may suggest that the arm be kept in a sling for a few days.

Growth-Plate Injuries: Understanding the Problem

Damage to a growth plate of a bone is always possible when a youngster experiences an injury near a joint. Each long bone of the body has at least two growth plates— one at each end of the bone. These growth centers determine the eventual length, as well as much of the shape, of the mature bone. Some bones have additional growth centers in the areas where muscle tendons attach to the bone.

Bone growth is controlled by several hormones. Bones grow at different rates, depending on the age and maturity of a youngster. Therefore, the amount of permanent damage a growth center sustains depends on both the type of injury and the age (maturity) of the youngster.

In a growing youngster, a serious injury to a joint is much more likely to damage a growth plate than the ligaments or tendons. Sprains (ligament injuries) are relatively uncommon in young children and active adolescents who have had trauma to a joint. For this reason, it is important that a youngster who has seemingly sustained a sprain be evaluated by a physician who is familiar with growth-plate injuries.

Fractures around the growth plate are particularly common in athletic youngsters. There are several possible types of fractures (breaks) that can affect the growth plate. Some involve only the growth plate itself, while others involve the growth plate and either the end (called the epiphysis) or the shaft (called the metaphysis) of the bone. The location and the type of growth-plate fracture will determine both how it is treated and the possible outcome.

Growth centers in areas where muscle tendons attach are susceptible to damage because of unusually pronounced pulling on the growth center by the muscles. This kind of growth-plate injury is most common in very active or athletic youngsters who start a new activity without easing into it gradually (conditioning). So-called *Osgood-Schlatter disease* is an example of this kind of injury. This condition occurs when the very strong thigh muscle and its tendon pulls on the growth plate on the front of the lower leg just below the knee. While it can occur in relatively inactive youngsters, Osgood-Schlatter disease is common in muscular young athletes who do a great deal of hard running and jumping. This problem causes pain in the leg just below the knee, especially with running or jumping. It heals itself in time, usually with little or no long-term damage. Rest and avoiding activities that cause pain seem to allow healing to take place more quickly. Similar growth-plate injuries can occur in other bones, such as the heel (called Sever's disease) and the elbow (called "Little League elbow").

Growth centers in bone have a very rich blood supply. Damage can occur if the blood supply is diminished or completely destroyed and leads to distortion of the growing end of the bone. *Legg-Calve-Perthes disease*, one of the most common examples of this kind of growth-plate problem, involves the hip joint, especially in young boys. It causes limping and hip or knee pain, which progresses over weeks or months and leads to permanent damage to the developing hip joint if it is not treated.

Slipped capital femoral epiphysis is another condition of the hip in preteenage boys. In youngsters with this problem, the growth plate in the hip is damaged, and the head of the femur (upper leg bone) slips out of place. Youngsters with this serious problem limp and complain of hip or knee pain. Its cause is unknown. Treatment is essential if permanent damage to the hip is to be prevented.

(For more information about Legg-Calve-Perthes disease and slipped capital femoral epiphysis, please refer to Chapter 14, "Swollen Joints, Limping.")

Fractures, Dislocations, and Growth-Plate Injuries: Signs and Symptoms

The signs and symptoms of serious bone and joint injuries are all similar. A doctor's evaluation (and often X rays) is necessary to determine the type and extent of injury. Suspect a fracture, dislocation, or growth-plate injury if a youngster experiences one or more of the signs and symptoms of such a problem (as listed in the Emergency Quick Reference) after a known injury.

Some signs and symptoms of fractures or growth-plate problems are more subtle and may develop over hours, days, or even weeks. The following signs and symptoms should prompt you to call the doctor for an evaluation:

561

RECOGNIZING
AND
MANAGING
SERIOUS OR
POTENTIALLY
SERIOUS
INJURIES

- Persistent pain in a bone or joint.

- Limping, whether or not the youngster says it hurts.

- Swelling over a joint that does not go away after a day or two.

- Stiffness or limited function of a joint.

- Persistent complaints of pain during play or a sports activity.

While these symptoms might signal nothing more than overuse of muscles or minor injury, they warrant evaluation to detect possible serious injury or illness.

Fractures, Dislocations, and Growth-Plate Injuries: What to Expect

The doctor's evaluation of a potential bone or joint injury starts with a detailed medical history and careful physical examination. He or she will want X rays to be taken of the injured area if there is a suspicion of a fracture, dislocation, or growth-plate injury. Often, X rays are taken of the noninjured side of the body also, in order that the doctor can compare the two sides. These "comparison views" may be necessary because of the many growth plates (which show as clear areas on X rays and can be misinterpreted as fractures) in the youngster's growing bones.

The treatment for fractures, dislocations, and growth-plate injuries depends on the type and severity of the damage to the bone and/or joint. In all but the most simple injuries, the doctor will recommend that the injury be treated by an orthopedic surgeon (a specialist in bone and joint problems). The orthopedist will first be sure the bone or joint is in the best possible alignment, then immobilize the bone and/or joint(s) to allow the injury to heal without the stress of constant movement.

Broken bones that are out of alignment and dislocations must be "set"—manipulated back into proper position—before they are allowed to heal. When this can be done by simple manual manipulation, the youngster will usually be given medication (either by mouth or by injection) for pain control and to relax him or her during the procedure. Complicated fractures, growth-plate injuries, and dislocations may require a surgical operation to put the bones or joints back into their proper position. Compound fractures and fracture-dislocations almost always are treated in the operating room.

After a fracture or growth-plate injury has been "set," the bone is immobilized while healing takes place. This is most often accomplished by using a cast that encloses the broken bone and the joints on both sides of it. The cast is left in place until the bone has healed. This process takes anywhere from three weeks for the most simple injuries to several months for more serious breaks. The doctor will check the youngster periodically during the healing process to be sure the bone has stayed in proper alignment and healing is progressing normally.

Certain fractures, especially those near the elbow and of the femur (thighbone) must be treated with traction for several weeks before a cast can be applied. This is because the strong muscles of the arm or leg will pull the broken bone out of alignment even if casted. Traction involves the use of weights to put a steady pull on the arm or leg, in order to keep the broken bone edges from overlapping or bending. This requires hospitalization until it is determined that the bone is healed or casting (or the use of crutches, a wheelchair, a sling, or whatever) is safe and effective.

After a joint dislocation, the doctor will recommend rest for several days or weeks before the youngster resumes her normal activities. This rest period allows the ligaments and tendons around the joint (which were stretched during the injury) to heal. Sometimes, a cast is applied to make sure that she does not further injure the damaged joint.

After a fracture, dislocation, or growth-plate injury has healed, the youngster will need to resume his regular activities gradually. The arm or leg that was immobilized during healing will be weaker than normal, and physical therapy and/or a prescribed exercise program might be recommended to hasten recovery.

THE DON'TS

Don't move a youngster with an obvious fracture without first immobilizing the injured bone or joint. Immobilization controls some of the youngster's pain and prevents further damage to the already injured bone or joint.

Don't hesitate to call the doctor if a youngster who had a seemingly minor injury has worsening pain or swelling after a few hours or even days—or experiences persistent pain and limited motion. Remember, some fractures and growth-plate injuries cause only minor symptoms at first. You always want to be sure that a growth-plate injury or other serious injury has not occurred—or if one has, that it is recognized so treatment can take place.

PLEASE NOTE: Now that you have a grasp of how to recognize and manage fractures, dislocations, and growth-plate injuries, it would be extremely helpful for you to go back to the Emergency Quick Reference With the Steps in Detail and review it carefully. The more familiar you are with that material, the more useful it will be to you when you need it.

563

RECOGNIZING
AND
MANAGING
SERIOUS OR
POTENTIALLY
SERIOUS
INJURIES

EMERGENCY QUICK REFERENCE

With the Steps in Detail

Genital Injuries

Genital Injuries in Boys

▶ MOST BLUNT INJURIES TO THE GENITALS IN BOYS (KICKS IN THE GROIN, FALLS ONTO BICYCLE CROSSBARS, AND SO ON) ARE NOT SERIOUS AND USUALLY INVOLVE BRUISING OF THE SCROTUM AND TESTICLE(S).

▶ INJURIES THAT INVOLVE THE PENIS MAY OR MAY NOT BE SERIOUS. TAKE TIME TO EVALUATE THEM BEFORE YOU CALL THE DOCTOR OR RUSH TO AN EMERGENCY ROOM.

▶ MOST INJURIES TO THE GENITALS ARE NOT SERIOUS AND CAN BE MANAGED AT HOME. TAKE THE FOLLOWING STEPS IF A YOUNGSTER HAS AN INJURY TO THE GENITALS.

- Have the youngster sit or lie down and rest until the pain has lessened. (Pain is usually severe for the first few minutes after an injury, often severe enough that he will lie down without needing much encouragement.)

- Have the youngster apply cool, wet cloths to the scrotum to help ease the pain and swelling.

- If there is bleeding from the penis, apply firm pressure over the place that is bleeding for ten minutes (by the clock), then check to see whether the bleeding has stopped. If not, apply pressure for another ten minutes and check again. (Remember, the penis has a very good blood supply and will bleed quite actively, even with minor cuts.)

- If the bleeding has stopped and the cut or scrape appears to be minor, you can continue your home treatment.

- Apply a cool, wet towel or cloth to the penis for twenty to thirty minutes to lessen swelling.

- You may give an appropriate dose of aspirin substitute if the youngster complains of pain.

- Have the youngster urinate into a glass container and check for signs of blood (cloudiness, pink or brown color, or obvious blood).

- If there is no blood in the urine, no pain with urination, and little or no swelling, you do not need to call the doctor or go to an emergency room right away. However, continue to check the youngster's penis or scrotum for worsening swelling, bruising, increased tenderness, or bleeding over the next one to two hours.

- Have the youngster support the genitals with an athletic supporter for several days after the injury.

- Ask the youngster to tell you about worsening pain—or any pain or discomfort when urinating.

- If the skin of the penis is caught in a zipper, you will probably need professional help to remove the zipper. Do *not* try to pull the skin from the zipper, since this could cause severe damage.

▶ **CALL THE DOCTOR OR TAKE THE YOUNGSTER TO AN EMERGENCY ROOM (IF YOU DON'T HAVE A DOCTOR OR CAN'T REACH YOUR DOCTOR) IF ANY OF THE FOLLOWING SYMPTOMS OR SIGNS ARE PRESENT:**

- There is marked or increasing swelling or bruising of the scrotum or penis for more than an hour after the injury.

- The injury involved known or possible penetration of the rectum.

- The youngster has severe or persistent pain, aching, or "drawing" in the scrotum or penis.

- Bleeding from an injury to the penis cannot be stopped with pressure after twenty minutes.

- You see blood coming from the opening in the penis.

- You suspect there is blood in the urine (obvious red blood, pink or brown color to the urine, or cloudy urine).

- The youngster is unable or unwilling to urinate after a genital injury or complains of pain or burning with urination.

565

RECOGNIZING
AND
MANAGING
SERIOUS OR
POTENTIALLY
SERIOUS
INJURIES

Genital Injuries in Girls

➤ **MOST BLUNT INJURIES TO THE GENITALS IN GIRLS CAUSE BRUIS-ING AND SWELLING OF THE GENITALS AND CAN BE MANAGED AT HOME. TAKE TIME TO EVALUATE THE YOUNGSTER BEFORE CALLING THE DOCTOR OR GOING TO AN EMERGENCY ROOM (IF YOU DON'T HAVE A DOCTOR OR CAN'T REACH YOUR DOCTOR).**

- Have the youngster lie down and try to keep her as calm as possible.

- Look at her genitals for any signs of swelling, bruising, or bleeding.

- If there is bleeding in the genital area, pat the area gently with a clean cloth and try to determine if the bleeding is coming from the outside or from inside the vagina.

- If the bleeding is coming only from the outside structures (the outer or inner lips of the genitals), apply firm pressure to the places that are bleeding for ten minutes. Check again for bleeding, and if it has not stopped, apply pressure steadily for another ten minutes.

- If the bleeding stops, apply cool, wet cloths to the genitals for twenty to thirty minutes.

- Look again at her genitals. Are there any open cuts or tears, or bleeding from inside the vagina?

- If there are no open cuts or tears, and swelling and pain are not severe, continue to have the youngster apply the cool cloths as long as it helps with the discomfort. You may give her the appropriate dose of an aspirin substitute to help relieve discomfort.

- Encourage her to urinate. If she is unable to do so, have her sit in a tub of water and try to urinate there.

- Ask her to tell you if she has worsening pain, continued or new bleeding, pain when she urinates, or cannot urinate.

➤ **CALL YOUR DOCTOR (OR GO TO AN EMERGENCY ROOM) IF ANY OF THE FOLLOWING SYMPTOMS OR SIGNS APPEAR AFTER A GENITAL INJURY IN A GIRL:**

- The injury involved known or possible penetration of the vagina, rectum, or other genital structures.

- There is bleeding that comes from inside the vagina, or you cannot be sure where the bleeding is coming from.

- You see cuts or tears in the genital area that are gaping open or bleeding heavily.

- Bleeding from an apparently minor cut or tear continues for longer than one hour.

- The youngster cannot or will not urinate, even in the bathtub of warm water.

- There is severe or increasing swelling or pain in the external genital structures (especially the labia).

- Bruising or tearing of the tissues between the vagina and rectum.

- A suspicion that the injuries were the result of sexual abuse or rape.

If You Suspect Sexual Abuse or Rape in Either a Boy or a Girl

▶ **IF THE SEXUAL ABUSE INCIDENT OR RAPE JUST OCCURRED:**

- Try to calm the youngster (and yourself) down.

- Do not have the youngster change clothes or take a bath.

- If the youngster has already washed, bathed, or changed clothes, take the clothing that was removed with you to the emergency room.

- Call your doctor or go to an emergency room so the youngster can be evaluated.

- Be sure to talk to the youngster about the fact that he or she will need to be examined, and encourage the youngster to tell you, the doctor, and/or a police officer (who will be called) what has happened.

▶ **IF YOU SUSPECT THAT A YOUNGSTER HAS BEEN A VICTIM OF SEXUAL ABUSE OR RAPE, BUT TO YOUR KNOWLEDGE THERE HAS BEEN NO RECENT INCIDENT** (nothing happened that day):

- Make an appointment for the youngster to see the doctor or call your local child abuse agency or "hotline" for help and instructions. If you are fearful the child may be in imminent danger of another incident, call the police for assistance.

- It's important to ask the youngster questions and get as much information about what happened as you can.

567

RECOGNIZING
AND
MANAGING
SERIOUS OR
POTENTIALLY
SERIOUS
INJURIES

- This entire situation is painful and stressful to the young person and you, but do all you can to encourage the youngster to be open and honest—not only with you, but also with any professionals who will need to talk with him or her. Remember, often the child or young person has been threatened (or a member of his or her family threatened) to prevent the child or young person from telling what happened—particularly if he or she knows the person who did it. (With sexual abuse the child usually knows the person and trusts him or her. With rape of an older youngster, the person may or may not be known to the youngster.)

▶ IT IS *VITALLY IMPORTANT* THAT THE CHILD OR YOUNG PERSON UNDERSTAND THAT WHAT HAPPENED *WAS NOT HIS OR HER FAULT.* BE LOVING AND SUPPORTIVE!

Genital Injuries: What You Should Know

Injuries to the genital organs are quite common in both boys and girls. While they are painful and frightening, they are usually not serious.

In boys, most injuries result from being hit in the genitals by objects such as balls, from falling onto bicycle crossbars, or from being kicked in the groin. Most often, this kind of injury causes momentary severe pain but no further injury. Preschool-aged boys can also be injured if a toilet seat falls down on the penis. In addition, many a youngster has caught the skin of the penis in a zipper—an event both painful and embarrassing.

In girls, most minor genital injuries occur because of falls onto such objects as bicycle crossbars or balance beams. Bruising and tearing can also result from doing the "splits" during play or gymnastics. The injuries caused by this kind of play are usually minor.

More serious damage can result from falling onto sharp objects or more forceful blunt injury. Serious damage to the genital structures themselves (the penis and testicles in boys and the vagina in girls), the rectum, and the urinary system are possible. Detecting these potential injuries should be your focus when you evaluate your youngster after a genital injury.

The problems of sexual abuse and rape have received increasing attention in the past few years. It is important to remember that genital injury might be the result of inappropriate sexual contact (in children of all ages) or rape (in older youngsters). A child or youngster who has been or might have been the victim of sexual abuse needs not only to be examined by a doctor experienced in recognizing this problem but also needs to be protected from further injury—both physical and emotional. A doctor (or any other person who works with children) who is aware or suspicious of possible sexual abuse is required by law to report this information to the police (who will then perform an investigation). Rape, a violent crime, should also be reported and steps taken to protect the young person—particularly if the rapist is known to the youngster (or he or she is able to identify the rapist). All children who experience sexual abuse or have been raped will more than likely benefit from psychological evaluation and care.

Genital Injuries in Boys: Understanding the Problem

Since the genitals in boys are relatively "exposed" to injury because they are suspended outside of the body, and because boys are usually quite active in both organized sports and free play, their genitals are quite susceptible to being hit, kicked, and crushed. Trauma to the genitals might involve the scrotum; the testicles and other structures inside the scrotum; the penis; or the urethra (the tiny channel that carries urine from the bladder outside the body), which runs through the penis.

All of the parts of the male genitals are richly supplied with blood, so bruising and bleeding are common with any injury. If there are no cuts or tears, the blood will collect under the skin, leading to bruising and swelling. If there are any open cuts or tears, especially of the penis, bleeding can be profuse.

The usual "kick in the groin" causes severe pain in the genitals. The injured boy usually doubles over in pain and may become pale, nauseated, and even collapse. He might vomit and feel quite bad for a few moments but then usually recovers without any continuing complaints except dull aching or soreness in the scrotum. With more severe injury, the scrotum and testicle(s) swell and appear bruised. Pain is more severe and lasts for several hours or days. Even then, the long-term effects are not serious.

If the scrotum is severely damaged, bleeding and direct injury can lead to problems with the blood supply to the testicle. This causes increasing pain, swelling, and tenderness of the testicle over several hours or days. More severe injury can also lead to the collection of fluid around the testicle (called a *hydrocele*) or even a *hernia* (so-called rupture).

In some boys and adolescents, a condition called *torsion of the testicle* mimics an injury to the scrotum or may actually follow such an injury. In this condition, the testicle twists inside the scrotum, narrowing or completely blocking the blood supply to the testicle. This is an emergency and must be treated promptly in order to prevent the testicle from being permanently damaged.

569

RECOGNIZING
AND
MANAGING
SERIOUS OR
POTENTIALLY
SERIOUS
INJURIES

Because of possible injury to the testicle and the other structures inside the scrotum, it is important that a youngster who has severe swelling or increasing pain in the scrotum be promptly evaluated by a doctor. The doctor will concentrate on whether or not there is damage to the blood supply of the testicle.

Injuries to the *penis* can cause severe swelling, bleeding, and bruising of the supporting structures of the penis, as well as damage to the tiny urethra, which passes through its center. Minor tears or cuts in the *urethra* usually heal rather quickly, without leaving serious permanent damage. However, with more severe injuries, the urethra can be completely cut. In this situation, emergency surgery would be needed to make a temporary opening from the bladder to the outside, and the urethra would have to be repaired through surgery.

Bleeding into the urine is a clue that damage to the urethra has occurred. When there is only a small tear, the urine might look pink, brownish, or cloudy. With some injuries, blood may be seen in the opening of the urethra (at the end of the penis) or in the urine. With the most serious injuries, the injured youth may not be able to urinate at all, or urination might cause the penis to swell because the urine leaks outside the tiny tube. It is important that a youngster with blood in the urine be evaluated by a doctor immediately, so the extent of the damage can be detected.

Unexplained swelling of the penis and its foreskin can be caused by inflammation and infection or might result from something tight being wrapped around the penis. If a boy is not circumcised (the foreskin of the penis has not been removed surgically), the foreskin itself can be the culprit that causes the swelling. If the foreskin is pulled back (for example, in order to clean the penis) and then not put back into its normal position, it can become stuck and cause this kind of swelling. In other boys, this kind of swelling has resulted from string or even hair being wrapped around the penis. It is important that a youngster with unexplained swelling of the tip of the penis be evaluated by a doctor. If the swelling becomes severe, the blood supply of the penis can be reduced, leading to permanent damage to the penis.

Trapping the skin of the penis in a *zipper* is common and causes both pain and embarrassment. When this happens, the skin around the zipper swells quickly, making removal of the zipper difficult. Usually, the skin cannot be "backed out" of the zipper, and attempts to pull the skin out lead to further damage and pain. In order to free the skin, the zipper must be popped open by inserting a sharp object between the two halves of the zipper. Usually, this must be done by a doctor or in an emergency room, so a local anesthetic can be given if needed. When it is obvious that you are not successful after a few tries, get help promptly, so the swelling does not increase unnecessarily.

Prevention of genital injuries in active boys should be a priority for you. If your youngster participates in contact sports, teach him the importance of protecting his genitals from injury. Insist that he wear an athletic supporter for comfort when he is active and a well-fitting protective cup for any sport that involves rough play, flying objects (such as baseball), or contact.

Genital Injuries in Boys: Signs and Symptoms

Most often, the major symptom of a genital injury in a boy is severe pain in the scrotum, penis, and groin. As noted, this pain can be severe enough to cause fainting, nausea, and even vomiting. Mild swelling of the scrotum, with or without minor bruising, and little or no discomfort after a short time signal a minor injury.

Be alert to the symptoms and signs of more serious injury, as listed in the Emergency Quick Reference. If you suspect serious genital injury, call your youngster's doctor, or take the youngster to an emergency room for evaluation. Since injuries to the testicle and to the urethra are potentially dangerous, it is important to err on the safe side with genital injuries.

Genital Injuries in Girls: Understanding the Problem

A girl's ovaries and uterus are protected by being inside the abdomen, but her external genitals are still susceptible to injury and are richly supplied with blood vessels. Therefore, falls and other injuries are likely to produce severe swelling, bruising, and bleeding. Being injured with sharp objects can cause damage to the structures of the perineum (the tissues around the vagina, urethra, and rectum) and can even lead to puncture of the abdominal cavity.

Most so-called *straddle injuries* (for example, falling on a balance beam, doing the "splits," or falling onto bicycle crossbars) cause little or no damage, although they certainly cause pain and bruising. There is usually swelling, bruising, and pain of the labia (the outer and/or inner lips of the genitals). If there is minor tearing or cutting of the delicate skin or lining of the genitals, bleeding can result. If swelling is more severe, the youngster might have pain or difficulty passing urine, because the swelling partially blocks the outlet of the urethra (the tiny tube from the bladder to the outside).

Most *lacerations* (cuts or tears) of the labia and other genital structures are minor and very shallow. They might bleed for a short time, then ooze tiny amounts of blood for several hours after a fall. Only a few of them require suturing (stitches), either because they are deep or because bleeding continues for more than a few hours.

Most often, parents worry about whether the hymen (the membrane at the entrance to the vagina) has been injured when their daughter has suffered a genital injury. Some blunt injuries can be severe enough to cause tearing of the hymen, but most do not cause any tearing around the vagina at all. Most often, bleeding comes from small tears in the labia rather than from the vagina itself.

The doctor may only be able to determine that there is no new tearing or bleeding from the hymen. He or she may not be able to tell if the hymen is "intact" or not. Part of the problem is that the hymen is different in each girl. Some girls have a rather tight, tiny ring of firm tissue around the vaginal opening, while others do not. Therefore,

571

RECOGNIZING
AND
MANAGING
SERIOUS OR
POTENTIALLY
SERIOUS
INJURIES

the vaginal opening can be normal, whether it appears large or small—even without injury or any past penetration into the vagina. The doctor will be more concerned about whether bleeding is coming from inside the vagina than whether the hymen has been torn.

If there is *bleeding from inside the vagina*, there is danger of damage to the internal structures of the body. This might be as minor as a small cut just within the vagina or as serious as perforation of the abdominal cavity through a hole in the vaginal wall. Because of the risk of internal injury and later infection, the doctor will want to do a careful internal examination if there is true vaginal bleeding after an injury. Sometimes, this kind of examination must be done in an operating room using a general anesthetic, so the doctor can be sure to see all of the important structures without the small child or youngster's experiencing severe pain or fighting the detailed examination.

Genital Injuries in Girls: Signs and Symptoms

Most often, genital injury is suspected when a young girl complains of pain in the genitals or has unexpected bleeding along with pain. Children who are able to talk can usually tell you what happened, but you are left with trying to decide whether the injury is serious or not.

Usually, straddle injuries cause pain and swelling, along with bruising and minor bleeding from the genital area. When you look at your youngster's genitals, you will see swelling, redness, and later bruising and some bleeding. If there are any small cuts or tears, she will also complain of pain or burning when she urinates, because the urine flows over the open cut(s). Therefore, she may not want to urinate.

Your role is to decide whether a potentially serious genital injury might have occurred. Call the doctor (or go to an emergency room) if there are signs and symptoms of more serious genital injury, as listed in the Emergency Quick Reference.

In girls who have had a genital injury, blood in the urine is not as helpful a sign as it is in boys. This is true because the urine normally flows over the external genital organs and will contain blood if there was any bleeding in the area at all.

Since there is a possibility of injury to the internal organs with severe genital trauma, it is important that you call the doctor or take your youngster to an emergency room for evaluation if you have any concern about possible severe injury.

Genital Injuries: What to Expect

When a boy has had a genital injury, the doctor will do a very careful examination of his external genitals, looking especially for possible injury to the testicles, penis, and urethra. He or she will check a urine sample, as well, if there is any question of injury to the urethra. The doctor might order a special scan of the testicles if he or she suspects torsion of the testicle or damage to the blood vessels of the testicle. The youngster might need to be admitted to the hospital for observation and treatment if the injury is severe.

A girl with a genital injury must be carefully examined to determine how extensive the damage is. At first, the doctor will look carefully at her external genitals and try to determine whether there is any bleeding from the vagina or tearing of the hymen. If the injury involves only the external genitals, no further examination may be necessary. If there is any bleeding from the vagina itself, or if there is new tearing of the hymen, an internal examination is necessary. As previously noted, sometimes this must be done in an operating room with a general anesthetic, so all of the internal structures can be carefully checked. Older youngsters and teenagers can sometimes cooperate with this kind of careful examination, but younger girls are usually too afraid to allow this procedure without an anesthetic. If any serious injuries are found, they will be repaired. If the youngster had a general anesthetic or the injuries are severe, she will be admitted to the hospital for observation and treatment.

You and the doctor will be concerned about the possibility of sexual assault or rape if genital injuries (to either a girl or a boy) are severe or cannot be explained. If sexual abuse is suspected, further examinations and testing might be needed. The doctor will also be concerned about the possibility of sexually transmitted disease if a youngster was attacked and about preventing pregnancy if a girl is sexually mature. Remember also that the doctor will be concerned about protecting the youngster from further abuse, and is required to report suspected sexual abuse to the appropriate authorities.

THE DON'TS

Don't overreact when a youngster has had a genital injury. Stay calm and try to calm the youngster, then evaluate the injury carefully.

Don't hesitate to call the doctor or go to an emergency room if you suspect a serious genital injury. Signs of potentially severe genital injury include the following: severe or increasing pain in the genitals after an injury; severe swelling or bruising; bleeding from the vagina in girls; bleeding from the penis in boys; inability or refusal to urinate.

Don't hesitate to have a youngster who was or might have been the victim of sexual abuse examined by the doctor or in an emergency room. It is important both to identify possible injuries and to protect the youngster from further physical and emotional harm.

PLEASE NOTE: Now that you have a grasp of how to recognize and manage genital injuries, it would be extremely helpful for you to go back to the Emergency Quick Reference With the Steps in Detail and review it carefully. The more familiar you are with that material, the more useful it will be to you when you need it.

573

RECOGNIZING
AND
MANAGING
SERIOUS OR
POTENTIALLY
SERIOUS
INJURIES

EMERGENCY QUICK REFERENCE

With the Steps in Detail

Head, Neck, and Back Injuries

▶ **TRY TO KEEP THE YOUNGSTER IN THE SAME POSITION IN WHICH YOU FOUND HIM—IF YOU THINK HE MIGHT HAVE A HEAD, NECK, OR BACK INJURY.**

- If you must move him because he is not breathing or has no pulse, do so as carefully as possible.

- Do your best *not* to bend her neck and back forward, twist them, or move them from side to side.

▶ **DETERMINE WHETHER OR NOT THE YOUNGSTER IS UNCON-SCIOUS.**

- Gently tap or squeeze his shoulder to see if he responds.

- Do *not* pick up a young infant or child to see if she wakes up or shake her vigorously.

If the Youngster Is Unconscious

▶ **CHECK TO SEE WHETHER HE IS BREATHING. THIS DETERMINES HOW YOU SHOULD PROCEED FROM HERE.**

If the Youngster Is Not Breathing

▶ **HAVE SOMEONE ELSE CALL THE PARAMEDICS OR AN AMBU-LANCE WHILE YOU TREAT THE CHILD. IF NO ONE IS WITH YOU, CONTINUE TREATING THE CHILD WHILE YOU PERIODICALLY SHOUT FOR HELP. WHEN HELP ARRIVES, HAVE THAT PERSON CALL THE PARAMEDICS.**

▶ **LAY THE YOUNGSTER ON A FLAT, FIRM SURFACE (USUALLY THE FLOOR OR GROUND) IF HE IS NOT ALREADY ON ONE. DO THIS CAREFULLY, AS MENTIONED PREVIOUSLY.**

▶ **OPEN THE AIRWAY.**

- Lift the young person's jaw so his head is in the "sniffing" position (chin jutted forward and head tilted slightly back, as people do when trying to smell something).

- Place a folded towel or other available material under the child's shoulders, taking care to keep her head as straight as possible.

- Clear the mouth of any vomited material or secretions.

▶ **BEGIN RESCUE BREATHING.** (If you are unable to remember the details of performing rescue breathing, turn to the Emergency Quick Reference on page 113, entitled "A Review of the Six Steps of CPR.")

▶ **CHECK FOR A PULSE.**

- If there *is no pulse*, begin full CPR (chest compressions with rescue breathing), as you learned in your CPR certification course. (If you are certified in CPR and are unable to remember the details of the procedure, turn to the Emergency Quick Reference on page 113, entitled "A Review of the Six Steps of CPR.")

- If there *is a pulse*, continue rescue breathing until the paramedics or ambulance personnel take over for you or until the youngster begins breathing on her own.

If the Youngster Is Breathing

▶ **HAVE SOMEONE ELSE CALL THE PARAMEDICS OR AN AMBULANCE WHILE YOU TREAT THE CHILD. IF NO ONE IS WITH YOU, CONTINUE TREATING THE CHILD WHILE YOU PERIODICALLY SHOUT FOR HELP. WHEN HELP ARRIVES, HAVE THAT PERSON CALL THE PARAMEDICS OR AN AMBULANCE.**

▶ **CHECK THE YOUNGSTER FOR SIGNS OF OBVIOUS INJURY.**

- Check the head for swelling, bumps, and bruises.

- Is there fluid or blood seeping from an ear or the nose?

575

RECOGNIZING
AND
MANAGING
SERIOUS OR
POTENTIALLY
SERIOUS
INJURIES

- Assess what happened (or what might have happened) and assume the youngster has a neck or back injury if there is a head injury. Likewise, assume there is a head injury if there is a neck or back injury.

▶ **CHECK FOR SIGNS OF SEVERE BLEEDING (BOTH OPEN WOUNDS AND INTERNAL HEMORRHAGING) AND TAKE STEPS TO TREAT IT.** (If you are unable to remember the details of managing this problem, turn to the Emergency Quick Reference on page 141, entitled "Managing Serious Bleeding," for a review.)

▶ **CHECK FOR SIGNS OF SHOCK:** PALE OR PASTY COLOR; COOL, CLAMMY SKIN; WEAK, THREADY PULSE; RESTLESSNESS; VOMITING; AND SO ON. (If you are unable to remember the details of managing this problem, turn to the Emergency Quick Reference on page 152, entitled "Managing Shock," for a review.)

- Keep the youngster warm by placing a blanket over her. (Do not try to overheat her.)

- Do *not* elevate his feet if there is a head, neck, or back injury.

If the Youngster Is Conscious or Wakes Up While You're Waiting for Help

▶ **KEEP HIM CALM AND DO NOT ALLOW HIM TO MOVE OR GET UP.**

▶ **ASK HER WHAT HAPPENED, AND USE THE ANSWERS TO HELP IN YOUR ASSESSMENT OF WHETHER OR NOT THERE IS A HEAD, NECK, OR BACK INJURY.**

- If he cannot remember, assume a potentially serious head, neck, or back injury has occurred.

- If she had a fall or was hit in the head, assume a head, neck, or back injury might have occurred.

▶ **CHECK TO SEE IF THE YOUNGSTER CAN FEEL YOU TOUCH HIM— ON THE LEGS AND THE ARMS.** (If you are unable to remember the details of how to systematically check the youngster, turn to the Emergency Quick Reference on page 503, entitled "Assessing Injury," for a review.)

- If he cannot feel your touch, assume a neck injury has occurred.

▶ **ALSO, ASK THE YOUNGSTER TO MOVE HER ARMS AND LEGS (SQUEEZE YOUR HAND, WIGGLE HER FINGERS AND TOES).**

- If the youngster cannot (or will not) move his arm(s) or leg(s), assume a neck or back injury has occurred.

If You Must Move the Youngster

▶ **IF YOU MUST MOVE A YOUNGSTER WITH A HEAD, NECK, OR BACK INJURY (BECAUSE HE IS IN DANGER OR YOU CANNOT GET PROFESSIONAL HELP), RECRUIT AS MANY PEOPLE AS YOU CAN TO HELP YOU.**

- Immobilize his head, neck, and back with anything you have available— pillows, boards, blankets.

Immobilize the head and neck if there is a known or possible head or neck injury.

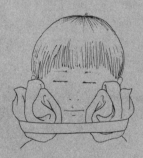

- Move her *as a unit*, keeping everything in alignment (as much as possible), so there is no further movement of the head, neck, or back.

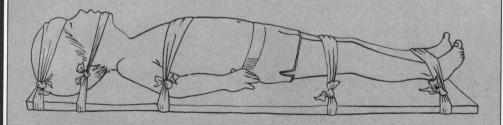

If you have no other choice but to transport an injured youngster, then carefully tie or strap him to a board to keep his head, neck and back in alignment and immobilized.

577

RECOGNIZING
AND
MANAGING
SERIOUS OR
POTENTIALLY
SERIOUS
INJURIES

- CPR should not be stopped to move a youngster, if at all possible, especially if the move is going to take more than a few seconds. If possible continue CPR while you transport the youngster to an emergency room.

- Transport him (lying down) to a hospital as carefully as you can.

- Be sure the youngster's airway is open, and monitor his pulse and breathing during the move. Be prepared to take action (rescue breathing and/or CPR—rescue breathing along with chest compressions) if the youngster's breathing and/or pulse stops.

- Your goal is to avoid doing further damage to the spinal cord (if damage has already occurred) or putting pressure on the spinal cord from any bones that have been injured (if damage has not yet occurred).

Head, Neck, and Back Injuries: What You Should Know

A neck, back, and/or head injury can be among the most potentially serious and frightening injuries any young person (or adult) can sustain. When it comes to these types of injuries, there are a few ''golden rules'' to follow:

- Remember that the initial damage has already been done and your job is to *ensure that no further damage occurs*.

- Never move a baby, child, youngster (or adult) who has or may have a head, neck, and/or back injury unless you have no other choice.

- If a head injury has or may have occurred, always assume that a neck and/or back injury may also have taken place.

- Always assume that there may be multiple injuries involved and use extreme care when evaluating the young person.

As we discussed in Chapter 15, when a youngster has a potentially serious injury, some people panic and try to quickly move the child or young person in order to get her to medical care. The problem is that movement—any movement—may mean the difference between a more serious injury and a more minor one or between a lifelong disability and a treatable problem. Therefore, whenever a neck, back, or head injury is *recognized or even suspected*, it is always best to have someone (if available) call the paramedics while you stay with the youngster. *Keep the young person absolutely still and in the same position in which she was found.* This rule applies regardless of the age or size of the youngster.

As a review, there are a few instances where this rule must be broken: if the youngster is not breathing and/or heart function has stopped, then CPR must be performed; if the young person's life is in imminent danger if he or she is not moved (for example, the youngster is threatened by fire, water, an oncoming train, car, truck, and so on); or if medical help cannot be summoned (because you are in an inaccessible locale or no phones are available, for instance) and you have no other choice but to move the young person. Even in these situations, you should take great care in moving the youngster (as discussed previously).

Often, people ask why it is so important to keep a child or youngster calm, still, and in the same position in which he or she was found when a neck, back, or head injury is recognized or suspected. Understanding the physical makeup of the head, neck, and back helps explain the reason behind such a rule.

As you know, the skull houses and protects the *brain*. In fact, it very much acts like a built-in helmet! The brain itself extends down to the base of the skull. This lower part of the brain is called the *brain stem*, which is a collection of complex circuits that work as conduits for the electrical impulses (signals) that move up and down the spinal cord—to and from the brain. The brain stem also controls heart function and breathing, as well as some other bodily functions.

The *spinal cord* extends from the brain stem down the back. This special structure acts as the pathway whereby sensory signals are transmitted to the brain (via the brain stem) from all parts of the body. From this same pathway, motor ''direction'' signals are sent from the brain to muscles. These impulses are responsible for motor function and reflexes (moving parts and areas of the body) and for ''sensations'' (being able to ''feel'' cold, hot, pain, pleasure, and so on). For example, when you want to move your big toe on your right foot, the command is sent by impulses from the brain through the brain stem down the spinal cord to the nerves that supply the right foot and toe— and you move your big toe! Impulses are then sent back to the brain telling it that the big toe moved as it was told. All of this happens unbelievably fast.

The spinal cord is located in the *spinal canal*—a tubelike space that runs down through the inside of the bones of the spine (the vertebrae). The spinal canal is lined by membranes called meninges. *Spinal fluid* fills the space between the spinal cord and the spinal-canal lining and acts as a protective cushion for the spinal cord. These structures are then protected by the *spinal column*—bony vertebrae with joints to allow for maximum motion in all directions while still guarding the spinal cord. These blocklike vertebrae support the weight of the head and torso and are separated by special cushions (called intervertebral discs) that absorb a great deal of the shock of motion and jarring.

Like other bones, the vertebrae are held together firmly by ligaments and their motion controlled by a complex group of muscles. These muscles, tendons, and ligaments and the spinal-column structure itself allow us to stand erect.

Damage to the Neck and Back: Understanding the Problem

579

RECOGNIZING
AND
MANAGING
SERIOUS OR
POTENTIALLY
SERIOUS
INJURIES

The severity of damage to the spine and spinal cord depends on many factors: the location of the injury (which will determine the areas and functions potentially affected); whether injury is to nerves, bones, discs, soft tissue, or the spinal cord itself; whether or not the structure(s) is (are) actually torn, severed, or has (have) pressure on it (them); if the injury is promptly recognized, managed, and treated; and if the youngster is prepared properly and transported safely. Damage can be temporary to permanent and can result in degrees of paralysis. If the spinal cord is severed, paralysis will result, and the extent of that paralysis will depend on the level (area) at which the spinal cord is severed.

Paralysis of the legs (lower limbs) is called paraplegia. Quadriplegia is paralysis of the arms and legs (all four limbs) and may also affect respiration (the ability to breathe). Hemiplegia (paralysis of one side of the body) most often results from damage to the brain itself rather than to the spinal cord. Essentially, the higher the injury is in the spinal cord (the closer to the brain stem)—then the greater the number of physical functions affected. Conversely, the lower the damage is in the spinal cord (the farther from the brain stem)—then the fewer the number of functions affected.

For example, if the spinal cord is severed in the neck, then the electrical impulses to and from the brain could not go any farther than the point in the neck where the spinal cord was severed (because there is now no pathway through which the impulses can carry their messages or receive information back). If the spinal cord was partially severed, then some signals might get through, but not all. The extent of permanent damage would depend on the areas of the body served by the part of the spinal cord that was partially severed. If, however, the cord was damaged by pressure from a broken vertebra, partial or full sensation and function may return with excellent treatment and rehabilitation.

There is a simple analogy to this complex system. Let's say you own a two-way radio with a very sophisticated antenna (spinal cord). This radio can transmit and receive information for five hundred miles in all directions. The electrical components inside the radio transmit and receive information. (They are essentially the "brain" of the radio.) The base of the antenna (nearest the brain) houses bundles of special wires that connect the antenna to the radio's brain, so the electrical impulses can be sent and received (doing the same job as the brain stem, found at the base of the skull).

If you damaged or severed part of the antenna farthest from the base of the antenna and radio, you might have some minor reception and transmission problems. You could find that the radio has more static or that the information is less clear. The closer the damage is to the radio's nerve center, the more problems occur and the fewer miles it could transmit or receive information. If the antenna was broken (severed) near the base of the antenna and radio, the brain of the radio could still keep sending electrical impulses—but they would stop right at the break. The pathway (antenna) has been destroyed, and the electrical information—although sent—has nowhere to go. If the base of the antenna (with all of its bundles of wires) was severely damaged, then the ability of the radio to function at all is seriously in doubt (since there is no way to get the information out of the radio's brain). The brain, brain stem, and spinal cord work in a very similar way.

As you can see, the spinal cord is a vital body structure. Even though it is surrounded by fluid and protected by the spinal canal and vertebrae, if a youngster experiences a great enough blow or falls or is thrown and lands in a certain way (on his or her head, neck, or back)—serious damage to one or all of these areas is possible.

Damage may be more minor, injuring muscles, ligaments, or other soft tissues. These usually heal with rest and proper treatment. A group of nerves can be temporarily or permanently damaged. An intervertebral disc can be herniated (pushed out of place) or even ruptured and can injure individual nerves that leave the spinal cord. Fractures (breaks) of the vertebrae can occur in many ways and in any area of the spine. A ''broken neck'' is a fracture of one or more of the vertebrae in the neck—called the cervical vertebrae. If just below the neck, the break is called a fracture of the thoracic (chest) vertebrae. If in the lower back, the fracture is of a lumbar vertebra. At the tail end of the spine are the sacrum (which is a platelike shield of vertebrae) and the coccyx (tailbone). Fractures in the cervical (neck) vertebrae and the lumbar (lower back) vertebrae are both the most serious and the most common.

At times, the fracture (whether in a cervical, thoracic, or lumbar vertebra) is *unstable*—meaning it can easily change position. If the spinal cord initially has *not* been permanently damaged, the youngster may experience problems but, with expert treatment and rehabilitation, fully recover sensation and function. However, even the slightest movement may push the fractured vertebra into the spinal cord—severing it or crushing it—and permanent paralysis will result. This is why it is so important that a youngster *not be moved* except by experts trained to prepare the youngster for transport, as well as transport him or her as safely and carefully as possible.

Also, injury may cause a slippage of the bones (of the spinal column) out of their normal alignment (called a dislocation or subluxation). This can occur with or without a fracture to a vertebra. A dislocation or subluxation may only put pressure on the spinal cord or permanently damage it. Again, improperly moving a youngster with this kind of injury may make a significant difference in the amount and/or permanency of the damage.

Since there is no way for you to know if the spinal cord has been permanently damaged when a young person (or adult) experiences a neck, back, or head injury—the best policy is to take no unnecessary risks and thereby guarantee no further damage.

Neck or Back Injury: Signs and Symptoms

581

RECOGNIZING
AND
MANAGING
SERIOUS OR
POTENTIALLY
SERIOUS
INJURIES

Suspect a neck or back injury if you find any of the following:

- The young person or child is unconscious.

- The youngster is found in an unusual position after an injury.

- The youngster is in shock, and you find no obvious serious bleeding.

- The baby, child, or young person cannot move a body part; complains of numbness, tingling, or a "funny feeling"; or is not able to feel you touch or pinch her.

- He complains of pain in the neck or back.

In all of the above situations, remember to keep the little one or older child as still as possible and call (or have someone else call) the paramedics (or an ambulance if you do not have paramedics in your area). In the meantime, assess the youngster as best you can for the extent or degree of his or her injuries.

If a youngster is found unconscious, *always* assume that a neck, back, and/or head injury could have occurred. As we discussed in Chapter 15 (How to Evaluate Your Injured Child), when a youngster is unconscious, check to make sure he or she is breathing and has a pulse. If not, perform CPR. If you must move the youngster to perform CPR, then do so with the greatest of care. If others can help you, move the injured youngster as a unit and be sure to support the head, neck, and back so *they do not move*.

If you actually see the young person become injured, determine quickly whether the fall or blow could have resulted in a neck or back injury. Falls onto the head that cause the neck or back to suddenly bend—forward or backward—often cause neck or back injuries. Remember that children have broken their necks by falling off of sofas, tabletops, fences, and playground equipment; or while doing somersaults, roller-skating, and bicycling; and while diving into ponds, pools, or the ocean. The list of possibilities is endless. The point is, if a youngster takes a nasty fall, never allow him to get up *until* you have determined that no serious injury has occurred—even if he says he's fine.

When a youngster is on the ground or floor—but conscious—tell her to hold perfectly still until you can make sure she is not seriously hurt. Even if the youngster argues with you or starts to cry, calm her down and start your assessment procedure.

As a review, here are the questions to ask: What happened (if you or someone else didn't see the injury)? How do you feel? Do you hurt anywhere? Is there tingling or a numb feeling (or a "funny" feeling) in your arm(s), leg(s), or on one side of your body? Can you wiggle your toes for me? Can you move your right leg for me? Now your left leg? Will you move your right arm for me? How about your left arm? Does your neck, back, or head hurt or feel different or funny? Are you nauseated (do you feel sick to your stomach), dizzy, or light-headed? Is your vision blurry? Do you have any abdominal pain (stomachache)? Are you having any trouble breathing?

Always make sure you have the youngster wiggle his toes and move his legs (in that order)—*before* asking him to move any part of the upper body. Also, if the youngster feels any numbness or tingling in the leg(s), arm(s), or on one side of the body, *do not allow* him to move and don't move him yourself. Call the paramedics and keep the young person as calm and still as possible.

If the youngster is unable to wiggle her toes or fingers or move her leg(s) or arm(s) *or* has any head, neck, or back pain—follow the same procedure (call the paramedics and keep the youngster calm and still). Also, if you are *not sure* whether there is a neck or back injury, or you feel there is a possibility of such an injury—*don't take a risk*. Call the paramedics and do everything you can to calm the young person and keep her still.

With a baby or a nonverbal child, there will obviously be no way to ask questions. Again, if the baby or child is unconscious, assume there is a real possibility of neck, back, or head injury (unless you know the youngster is unconscious because of airway obstruction, poison ingestion, or a convulsion, for example). But remember that the child could have been injured if he fell after experiencing an airway obstruction, convulsion, poisoning, and so on).

If the baby or little child is conscious, be very warm and reassuring and tell him to please hold "very still" for you for just a moment. The child can also "feel" this message if you firmly but carefully put your hand on his arm or shoulder and hold him in place. You don't want this to be strong enough to cause any movement or forceful enough to have the youngster fight you—you're just trying to say, "You're hurt, and please be really still." Look at the child's feet. Is he wiggling his toes or moving his legs? If there is no movement, pinch the bottom of each foot. If the child doesn't cry or move the foot, then pinch each leg. If there is still no reaction, don't move the child and call the paramedics. Remember, *no child is too small* to sustain a neck or back injury and must be treated in the same manner as you would an older child, teenager, or adult.

Neck and/or Back Injury: What to Expect

When the paramedics or ambulance attendants arrive, they will usually place a C-collar (cervical or neck collar) around the young person's neck so it does not move. They will also secure the youngster in the position in which they find her, so there is no movement of the neck or back, then move her as a unit onto a stretcher.

Once at the hospital, X rays (and other sophisticated diagnostic tests) will be ordered after the doctor examines the youngster, in order to identify what is damaged and the possible extent of the damage. If damage has occurred, the youngster will be put into one of several different kinds of traction (devices to pull on the head, neck, and back)

583

RECOGNIZING
AND
MANAGING
SERIOUS OR
POTENTIALLY
SERIOUS
INJURIES

to keep the spinal column in alignment and to relieve pressure on the spinal cord. In some situations, surgery is necessary to realign the spine or to put special devices for traction in place.

Since damage to the neck and back is so diverse, it is not possible to describe "what to expect" in every situation. Further treatment and rehabilitation will depend on the kind and severity of damage sustained. Recovery can be complete or partial and take a short or long period of time.

There is one thing you should keep in mind if there is damage to the spinal cord. When the spinal cord is damaged, a phenomenon called *spinal shock* can occur. This is a temporary reaction to the injury and often confuses the overall picture. With spinal shock, the young person's blood pressure may drop, he or she may collapse, and various functions (including breathing and bladder function) may be affected. Because of spinal shock, it is often difficult to determine the *true* extent of damage or its long-term effects. This (and the fact that temporary swelling around the spinal cord can also occur) is why doctors in many situations are ambiguous about the extent of damage or degree of disability (if any) a youngster has sustained. Once spinal shock and swelling have subsided (it can take days or weeks), then much more can be evaluated and more information given to you.

Damage to the Head: Understanding the Problem

As discussed in Chapter 9 (Unconsciousness), for our brains to work properly, we must have a normal flow of blood (and thereby oxygen and nutrients) to all areas of the brain. Anything that disturbs this natural flow of oxygen and nutrients will result in faulty function of our brain cells. This faulty function can be permanent or temporary and mild to severe—depending on the degree of damage to the brain cells.

Unlike most other cells of the body, brain cells do not reproduce themselves. Therefore, if the brain is injured and a limited number of cells are damaged, then the visible damage is usually temporary, or there may be some minor permanent damage. If, however, the injury is severe and a significant number of brain cells are destroyed in a certain area of the brain, then permanent damage is very likely, and the function(s) affected will depend on the area of the brain that was injured.

As a review, there are really *two injuries* that can occur with a head injury. The first is the one we can often feel and see—the injury to the skull and scalp. The second injury—the one that is actually the real problem—occurs when the brain bounces against the inside of the skull. Remember, the skull is very much like a helmet—a hard, protective covering. But when the head experiences a great enough blow, the brain can hit the skull just where the blow occurred *or* can bounce back and forth against the skull/helmet.

If the force of the brain hitting the skull is great enough, unconsciousness will occur.

Unconsciousness, even for a second, always signals the need for the youngster to be evaluated by a physician. (With a potentially serious injury, a very young child may appear "stunned" rather than truly unconscious.) This whack against the skull may also result in swelling and bleeding of the brain—either in the area of the blow or over a larger area of the brain if the blow was severe enough.

A *concussion* is essentially a brain bruise. The child will either experience loss of consciousness (for seconds to minutes) or an alteration of consciousness. (Review Chapter 9 for detailed information on the various degrees of loss of consciousness.) In response to the injury (the bruise to the brain), the brain cells begin to swell. It is both the bleeding and (in particular) the swelling that can cause very serious problems.

When an area of the brain or the entire brain swells and bleeds, the pressure inside the skull (intracranial pressure) increases. This increased intracranial pressure, if severe and uncontrolled, can damage the brain more than the original blow did. The reason? There is only a limited amount of space in which the brain can expand before the skull puts pressure on it. Fortunately, the swelling and bleeding due to a concussion disappear in a few hours or a day, and the young person returns to normal within a few days or a week.

A *contusion* of the brain, on the other hand, is a more serious injury. With a contusion, a part of the brain is damaged permanently, and there is local bleeding, as well as tearing of the brain structures in that localized area. Brain swelling in this case is much more severe and long-lasting. Recovery from a contusion is slower and depends on the extent of the damage. When fully recovered, the youngster will have some permanent damage. What functions are affected and the degree to which they are affected will depend on what area of the brain experienced the injury. Therefore, permanent damage from a contusion can be very slight (almost undetectable) to quite severe.

Bleeding itself can be a serious problem with a head injury. If a medium to large blood vessel—a vein or artery—is torn, then bleeding occurs, and the accumulated blood (called a hematoma) puts pressure on the brain.

An *epidural hematoma* occurs when an artery on the surface of the brain is torn. This is very dangerous, since blood flow in the arteries is rapid (the heart pumps blood through the arteries *with force*). The youngster may experience a momentary loss of consciousness, then wake up for minutes to several hours, acting relatively or perfectly normal. Suddenly, the youngster's condition will begin to deteriorate rapidly, and he or she will lose consciousness again. In this situation, the youngster could die quickly.

Therefore, it is vitally important to remember that if a youngster has experienced a head injury and appears fine (and has even been medically evaluated and released) but later lapses into unconsciousness, immediate medical care is imperative. Call the paramedics or an ambulance and be sure to tell them, as well as the emergency physicians, about the head injury, the previous evaluation, and the sudden loss of consciousness. An epidural hematoma is much more likely if the injury involved the temple area.

585

RECOGNIZING
AND
MANAGING
SERIOUS OR
POTENTIALLY
SERIOUS
INJURIES

A *subdural hematoma* (a blood clot) occurs when the veins of the brain bleed. Usually, blood seeps from the injured veins rather slowly and causes progressive deterioration (or not as quick a recovery as expected) over a period of several hours or days. Observation (in the hospital or at home) after a serious head injury (with loss of consciousness) is performed to detect this kind of gradual deterioration—as well as the sudden deterioration caused by an epidural hematoma. If a subdural hematoma is suspected, special tests (usually a CT—Computerized Tomography—scan or ultrasound test of the head) are performed. If a youngster is at home and you notice that he is not responding as well as before or begins to show other signs of more serious brain injury (listed below), go to the emergency room immediately so he can be evaluated again.

Both epidural and subdural hematomas form over the surface area of the brain and apply pressure to the brain from the outside. If, however, bleeding occurs internally (inside the brain itself), called an intracerebral hemorrhage, the problem is somewhat different, although still very serious. You and the doctor will not usually be able to tell the difference without special tests.

A *skull fracture* is an actual break in one or more of the bones of the head (skull). Although the idea of a skull fracture frightens people, unto itself, it is relatively unimportant. The damage to underlying brain structures as a result of the injury is what should concern you. What the fracture tells you (and the doctor) is that the blow to the head was forceful and could have been severe enough to damage the brain underneath.

There are several types of skull fractures—ranging from a simple linear fracture (a single-line break) to a depressed skull fracture (the bone is pushed inward against the brain). Some youngsters with skull fractures do not even lose consciousness, while others show obvious signs of brain injury. Suspect a skull fracture if: there is very severe swelling of the scalp after a head injury; the swelling continues to increase several hours after the injury occurred; you can feel a depression (''dent'') in the skull under a bump; or you notice bruising behind the ear(s) or of the eye(s) after a head injury. Call your doctor or go to an emergency room if you notice these later signs of a skull fracture, even if the original bump did not seem particularly severe.

A *laceration* (cut) on the scalp may mean there is a more serious underlying injury to the brain, but most often it is just a superficial injury to the scalp alone. Again, if the youngster was unconscious, even for a moment, or experiences changes in consciousness, then he or she needs immediate medical attention. If, however, the youngster seems fine (except for the laceration), apply pressure to the cut for fifteen to twenty minutes, then look at it carefully. If the laceration is small (shorter than an inch) and the edges lie together easily, without gaping open, you can treat it at home. Wash it carefully with soap and water, be sure the bleeding has stopped, and apply a sterile adhesive bandage (if you can).

Because the scalp has a very good blood supply, cuts often bleed a great deal. Don't let this alarm you. However, a scalp laceration usually needs sutures (stitches) if you are unable to stop the bleeding or if it is very deep, longer than an inch, or has jagged edges. Call your doctor or take the youngster to an emergency room or urgent-care center if you think a scalp laceration needs sutures.

Serious Head Injury: Signs and Symptoms

When a youngster has a head injury, your first question will be "Is it serious?" You may also wonder if his or her skull is fractured, but this is of slightly less concern, in that a serious head injury can occur without the skull's being fractured.

Of course, if the youngster is still unconscious, the likelihood of serious head injury is high. You will need to get help. Call the paramedics or an ambulance (or get others to help you move the youngster *carefully*, if you have no other choice, and take him to an emergency facility). If you can, try to determine whether the youngster might have been unconscious *before* he fell or was injured.

Most people don't quite know what to do if a youngster was injured but *is* conscious. They often feel all is well just because she is conscious or react in totally the opposite way and feel that any fall means a serious head injury. A serious head injury is likely if any of the following has occurred or does occur:

- The youngster lost consciousness, even for a moment. (A young infant or toddler's seeming stunned should also raise your suspicions that the injury may be serious.)

- There is bleeding and/or clear drainage from his ear(s).

- There is bleeding and/or clear drainage from the nose (if there is no obvious nose injury). Try to distinguish the runny nose that follows crying in a young infant or child from a clear runny nose that persists long after crying has stopped.

- The youngster is not fully awake and acting like himself—is sleepy, lethargic, irritable, or talking nonsense.

- She cannot remember what happened or seems disoriented.

- He has vomited more than once, or vomiting occurs hours after a head injury. (Many youngsters vomit or are nauseated immediately after any injury—a shock-like reaction to the pain.)

- She seems uncoordinated or staggers when she walks.

- He seemed fine for a few minutes but now seems much worse.

- She complains of problems seeing or tells you she sees "double."

- He has trouble moving one side of the body or seems weak.

- Her eyes are crossed (and they usually aren't), or her eyes move in an unusual way.

587

RECOGNIZING
AND
MANAGING
SERIOUS OR
POTENTIALLY
SERIOUS
INJURIES

- One pupil is larger than the other.

- The youngster has a convulsion (seizure) after a head injury.

- You can feel a depression (''dent'') in the bone of the skull when there wasn't one before, especially if it's under a bruise.

- Swelling of the scalp is very severe or continues to increase even hours after a head injury.

If your child seems fine at first, watch him closely for twelve to twenty-four hours after the injury. You can allow him to sleep, but wake him every two hours to check him. Make sure he wakes up or stirs around as he usually does, but you don't have to wake him completely. For example, if he's usually difficult to wake up and cranky, then his doing this should not worry you. If he's usually groggy when awakened, or a bit incoherent for a few minutes, then his doing that should not alarm you either. *However*, if he's usually easily awakened, alert, and up quickly but this time won't wake up or move around at all, you may have a problem. Check to see whether his pupils are the same size and that they get smaller when a small light is shined into them. (See Chapter 9 for details on how to do this.) Call your doctor (or go to an emergency room) if any of the previously listed symptoms occur—whether you notice them at the time of the injury, a few hours later, or even a few days later.

A child with a *skull fracture* can show any of the symptoms of a serious head injury—or none at all. If the skull took most of the force, then there might be no significant brain injury. Most of the time, however, there are at least signs of a concussion. Once in a while, though, the only clue you might have is continued enlargement of a bruise on the head—because the blood vessels located in the skull bone itself continue to ooze for as long as twenty-four hours. If you notice that the swelling continues to develop, you might be dealing with a fracture.

Sometimes, a youngster will suffer a *depressed skull fracture* and show few, if any, signs of brain injury right away. This kind of fracture, in which the bone is broken enough to push inward, most often results from being hit by or falling onto a relatively small object (for example, being hit with a golf ball or falling on a rock). You may be able to feel the depression as a ''dent'' in the head.

Head Injury: What to Expect

When your child goes to an emergency room or is seen by his or her doctor because of a potentially serious head injury, the doctor will first do a detailed examination, including a neurological (nervous system) assessment. If there is suspicion of serious bleeding inside the skull (called intracranial hemorrhage), the doctor will want to do special tests right away. Most often, the doctor will do a CT scan (a special computerized X ray that will quickly help make the diagnosis of intracranial bleeding). If there is time, X rays of the skull (and often the neck) might also be done. In certain circumstances, special X rays in which "dye" is injected into the blood vessels (called arteriograms) might also be recommended or needed.

If the little one, child, or teenager has had a concussion or skull fracture, she will most often need to be in the hospital for a day or two, although there might be situations in which you will be able to watch her closely while at home.

If there is bleeding within the skull, your child might need surgery in order to remove the blood, as well as release the pressure that swelling and bleeding place on the brain. If there is increased intracranial pressure because of swelling, special treatments and intracranial pressure monitoring will be needed—and the youngster would have to stay in an intensive-care unit for this observation, monitoring, and treatment.

A Note About "Bumps on the Head"

Children of all ages experience countless "bumps on the head": a crawler or toddler may hit his head on a coffee table; the preschooler may fall off a swing set and hurt her head; the school-aged child may slip on the playground; and the older child or adolescent may be hit by a tennis ball, baseball, or basketball or run into a fence, post, or tree. The possibilities are endless. The point is, the good old bump on the head *should not* be confused with a serious head or neck injury.

Your assessment process is invaluable in these most often minor occurrences. *One excellent rule:* If the youngster is up and moving right after the injury occurred and did not lose consciousness even for a second—then he is usually fine. Most often, you'll see a toddler fall, hit her head and get up yelling and screaming before you can even reach her. (Often, the youngster rubs the area that hurts.) A little one might even cry so hard that she holds her breath, turns blue, and momentarily loses consciousness, then starts to breathe again right away—a scary but not serious situation!) *A second rule:* If the youngster does not seem to experience any changes in behavior for twelve to twenty-four hours (as previously discussed) when a head injury or other injury that may have involved the head has occurred, then you have verified the injury as minor. In other words, watch the child's response at the time of injury and keep an eye on him for twelve to twenty-four hours to ensure that more serious damage did not take place.

A bump on the head will often swell, bruise, and be quite tender to the touch. As long as it appears within one hour or so after the injury and gradually goes down or at least *doesn't enlarge* over a twelve- to twenty-four-hour period, then there's almost never a serious underlying injury. Icing (placing an ice pack on) the area (if the youngster will let you) reduces pain, swelling, and bruising. Some children will put up a terrible fuss if you try to ice the injured area. In this situation, forget about the ice pack and let the child resume his normal activity.

It is also not uncommon for a small child to vomit *once* immediately after experiencing a minor bump on the head. If, however, she vomits again or acts differently (as previously discussed), then call the doctor for advice.

A note about bruises on the forehead in small children: Forehead bumps often swell a great deal at first, then leave a small bump and red spot. As the blood in the bruise changes color, it will turn to blue and purple and may even cause a black eye. Look for a forehead bruise if your youngster wakes up with some bruising and discoloration of the eyelid several hours after a bump on the forehead. However, deep bruising of the eyelid(s) that looks a bit like "raccoon eyes" should prompt you to call the doctor, since it can signal a skull fracture.

THE DON'TS

Don't ever move a youngster—no matter what age or size —if there is any possibility of a serious neck, back, or head injury. Remember, it's better not to take the risk unless you are absolutely certain this type of injury could not have occurred.

Don't hesitate to call the paramedics when you suspect a serious neck, back, or head injury.

Don't forget to move the youngster as a unit (supporting the head, neck, and back) if you have no choice but to move her. Obviously, you may have to move the youngster if CPR needs to be performed, if the young person's life is in imminent danger if she is not moved, or if there is no other way to get the young person to medical help. In each of these situations, use extreme care.

Don't forget to watch for signs and symptoms of underlying damage for twelve to twenty-four hours after a head injury—even if the child feels and appears fine at the time of the injury.

PLEASE NOTE: Now that you have a grasp of how to recognize and manage head, neck, and back injuries, it would be extremely helpful for you to go back to the Emergency Quick Reference With the Steps in Detail and review it carefully. The more familiar you are with that material, the more useful it will be to you when you need it.

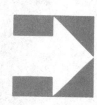

EMERGENCY QUICK REFERENCE

With the Steps in Detail

Heatstroke, Heat Exhaustion, and Heat Cramps

▶ **HEATSTROKE IS A LIFE-THREATENING EMERGENCY. BE ALERT TO ITS SIGNS AND SYMPTOMS, ESPECIALLY DURING VERY HOT, HUMID WEATHER AND IF A YOUNGSTER HAS BEEN VERY ACTIVE DURING HOT WEATHER:**

- Sudden rise in the youngster's body temperature to 105 degrees or more.

- Hot, dry skin.

- Pale or gray appearance (or occasionally very red and sweaty).

- Confusion, delirium, or irritability.

- Convulsions.

- Coma.

▶ **IF YOU SUSPECT HEATSTROKE, BEGIN COOLING THE YOUNGSTER IMMEDIATELY:**

- Remove him from the hot environment and take off his clothes.

- Put him in a tub of cold water. As the water warms up, add more cold water or even ice.

- Rub his skin with ice cubes if they are available, and use a fan if you have one.

- Have someone else call the paramedics while you treat the child. If no one is with you, continue treating the child while you periodically shout for help. When help arrives, have that person call the paramedics.

- If you cannot get the paramedics or an ambulance, take the youngster to an emergency room for evaluation and treatment. If you have to transport him yourself, use your air-conditioning if you have it, or open the windows and use the fan.

591

RECOGNIZING
AND
MANAGING
SERIOUS OR
POTENTIALLY
SERIOUS
INJURIES

▶ **HEAT EXHAUSTION OCCURS WHEN A CHILD LOSES TOO MUCH WATER AND/OR SALT DURING HEAVY EXERCISE OR EXCESSIVE HEAT. ITS SIGNS AND SYMPTOMS ARE AS FOLLOWS:**

- Severe fatigue and weakness.

- Extreme thirst.

- Headache, dizziness.

- Loss of appetite, nausea, and vomiting.

- Lethargy, incoordination, and irritability.

- Rapid, uncomfortable breathing.

- Rapid, weak pulse.

- Muscle cramping can occur.

▶ **IF YOU SUSPECT HEAT EXHAUSTION, BEGIN TREATING THE YOUNGSTER:**

- Insist that she rest in a cool environment.

- Offer him large amounts of cold liquids to drink. Start with liquids that contain salt, such as commercial salt-containing beverages (Gatorade, Pedialyte, Lytren, Lyte-Pop and so on), tomato juice, orange juice, or carbonated drinks. Later, you can offer water, popsicles, Kool-Aid, and so on.

- Contact the doctor if the youngster does not improve after several hours or if she seems to feel worse, in spite of your treatment.

▶ **HEAT CRAMPS ARE SUDDEN, SEVERE MUSCLE CRAMPS THAT OCCUR AFTER OR DURING VIGOROUS EXERCISE BECAUSE OF SALT DEPLETION.** (THEY MAY INVOLVE THE MUSCLES OF THE ABDOMEN, MAKING YOU THINK OF APPENDICITIS OR ANOTHER EMERGENCY.) **YOU CAN TREAT HEAT CRAMPS AT HOME:**

- Have the youngster rest in a cool environment. Tell him to avoid sudden movements, especially stretching.

- Offer her plenty of salty foods or drinks, such as tomato juice, salted snack foods, and commercial beverages like Gatorade.

- Offer water and other liquids if he is thirsty after eating the salty things, but don't overdo them.

Heat Injury: What You Should Know

Heat exhaustion and heat cramps are fortunately much more common than heatstroke (which is a life-threatening emergency). However, heat injury is a serious risk for infants, children, and older youngsters (as well as the elderly, who are also at great risk).

Heat exhaustion and heat cramps happen when a child loses a great deal of perspiration (sweat), which contains both water and salt, and does not take in enough water and salt to replace the losses. Heatstroke, on the other hand, results from a faulty heat "thermostat"—the body's normal temperature-regulating system fails, and body temperature rises to very high levels.

While it's very important to recognize and treat the symptoms of heat-caused injury, it's even more important to know about the situations in which the risk of heat injury is greatest. In this way, you can *prevent* problems rather than treat them after they occur.

Heatstroke, Heat Exhaustion, and Heat Cramps: Understanding the Problem

Under normal circumstances, the body has an amazing ability to maintain a steady temperature under a variety of environmental conditions. Its "thermostat" regulates body temperature to stay within one degree Fahrenheit most of the time (through several mechanisms). This temperature-regulating system depends on a youngster's having normal blood vessels, a normal amount of blood (not being dehydrated), the right balance of salt and water in the body, the ability to shiver, and the ability to sweat normally.

Body heat is produced by muscle activity, as well as general bodily functions that "burn" nutrients to produce heat and energy. Normally, the inside of the body is warmer than the outside, and the blood carries heat as well as nutrients to the surface tissues of the body. The skin, with its blood vessels and sweat glands, helps to regulate body temperature.

Outside temperature has a great deal to do with the body's temperature-regulating system. At cold temperatures, we "feel" cold and tend to become more active. We try to get shelter, put on more clothing, and shiver. Sweating is reduced or eliminated altogether. In addition, cold sets into play a reflex that narrows the blood vessels to the skin, so less heat is lost to the outside. At neutral temperatures, we feel "comfortable"—our skin temperature is pleasantly warm, we don't shiver, and we sweat very little.

593

RECOGNIZING
AND
MANAGING
SERIOUS OR
POTENTIALLY
SERIOUS
INJURIES

At very warm temperatures, the body acts to increase its heat loss. Blood circulation to the skin increases, so we look pinker or redder than usual. Sweating increases dramatically, because evaporation of sweat is a cooling process for the body. We "feel" warm, so we usually slow down our activities, remove as much clothing as possible, and try to get into a more comfortable environment. Because the increased sweating means we need more water (and salt, which is lost in the sweat), we feel thirsty and try to drink more liquids. The kidneys also play a role, by reducing the amount of urine that is produced and by cutting down on the amount of salt that is lost in the urine. If this cooling process is effective, body temperature stays normal, and no problems occur.

Several factors can make the body's heat-losing system malfunction, leading to problems like heat exhaustion, heatstroke, and heat cramps. Heavy exercise in the heat not only produces more body heat but leads to loss of a great deal of water and salt. If a youngster does not drink enough liquid or take in enough salt to replace the losses, the body's chemical balance is disturbed. Less and less blood can be circulated, and body tissues and cells do not function as efficiently as they should. Clothing also plays a role. Too much clothing or clothing that does not allow sweat to evaporate traps heat and sweat underneath the clothing. In addition, if the humidity is high on a warm day, less heat can be lost through sweating, because less sweat evaporates into the air.

Heatstroke occurs when the body's "thermostat" malfunctions and the normal heat-losing mechanisms fail to function. Sweating is ineffective or stops altogether, so body temperature rises dangerously, to levels over 105 degrees. If the temperature is not reduced quickly, death can occur within a very short time. Heatstroke can follow a long period of sweating, because the person becomes dehydrated, or can happen "out of the blue," without warning or explanation. It is also a problem for children with a rare hereditary lack of sweat glands. Regardless of the cause, it must be treated immediately.

Heat exhaustion is much more common than heatstroke and happens when a youngster does not drink enough water to replace all that he or she is losing through sweating. Salt depletion also plays a role, especially in young infants and children who are not used to heavy exercise and/or are not able to "tell" you that they are thirsty (essentially, that they need water and/or salt) or in those who have cystic fibrosis (a congenital disease in which an abnormal amount of salt is lost in the sweat). While heat exhaustion usually results from heavy exercise, young infants and children can also suffer heat exhaustion without abnormal amounts of exercise (but due to a heat wave or chronic health conditions).

Heat cramps usually occur in youngsters or teenagers who are very physically fit. When they exercise, they sweat a great deal and often drink enough water to replace the fluid that was lost but may not replace enough salt. Salt depletion leads to severe muscle cramping, usually *after* a long period of exercise or work when youngsters are resting.

Heat Injury: Signs and Symptoms

Heatstroke generally gives little warning. An infant, child, or toddler might act very irritated or confused, then suddenly lose consciousness. An older youngster might tell you she has a headache and feels dizzy or odd. When you touch her, she feels very hot and usually has either pink or white, dry skin. (Most often, sweating has stopped before heatstroke occurs.) She might have convulsions or repeated stiffening of her arms or legs. Her pulse at first is fast and very strong, then becomes fast and weak.

With *heat exhaustion*, a youngster will become too exhausted and weak to continue to play or exercise. He will complain of terrible thirst and have a severe headache. He may be dizzy or wobbly when he stands up or walks. You will notice that he is breathing very fast and his pulse is also fast. He may be willing to drink water or other liquids but might complain of nausea or lack of appetite. Later, he may vomit and have diarrhea. His behavior is most often unusual—he seems "out of it" and uncoordinated. Heat exhaustion can lead to heatstroke, so you must promptly treat any signs of heat exhaustion to prevent heatstroke.

Heat cramps are a less serious problem than either heatstroke or heat exhaustion. A youngster with this problem usually feels fine during exercise but develops excruciating cramps in her muscles minutes to hours after stopping to rest and relax. Most often, the cramps occur in the arms or legs, but sometimes they attack the muscles of the abdomen. If this occurs, you might think she has a very serious problem like appendicitis. Heat cramps usually are brief, with each one lasting only a minute or two. If you touch the cramping muscle, it will feel as hard as a rock. Sudden tightening of a muscle, stretching, or contact with cold water can set off a new cramp.

Preventing Heat Injury

Most heat injury—whether heat exhaustion, heat cramps, or heatstroke—can be prevented if you pay attention to the kinds of situations in which an infant, child, or older youngster is at risk for these problems. Because young infants, toddlers, and preschoolers *are dependent on you* to recognize the risks and protect them when it is hot, be especially careful to take steps to meet their needs and be watchful of them when the weather is hot or they have been very physically active.

- Do not overdress infants and young children, especially in hot or humid weather.

- Pay attention to signs that the little one is too warm—hot, pink, or red skin; sweating; panting; heat rash.

- Use a cool, wet washcloth to sponge a baby or toddler frequently when she is hot. It feels as good to her as it does to you when you're hot!

595

RECOGNIZING
AND
MANAGING
SERIOUS OR
POTENTIALLY
SERIOUS
INJURIES

- Offer extra juice, water, or commercial electrolyte beverages (Gatorade, Pedialyte, and so on) to your infant or child. If you don't offer it, you may not know that he is thirsty!

- Dress active youngsters in lightweight, cotton clothing in hot weather, so sweat can evaporate. If you use layers, you can remove clothing as a youngster gets warm.

- Enforce a rest period during the hottest part of the day, and encourage quiet play, even for older youngsters.

- *Never* leave an infant or child in a closed or partly closed car, van, or truck— even for a few minutes. The temperature inside the motor vehicle can rise above 100 degrees in a matter of minutes, and babies and small children can die very quickly.

Teach your older children and teenagers how to prevent heat injury, as well as how to recognize the early signs of a problem. Encourage them to stop their exercise or play at the first sign of a problem even if their friends continue to play. Remind them that heat exhaustion and heatstroke often give them a feeling of euphoria—as if they could play on forever—when, in reality, they will eventually collapse. Being very hot and almost euphoric is a sign to stop and cool down.

- Make sure that active youngsters rest and cool off frequently during vigorous play or exercise.

- Be sure that there is plenty of juice, commercial electrolyte beverage (Gatorade, for example), and water available for active youngsters and that they know to drink whenever they feel thirsty.

- Be sure that your young athlete conditions gradually when he is exercising in the heat. The youngster should start slowly and gradually increase the amount of time he spends working out.

- Pay particular attention to the philosophy of coaches and trainers of sports programs for youngsters who are training in the summer and early fall. Be sure that water and commercial electrolyte solutions are available and that coaches and others do not think it is "silly" or "weak" to drink while exercising.

- Encourage your teenager to avoid drinking alcohol before or during vigorous exercise. Alcohol not only impairs his judgment but also increases the risk of heat injury. (This is something that adults should be aware of, as well.)

- Be sure that youngsters who are well conditioned know that they must eat or drink things that contain salt in order to avoid salt depletion during exercise or excessive sweating.

• Most professionals agree that the use of salt tablets is not a safe practice, since there is no way to evaluate the amount of salt loss and regulate proper intake through the tablets. One's thirst is the best barometer and electrolyte and other fluid replacement the best answer, along with proper rest and cooling. Therefore, do not give babies, children, or teenagers salt tablets.

THE DON'TS

Don't ignore the early signs and symptoms of heat exhaustion, heatstroke, or heat cramps in your child. Enforcing rest, cooling down, and drinking liquids at the earliest sign of a problem can prevent serious injury.

Don't use salt tablets to replace salt that is lost through sweating. As noted previously, it is easy to give too much salt this way. Youngsters who are playing or exercising need water as well as salt (through electrolyte solutions and fruit juices) to replace what their bodies have lost.

Don't hesitate to insist that your child or youngster stop activity immediately and cool down. Remember, she often feels "just fine" and almost euphoric—and can suddenly collapse. If in doubt, take her temperature to see how high it is. If over 100 degrees, it's best for her to rest and cool down before continuing activity. If up to 103 degrees or greater, immediately treat the youngster and have her stay out of the heat and remain inactive for several hours.

PLEASE NOTE: Now that you have a grasp of how to recognize and manage heatstroke, heat exhaustion, and heat cramps, it would be extremely helpful for you to go back to the Emergency Quick Reference With the Steps in Detail and review it carefully. The more familiar you are with that material, the more useful it will be to you when you need it.

597

RECOGNIZING
AND
MANAGING
SERIOUS OR
POTENTIALLY
SERIOUS
INJURIES

EMERGENCY QUICK REFERENCE

With the Steps in Detail

Smoke Inhalation and Carbon Monoxide Poisoning

▶ **BE ALERT TO THE SIGNS OF SMOKE INHALATION OR RESPIRATORY BURNS:**

- Burns or soot around the face and head.

- Burning or singeing of the eyebrows, eyelashes, or nose hairs.

- Swelling or redness inside the mouth or nose or around the eyes.

- Soot-tinged saliva or coughed-up mucus.

- Breathing difficulty, coughing, or hoarseness.

- Unusual behavior, including excitability, irritability, lethargy, or coma (due to lack of oxygen).

▶ **BE ALERT TO THE SIGNS AND SYMPTOMS OF CARBON MONOXIDE POISONING, WHICH CAN OCCUR WITH OR WITHOUT A FIRE:**

- *Mild poisoning:* headache, dizziness, mild difficulty breathing, and vision problems.

- *More severe poisoning:* unusual sleepiness or lethargy, nausea and/or vomiting, clumsiness or lack of coordination, and unusual behavior.

- *Serious poisoning:* extreme weakness, incoordination, coma, convulsions, cardiac arrest, and death.

▶ **ALWAYS ASSUME THERE IS A POSSIBILITY OF SMOKE INHALATION, INHALATION OF POISONOUS FUMES, AND/OR CARBON MONOXIDE POISONING IF YOU OR YOUR CHILD IS INVOLVED IN A FIRE—EVEN IF HE HAS NO BURNS.**

- Remove the youngster (and yourself) from the area of the fire and into fresh air as quickly and safely as possible. Cover your face with a wet towel if you must try to reenter a smoky area or are escaping from a smoky area. Stay as close to the floor as possible.

- If the youngster is not breathing, begin rescue breathing. If his heart has also stopped, begin full CPR (rescue breathing with chest compressions). (If you are certified in CPR and are unable to remember the details of the procedure or how to perform rescue breathing, turn to the Emergency Quick Reference on page 113, entitled "A Review of the Six Steps of CPR.") Continue your efforts until emergency help arrives.

- If the youngster is coughing but otherwise seems fine, keep him in the open air (and be sure he uses the oxygen that the paramedics bring) until he can be evaluated in an emergency room.

- *Always* have the youngster evaluated in an emergency room if she showed signs of possible smoke inhalation or carbon monoxide poisoning (coughing, hoarseness, difficulty breathing, noisy breathing, unusual behavior), even if the problem seems minor.

▶ **ASSUME THAT CARBON MONOXIDE POISONING MIGHT HAVE OCCURRED IF A YOUNGSTER IS FOUND UNCONSCIOUS OR SHOWS UNUSUAL BEHAVIOR AFTER BEING IN AN ENCLOSED SPACE WHERE SUCH POISONING IS POSSIBLE.**

- Get the child into fresh air as quickly as possible.

- If breathing has stopped, begin rescue breathing at once. Begin full CPR (rescue breathing with chest compressions) if you cannot feel a pulse. (If you are certified in CPR and are unable to remember the details of the procedure or how to perform rescue breathing, turn to the Emergency Quick Reference on page 113, entitled "A Review of the Six Steps of CPR.")

- Call the paramedics or get the youngster to an emergency room as quickly as possible, even if he or she seems better after being in the fresh air.

599

RECOGNIZING
AND
MANAGING
SERIOUS OR
POTENTIALLY
SERIOUS
INJURIES

Smoke Inhalation and Carbon Monoxide Poisoning: What You Should Know

Each year, smoke inhalation, carbon monoxide poisoning, and poisoning due to toxic fumes from fires cause more deaths than the burns from the same fires. This problem and its magnitude have been understood for only about forty years, and each year, advances are made in providing better care for infants, children, and adults who suffer these serious injuries.

Carbon monoxide poisoning can occur without a fire, as well. Each year, children (and adults) are poisoned by being in unsafe environments where this odorless gas collects. This kind of carbon monoxide poisoning can be very difficult to detect unless you are quite suspicious that it has occurred.

Smoke Inhalation: Understanding the Problem

When a youngster inhales smoke during a fire, there are several possible kinds of injury. The damage that results depends on multiple factors: what kinds of materials are burning; whether the youngster was trapped in an enclosed space; how hot the fire is; whether or not the heat and smoke are very dry; and the amount of time the youngster breathed the smoke.

Smoke contains many kinds of particles, gases, and chemicals. Many of these irritate the linings of the nose, mouth, throat, trachea, and airways of the lungs. This irritation causes swelling of the linings of the airways, and the damaged cells pour out large amounts of mucus and fluid. This swelling and the extra fluid cause the youngster to have difficulty in breathing air in and out and prevent oxygen from entering the bloodstream as well as it should. They also set up the perfect conditions for infection. If the smoke contains particles that continue to burn after they are inhaled, the delicate tissues of the airway can be burned directly, worsening the problem.

Many toxic gases are found in smoke, and these add to the problem of smoke inhalation and the injury it causes. All smoke contains large amounts of carbon monoxide, because burning is usually incomplete. Other toxic gases are produced, as well, and this risk is increased when plastics or other human-made materials burn. These toxic materials cause damage to the lungs and can also have damaging effects on other body organs when they are absorbed. Therefore, the kinds of materials being burned in the fire have a great deal to do with how bad the smoke injury will be.

When a child inhales smoke and toxic fumes, he or she may show signs of damage immediately (for example, coughing, difficulty breathing, or unconsciousness) or may appear to be fine at first, then develop problems after several hours. For this reason, it is imperative that any youngster who has been in a fire be evaluated in an emergency room.

Smoke Inhalation: What to Expect

Whenever smoke inhalation is a problem, your goal and that of any professionals is to make sure a youngster gets as much oxygen as possible. Paramedics who go to the scene of a fire will insist on administering oxygen to anyone who might have had serious smoke inhalation, even if they seem to have only minor injury. They will also insist that the child be evaluated in an emergency room.

Because the damage from smoke inhalation may not be obvious immediately afterward, emergency-room physicians and others familiar with the potentially deadly effects of smoke inhalation are very careful in evaluating children (and adults) who may have been injured. The evaluation includes a careful physical examination, chest X ray, and blood tests to determine whether there is enough oxygen in the blood and how much carbon monoxide is present. Oxygen is administered, and the youngster is usually admitted to the hospital for observation.

Serious smoke inhalation often leads to severe enough damage that a youngster needs to have assistance with breathing for hours or days while the damage heals. Infection in the lungs (pneumonia) and airways is also very common, so care is taken to recognize and treat it as soon as possible.

Carbon Monoxide Poisoning: Understanding the Problem

Carbon monoxide is a colorless, odorless gas that is produced when materials are incompletely burned. It is particularly deadly because it is impossible to detect. It is always present in high concentrations when there is a fire, especially in an enclosed space. However, it can build up in other situations and be a "silent killer." The risk of carbon monoxide poisoning is very great when wood or other materials are burned in poorly ventilated stoves or in closed homes, when car engines are running in closed garages, and in closed cars with faulty exhaust systems. In addition, children are at particular risk if they ride in the backs of trucks, vans, or station wagons with their exhaust pipes at the back rather than at the side.

All people normally have some carbon monoxide in their blood, but at high levels it is extremely dangerous. The reason? It prevents oxygen from reaching tissues. It attaches to hemoglobin, the substance in the red blood cells that carries oxygen two hundred to three hundred times as easily as oxygen does. It also "hangs on" to the hemoglobin much more tightly than oxygen does. So, in effect, the red blood cells are prevented from carrying oxygen, and all of the vital tissues and organs of the body are starved of oxygen.

Carbon Monoxide Poisoning: What to Expect

601

RECOGNIZING
AND
MANAGING
SERIOUS OR
POTENTIALLY
SERIOUS
INJURIES

The treatments for carbon monoxide poisoning all revolve around ways to provide oxygen to the starving cells. Breathing 100 percent oxygen for several hours is one way to eliminate carbon monoxide from the system and provide as much oxygen to the cells as possible. In some situations, oxygen must be given under high pressure (called hyperbaric oxygenation). While the youngster is undergoing oxygen treatment, he may also need intravenous fluids, to ensure that his kidneys continue to function.

THE DON'TS

Don't assume that an infant, child, or older youngster has escaped injury from smoke inhalation just because he seems to have very little trouble breathing right after the incident. The damage from inhaling smoke and toxic gases can appear several hours afterward.

Don't overlook the symptoms of carbon monoxide poisoning if a youngster has been found in a high-risk situation. Be alert to signs of headache, confusion, lack of coordination, nausea and vomiting, lethargy, or unusual behavior, and take action. Be sure the youngster is evaluated by a doctor as soon as possible.

PLEASE NOTE: Now that you have a grasp of how to recognize and manage smoke inhalation and carbon monoxide poisoning, it would be extremely helpful for you to go back to the Emergency Quick Reference With the Steps in Detail and review it carefully. The more familiar you are with that material, the more useful it will be to you when you need it.

C H A P T E R   17

Recognizing and Caring for Common Injuries

Included in this chapter is information on how to recognize and care for the common injuries listed below. The page numbers in parentheses indicate where the Quick Reference for each type of injury can be found.

QUICK REFERENCE

With the Steps in Detail

Blisters and Chafing

Treating Blisters

▶ **CLEAN THE AREA WITH SOAP AND WARM WATER. THESE ARE YOUR BEST WEAPONS AGAINST INFECTION.**

- Keep the blister(s) clean in order to avoid infection.

- Some people prefer to use antiseptic creams, lotions, sprays, or ointments, but these are not necessary.

- A bandage or adhesive strip (particularly in active youngsters) will help keep the blister(s) clean and better protect against infection. Petroleum jelly applied to the open blister(s) reduces the rubbing and irritation.

- Do not break the blister(s), since you would be opening the raw area underneath to infection.

- If the blister(s) become(s) inflamed, red, and very tender—soak repeatedly in warm water (for ten to fifteen minutes each time).

- If this treatment does not reduce inflammation and redness, then call the doctor for advice.

Preventing Blisters

▶ **PETROLEUM JELLY (VASELINE) OR A SIMILAR LUBRICATING OINTMENT MAY HELP PROTECT ALREADY FORMED BLISTERS ON THE HANDS OR FEET.**

▶ **SPECIAL CARE SHOULD BE TAKEN TO ENSURE THAT SHOES AND GLOVES FIT CORRECTLY.**

▶ **SOMETIMES, WEARING TWO PAIRS OF SOCKS HELPS PREVENT BLISTERS ON THE FEET.**

▶ **IF THE YOUNGSTER IS INVOLVED IN SPORTS, TAKE CARE TO EN-SURE PROPER SIZES, WEIGHTS, AND GRIPS ON BATS, RACKETS, CLUBS, HANDLEBARS, AND SO ON. GLOVES CAN BE WORN TO PROTECT SENSITIVE HANDS.**

Treating Chafing

▶ **CLEAN THE AREA WITH SOAP AND WARM WATER.**

● Applying cool water or a cool, water-soaked towel will help ease the discomfort.

▶ **AVOID FURTHER RUBBING OF THE AREA (IF AT ALL POSSIBLE) UNTIL THE CHAFING HEALS.**

▶ **THE USE OF PETROLEUM JELLY OR A SIMILAR LUBRICATING OINTMENT PROTECTS THE CHAFED AREA AND HELPS LESSEN THE EFFECT OF CONSTANT RUBBING ON THE SKIN.**

Preventing Chafing

▶ **ALTERATIONS IN CLOTHING ARE OFTEN HELPFUL.**

● For babies, for example, removing plastic pants or even diapers for short periods of time will help alleviate chafing around the waist and legs.

● If a piece of clothing—shorts, pants, shirt or blouse, and so on—is causing chafing, it may be too tight or improperly fitted. It should not be used if the problem occurs each time the youngster wears it.

● Light, smooth clothing helps prevent chafing due to clothes rubbing against skin and should be worn when youngsters are playing.

● Prevent excessive moisture in areas where skin rubs together. Use a bland powder or cornstarch. If excessive perspiration is a problem, try an antiperspirant (deodorant) or ask your pharmacist to prepare a special solution for you.

Blisters and Chafing: What You Should Know

Blisters as well as chafing are caused by constant rubbing of the skin—by clothing, shoes, another object, or even skin against skin. A shoe may rub against the heel or elsewhere on the foot; a diaper or plastic pants may rub around the waist or upper leg; the bicycle handlebars may rub against the hands; a pair of shorts may rub against the inside of the legs; and the skin on the inside of the thighs may rub together, especially when running. The list goes on and on.

Chafing can occur almost anywhere on the body. It results from a combination of moisture (perspiration or water) and constant rubbing. This continual irritation actually wears off the top layer(s) of skin, leading to redness and pain. Many children will tell you that the area feels "hot" or "burns."

Blisters, on the other hand, most commonly form on the feet and hands. Blisters occur when there is enough friction and pressure applied to an area that underlying layers of skin rub against each other. As a response to this, fluid forms, pushing the skin out. Blisters can be quite painful and have the potential to become infected if the surface skin breaks. Therefore, care should be taken to treat blisters properly if they have formed and prevent new ones from forming.

THE DON'TS

Don't forget to carefully clean blisters and chafed areas. Infection can occur if blisters, in particular, are not properly cleaned.

Don't forget to leave the blister alone and NOT intentionally break it. This opens up the area to infection.

Don't hesitate to use Vaseline (or a like product) to protect against further blistering or to prevent blisters from forming.

Don't allow youngsters to wear shoes too small or too large for them. This usually results in constant friction and blister formation.

Don't forget to call the doctor if a blister or chafed area looks infected and your treatment has not resolved the problem.

PLEASE NOTE: Now that you have a grasp of how to recognize and manage blisters and chafing, it would be extremely helpful for you to go back to the Quick Reference With the Steps in Detail and review it carefully. The more familiar you are with that material, the more useful it will be to you when you need it.

QUICK REFERENCE

With the Steps in Detail

Bruises

▶ **EVALUATE THE INJURY:**

- Ask the youngster (if old enough) how the injury occurred and where he or she hurts.

- Try to determine whether there are other more serious injuries and deal with them first. Be attentive to hidden areas—abdomen, chest, genital region—and check the child's head carefully, especially if a serious fall or blow was involved.

- If there are no serious injuries, treat the bruise(s).

▶ **TREATING THE BRUISE(S):**

- Place an ice pack over the bruised area. (You can easily make an ice pack by placing ice cubes or crushed ice in a plastic bag, then wrapping this with a thin, soft towel. If ice is not available, soak a towel in cold water and apply to the bruised area. Resoak the towel as needed to keep it cold.)

- Keep the ice pack or towel on the bruised area for thirty minutes, then remove it for fifteen minutes. Repeat this routine until pain and swelling are reduced. Serious or deep bruises will benefit if this is continued for as long as twenty-four hours after the injury.

- An aspirin substitute, acetaminophen (such as Tylenol, Tempra, Liquiprin, or other brands), may be helpful in relieving pain or discomfort. Do not use aspirin unless your doctor recommends it. Give only the proper dosage for the youngster's age and weight.

▶ **WHEN TO CALL THE DOCTOR:**

- There are other injuries more serious than the bruise.

- Severe pain or discomfort, loss of motion, or weakness persist after a few hours, or the youngster experiences persistent nausea, vomiting, inactivity, or loss of sleep.

Bruises: What You Should Know

A bruise (also called a contusion) is probably the most common type of injury children (and adults) experience throughout their lifetimes. A bruise occurs when some type of object hits a part of the body, or an area of the body strikes an object. If the force is great enough, blood vessels are broken, and bleeding occurs. Bleeding can take place in any type of tissue—the various layers of the skin, muscles, bones, or even deep organs.

Pain, swelling, and surface redness usually occur immediately. A "black-and-blue mark" (called an ecchymosis) may appear within a few minutes if the broken blood vessels are close to the skin. However, this discoloration more often appears several hours later or even a few days later if the injury is deeper (because the blood slowly seeps to the skin surface). If the injury is quite deep, you may never see a "black-and-blue mark," even though there is a bruise beneath the skin. You may notice a lump (called a hematoma—which is a collection of blood) whether or not there is discoloration of the area.

Most bruises—even the small, "minor" ones—continue to get larger over an hour or two after the injury. This is due to oozing of small amounts of blood from the injured blood vessels. Do not let this alarm you—unless the swelling is very great. *If, however, the bruise is near or in a joint, or there appears to be loss of motion or deformity, the injury may be more serious than a simple bruise.*

If the blow was to the trunk of the body or to the head and the youngster experiences *persistent or severe pain, nausea, vomiting, inactivity, or loss of sleep—call your doctor for advice and instructions.* These symptoms may signal damage to an internal organ and should prompt you to seek immediate medical evaluation.

Although a child or youngster may complain about a bruise hurting, most bruises are minor and nothing to worry about. They do, however, cause discomfort if they are large. Therefore, it is best to treat large bruises. Treatment involves ice (and elevation if a leg is bruised). Minor bruises may require only one or two ice-pack treatments, while larger, more painful bruises often require many ice-pack treatments over a twenty-four-hour period. Very young children usually object to ice packs, so use your judgment as to whether a bruise is big enough to warrant the fight. When an older youngster refuses to have the ice pack put on again, it usually means that the bruise is no longer as painful to him or her.

Finally, many parents express concern over the color changes they see in a bruise. Sometimes, this leads to a call to the doctor because the parents feel some other problem is occurring with the bruise. These color changes are simply *part of the healing process*. First the bruise may be faint blue, then a deeper blue or purple. It may later go through a whole range of color changes: purple, then blue, then greenish, then brown or yellow—then gone! These color changes are the result of the body's natural processes of breaking down the trapped blood and carrying it away. Healing time can be as short as a few days or as long as two or three weeks—depending on the size and depth of the bruise.

THE DON'TS

Don't apply heat to a bruise. This may increase the bleeding in the injured area, causing greater pain and swelling. Mild heat can be applied twenty-four hours after the injury occurred. At this time, a warm bath may also help ease soreness.

Don't give the youngster aspirin for relief of pain or discomfort of a serious bruise unless your doctor recommends it. Many doctors prefer that an aspirin substitute be used because one of aspirin's usual effects is a mild interference with blood clotting.

Don't ignore signs and symptoms of a deeper or more serious injury. These include severe pain, severe swelling, deformity, or inability to move an arm or leg, as well as persistent nausea, vomiting, inactivity, or loss of sleep (if the blow was to the trunk of the body or head).

Don't overreact to the situation. A minor bruise will cause little damage and will heal rapidly, so the youngster can go back to his or her usual activities almost immediately.

PLEASE NOTE: Now that you have a grasp of how to recognize and manage bruises, it would be extremely helpful for you to go back to the Quick Reference With the Steps in Detail and review it carefully. The more familiar you are with that material, the more useful it will be to you when you need it.

QUICK REFERENCE

Calluses

▶ **SOAK THE CALLUSES IN WARM WATER TO SOFTEN THEM.**

▶ **USE ONE OF THE CREAMS OR LOTIONS AND A PUMICE STONE OR OTHER ABRASIVE AVAILABLE ON THE MARKET TO THIN OR REMOVE THE CALLUSES.**

▶ **DO NOT ATTEMPT TO REMOVE VERY THICK AND HARD CALLUSES WITH A KNIFE OR RAZOR BLADE. IF FOOT CALLUSES HAVE DEVELOPED TO THIS STAGE, THE YOUNGSTER SHOULD BE SEEN BY A PODIATRIST (A DOCTOR WHO SPECIALIZES IN PROBLEMS OF THE FOOT).**

Calluses: *What You Should Know*

When an area (usually of the feet or hands) is subjected to significant pressure, layers of skin harden to protect that area. These layers of hardened skin are called calluses. While developing, calluses can be painful and bothersome. When they occur on the ball of the foot, they occasionally cause pain and can interfere with walking.

Calluses are most often easily removed with one of the many peeling products or abrasive gadgets available on the market today. However, when calluses on the foot become very thick, it is best to have a podiatrist evaluate the problem. In these cases, he or she usually removes the hard, thick layers of dead skin with a scalpel (this does not hurt, and there is no bleeding involved). The youngster may benefit from special shoe inserts or a different type of shoe to prevent the recurrence of calluses. The podiatrist can fit these inserts or recommend proper shoes based on the youngster's needs.

THE DON'TS

Don't try to remove thick calluses yourself. Many people get hurt or hurt others while trying to remove thick calluses with a knife or razor blade. This is a dangerous practice. A podiatrist is skilled and trained to remove thick calluses carefully and painlessly.

Don't forget to have the youngster seen by a podiatrist if he or she continues to form thick calluses in the same area. Often, steps can be taken to alleviate the problem with special shoe pads and to make the youngster more comfortable.

PLEASE NOTE: Now that you have a grasp of how to recognize and manage calluses, it would be extremely helpful for you to go back to the Quick Reference and review it carefully. The more familiar you are with that material, the more useful it will be to you when you need it.

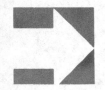

QUICK REFERENCE

With the Steps in Detail

Cuts and Scrapes

Your goal is to perform the "three Cs of cuts and scrapes": *c*alm the child, *c*ontrol the bleeding, then *c*lean the wound to avoid possible infection. You can treat most cuts and scrapes yourself but may need professional help with some.

▶ **CALM THE CHILD. ASSURE THE CHILD THAT EVERYTHING IS OK AND THAT YOU CAN MAKE THE CUT OR SCRAPE "ALL BETTER" RELATIVELY FAST.**

- Sometimes, it's helpful for the youngster to take part in the treatment process. For example, he can hold the gauze pad or cloth on the cut or scrape and apply pressure or help you clean and dress the wound. This makes the youngster turn his attention away from the "hurt" and direct it to helping himself fix the problem. This not only teaches the youngster how to take care of these more minor problems but helps him to feel *capable* of handling "little" emergencies.

- Take the time to explain how important it is for the youngster to help keep the cut or scrape clean and to keep the bandage on until it "gets better."

▶ **CONTROL AND STOP THE BLEEDING. DO THIS BY APPLYING FIRM AND STEADY PRESSURE DIRECTLY OVER THE CUT OR SCRAPE.**

- If possible, use a sterile gauze pad or clean cloth.

- It usually takes no more than five to ten minutes of steady pressure (often less) to totally stop a cut (even a large one) or scrape from bleeding.

▶ **CLEAN THE CUT OR SCRAPE.**

- Use warm water and soap to carefully and thoroughly clean the area.

- Make sure you remove all debris by gentle scrubbing, or an infection may occur. You may need to apply pressure to stop the bleeding again after the cleaning process.

- Soap and water are your best allies in cleaning minor injuries. There is no special reason to use the fancy cleaners or antiseptics you'll find on the shelves in the drugstore or market.

- Rinse the area for a few minutes under warm, running water to remove all soap and pat the area dry with a sterile piece of gauze (if available) or a clean, dry cloth.

- Look carefully at the injury to decide whether you need professional help.

▶ **WHEN TO CALL THE DOCTOR (OR GO TO THE EMERGENCY ROOM IF YOU HAVE NO DOCTOR OR CANNOT REACH YOUR DOCTOR):**

- A cut is very large or deep.

- Bleeding will not stop after twenty to thirty minutes of pressure, or blood appears to be pumping out.

- The edges are gaping wide open, or you see fat in the cut (this means the cut is deeper into the tissue).

- The cut is over an inch or so long, unless the edges stay right next to each other.

- There is something embedded in the cut, and you can't get it out by carefully using tweezers.

- The cut is on the hand (especially the palm) and is deep. Or you are not absolutely sure the youngster can move his or her hand and fingers completely normally.

- The cut is located on the face, and the edges are even slightly gaping.

- The cut is on the lip and extends past the edge of the lip onto the skin.

- The scrape is large and has dirt, sand, glass, or other debris in it, and you are unable to get the debris out (without causing further damage). *Please note:* This is important, not only to prevent infection but also to avoid permanent discoloration of the skin after healing (called "tattooing"). Also, when vigorous scrubbing is necessary, the youngster might need to be sedated or given a local anesthetic (since scrubbing can be painful).

- Your child has a fairly serious, dirty cut (or puncture wound) and has had fewer than *two* tetanus immunizations (as DTP, DT, or tetanus); has not had a tetanus booster (as DTP, DT, or tetanus) at age four to six (if older than six); or has not had a tetanus booster (as DT or tetanus) in the last ten years (if over ten years old). (For further information on tetanus immunization and the recommended immunization schedule, refer to Chapter 3.)

▶ DRESS THE CUT OR SCRAPE:

- You may apply antiseptic cream or ointment to the area if you wish, but this is not essential for healing or infection prevention—if you were careful to thoroughly wash the cut or scrape and surrounding area with warm water and soap. You may wish to use an ointment on a large scrape to keep the bandage from sticking.

- Cover the area with a sterile gauze pad and tape or an adhesive strip (if a smaller cut). This will lessen the risk for infection by keeping the area clean. You'd be surprised how a bandage also has the power to serve as a "badge of courage" for the little ones. It is often helpful to cut the strip to fit in certain more difficult areas—for example, on the chin. (See the accompanying illustration.)

▶ SOME CUTS WILL NEED A LITTLE EXTRA CARE FROM YOU:

- If there is a small amount of gaping, try to hold the edges together using a "butterfly" bandage or sterile paper tape (such as Steristrip) pulled across the edges. Keep this in place until a firm scab forms. This may save you a trip to the doctor or emergency room for stitches.

It is easy to tailor an
adhesive strip to fit the
area that is injured. Cut
the adhesive and mold the
strip to fit difficult areas
such as the chin or
fingertip.

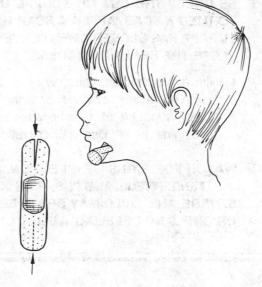

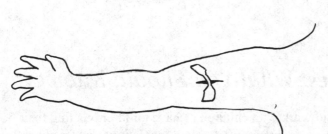

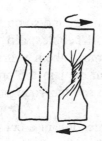

Pull the edges of a small cut together using a "butterfly"
bandage that you make with adhesive tape.

● If there is any dead skin at the edge of a cut, you can trim it off carefully
using a pair of small, sharp scissors. If this is painful, stop! You are
not trimming away dead skin if there is pain.

▶ **RE-DRESS THE CUT OR SCRAPE UNTIL IT IS CLOSED OR HAS FORMED A SCAB. AFTER A SCAB HAS FORMED OR THE CUT OR SCRAPE HAS CLOSED, THEN LEAVE IT OPEN TO THE AIR TO COMPLETE THE HEALING PROCESS.**

- With active children, you may need to rewash and re-dress the area daily. Others are notorious for going through half a box of adhesive strips in a couple of days because they keep reopening the cut and grinding dirt into it. Use your discretion.

▶ **WATCH FOR SIGNS OF INFECTION, SUCH AS REDNESS, SWELLING, TENDERNESS, AND PUS. IF AN INFECTION IS BECOMING MORE SEVERE, THE CHILD MAY BE FEVERISH OR MAY SIMPLY SAY HE OR SHE IS NOT FEELING WELL.**

Cuts and Scrapes: What You Should Know

Most parents and others who work with children or have children visiting their homes a great deal will have treated countless cuts (called lacerations) and scrapes (called abrasions) before the youngsters even reach their teenage years. These problems are easily treated at home and rarely need medical intervention—unless the cut or scrape becomes infected or the cut needs stitches. The point of treatment, then, is to promote healing and avoid infection.

Therefore, it is vital that any dirt, pebbles, pieces of clothing, and so on be washed out of a cut or scrape immediately after the injury occurs. If pebbles, dirt, splinters, or glass are deeply embedded in the skin, do not try to remove them yourself, since you could cause further tissue damage. Call the doctor and explain the problem, so proper action can be taken. (The doctor will either wish to see the youngster or may prefer that he or she be treated in an emergency room.)

After early treatment, you need to watch for signs of infection in a cut or scrape. If the area becomes inflamed, red, swollen, and tender, or pus seeps out, soak the cut or scrape in very warm water for ten to fifteen minutes. Do this a few times. If the child gets feverish or starts ''not feeling well,'' call the doctor for advice. Most often, frequent soaking of a cut or scrape that may be becoming infected or is infected will resolve the problem. But call the doctor if these steps aren't successful.

THE DON'TS

Don't hesitate to call the doctor if there are pebbles or other objects deeply embedded in the skin, the cut is deep enough that you wonder whether it might need stitches, or if the cut or scrape becomes infected.

Don't rush to an emergency room only to get a tetanus booster. The youngster may not need one. Refer to Chapter 3, and call your doctor's office if you're not sure whether your child is adequately protected or whether a tetanus booster is necessary.

Don't feel you need to use special antiseptics and creams or ointments to prevent infection. Soap and water, along with natural healing, are your best weapons against infection.

Don't use sprays, creams, or other products that contain anesthetics (meant to numb a sore). They're not needed and can potentially lead to an allergic reaction or sensitivity to the anesthetic.

Don't forget to include the youngster (particularly the young child) in the treatment process. Including children in the treatment process helps to teach them how to care for minor injuries and gives them self-confidence.

PLEASE NOTE: Now that you have a grasp of how to recognize and manage cuts and scrapes, it would be extremely helpful for you to go back to the Quick Reference With the Steps in Detail and review it carefully. The more familiar you are with that material, the more useful it will be to you when you need it.

QUICK REFERENCE

With the Steps in Detail

Muscle Cramps

▶ **IF IN THE CALF:**

- Grab the front part of the foot, including the toes, and *push* the foot up toward the youngster's body (the opposite of pointing the toe). If the youngster were to do this, she would grab the front part of her foot and toes and *pull* her foot up toward her.

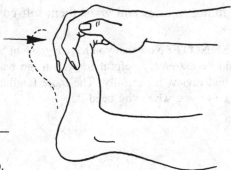

A cramped muscle in the calf can be stretched by pulling the foot up.

- You can also have the youngster stand with his feet flat and knees straight—which will stretch the cramped muscle.

- Pointing the toes when the muscle cramp is in the calf will only *make it worse.*

▶ **IF IN THE THIGH:**

- Bend the knee as far as possible if the cramp is in the large muscle at the front of the thigh. Have the youngster kneel down, then sit back on his heels.

- Straighten the knee and leg completely if the cramp is at the back of the thigh (below the buttocks). It may help to have the youngster sit down on the ground or floor with his legs straight, then bend and touch the toes.

▶ **IF IN THE FOOT:**

- Have the youngster stand on the foot, keeping it flat or even bending the toes upward.

▶ **IF IN THE NECK:**

- Turn the head away from the side of the cramp. (For example, if muscle cramp is in the left side of the neck, turn the head to the right.)

▶ **IN ALL CASES, YOU ARE TRYING TO RELAX THE CRAMPED MUSCLE BY STRETCHING IT. IF ONE MOVEMENT SEEMS TO MAKE THE CRAMP WORSE, HAVE THE YOUNGSTER TRY THE OPPOSITE MOVEMENT OR POSITION.**

Muscle Cramps: *What You Should Know*

A muscle cramp can occur in any muscle of the body but is more frequently experienced in the legs, arms, neck, and back. If you've ever had one, you know it really smarts! In fact, a muscle cramp usually hits suddenly (without warning) and is totally debilitating for a moment. However, muscle cramps can be alleviated rapidly, and the youngster can go on with his or her activity.

Essentially, a muscle cramp occurs when a muscle contracts (shortens) as much as it can—but then does not relax. The muscle experiences a tight spasm. A muscle cramp often results because of muscle fatigue, wearing clothing that binds the muscle, excessive cold, or various other reasons.

Muscle injury can also be the culprit—and is the one problem of which you need to take notice. If the same muscle cramps continuously or repeatedly over a short period of time, then the area should be iced (with an ice pack or a cold, wet towel) and rested. If there is no substantial improvement after rest and icing, then call your child's doctor for advice (since an injury to the muscle rather than a simple muscle cramp may have taken place).

THE DON'TS

Don't forget to rest and ice the area if muscle cramping recurs.

Don't hesitate to call the doctor if icing and rest do not significantly improve the pain or spasm. This may signal a more serious injury and would require evaluation.

PLEASE NOTE: Now that you have a grasp of how to recognize and manage muscle cramps, it would be extremely helpful for you to go back to the Quick Reference With the Steps in Detail and review it carefully. The more familiar you are with that material, the more useful it will be to you when you need it.

QUICK REFERENCE

With the Steps in Detail

Overuse Syndrome

▶ **THE YOUNGSTER SHOULD REST FROM THE ACTIVITY OR SPORT THAT CAUSED THE PAIN OR DISCOMFORT.**

- Rest means using the injured area as little as possible and not participating in the sport or activity until *all* pain or discomfort subsides.

▶ **ICE THE PAINFUL AREA.**

- If swelling or inflammation is present, placing an ice pack (or cold, wet towels) on the area for thirty minutes, then off for fifteen minutes may lessen the discomfort.

- You can continue icing (thirty minutes on, fifteen minutes off) for twenty-four hours if the youngster is quite uncomfortable.

▶ **WHEN TO SEE THE DOCTOR:**

- If pain persists after adequate (several days) rest and nonuse of the injured area, call the doctor for advice.

- If the young person experiences repeated overuse syndrome of the same area, make an appointment for evaluation.

- Persistent joint pain, swelling, or limping should signal a potentially more serious problem and should prompt you to call the doctor for evaluation.

Overuse Syndrome: What You Should Know

Overuse syndrome is exactly that—overuse of muscles, tendons, ligaments, and joints. Most often, overuse syndrome is the result of too-strenuous activity or sports training programs that progress too rapidly. Most very young children will rest when they are tired unless they are being pushed. Therefore, it is rare that they will experience overuse syndrome. However, when a youngster starts to become active in organized sports, he or she is more susceptible to experiencing overuse syndrome. All parents should be aware of this potential and make sure that youngsters are not increasing their level of activity in a sport too rapidly. You'll need to be able to distinguish between the normal achiness that everyone experiences when using muscles in a new way—and real pain from overuse or abuse.

No child, youngster, or teenager should be allowed or encouraged to play *any sport* if he is in pain. If the youngster is pushed to play the sport while hurting, he may experience serious or permanent damage to a muscle, ligament, tendon, bone, or joint. Therefore, anytime the young person experiences real pain from an activity or sports participation—it is imperative that he rest until pain and discomfort have been alleviated.

If pain persists even after adequate rest and nonuse of the area, the young person should be evaluated by a doctor. Also, if you notice that she has constant joint pain, is persistently limping, or one area is swelling repeatedly with activity, she should be evaluated. This should be done to ensure that a slow but destructive process has not occurred or a growth-plate injury has not taken place.

THE DON'TS

Don't allow your child or teenager to participate in a sport or physical activity if he or she is in pain. It is situations like this that can result in permanent damage or serious injury.

Don't hesitate to call the doctor if you're not sure whether the problem is overuse syndrome or something more serious. This is particularly true if the young person experiences persistent joint pain, swelling, reinjury, or limping.

PLEASE NOTE: Now that you have a grasp of how to recognize and manage overuse syndrome, it would be extremely helpful for you to go back to the Quick Reference With the Steps in Detail and review it carefully. The more familiar you are with that material, the more useful it will be to you when you need it.

QUICK REFERENCE

With the Steps in Detail

Shin Splints

▶ **HAVE THE YOUNGSTER GET OFF HIS OR HER FEET.**

- Elevate the injured leg(s).
- Sometimes, a heating pad or warm towels reduce the discomfort or pain.

▶ **IF THE YOUNGSTER HAS SERIOUS TROUBLE WALKING OR IS IN SEVERE PAIN, CALL THE DOCTOR FOR ADVICE.**

Shin Splints: What You Should Know

The shin is the front part of the leg between the knee and the ankle. Frankly, no one really quite knows the exact cause of a shin splint or at what location on the shin the injury occurs. But shin splints do cause pain up and down the shin—particularly when walking or running.

With so much emphasis on athletics today, many young people may experience shin splints, so it's actually easier to prevent shin splints than to treat them. Well-cushioned and properly fitted athletic shoes are vital. Some youngsters have problems if they are running a great deal on *hard surfaces*, such as concrete or asphalt—while others seem to have problems on soft surfaces, such as grass, soft dirt, and sand.

If the youngster is involved in athletics, he should be doing stretching exercises before playing or practicing. If she is a runner, it is vital that distance be increased slowly as the body and legs are conditioned to meet the stresses. Care should be taken never to overdo early training.

If the youngster continues to have a problem with shin splints, he or she should be evaluated by a doctor. The only real treatment for shin splints is resting the legs by literally staying off them until the injury heals. Sometimes, crutches are used so youngsters can still go to school and get around. After that, properly fitted footwear and altering the running surface might prevent further injury. If shin splints become a real problem, seek professional advice from a doctor interested in sports problems.

THE DON'TS

Don't allow the young person to continue playing if she is experiencing shin pain. Have the youngster get off her feet and rest the injury.

Don't forget that well-cushioned and properly fitted athletic shoes (specifically designed for running) are very important in preventing shin splints.

Don't hesitate to call the doctor if you are unsure of the seriousness of the injury, if the youngster is in severe pain, or if shin splints recur.

PLEASE NOTE: Now that you have a grasp of how to recognize and manage shin splints, it would be extremely helpful for you to go back to the Quick Reference With the Steps in Detail and review it carefully. The more familiar you are with that material, the more useful it will be to you when you need it.

QUICK REFERENCE

With the Steps in Detail

Sprains and Strains

▶ **SUSPECT A SPRAIN OR STRAIN IF:**

- There is pain and swelling around a joint after an injury—but no deformity of the joint.

- The youngster or teenager experiences pain when moving or using the joint. (Toddlers and small children are more likely to have growth-plate injuries with these symptoms, as discussed previously in Chapter 16.)

▶ **DO NOT ALLOW THE YOUNGSTER TO USE THE INJURED AREA.**

- If the injury is to the leg, hip, or groin (pelvic area), have the youngster stay off his or her feet and elevate the injured area.

- If the injury is to the hand, wrist, arm, or shoulder, have the youngster rest the area.

▶ **APPLY AN ICE PACK TO THE INJURED AREA:**

- You can easily make an ice pack by placing ice cubes or crushed ice in a plastic bag, then wrapping this with a thin, soft towel.

- If ice is not available, soak a towel in cold water and apply it to the injured area. Resoak the towel as necessary to keep it cold.

- Keep the ice pack or towel on the injured area for thirty minutes, then remove it for fifteen minutes. Repeat this routine until pain and swelling are reduced. A more serious sprain or strain may require this treatment for twenty-four hours.

▶ **IMMOBILIZE THE AREA IF THERE IS EXCESSIVE DISCOMFORT OR PAIN.**

- An elastic wrap (not applied too tightly) often helps control pain and "reminds" a youngster not to overdo it.

- Use aspirin substitute (in the correct dosage) to reduce pain and in-flammation—unless the youngster is sensitive to it.

▶ **WHEN TO CALL THE DOCTOR:**

- If there is deformity, severe pain or discomfort, severe swelling, loss of motion, or loss of sleep—call the doctor for advice and/or evaluation.

- If the injury is not substantially improved in twenty-four to forty-eight hours—call the doctor for evaluation.

Sprains and Strains: *What You Should Know*

A *sprain* is an injury to a ligament. Ligaments connect bone to bone and stabilize the joints (elbows, knees, hips, ankles, and so on) of the body. When a ligament is damaged, the joint becomes unstable and loose. A ligament is similar to a rubber band. It sustains injury when it is stretched beyond its proper point or, worse yet, stretched to the point where it tears apart.

A *strain* is an injury to a muscle–tendon unit (the unit that provides power and strength to the joint). It is this strength and power that translate into movement. This unit can be damaged in many ways. If the muscle fibers tear, then it's called a *muscle strain. Tendon strains* occur when the tendon fibers tear, either within the tendon itself, at the junction where the tendon meets muscle, or where the tendon attaches to bone. A very severe (but less common) problem occurs if both the muscle–tendon unit of a joint and the ligaments of a joint are injured.

Although a sprain and a strain are different injuries, the severity of each one is based on the same criteria. The severity of a sprain or strain can usually be determined by the degree of disability experienced by the youngster. Swelling and inflammation stabilize twenty-four to forty-eight hours after the injury occurred. At this time, if the young person can walk without a limp and rise up on his or her toes or can use the injured arm, shoulder, or wrist—then the sprain or strain is a minor one.

Minor sprains and strains can usually be cared for at home. It's important for the youngster to rest the area (as much as possible) and elevate the injury if in the leg. A *minor sprain* will normally heal in seven to ten days. A *minor strain* will usually take five to ten days to heal.

If, however, the young person has trouble putting weight on the area or using it twenty-four to forty-eight hours after the injury, then it is more than likely that the sprain or strain is a moderate injury. Moderate sprains and strains should be evaluated by a doctor, since immobilization may be necessary. The doctor may also want to take an X ray to rule out the possibility of a growth-plate injury (discussed previously in Chapter 16). With proper care, *a moderate sprain or strain* will take two to three weeks to heal.

If the youngster cannot put any weight on or move the injured area twenty-four to forty-eight hours after the injury occurred, it is likely that he or she sustained a severe sprain or strain. It is vital that the doctor evaluate a possible severe sprain or strain because: treatment (splinting, casting, bracing, and so forth) may be needed; the doctor would want to rule out a possible growth-plate injury, as well; and a rehabilitation program may need to be prescribed. In some cases, surgery is necessary to repair the damage, but this occurs only infrequently.

Because it is difficult to evaluate the extent of damage until swelling and inflammation stabilize (twenty-four to forty-eight hours after the injury), doctors will often have you wait at least twenty-four hours before seeing the youngster. However, if you feel the injury is really severe *or* there is any deformity associated with the injury *or* the pain is so severe that the youngster finds it unbearable—have him or her seen immediately, either by your doctor or in an emergency room.

THE DON'TS

Don't put heat on a possible sprain or strain for at least twenty-four hours, since this will only cause increased blood flow to the area, swelling, inflammation, and pain.

Don't hesitate to call the doctor if you are unsure of the possible seriousness of the injury.

Don't allow the youngster to use the injured area if there is pain, limited motion, or severe swelling.

PLEASE NOTE: Now that you have a grasp of how to recognize and manage sprains and strains, it would be extremely helpful for you to go back to the Quick Reference With the Steps in Detail and review it carefully. The more familiar you are with that material, the more useful it will be to you when you need it.

QUICK REFERENCE

Sunburn

Minor Sunburn

▶ **PREVENT FURTHER SUN EXPOSURE AND BURNING. GET THE YOUNGSTER OUT OF THE SUN—OR COVER HIM WITH LONG-SLEEVED CLOTHING, LONG PANTS, HAT, TOWEL, UMBRELLA, OR WHATEVER.**

▶ **KEEP THE BURNED AREA COOL.** IF YOU ARE STILL AT THE BEACH, FOR EXAMPLE, THEN COLD, WET TOWELS PLACED OVER THE SUNBURNED AREA WILL NOT ONLY LESSEN SOME OF THE DISCOMFORT BUT ALSO PROTECT AGAINST FURTHER EXPOSURE.

▶ **ONCE AT HOME, THE CHILD OR YOUNGSTER MAY FEEL MORE COMFORTABLE IF SHE TAKES A FEW COOL BATHS—PARTICULARLY IF THE SUNBURN IS OVER A LARGE AREA OF THE BODY.**

▶ **YOU MAY WISH TO USE A SUNBURN CREAM OR OINTMENT THAT CONTAINS AN ANESTHETIC MEDICATION TO HELP LESSEN DISCOMFORT.** HOWEVER, SOME PEOPLE BECOME SENSITIVE (ALLERGIC) TO THE ANESTHETIC AGENT IN THESE PREPARATIONS. IF YOU SEE ANY RASH, DISCONTINUE USE OF THE PRODUCT. CALL THE DOCTOR IF THESE REACTIONS SEEM SEVERE.

More Severe Sunburn

▶ **USE COLD, WET TOWELS OR COOL WATER TO RELIEVE SOME OF THE DISCOMFORT AND COOL DOWN THE SKIN.**

▶ **NEVER PUT ANYTHING (OTHER THAN COOL WATER OR COLD, WET TOWELS) ON A MORE SEVERE SUNBURN.**

▶ **DO NOT RUB OR BREAK BLISTERS IF THEY OCCUR.** INSTEAD, COOL THE AREA DOWN AS PREVIOUSLY NOTED, THEN WRAP THE SUNBURNED AREA WITH A DRY, STERILE, NONSTICK GAUZE WRAP OR LARGE STRIPS OF A CLEAN, WHITE SHEET.

▶ **USE ASPIRIN SUBSTITUTE FOR CHILLS, FEVER, OR PAIN.**

▶ **CALL THE DOCTOR FOR ADVICE IF THE SUNBURN INCLUDES A LARGE AREA OF BLISTERING OR COVERS A LARGE PART OF THE BODY, ESPECIALLY IN AN INFANT OR YOUNG CHILD.**

Sunburn: What You Should Know

Sunburn occurs when the invisible ultraviolet rays of the sun burn layers of the skin. With increasing exposure, more layers of the skin are burned. Depending on the intensity of the ultraviolet rays and the length of exposure, a sunburn can be either a bothersome, uncomfortable skin injury or very serious and painful.

Sunburn is first noticed when the skin becomes red, swollen, and feels hot. However, these symptoms may not be evident until hours after the exposure. The skin may then become dry and shiny, and blisters may form. The internal body temperature can also rise with a severe sunburn. If it does, the youngster may feel hot, nauseated, shivery, and sickish overall.

Some sunburns are so severe that they are classified as second-degree. Severe burns occur more often when a youngster is exposed to overcast weather, higher altitudes, wind, water, or snow. They also occur in very young infants or very fair (blond, redheaded) youngsters who are exposed to the sun for longer than they should be. In these conditions or for these more susceptible youngsters, it's easy to forget how quickly a severe sunburn can occur; therefore, we often do not take appropriate preventive measures. With young children, care should be taken to ensure that they are well protected if they fall asleep in the sun or even in overcast weather at a park, beach, or on a boat (where reflections of the sun's rays can also lead to burns).

A first-degree burn is red with minor swelling and pain. A second-degree burn is also red but may be blotchy at first and blistered later. The skin looks almost wet, and there is severe pain and swelling. (For information about the treatment of second-degree burns, review Chapter 16.)

Preventing Sunburn

Prevention of sunburn is always best and is fairly easy to do. Two commonsense approaches are available. The first approach involves gradual exposure to the sun— especially of small infants and children and those most susceptible to burning (fair-skinned youngsters, those with freckles, and redheads). The second approach is to protect the skin (during unavoidable, lengthy exposure) with chemical sunscreen products (available in markets, drugstores, and so on), as well as with light, reflective clothing and hats or other shades.

Limit exposure (especially that of young infants and toddlers) to five to ten minutes when first exposed to the sun. Then gradually increase the exposure time each day by five to ten minutes if you eventually intend to allow youngsters to play in the sun for long periods of time. When their exposure time is up, protect them with hats and sunscreen products for the remainder of sun exposure. Monitor the youngsters' time in the sun by watching the *clock*—not by evaluating their redness. (Remember, the full extent of a sunburn will not be visible for four to six hours.)

Take care to apply a sunscreen on all exposed areas of a young child's or older youngster's body (including often-forgotten areas, like the ears, neck, head, and hands)—if he or she will be in the sun longer than fifteen to thirty minutes. Reapply the sunscreen frequently (especially after *each time* the youngster gets wet or perspires enough to wash it off). Make sure you read the product label carefully so you *know* you are buying a sunscreen and *not* a suntanning lotion.

Sunscreen products provide varying degrees of protection, so you need to determine the amount of protection desired. Products carry numbers from 1 to 15, depending on the amount of screening protection they provide. For maximum protection, the sunscreening product would be designated 15. The lower-numbered products provide less and less sunscreen protection. Many people purchase a sunscreen that will allow for some exposure and therefore some tanning (for example, number 6 or 8 sunscreen). They then apply number 15 sunscreen when exposure will be lengthy or after children have slight tans.

It should be noted that sun exposure (particularly repeated deep tanning) has been directly related to serious skin wrinkling and skin cancers. It is therefore best not to start a child or youngster out early in getting deep tans and bad sunburns. It may have little significance at a young age, but the number of exposures and skin damage accumulating over many years may cause trouble in adult life.

One special note: There are medications—for example, some antibiotics (especially tetracyclines, sometimes used by teenagers with acne) and tranquilizers—that make a youngster (or adult) more susceptible to sunburn or other reactions to the sun. This information is usually noted on the prescription bottle. If sunburn or other reactions occur and the youngster must be in the sun—then ask your youngster's doctor whether there is another medication that can be substituted for the original one. If a substitute medication is not possible, make sure the youngster uses a number 15 sunscreen and wears cool, light, and protective clothing, as well as a hat.

Certain youngsters are sensitive to one or more of the ingredients in sunscreens. Suspect this reaction if you notice that your child develops a fine, red rash in the areas that were treated with the sunscreen. This reaction usually appears after the sun exposure and might progress to be an itchy, slightly bumpy rash. Stop using the sunscreen and try a product with different ingredients the next time, or contact your doctor for his or her recommendations.

Also, if a child or youngster is susceptible to having *fever blisters or cold sores* (herpes simplex 1 infections), he or she is likely to develop blisters with sun exposure. It is a good idea for these young people to use a zinc oxide preparation (or a similar sun blocker) on the lips whenever in the sun, snow, or sand. This does not provide total protection but is helpful.

THE DON'TS

Don't hesitate to call the doctor for advice if sunburn appears severe and the youngster is in a great deal of pain. It's easy to forget that the sun can cause second-degree burns. An extensive sunburn with blistering in a young infant or toddler always warrants a call to the doctor.

Don't forget to purchase a sunscreen and have your children use it. This is particularly important when there is overcast weather or wind or when young people are playing in or lying on sand or are near or in water or snow. In these situations, the sun's reflection off these surfaces intensifies the ultraviolet rays.

Don't put anything (except cool water or a cold, wet towel) on a sunburn that appears to be severe. Only a minor sunburn can be treated with anesthetic sunburn sprays, creams, or lotions. These products are not necessary even with mild burns and may actually be harmful if an allergic reaction occurs or the youngster is sensitive to the product.

PLEASE NOTE: Now that you have a grasp of how to recognize and manage sunburn, it would be extremely helpful for you to go back to the Quick Reference and review it carefully. The more familiar you are with that material, the more useful it will be to you when you need it.

SECTION 5

Helpful Hints About Home Treatment

It's always the same dilemma—what can we do to make our children more comfortable when they are sick and at home? The questions are endless: What should or shouldn't they eat? Should their activity be limited? Is there any equipment that can help make them feel better? How best can we provide both comfort and diversion while they're getting well?

There are other questions, too: What medications are safe and helpful? What medicines should be avoided? How do we choose the correct dosage? What are common misunderstandings about both prescribed and over-the-counter drugs? Are there ways to prevent the spread of infection to other family members? All are common concerns of parents—particularly when an illness or recovery period is rather lengthy.

Section 5 (Chapters 18, 19, and 20) covers useful information about what you can do to help your child feel more comfortable, what you should know about prescribed and over-the-counter medications, and ways you can better prevent or control the spread of infection. With this information, you will feel more confident about the decisions you make while your child is ill or recovering from an illness or injury because you will be better equipped to make those decisions.

629

C H A P T E R **18**

Helping Your Child
Feel More Comfortable

QUICK REFERENCE

With the Steps in Detail

Helping Your Child Feel More Comfortable

Feeding Your Baby or Toddler When Ill

▶ **IF THE BABY IS BREAST-FEEDING ONLY, CONTINUE TO NURSE AS OFTEN AS HE WISHES TO BE FED.**

▶ **IF THE BABY IS FORMULA-FED ONLY, THEN GIVE HER A BOTTLE AS USUAL.**

- If the baby refuses the bottle, try diluting the formula with water (half formula and half water).

▶ **IF THE BABY NORMALLY EATS SOLID FOODS (WHETHER HOME-MADE OR COMMERCIAL), AS WELL AS BREAST MILK OR FORMULA, FIRST TRY FEEDING HIM AS USUAL.**

631

- He will generally be more willing to accept bland foods, such as cereal and fruit, than vegetables, meats, and so on.

- Try the baby's favorite foods, and don't introduce new foods during illness.

- If the little one turns down most or all of his solids, offer breast milk, formula, or diluted formula, as suggested above.

▶ **IF THE INFANT REFUSES TO NURSE OR DRINK HIS OR HER FOR-MULA, TRY OFFERING ONE OR MORE OF THE FOLLOWING:**

- Plain water.

- Sweetened water.

- A commercial electrolyte solution such as Pedialyte. (Ask your doctor or pharmacist for help if you need it.)

- Dilute fruit juices (half water and half juice), but only if the baby already takes fruit juices.

▶ **OFFER THE ABOVE-LISTED "CLEAR LIQUIDS" TO A SICK BABY IN ADDITION TO REGULAR FEEDINGS, ESPECIALLY IF THE LITTLE ONE HAS FEVER.**

▶ **OFFER SMALL, FREQUENT FEEDINGS.** Babies who are not feeling well are more likely to readily accept them.

▶ **DO NOT ADD NEW LIQUIDS** (ONES THE BABY HAS NOT HAD BE-FORE), **EXCEPT FOR PEDIALYTE OR SIMILAR ELECTROLYTE SO-LUTIONS.** You do not want to compound the problem by adding the risk that the baby may be sensitive or allergic to the "new" liquid.

▶ **IF THE BABY HAS DIARRHEA AND/OR IS VOMITING, YOU WILL NEED TO LIMIT THE TYPES OF LIQUIDS AND SOLIDS YOU OFFER TO HIM OR HER.** If you need more information about managing these problems, turn to the sections entitled "Diarrhea" on page 399, and "Vomiting," on page 489.)

Feeding Your Child or Teenager When Ill

▶ **OFFER SIX TO EIGHT LIGHT MEALS (SNACK-SIZE) PER DAY, IN-STEAD OF THREE LARGER MEALS.**

● Try to give the youngster choices at each snack.

▶ **ENCOURAGE THE YOUNGSTER TO DRINK ADDITIONAL LIQUIDS, ESPECIALLY "CLEAR" LIQUIDS (SUCH AS FRUIT JUICES) OR COMMERCIAL ELECTROLYTE SOLUTIONS (SUCH AS GATORADE).**

▶ **FIX THE YOUNGSTER'S "MOST FAVORITE" FOODS RATHER THAN INSISTING THAT HE OR SHE EAT A WELL-BALANCED DIET (UNLESS THE DOCTOR HAS PRESCRIBED A SPECIFIC DIET).**

● Children (and adults) tend to tolerate foods that consist of more carbohydrates (such as potatoes, rice, bread or toast, noodles, crackers, and Jell-O) better than those foods that consist of more proteins (such as meats, dairy products, and eggs).

● Sweet foods are usually preferred over salty or highly seasoned foods.

▶ **CARBONATED DRINKS ARE HELPFUL IN TREATING NAUSEA BUT SHOULD BE TAKEN IN SMALL AMOUNTS.** Do not give them if a youngster has sores in his mouth or a sore throat.

▶ **COLD FOODS AND DRINKS HELP SOOTHE A SORE THROAT AND/ OR SORE MOUTH AND MAKE A YOUNGSTER FEEL MORE COMFORTABLE IF SHE HAS A FEVER.** (These include such things as fruit pops, fruit juices, yogurt, Jell-O, ice cream, and puddings.)

▶ **IF THE YOUNGSTER HAS DIARRHEA AND/OR VOMITING, YOU NEED TO LIMIT THE TYPES OF FOODS AND LIQUIDS YOU OFFER.** (If you need more information about managing these problems, turn to the sections entitled "Diarrhea," on page 399, and "Vomiting," on page 489.)

▶ **IF THE YOUNGSTER IS CONFINED TO BED OR MUST BE VERY INACTIVE, AVOID CONSTIPATING FOODS** (SUCH AS EXCESSIVE MILK OR MILK PRODUCTS). **OFFER LARGE AMOUNTS OF WATER, FRUIT JUICE, FRUIT, AND HIGH-FIBER FOODS** (RAW VEGETABLES, WHOLE-GRAIN PRODUCTS).

Activity Level When Ill or Injured

▶ **BABIES, TODDLERS, AND YOUNG CHILDREN WILL USUALLY LIMIT THEIR OWN ACTIVITY WHEN ILL OR INJURED, BASED ON HOW THEY FEEL.**

- Let the little one be the judge as to the extent of his activity. However, you might encourage additional quiet time or nap time.

- If you feel the child is not regulating his activity level well, then step in and limit the amount or duration of play activity.

▶ **OLDER CHILDREN AND TEENAGERS MAY NEED TO BE MONITORED AND HAVE SOME LIMITS SET ON THEIR ACTIVITY, SINCE THEY TEND TO OVERDO OR WANT TO PROVE THEY ARE JUST FINE.**

- Rest is an important part of recovery, so where necessary, talk to the youngster about "taking it easy," and if necessary, set limits.

▶ **CHILDREN (OF ALL AGES) SHOULD NOT BE ALLOWED TO PLAY WITH (OR BE AROUND) OTHER CHILDREN FOR AT LEAST TWELVE TO TWENTY-FOUR HOURS AFTER THEY HAVE BEEN WITHOUT FEVER OR UNTIL TWENTY-FOUR HOURS AFTER THEY HAVE TAKEN MEDICATIONS TO TREAT INFECTION, IN ORDER TO PREVENT THE SPREAD OF INFECTION.**

▶ **SUGGEST QUIET GAMES TO PLAY, PROVIDE A CHANGE OF ENVIRONMENT WHENEVER POSSIBLE, AND THINK OF DIVERSIONS FOR THE YOUNGSTER.**

- Remember, it's the little things you do that make the difference.

- Playing music, reading stories, working with arts and crafts, and even helping you cook can be entertaining.

- Taking a ride in the car or going to the market with you (if the child is not contagious or seriously ill) can provide a diversion.

- In good weather, sitting or playing quietly in the backyard is almost never harmful.

▶ **ALLOW OLDER CHILDREN AND TEENAGERS TO TALK ON THE TELEPHONE, SO THEY CAN STAY IN CONTACT WITH THEIR FRIENDS.**

- Arrange for them to get and complete schoolwork as soon as they are able to concentrate, even for short periods of time.

▶ **TAKE THE TIME TO TALK WITH THE YOUNGSTER AND PARTICIPATE IN GAMES OR ACTIVITIES WHENEVER YOU CAN.**

Providing Comfort to a Sick or Injured Youngster

▶ **IF A YOUNGSTER WANTS A SPECIAL TOY, BLANKET, OR SOME OTHER OBJECT OF ENDEARMENT FROM OUT OF THE PAST, BE SURE YOU ALLOW HIM OR HER TO HAVE IT.**

- Everyone regresses a bit when ill, and having an object that has always represented comfort, love, and safety helps.

▶ **DON'T PROMISE THE YOUNGSTER ANYTHING YOU CAN'T DE-LIVER.**

- Be sure to tell the youngster what's wrong in terms she can understand.

- Be honest about how long the problem will last or what to expect at the doctor's, for example. If you don't know the answers about her illness, tell the youngster that rather than guessing incorrectly.

▶ **REMEMBER THAT SHOWING AFFECTION IN LITTLE WAYS HELPS A GREAT DEAL WHEN ANYONE IS NOT FEELING WELL, AND YOUR ATTENTION IS PART OF THE "MEDICINE" THAT A SICK OR IN-JURED CHILD NEEDS.**

Equipment That Is Helpful

▶ **IF A YOUNGSTER IS RESTRICTED TO BED REST, ASK THE DOCTOR WHETHER THERE IS SPECIAL EQUIPMENT THAT WOULD BE USE-FUL TO YOU OR HELPFUL IN MAKING THE YOUNGSTER MORE COMFORTABLE.**

▶ **IF THE CHILD IS INJURED, ASK THE DOCTOR ABOUT EQUIPMENT SUCH AS CRUTCHES, A WHEELCHAIR, AND THE LIKE THAT WOULD BE HELPFUL TO THE CHILD.**

▶ **SOME EQUIPMENT IS HELPFUL TO HAVE IN ANY HOUSEHOLD FOR MINOR OR MODERATE ILLNESSES:**

- Humidifier (the cool-mist type) or vaporizer.

- Hot water bottle.

● Heating pad (for use only if a youngster is over five years old, and not to be used during sleep).

● Ice packs or ice bags.

▶ **DON'T FORGET THE "LITTLE" CONVENIENCES, SUCH AS:**

● Tissues and a basket or bag for their disposal.

● Cool, damp towels (for sponging during fever or for comfort after vomiting).

● A bucket or pan near the youngster (if vomiting is likely).

● A small tray with a pitcher of water or juice and a glass or cup—to encourage the youngster to drink liquids.

If Someone Else Has to Care for the Youngster

▶ **MAKE SURE THE CARE-GIVER IS SOMEONE WHO IS ABLE TO MEET THE YOUNGSTER'S NEEDS—BOTH PHYSICALLY AND EMOTIONALLY—DURING ILLNESS OR RECUPERATION FROM AN INJURY.** Look for someone who is reliable in giving medication correctly, observing the youngster carefully, providing comfort, being kind and sensitive. Above all, the person should have common sense!

▶ **CALL FREQUENTLY FOR REPORTS IF THE YOUNGSTER IS FEELING REALLY BAD, AND TRY TO TALK DIRECTLY WITH YOUR CHILD OR OLDER YOUNGSTER WHENEVER POSSIBLE.**

▶ **IF THERE IS NO ONE TO STAY WITH AN OLDER YOUNGSTER OR TEENAGER, BE SURE THAT SOMEONE CAN CHECK ON HIM OR HER FREQUENTLY (IN PERSON) AND THAT YOU PERSONALLY CALL THE YOUNGSTER OFTEN.**

When to Let the Youngster Go Back to School

▶ **ALLOW YOUR YOUNGSTER TO RETURN TO SCHOOL UNDER THE FOLLOWING CIRCUMSTANCES:**

● The youngster is not contagious and is feeling normal or nearly normal.

● She is able to participate in all or nearly all of the usual activities.

- She does not require too much extra care or attention.

- The doctor has given permission (when a long or serious illness or injury is involved).

The Gift of Giving

One of the most common errors we make is to expect our children to behave pretty much the way they normally do—even when they're sick. It's important that we use ourselves as examples of how a person feels when sick. We feel cranky, upset, angry, frustrated, convinced no cares or knows how badly we feel. We regress a little, become more dependent, and want a touch of special care and attention. But when our children are sick, we often expect (by some miracle) that they should act or feel differently. When most children are sick, they regress a little, just as adults do. They become more infantile and more dependent on others. For some children, this means they are more subdued and quiet and need to be cuddled more. For others, it means they are more irritable, difficult to entertain, harder to keep calm, and cranky.

We also feel quite helpless, at times, because we don't really know *how* to help the youngster. The fact is, there are times when nothing we do makes a child more comfortable (no one feels comfortable vomiting, for example). But in those situations, we can, by our actions and words, let the youngster know that we understand he feels bad, really care about him and what he's going through, and love him. Most often, though, there are things we can do to make a youngster more comfortable and secure when he is sick. In other words, when our children are ill or injured, it is a time when we can make a significant difference—not only by providing for their physical needs, but by giving of ourselves (our time, our participation, and our love).

Feeding Your Sick Child

Most children (and adults) who are mildly to moderately sick don't eat as well as they usually do. They tend to be more finicky about what they eat and are more likely to accept their "most favorite" foods rather than a wide variety of foods. It's important to remember that there is a point at which youngsters may reject even the foods that normally make them feel good. This does not always mean the young person is seriously ill—unless he or she refuses to eat *or* drink anything at all (as discussed in detail in Chapter 12).

It's fascinating to realize that most people associate certain foods with comfort and warmth. If you asked a roomful of adults what they eat when sick—almost inevitably the foods will be those that were given to them as children when they were sick. These are "special" foods with "special" significance. Most families have favorite "comfort foods" that are associated with being sick and being comforted by mothers and/or fathers. Whether chicken soup, Jell-O, tapioca pudding, ice cream, mashed potatoes, cream of wheat, or popsicles—these foods symbolize specialness. This is not a bad thing for children to learn. In fact, it's probably a good experience, because serving these "special" foods tells the youngster that you love him and that you really do understand that he doesn't feel well.

However, we also need to remember that there's nothing really magical about any one of these "comfort foods"—except that they tend to be among the more acceptable foods when children or adults don't feel well. What we mean by "magical" is that we often think that food makes the child well—that it has a healing quality. Many parents find themselves caught in a dilemma: "Do I let her eat what she wants to eat, or do I prepare very healthy, well-balanced meals and make her eat them?" It is true that children need to consume some calories when they are sick, and it would be nice if their calories were "healthy" calories. Although this sounds good in theory, it often doesn't work in practice.

If a breast-fed baby (not yet on solid foods) is ill, it is always best to continue to nurse the baby as she wishes to be fed. If the baby won't accept the breast, then try offering small amounts of water, sweetened water, or a commercial electrolyte solution, such as Pedialyte.

If your sick baby is formula-fed, try feeding his bottle as usual. If the baby won't accept the formula, try diluting the formula with water to half its usual strength (make the bottle with half formula and half water). If this does not work, offer Pedialyte or a similar commercial electrolyte solution. If the baby is already taking juices, you can also give him diluted juices, either in addition to or as an alternative to formula, diluted formula, and/or electrolyte solution.

If the baby or toddler is on solids as well as being breast-fed or formula-fed, see if she will tolerate normal feedings. If not, try giving liquids, as well as her favorite solid foods (usually cereals, yogurt, and fruits). If the baby does not accept the solids, don't worry as long as she is drinking well. If you think about it, *your* appetite for food is usually reduced with illness also!

Number one premise: It is more important for a youngster to drink liquids than to eat solid foods. That's not to say that you should not offer solid foods, but only that you should *not* panic if the youngster refuses to eat solid foods at all, eats only a little, or will only eat certain types of foods.

Here are a few guidelines that might be helpful. Try to restrict solid foods to those that are fairly *bland and simple*. This keeps the food easy to digest with almost any illness. Avoiding greasy and highly spicy foods is always wise. Offer the youngster *six to eight light meals (snack-size) per day* instead of three larger meals.

For example, a youngster might accept: a little hot cereal for breakfast; a piece of toast with jelly two hours later; a few soda crackers with cheese and a piece of fruit for lunch (fruit and cheese are acceptable as long as he or she doesn't have severe diarrhea or vomiting); a little Jell-O a few hours after lunch; a small serving of macaroni and cheese with a piece of toast for dinner; and ice cream a few hours after dinner. Available throughout the day should be water and fruit juices (and sodas if that's all the youngster will drink). If you add up all the little bits of food eaten here and there, you realize that the young person has actually consumed a reasonable amount.

Another fact: Most youngsters will tolerate carbohydrates (potatoes, rice, and macaroni) better than proteins (meat, pork, chicken, and fish). When sick, children (and adults) prefer sweet things to salty things. Fancy gourmet foods are usually not appreciated or readily eaten—simply because they don't taste good. Medications and/or the inability of the youngster to smell normally change the taste of foods; therefore, things often taste sour, bland, or unusual.

If the youngster refuses all solid foods—then *encourage him or her to drink liquids.* Try to entice the young person to accept liquids that are relatively healthy or have some protein content. Fruit juices contain vitamins and natural sugars and are generally more desirable than sodas and carbonated drinks. However, if the youngster has diarrhea and/or vomiting or simply refuses plain water or fruit juices—then sodas and other carbonated drinks are fine. With infants and young children, it's best to dilute fruit juices (one-half water to one-half juice). Gatorade can also be given (it's an electrolyte replacement that gives the youngster a little of the special body salts that he or she needs).

Be ingenious about what you offer. Gelatin products "count" as liquids and contain some protein, as well as sugar. Frozen fruit pops (make your own with fruit juice) are also liquids and tasty. Ice cream, sherbet, and milk shakes are further good sources of nutrition during an illness, but they offer less "actual" liquid than the "clear" fruit pops. It's important to remember, however, to use milk products only if the youngster doesn't have diarrhea and/or vomiting.

A few other points to remember: If the young person has a sore throat, sore mouth, or fever—cold things (cold drinks, ice cream, frozen fruit pops, and so on) will usually be soothing to her. Often, carbonated sodas are helpful in treating nausea. (Open the can or bottle and let it sit for ten minutes or so before giving it to the youngster, so it isn't too cold or too fizzy.) Give the youngster choices at each snack or meal instead of just serving something to him. For example: Would you prefer macaroni and cheese or chicken soup? Do you feel like having some ice cream or Jell-O right now? Do crackers sound good to you, or would you like some mashed potatoes? Also, serve the food on a nice little plate or serving tray so it looks special.

Many parents run into a pitfall when they call the doctor and say the child isn't eating or drinking. Often, they tend to discount what the youngster has eaten or drunk all day long and focus their attention on what the child didn't eat or drink at a main meal. Therefore, carefully watch what the child eats and drinks *throughout the entire day*.

One baseline value to use is this: if the child or young person is urinating at least two to four times a day, then he or she is not seriously dehydrated (has had enough fluids and/or food for you not to worry excessively). If the child or young person is urinating normally—then you have nothing to worry about in terms of liquids and food intake. If you become concerned and are truly convinced the youngster isn't eating or drinking enough—call the doctor for advice and/or evaluation. Be sure to tell the doctor *exactly how much of what* the child has been taking throughout the last few days. If a child or youngster *totally refuses* to eat or drink over a twelve- to twenty-four-hour period, call the doctor for evaluation.

In the final analysis, unless the doctor has prescribed a special diet or the youngster has a chronic problem (such as diabetes) and must follow a carefully planned menu, the youngster should be free to eat or drink what helps him feel better and what is most tolerable to him. It's futile to try to force-feed a young person. This will only make you and the youngster miserable (and it's unnecessary). As long as the youngster was well nourished and growing normally before he got sick, then allowing him to choose what he will eat and drink while sick will not be harmful. You will notice that as the young person feels better, he will increase not only the amount but the variety of foods eaten. Therefore, appetite is a good gauge of how the youngster is feeling. As the child's appetite picks up, you will know that he is feeling better.

Should You Limit His or Her Activity?

There are very few circumstances that would require a child or teenager to totally limit his or her activity. In all situations of illness or injury, common sense plays the most important role. When young people are truly sick, they will *not want* to do the things they normally do. Most children will be more sedentary than usual. Younger children will want to be held more, cuddled, pampered, and soothed. They may want to watch television and play quiet games rather than run around the house or ride their bicycles. They may show some bursts of energy but then want to rest again. Older children will also want some special attention, shows of affection and love, and some pampering. They'll prefer watching television, playing video games, reading, and probably talking on the telephone.

There are some basic premises, however, that you can use to protect the energetic older child or teenager who responds to illness or injury either by pretending to feel fine or by staying active because he thinks that will make him feel better. If the youngster has a fever, he shouldn't be doing his normal activities! Rather, he should be staying quietly around the house. If she is sick enough to stay home from school, then she is sick enough not to run around and be involved in physically tiring activities.

Interestingly, infants, toddlers, and younger children usually restrict their own level of activity—based on how they feel. If a preschooler is running around the house, playing normally, and refuses to stop to take a nap or rest—then he is not very sick or he wouldn't be doing this. In fact, trying to limit a young person when she feels well enough to do something will only frustrate you and the youngster. Ironically, both of you will exert more energy trying to hold down the youngster's activities than if you allowed her to go ahead and play!

We also need to remember that there's nothing magical about lying in bed. Permitting children to play quiet games in the living room, watch television, color, paint, or read can be just as restful as being in bed (unless the doctor has specifically instructed you to keep the youngster in bed with no diversions). In fact, some children will rest better when allowed to do a few things, change their environment from time to time, even go out in the backyard to play quietly and take advantage of sunshine and fresh air.

Most professionals feel that a child should not be with other children until he has been free of fever for at least twelve to twenty-four hours or until twenty-four hours after starting medication that attacks the infection and prevents it from spreading. But this *does not mean* the child should feel a prisoner of his illness. He may want to play quietly in his backyard sandbox or play with the dog—or even play quiet games with brothers and sisters (who have more than likely already been exposed to the illness long before the child showed signs of it). Permit these activities unless the doctor specifically instructs you to keep all children and others away from the ill child (which is an unusual occurrence).

The main thing to remember is that there are few illnesses where reasonable activity will make a youngster worse. (The exceptions are wheezing and similar problems, but with these, the doctor will be very specific about what a youngster can and cannot do.) A child should learn early on that rest is an important aspect of getting well— but that rest may include a variety of quiet activities, as well as sleeping and lying down.

Equipment That Is Helpful

There really isn't much equipment that you need when caring for your sick or injured child—other than those very obvious items we tend to forget about. For example, having tissues within reach (and a container for the used ones) when the youngster has a cold—whether he or she is in bed, lying on the couch, or playing on the floor— is not only useful but makes the youngster more comfortable. A small tray with a pitcher of cold water and a glass are always pleasant and useful when a youngster is ill.

Other helpful items to have available are a cool, damp towel and a dry towel— particularly if the youngster has a fever or is nauseated. If the youngster is vomiting or feels nauseated, then a pan or bucket next to the bed or couch will make him feel secure if he suddenly gets sick and knows it's impossible to get to the bathroom on time. A humidifier or vaporizer also makes the room a little more comfortable for the youngster who is congested. (For safety reasons, a "cool-mist" type is best.)

One warning: Heating pads should *not* be used for children under five years old because of the possibility of burns. Care should be taken in using heating pads in children over five, as well. No matter what the child's age (and this should apply to adults, too), he or she should not use a heating pad when sleeping—unless an adult is right there (and awake) to watch the youngster. These are simply precautions in the event a fire breaks out (if an electrical short takes place in the heating pad). Precautions should be taken with *all* electrical appliances and equipment.

If the young person is injured, you should ask the doctor whether crutches, a cane, a wheelchair, or other devices would be helpful. If the child is restricted to total bed rest (due to either injury or illness), then ask the doctor or nurse for ideas about items, equipment, or things that you can do that would be useful, helpful, or make the young person more comfortable. Hospital supply stores have many kinds of equipment for rent or purchase (and can be a good source of information or ideas, as well). The environment doesn't need to be elaborate. Remember, convenience and comfort are the goals.

Providing Comfort and Diversion

It's often difficult to remember that young people—even those with the best disposition (cheerful, easygoing, and intelligent)—can become more demanding, a little cranky, or hard to please when sick. Or they may pretend that all is well and they're just fine—because they don't want to worry you or make demands on you. In either case, these young people want to know that you care and that you *really* understand that they don't feel well.

In fact, it's the little things you do that can make the difference. For example, making meals (snacks) look attractive and appealing shows that you've added a special touch and gone to a little trouble. This makes youngsters feel special (even if they never say so) and encourages them to eat. As mentioned previously, offer youngsters choices about what they would like to eat. This tells them you're trying to please them and also gives them a special role in their recovery. In other words, it gives them some "say" in taking care of themselves—with your help.

Little niceties—like extra pillows or a favorite comforter or quilt—always make people (of any age) feel special and cozy. Watch, however, that the youngster doesn't get overheated. Some people feel that they need to bundle the youngster up in order to sweat out a fever or keep a child well covered with extra blankets so he or she doesn't "catch" a chill. It's true that when we are less active, more quiet, and restful, we don't produce as much of our own body heat—so we usually need an extra cover. The same is true of young people. However, overheating is never a good idea, does *not* contribute to breaking a fever, and will only make the youngster uncomfortable. It's also a fallacy that anyone gets a "cold" by being cold!

Another fallacy about colds needs to be corrected. Many people don't allow an ill youngster to take a bath—for fear that he will get a chill and then pneumonia. In reality, a nice, warm bath can be very pleasant, relaxing, and comforting for youngsters who are sick. You've often heard that allowing already sick youngsters to wash their hair or get their ears wet can cause a chill, cold, or even an ear infection. Not true! Unless the doctor specifically instructs you not to allow a child to take a bath or get his ears wet (a prohibition that is usually needed only when there is a hole in the eardrum, because of infection or because the youngster has ventilation tubes in the ears), then soaking in a tub and getting clean is perfectly acceptable and helps a youngster feel good all over.

A rubdown with lotion (particularly a back rub) will relax the young person and also gives her a feeling of being loved and comforted. These little expressions of love also tell the youngster that you are giving of your own personal time to help her feel better. Simple little things like fluffing up pillows, changing the bed sheets, fluffing up the couch, opening the curtains or shades so sunlight flows into the house, and changing the environment (having the youngster move around the house if she feels like it) make recovery more pleasant.

Essentially, then, you need not be elaborate or expensive. Playing music, playing a quiet game, reading a book with a younger child, or having him or her draw pictures for you or "create" something special with paper, colors, cloth, and so on can entertain children for a long time. Older children may want to help you cook (which is fine unless they are terribly contagious) or help you with another chore. Teenagers may want some special time with you—to talk and share ideas and feelings.

If the youngster is mildly ill and feeling fairly well, he may enjoy a ride in the car or a trip to the market—just for a change of scenery. He may enjoy sitting in the backyard for a while—or just getting dressed instead of staying in pajamas and robe all day.

If a younger (or even older) child suddenly wants a teddy or blanket or special toy that she hasn't played with for a long time (or even years)—take care not to make fun of the youngster or make her feel foolish or like a baby. Comfort and security are important, and regression is perfectly normal. Be happy to find the special object for the youngster, and don't make a big deal out of it.

Finally, try to explain to the young person what is wrong with him in words he can understand. Never lie about what is happening. Children are bright and sensitive and will eventually catch you in a lie. More important, they may not trust other things you tell them later—if they feel you were not truthful before.

For example, often the youngster wants to know when she'll be well. Until children are seven or eight years old, they really don't understand "time." With them, it's best to be general but honest. "Johnny, you're going to feel better tomorrow and even better the day after tomorrow. It won't be too long, but why don't we wait and see how you feel each day, OK?"

With older children, you can tell them approximately when they will be well—if you know. "Well, Valerie, this kind of flu lasts about a week. Today is Wednesday, so you'll probably feel really good by next Wednesday. But if you're feeling much better on Sunday—that's four days from today—maybe you can go back to school on

Monday.'' Teenagers will be more blunt—wanting to know specifically ''when this will be over!'' Ask the doctor, and make sure you relay the message exactly. Or even better, tell the teenager to ask the doctor before she leaves the office, so she becomes more involved in her own care.

Most important, *never* promise anything you can't deliver. Don't tell the child that if he takes this medicine, he'll feel all better afterward. (He'll feel all better in a few days if he continues to take his medicine!) Don't promise the young person that she can go back to school tomorrow if you know that just isn't possible. Never promise that his friends can visit later today when you know that won't happen because he's still contagious.

Comfort and diversion encompass a great many things, but all in all, you can make a youngster's illness or injury less difficult if you spend some time with the child, go out of your way to make him feel special, and treat him with both respect and understanding. These kindnesses are remembered long past the illness or injury—even into adulthood.

A Word About Child-Care Problems During Illness

In this age of working parents, a child's illness often places an unusual burden on a parent to arrange for quality child care. Your choices may be quite limited, and you may not be able to be with your sick child—even though you wish to be. Many times, parents are tempted to send their children back to school or the child-care center too early—because they just don't know what else to do.

This is a difficult situation for everyone. Obviously, the youngster would feel better if you were home—and so would you. When this is simply not possible, you really need to be sure that the youngster is in competent hands—with a neighbor, a grandparent or other relative, or another trustworthy person. You need someone who can *watch* the child for unexpected (or expected) problems, report things to you accurately, give medication(s) reliably and correctly (if needed), provide comfort, be kind and understanding—and generally use common sense. You can also suggest that the person who is going to care for the child take some of the measures we've discussed to help the youngster feel more comfortable.

Even an older youngster or teenager who is sick needs someone who cares. He may feel very lonely and afraid when ill but be hesitant to tell you if saying so would mean you'd miss work or he'd be made fun of or would feel embarrassed by making this admission. Don't force the youngster to make the decision. If you must leave her alone, arrange for someone who can frequently check (in person) on the young person and keep in touch yourself with frequent phone calls.

Use common sense before sending a youngster back to school or group child care (this applies to mothers and fathers who work in the home, as well as to those who work out of the home). He or she should be (1) not contagious, (2) able to participate in activities fully or with only minor modifications, and (3) well enough not to require too much extra care and attention. Each school or center, however, has its own rules—designed for the protection of both the injured or ill child and the group of children. While some rules may not always be to everyone's liking (and occasionally don't even make sense), they were made with the youngsters' well-being in mind. If the rules don't seem right and reasonable, discuss them with those in charge. If other parents are also in agreement with you, then together you may be able to institute changes in the rules—based on sound and safe health principles for *all children*.

THE DON'TS

Don't forget that it's the little things that make a youngster feel more comfortable. You do not have to go to great expense to help your child feel a little better.

Don't forget to ask the doctor about any equipment or other things that might be helpful to your child if his illness or injury will require a long recovery period or be quite restrictive.

Don't hesitate to let the youngster eat what she wants when ill or injured (unless the doctor has prescribed a specific diet).

Don't worry that a youngster "will not eat" during an illness. Remember, his activity level is lower than usual, and he will not starve. Just be sure to offer plenty of nourishing liquids.

Don't hesitate to be creative and inventive when finding diversions for the ill or injured youngster. Remember that doing something is usually better than doing nothing other than just lying there.

Don't forget that affection and understanding go a long way. Talking to the youngster, taking time to spend with him or her, and showing affection are all very important to a sick or injured child.

PLEASE NOTE: Now that you have a grasp of how to make your child feel more comfortable during an illness, it would be extremely helpful for you to go back to the Quick Reference With the Steps in Detail and review it carefully. The more familiar you are with that material, the more useful it will be to you when you need it.

CHAPTER 19

What About All Those Over-the-Counter and Prescribed Medications?

QUICK REFERENCE

With the Steps in Detail

Prescribed and Over-the-Counter Medications

▶ **ALWAYS WEIGH THE RISKS VERSUS THE BENEFITS BEFORE GIVING A CHILD OR YOUNGSTER ANY OVER-THE-COUNTER MEDICATION.**

▶ **GIVE OVER-THE-COUNTER MEDICATIONS ONLY WHEN ABSOLUTELY NECESSARY.**

▶ **ALWAYS ASK YOUR DOCTOR ABOUT THE RISKS VERSUS THE BENEFITS OF ANY PRESCRIBED MEDICATION RECOMMENDED FOR YOUR CHILD.** You should know the possible minor side effects and adverse reactions of any medication—and what action you should take if the child experiences any of them.

647

WHAT ABOUT
ALL THOSE
OVER-THE-
COUNTER AND
PRESCRIBED
MEDICATIONS?

▶ **BE EXTREMELY CAUTIOUS ABOUT GIVING MEDICATIONS ONLY AS DIRECTED.**

- **Measure all liquid medications carefully by using a measuring device**—*not* a common table-use teaspoon or tablespoon, a bottle lid (unless marked for such use), or drinking from the bottle.

- With over-the-counter medicines, be sure to read the directions and carefully follow the instructions as to how to determine the amount of medicine to give the youngster.

- If the medication is in tablet or capsule form, give only the amount prescribed (or directed on the label). **Don't double up on any medicine,** thinking this will help the child get well sooner (it won't and may, in fact, cause serious problems), **or cut the amount of the prescribed medication in half** (for example, because the child seems to be getting better and you think he or she may need less).

- **Always give medicines at the time intervals prescribed or directed.**

- Whether a prescribed or over-the-counter medication, write down the time given and the amount. In this way, you will know *for sure* when and how much was given. This is especially important if more than one person is responsible for giving the medicine.

▶ **IF THE DOCTOR HAS EXPLAINED THAT ALL OF THE MEDICINE SHOULD BE USED, MAKE SURE YOU DO SO, EVEN IF THE YOUNGSTER SEEMS WELL TO YOU.** Some medications (in particular, antibiotics) must be given for a certain number of days to effectively destroy the microorganism that is causing the illness. If the medicine is stopped early, the microorganism can multiply again, and the youngster may experience a relapse (get sick again).

▶ **NEVER GIVE A CHILD OR YOUNGSTER (OR ANYONE, FOR THAT MATTER!) A PRESCRIPTION MEDICATION NOT PRESCRIBED FOR HIM OR HER.**

Drugs: What You Should Know

Thirty or forty years ago, rest was the major ingredient in treating illness or injury. In addition, a youngster with a stomachache might have been given baking soda and water. A child with a cold could have been asked to gargle with warm salt water or breathe steam to clear the sinuses. Cod liver oil and laxatives were turned to regularly for almost every ailment. Sulfa drugs were part of the treatment regimen for pneumonia. Boiled eucalyptus leaves were used to help relieve congestion. Aspirin was taken sometimes for headaches, but mostly for fevers, and usually only by adults. It's amazing to consider the fact that penicillin was given experimentally only in 1943. That's not very long ago!

Although some drugs were available, few people reached for the medicine cabinet every time a youngster (or adult) experienced an illness or injury. It was accepted then that minor illnesses and even a few more serious ones were simply part of life.

Today it's an entirely different story. Just go into any pharmacy or drugstore and you will see row after row of over-the-counter drugs and countless prescription medications. In fact, so many different medications are available in various forms (liquid, capsule, tablet, or injectable) that each year a new *Physician's Desk Reference* (*PDR*) is released so doctors can stay updated as to what medications are available (including the new ones approved by the time of publication); what their potential benefits, side effects, and adverse reactions are; and what dosages are recommended by the manufacturers. Update inserts are sent out as new drugs are developed or existing drugs recalled, or when new information is found out about certain medications.

The fact is, there are literally thousands and thousands of approved prescription and over-the-counter medications in the United States today—quite a contrast to thirty years ago. And new medications are being discovered or developed and tested almost daily in research laboratories all over the world.

As with almost everything in our lives, there are both pluses and minuses associated with advances in medical technology and knowledge. Some medications have, in countless cases, saved lives or improved the quality of life. Some are truly miracle drugs, such as antibiotics, synthetic hormones, certain anticancer (chemotherapeutic) agents, immunizations, heart medications, and a whole host of others.

On the flip side, we have very much become a medication/drug-oriented society. The concept of ''there's a pill for every ill'' is constantly advertised on television and radio, in newspapers and magazines, and on billboards, buses, bus stops, and the like. Unfortunately, our children are being exposed to this philosophy at quite young ages. They hear that you take a pill for a headache, a stomachache, a cold, the flu, and a sore toe; there are medicines for diarrhea, constipation, coughs, congestion, and a bad day. It's not that medications should not be used when necessary, but often children learn to ask for a pill or are given something before anything else is tried first.

For example: How many people teach their children stress-management techniques? When your child or teenager initially complains of a headache, upset stomach, or being

649

WHAT ABOUT
ALL THOSE
OVER-THE-
COUNTER AND
PRESCRIBED
MEDICATIONS?

tired or achy, do you have her lie down and relax for a half hour or an hour? Have you tried having the youngster lie down or sit down in a darkened room, listening to quiet music? How about teaching him to close his eyes and concentrate on his favorite peaceful scene—like the ocean, the trees at the park, the lake, a piano or violin being played, or even a perfect circle? The point is, some complaints are due to stress, overexertion, or fatigue. If we could begin teaching our children at very young ages methods of relieving common complaints (and thereby teaching them how to relax, as well), then they might not reach for a pill as a first response to every discomfort.

If, indeed, the relaxation doesn't alleviate the headache, stomachache, or other problem, then the child or teenager may be coming down with something. You'll be able to determine this based on the set of symptoms that develop, as discussed in previous chapters. On the other hand, if the headache (or the stomachache or slight diarrhea or whatever) remains the only symptom, and relaxation (stress management) does not alleviate the problem, and it's very bothersome, then going to the medicine cabinet is a reasonable next move.

It may seem rather strange or out of place to discuss stress and stress management in a chapter on over-the-counter and prescribed medications. The fact is, it's the best place for us to point out the need for alternatives to using medications—and the importance of using medications only when necessary. Just think if you were taught—beginning at two years of age—that the best "medicine" for a headache or a long, stressful day was to lie down and concentrate on relaxing your big toe on your right foot, then all the little toes, then your entire right foot, then the same with your big toe on your left foot—all the way up to relaxing the scalp and hair on your head? Or if you were taught at age two to lie down each afternoon and listen to quiet music for half an hour—what would your life be like today?

The point is, each of us would have learned how to better manage our stresses and how to relax. We would have been given ammunition for dealing with common complaints instead of reaching for a drug. And we would have established a built-in stress-management technique for a lifetime.

No one can say for sure that there is a direct cause-and-effect relationship between our society's attitude about medication use and illegal drug use by so many young children. However, if we teach our children at very young ages that drugs/medications are good for them—and take away all their problems—then some children may carry this attitude one step further. If drugs are the answer to almost everything, then why aren't they the answer to feeling good all the time—even if they're illegal drugs and even if they've been told some drugs are dangerous? What's so dangerous about feeling good?

If we teach our children a healthy respect for medications/drugs—and teach them early on about other means of managing common complaints—then they won't have a built-in "drug-dependent" attitude. For them, there won't be "a pill for every ill" but rather an understanding that medicines should only be used when absolutely necessary.

Teaching children stress-management techniques can actually be made into fun games, at first, when they are very young. Playing together is even more fun for them. Every day, when mother or dad or both get home from work, everyone can lie on the floor (on their backs) with a pillow under their heads. Now everyone tries to lie very still with their eyes closed. You can start by wiggling your toes—then make your toes rest, then your feet, and so on up the entire body. Now every part of your body should feel "really good" and be resting. Next, we're all going to imagine our favorite place and try to see it in our minds and just rest and relax for ten minutes.

Again, the point is for us to do everything we can to teach a healthy respect for medicines—to teach our children that they are used only when absolutely necessary and then carefully taken as directed. In addition, we can do our children a great service if we teach them ways to eliminate minor complaints and enhance their lives overall by learning stress-management techniques at an early age, and encourage the practice of these techniques throughout their lives. In this way, they may learn to look to *themselves* for the answers rather than to drugs—legal or illegal—as they grow older.

Drugs: Terms You Need to Understand

A drug is a chemical substance used to control a body function or symptom. The words *drug, medication*, and *medicine* are interchangeable.

All drugs are classified as to how they may be obtained. For example, *over-the-counter* (OTC) drugs can be purchased without a prescription from a doctor. Most (but not all) over-the-counter drugs treat the symptoms of illnesses (how we feel) but not the illnesses themselves. Some over-the-counter drugs are useful and safe, while others have very little benefit and may cause problems in some youngsters.

A *prescription* drug is one that must be ordered by a physician (or in some cases, a dentist), either in writing or by telephone. *Narcotics* form one class of prescription drugs. These are powerful drugs that have effects on the brain, as well as other organs of the body. Narcotics (painkillers, sedatives, and so on) have the ability to produce physical addiction if used for extended periods of time. *Controlled substances* are drugs whose use and prescriptions are specifically regulated by the federal and/or state governments. These are drugs that have a strong potential for abuse and/or produce chemical dependency or addiction.

Combination drugs are medications/products that contain two or more separate drugs. Most of these drugs were combined in the belief that they would act together to have a better overall effect. However, some combination drugs, especially those available without a prescription, are put together irrationally. Some contain ineffective or even potentially dangerous drugs, and others are mixed so that dosages of the ingredients are incorrectly balanced (too little of one, too much of another). They can also be dangerous because people tend to take more than one kind of medicine without realizing that they may be duplicating one or more of the ingredients in the combination drug.

651

WHAT ABOUT
ALL THOSE
OVER-THE-
COUNTER AND
PRESCRIBED
MEDICATIONS?

A *generic* drug is a non–brand-name product that is usually less expensive than the same brand-name product. Most generic drugs are as effective as the higher-cost brand-name drug. You should always ask the doctor if he or she can prescribe the generic drug. At times, the doctor will prefer a specific brand, since a particular brand-name drug may be more effective than the generic version or have other desirable characteristics (such as better taste).

Antibiotic is a term used to refer to a group of drugs that are effective in destroying bacteria. Antibiotics are *not* effective against viruses, although a few antiviral drugs are presently available, and additional research is being performed each year to develop more antiviral drugs.

Drugs: The Risks Versus the Benefits

Drugs cause predictable effects—some that are desirable and others that are not. Although most people think that over-the-counter drugs are safer than prescribed drugs (and that is why they are sold over the counter), some over-the-counter drugs can be just as dangerous as some prescribed drugs. This is very important to keep in mind.

Most drugs have been tested for both their effectiveness and their safety—first in laboratories, then in animals, and finally in humans. However, many products on the market for years have never been tested scientifically until recently. Some were found to be ineffective. These drugs—most of them a combination of medications (irrational combinations, generally)—have for the most part been removed from the market, but a few are still available. Still others have been relabeled to tone down the "promises" they make.

In order to weigh the risks against the benefits of any drug, you must be able to understand its potential therapeutic effects, side effects/cautions, and possible adverse reactions (including allergic reactions, idiosyncratic reactions, and toxic effects). Let's look at each of these in turn.

Therapeutic effects are the expected "good" things that result from taking the drug and the reason(s) the drug is recommended, used, or prescribed. For example, the therapeutic effect of ampicillin (an antibiotic) is to destroy bacteria that cause certain common infections. One of the therapeutic effects of theophylline is that it stops wheezing.

Side effects/cautions are common symptoms or signs that can occur when using a particular drug. These can be minor, but bothersome, and are expected to be experienced by many people who use the drug. Ampicillin, for example, can cause diarrhea, a nonallergic rash, or a tendency to get thrush (yeast infection). Theophylline can cause shakiness, nausea, hyperactivity, or a rapid heartbeat.

Adverse reactions are more serious reactions that occur in a number of people who use a drug. They are serious or bothersome enough that the drug must be stopped and/or never used again.

- For example, in some children, ampicillin may cause an *allergic reaction* (hives or a full-blown anaphylactic reaction). Allergic reaction implies a true immune-system response against the drug and can be life-threatening if the drug is used again. Anaphylactic reactions and hives are signs of true allergy to a medicine. It's important to distinguish this from other reactions to medicines, since having an allergic reaction means the youngster should *never* take that medicine again.

- *Idiosyncratic reactions* are unusual reactions to a medicine that are not real allergy but are quite unique to the individual. In fact, the reaction may be the exact *opposite* of the expected reaction. For example, a youngster may experience hyperactivity from phenobarbital, which usually acts as a sedative.

- The *toxic effect* of a drug is predictable if the dose of a medicine is too high or its level in the blood is too high. The toxic level can be reached by a single high dose or, with some medications, because of a gradual buildup over time.

When a doctor prescribes a medication, he or she thinks carefully about what problem a child has and about the drugs available to treat the problem. The doctor weighs the possible risks and benefits, then prescribes the medication(s) that are likely to produce the best benefit with the least risk. For example, if a youngster has a middle-ear infection, an antibiotic is needed to cure the infection. The doctor must know which antibiotics will kill the bacteria that are most likely to be causing the infection. Then he or she chooses the one that seems best for that child. Many times, ampicillin or amoxacillin (a relative of ampicillin) is chosen because it is safe, effective, and relatively inexpensive. However, if a youngster has had many ear infections in the past, for example, ampicillin might not be as effective as another drug. Likewise, if a youngster has had a problem with ampicillin in the past, the doctor will prescribe a different antibiotic.

You should exercise the same kind of care in choosing over-the-counter medicines for your child. Let's use an example to show how you might compare the risks and benefits of over-the-counter drugs to help you decide whether using a particular drug is a good idea.

Suppose your two-year-old son has a cold. He is miserable, with a mild fever, sniffling, nose congestion, and a cough. You know that if you treat his fever, he will probably feel much better. If you talk to the doctor, ask your pharmacist, or read the labels on various medicines for fever, you'll find that acetaminophen (Tylenol, Tempra, Panadol, and so on) is helpful in reducing fever and has very few serious side effects if given in the correct dosage. It makes sense to use it for your miserably ill little child.

Now you are faced with whether or not to treat any of his other symptoms. When you go to the pharmacy, you find many medicines you could use for congestion and cough. All of them look about the same when you read the labels or talk to the pharmacist. You decide that the chance of their helping is worth taking, so you choose one of them and give your child one dose. You notice that his nose really doesn't seem much better, but the medicine has made him very irritable and hyperactive. You would probably now decide that you won't give any more doses, because the tiny amount of improvement in his congestion isn't worth causing him to be more miserable from the drug.

Try to use this principle of weighing the benefits against the risks of over-the-counter drugs, and ask your doctor to explain the risks and benefits of any prescription drugs. By doing this, you will have done all you can to ensure your child's safety when you must give medicines.

653

WHAT ABOUT ALL THOSE OVER-THE-COUNTER AND PRESCRIBED MEDICATIONS?

General Principles of Drug Use

DRUGS TO RELIEVE SYMPTOMS

When you are giving a youngster a medication to improve how he or she feels or to relieve particularly bothersome symptoms, use common sense and your knowledge of the drug you want to give:

- *Use ONLY the medications that are really needed, and use them only when the symptoms are especially uncomfortable for your child.*

  Weigh the risks of side effects against the possible benefits.

  Remember that the *other* things you can do to help a youngster feel better can be just as effective as a drug. For example, tissues are just as useful as medicines in treating colds.

- *Use a single drug and not a combination whenever you can.*

  If you don't know which choice to make, check with your doctor or pharmacist for the types of over-the-counter medications he or she recommends.

  Be aware that many over-the-counter drugs are just as effective in treating symptoms as some prescription drugs and usually cost less.

  If you use a combination drug, you may risk added side effects and increase the possibility of overdosing drugs unexpectedly. (For example, many over-the-counter "cold medicines" contain aspirin or acetaminophen. If you give both the cold medicine and separate aspirin or acetaminophen, you are giving too high a dose.)

- *Use the correct dose—no more and no less.*

  Read the label carefully, or check with your doctor or pharmacist if you are not sure how much to give.

• *Don't hesitate to use a store brand or generic drug, as long as you are sure of the dose. (Ask the pharmacist to help you.)*

DRUGS THAT ARE PRESCRIBED BY THE DOCTOR

When the doctor orders a prescription drug, the label will tell you how to use the medicine. Be sure you understand the instructions and follow them carefully. Prescription drugs might be used to cure the problem or to treat particularly troublesome symptoms:

• *Ask for generic drugs unless your doctor prescribed and meant a specific brand. Ask the pharmacist about this.*

• *Use ALL the medication that was prescribed, unless the doctor clearly told you that you could stop when the youngster felt better.*

This is particularly important if the medication is an antibiotic. The youngster will probably feel and act well before the infection is completely cured.

Don't save antibiotics or other drugs for another illness or another person unless the doctor tells you to do so.

• *Be sure to follow the directions to the letter.*

If medication is ordered four times a day, give four doses a day.

If the drug is to be given every so many hours, do that, too. Usually, this direction means that you must give the medicine *around the clock*. Check with the doctor if you're not sure.

Be sure you understand whether the medicine is to be used as needed or until it is gone.

CHOOSING THE CORRECT DOSAGE

Whenever you use a drug, whether prescribed or over-the-counter, be sure to give the correct dosage, based on your child's size. The correct dose is enough to cure the illness or improve the symptoms, but not enough to cause harm. For prescribed medicines, this information will be written on the label and is based on the doctor's orders. If you are using over-the-counter medicine, you must choose the appropriate dose, based on the directions on the package.

• *With prescribed medicine, follow the directions on the label exactly. Ask the pharmacist to explain the directions to you if you don't understand, or call the doctor if you become confused.*

655

WHAT ABOUT
ALL THOSE
OVER-THE-
COUNTER AND
PRESCRIBED
MEDICATIONS?

- *When possible, give medicine based on your youngster's weight rather than on his or her age. As you know, children of the same age can vary a great deal in size.*

- *With certain medicines, it is important for you to know the actual milligram dose the doctor recommends. This is particularly important and helpful with acetaminophen (aspirin substitute) since you will then be able to change brands or forms without difficulty.*

- *Many over-the-counter drugs have warnings on the label about not using them for children under a certain age. Others instruct you to use them only with a doctor's recommendation.*

  Do not "guess" about the dosage when you see this kind of warning. Call the doctor for advice, or avoid using the medication.

  You should be aware that many of the drugs that are labeled in this way are actually safe for young children *if they are used under a doctor's supervision.* If the doctor recommends them and tells you how to use them, you should feel comfortable with them.

- *Be aware that some over-the-counter drugs have labels that give doses that are too low to be fully effective. This is done to prevent overdosage, but it makes it difficult for you to judge which label shows the correct dosage.*

  Do not automatically increase the dose of a drug without checking with your doctor.

- *If you are giving an infant or young child a liquid medicine, use an appropriate measuring device.*

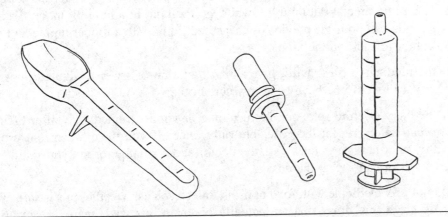

All medicines should be measured precisely by using one of several different plastic devices available.

Medicine syringes, medicine cups, and test-tube–like spoons can be purchased in any pharmacy and are both accurate and easy to use. Try to find one that is marked in both teaspoons and milliliters.

Do not use unmarked droppers or household teaspoons or have a youngster drink from the bottle. Household spoons vary a great deal in how much they hold, and spillage is a problem.

Giving Medicine to Children: Helpful Hints

As you might imagine (or know from experience!), giving medicine to a child can be a great challenge, especially if the drug is a foul-tasting liquid. Prepare yourself ahead of time by having everything available and by being ready to be firm if you must.

INFANTS AND YOUNG CHILDREN

Medicines for infants and young children should almost always be in liquid form. It is very unsafe to put a tablet (even a small one) in the child's mouth and let it melt, and crushing tablets can be a problem if the powder is especially bitter or foul. There are several "tricks of the trade" for giving medicines to unwilling children:

- Hold the baby or toddler securely. Be gentle but firm, and make sure she cannot jerk away or hit your hand. It is better to be firm the first time than to have to repeat doses or have a battle. You will have less of a problem if the little one knows you mean business.

- Use a proper, convenient measuring device, as discussed previously. Pour or squirt the medicine into the side of the little one's mouth or under his tongue, a little bit at a time. Wait until he swallows, then put in a little bit more. Or if you wish, you can pour the previously measured liquid into a rubber nipple and allow an infant to suck on the nipple.

- If the medicine tastes awful, give a *small* amount of water or diluted juice right afterward unless you have been instructed otherwise by the doctor.

- If the baby or child spits out the medicine or vomits immediately after taking it, you can safely repeat the dose, but only once. If you have a constant problem with your youngster, check with the doctor about whether or not you should keep giving it or can repeat the dosage.

- Do not mix medicine with food or drink unless you ask whether this is safe. While there are a few drugs that are actually given in this way, many are inactive if mixed or do not absorb into the youngster's system well unless they are given on

657

WHAT ABOUT
ALL THOSE
OVER-THE-
COUNTER AND
PRESCRIBED
MEDICATIONS?

an empty stomach. Besides, you may not be able to cajole the youngster into finishing all the beverage or food!

OLDER CHILDREN AND TEENAGERS

Older children usually would prefer to take tablets, chewable medications, or capsules whenever possible. Liquids tend to taste bad to them, and they usually need to take large amounts of liquids in order to get the correct dose for their weight. Fortunately, more and more medications are available in forms that are easy for young children to take. However, it is both possible and a good idea to teach youngsters how to swallow pills:

- Have the child stand up or sit up straight.

- Have her put the tablet as far back on her tongue as she can reach, then take a drink of water and swallow "as if you're swallowing just the water."

- You can also put the tablet on a spoonful of applesauce, jelly, or gelatin and have her swallow it that way.

- If medicine comes in a large capsule, pour out the contents of the capsule into applesauce, jelly, or gelatin and have the child swallow it that way.

- Certain tablets and capsules have medicine in timed-release form. That is, not all of the medicine is supposed to be absorbed into the body at the same time. With these drugs, it is important that your child *not chew* the tablet or the little beads from inside the capsule.

Encourage your older children and teenagers to assume responsibility for taking their own medicines. However, be sure to supervise them so they take the medicine properly and on time and thereby get the treatment they need, especially for infections or chronic illnesses. It's often difficult not to cross the fine line between gentle encouragement and nagging!

- Be sure the youngster understands why it's important to take the medication, especially if she feels it isn't necessary. If you are having problems, be sure to ask the doctor to help with the explanation and encouragement.

- Be sensitive to the young person's need to be "just like the other kids," especially if he has a chronic illness and must take medications frequently or every day. Work with him to make the task of taking the medicine as "painless" as possible.

- Try setting up a chart or schedule in the teenager's bedroom or bathroom. As you know, it is hard for anyone to remember to take medicine, especially if there are few if any symptoms of feeling sick.

- Try to convey the message that you trust the young person to be independent, and avoid saying (or implying) ''I told you so'' if the youngster becomes more ill because of not taking the prescribed medicine. Usually, she is fully aware of the consequences but is ''hoping'' it won't happen this time.

Common Misunderstandings About Medications

Through the years, quite a few misunderstandings have developed about medications, both prescription and over-the-counter drugs. Because of these misunderstandings, many children (and adults) suffer needlessly or are given drugs they should never receive. Some of these misunderstandings are as follows:

- ''If a little bit is good, a little more is better.'' This is definitely not true when it comes to drugs. Always use the correct dosage, especially when infants and children are involved.

- ''If a youngster has a 'little' something, then a 'little' medicine should be enough.'' If a drug is needed at all, especially to relieve an uncomfortable symptom, then use the full, correct dose. One of the most common causes for a fever's not coming down is using too little acetaminophen. (Of course, using too much is dangerous— check to be sure you are giving the right amount based on a youngster's size.)

- ''One antibiotic is as good as another.'' Not so. Each antibiotic is effective against only some of the many bacteria that cause infection, and many bacteria develop ''resistance'' to antibiotics that are frequently used.

- ''A little antibiotic can 'nip a cold in the bud.' '' Colds are caused by viruses, and viral infections are not cured by antibiotics. In addition, it has been proved that antibiotics given for a cold do not usually prevent the bacterial infections that can complicate colds. Rather, the infections that develop often require more powerful antibiotics than might be needed otherwise.

- ''The 'all-in-one' or 'all-purpose' medicines (for colds, for example) are better than single-ingredient drugs.'' Wrong. In fact, the more ingredients a drug has, the more suspicious you should be that it will *not* be effective. In addition, you are multiplying the chance of unwanted side effects.

THE DON'TS

Don't hesitate to ask your doctor about the risks versus the benefits of any medication prescribed for your child. You should also be aware of the expected side effects (if any) and the possible adverse reactions, as well as what to do if they occur.

659

WHAT ABOUT
ALL THOSE
OVER-THE-
COUNTER AND
PRESCRIBED
MEDICATIONS?

Don't forget to ask yourself "Does my child really need this over-the-counter medication?" before giving it to the youngster. Remember, medications have their place and their purpose but are not the answer for every ache, pain, or minor discomfort.

Don't forget to give any medication exactly the way it is prescribed by the doctor or according to the directions on the bottle (for over-the-counter medications). Be sure to measure all liquid medicines carefully, using a marked measuring device. Always write down the time the medication was given. If you are to give the youngster the medicine until it is totally gone, be sure to do so, even if he or she gets better in a few days.

Don't forget that giving too much medicine may cause a very serious problem, and giving too little may not help the child. It is important to follow the instructions carefully and to remember that, to be effective, medications must be given precisely as instructed.

Don't ever give a youngster a medication prescribed for another youngster (or adult). Even if you feel it is the right type of medication, you really can't be sure it is, and you don't know whether the amount is correct or whether the medicine would be the one the doctor would prescribe or recommend.

Don't forget to teach your children that not all illness—or discomfort—can or should be "cured" by taking a medicine. If children learn this early, we might then raise a generation of people who would be more tolerant of not feeling perfect all the time and who would be less likely to overuse or abuse over-the-counter, prescription, or street drugs.

PLEASE NOTE: Now that you have a better understanding of over-the-counter and prescribed medications, it would be extremely helpful for you to go back to the Quick Reference With the Steps in Detail and review it carefully. The more familiar you are with that material, the more useful it will be to you when you need it.

(*The Children's Pharmacy* by Ann Carey, R.N. [Warner Books, 1985] is an excellent resource that details the risks, benefits, and doses of more than two hundred prescribed and over-the-counter medications used for children. We, as well as the author of *The Children's Pharmacy*, recommend that your child's doctor be consulted when it comes to giving a child any medication, but the book provides excellent information and is an invaluable resource.)

C H A P T E R 20

Preventing or Controlling the Spread of Infection

QUICK REFERENCE

With the Steps in Detail

Preventing or Controlling the Spread of Infection

Preventing or Controlling the Spread of Infection Overall

▶ **COLDS, FLU, AND OTHER CONTAGIOUS DISEASES ARE OFTEN SPREAD BY SALIVA (DROPLET SPREAD). THEREFORE, CHILDREN SHOULD BE TAUGHT TO COVER THEIR MOUTHS WHEN THEY COUGH OR SNEEZE AND AVOID CONTACT WITH ANYTHING THAT COULD BE WET WITH SALIVA OF ANOTHER CHILD (OR ADULT).**

- Teach children not to drink from another person's glass or cup, and don't let babies share bottles.

- Teach children to use their own tableware/silverware and not to share with others.

- Teach youngsters (when old enough) to wash their hands after using the bathroom, before eating, and after playing with or holding a baby or toddler.

- Older children should be told not to kiss younger children on the mouth.

- Remember to wash toys, stuffed animals, washable books, and other items a baby, toddler, or small child drools or chews on. Anything wet with saliva is a breeding place for microorganisms.

▶ **TEACH YOUR CHILDREN TO AVOID CONTACT WITH OPEN SORES, WOUNDS, RASHES, AND PARASITES ON THE SKIN OF OTHER CHILDREN.** This helps prevent skin infections.

- Teach your child never to share hats, scarves, combs, and brushes with other children.

▶ **CAREFUL HAND-WASHING AFTER USING THE TOILET, CHANGING DIAPERS, CHANGING CLOTHING, AND BEFORE HANDLING FOOD HELPS PREVENT INFECTIONS SPREAD BY CONTACT WITH STOOL (FECES, BOWEL MOVEMENT) AND SALIVA.**

- Children should be taught good hygiene as early as possible.

- Remember that babies can get feces on their hands, legs, feet, face—in fact, everywhere—by reaching into their diapers. They can spread infection to another child (or adult) who comes into contact with the bowel movement.

▶ **EAT IN RESPECTABLE EATING ESTABLISHMENTS AND BE CON-SCIENTIOUS ABOUT HANDLING FOOD AT HOME IF YOU OR A MEM-BER OF THE FAMILY HAS AN INFECTION.**

- Food can become contaminated by sick food handlers or those who are carriers of disease, so it's important to go to restaurants where conditions are excellent.

- Water can be contaminated by sewage. Boil or chemically treat any water you suspect has been contaminated before you use it for drinking, cooking, or washing.

- Follow health regulations if you have your own sewer system or are doing your own plumbing work.

- Diseases can also arise from improper preparation of food, food left out of the refrigerator too long, or certain foods contaminated by the environment.

▶ **BE SURE TO DISPOSE OF ALL ANIMAL WASTE PROMPTLY AND SAFELY, AND BE SURE TO PROVIDE ANIMALS WITH GOOD HEALTH CARE.**

- All pets should receive proper immunizations and have booster immunizations on schedule.

- Take your pet to a veterinarian if you see any signs of illness. Pets should also have periodic evaluations to check their overall health and to detect intestinal and skin parasites.

- Purchase pets only from reputable sources.

▶ **IF YOU ARE GOING ON A VACATION OR WILL BE VISITING AN UNFAMILIAR AREA, INVESTIGATE THE AREA AHEAD OF TIME. FIND OUT WHETHER THERE ARE CERTAIN INSECTS OR ANIMALS THAT ARE KNOWN TO SPREAD DISEASE OR WHETHER THE AREA HAS ENVIRONMENTAL HAZARDS OR RISKS (CONTAMINATED LAKES OR RIVERS, POOR SEWAGE, AND SO ON).**

- Take precautions when camping or during other recreational activities.

- Use effective insect repellents.

- Be alert for signs of a problem.

- Teach your children to stay away from wild animals.

- Follow health department recommendations about immunizations and other precautions if you will be traveling to areas of the world where infectious diseases present a risk to travelers.

- Also take care to control insects in your own area, property, and/or home.

▶ **TEACH YOUR CHILDREN GOOD HEALTH HABITS IN ORDER TO KEEP THEIR RESISTANCE AT ITS PEAK, THEREBY PERHAPS HELPING THEM AVOID SOME CONTAGIOUS DISEASES OR REDUCING THEIR SEVERITY. THESE GOOD HEALTH HABITS INCLUDE THE FOLLOWING:**

- Excellent nutrition.

- Adequate sleep and rest.

- Adequate exercise.

- Stress-management skills.

▶ **IF YOUR CHILD REQUIRES GROUP CARE (DAY-CARE CENTER, NURSERY SCHOOL, PRESCHOOL, AND SO ON), BE SURE TO VISIT THE FACILITY AND SEE HOW CARE IS PROVIDED.**

- Check policies, procedures, and philosophy of care.

- Review health policies and procedures.

When You Know a Child Has an Infection

▶ **DO NOT SEND YOUR CHILD TO SCHOOL OR DAY CARE OR ALLOW HIM TO PLAY WITH OTHER CHILDREN IF YOU SUSPECT OR KNOW HE HAS AN INFECTIOUS DISEASE.**

- Keep him away from others for at least twenty-four hours after the signs of the infection are gone or for twelve to twenty-four hours after starting medication to treat the infection.

▶ **TAKE REASONABLE CARE NOT TO SPREAD INFECTION WITHIN YOUR HOME IF YOUR CHILD IS SICK.**

- If possible, separate the sick child from your other children, especially for sleeping.

- Have the youngster use separate towels, washcloths, pillowcases, blankets, clothing, and tableware/silverware, and wash these carefully and frequently.

- Remember that toys and cloth items that an infant or toddler chews on or drools on should be washed or laundered frequently during the illness.

- Emphasize hand-washing for all family members, especially after caring for the sick child, but also after using the toilet, before eating, and before and after playing with young infants and toddlers.

- Reemphasize that youngsters not kiss each other on the mouth, especially when one or more of them are ill.

Infections: What You Should Know

Have you ever been told that you will get a cold or the flu if you get your feet wet or go out into the night air with damp hair or simply stand in a draft? Have you ever heard someone say that he had to get out of these wet clothes before pneumonia set in? Ever hear a mother say her daughter or son got an ear infection because the youngster forgot to wear a hat? The list of old wives' tales is endless. And unfortunately, most are still accepted as fact—not recognized as fiction!

"But," you say, "I remember the time I got wet in the rain and did get a cold." You may also remember a friend's getting pneumonia after being in the snow—without being dressed properly. Or the time your child didn't wear a hat and ended up with an ear infection. Here, you see, is where the problem lies.

Because these associations can be made, most people feel they are proof positive of "cause and effect." The fact is, until medical science learned more about what really causes infectious or contagious diseases (any disease that can be transmitted to a person) and how these diseases are spread, such incorrect associations of cause and effect were actually quite reasonable to make.

In order to dispel these myths, we first need to understand what causes infection and how it is spread. Here are a few basic premises to remember (which we will explain in more detail):

- Infections are caused by microorganisms (bacteria, viruses, fungi, or parasites).

- If one of these various microorganisms invades the body and isn't destroyed by the body's defense system—the person will get an infection.

- The same microorganism can cause more or less severe or serious symptoms and illnesses in different people.

- Infections are spread by transmission of the organism from one person to another or from an animal or insect (dog, cat, flea, mosquito, and so forth) to a person.

- Poor nutrition, poor sleep habits, lack of adequate exercise, and stress may make us more susceptible to infection, once exposed.

The fact is, all infectious diseases are caused by microorganisms—tiny "germs" such as viruses, bacteria, parasites, or fungi. Most of the time, the culprit is a virus or bacteria. The problem is, there are countless numbers of these microorganisms that can potentially cause infection in humans. That is why a youngster (or adult) can get many colds or flus—each caused by a *different* microorganism.

These germs can enter the human body through a tiny cut or scratch in the skin or through the nose and respiratory tract or the mouth and digestive tract. Once in the body, the microorganisms either establish themselves in the tissues and multiply rapidly, causing mild to severe illness, or the body's immune system (defense system) attacks the microorganisms before they can become established and destroys them.

If not destroyed, the microorganisms may: cause a mild infection (for example, at the site of the cut or scratch); be limited to a small area of the body or a single organ and/or organ system; or involve many or all of the body systems (to a greater or lesser degree).

If limited to only one area of the body, one organ and/or organ system, then the infection is called a localized infection. An infection that involves several or all areas and organ systems is called a generalized, or systemic, infection. Sepsis, or septicemia (commonly known as "blood poisoning"), is one of the most potentially devastating forms of infection. In this type of infection, the microorganism invades the bloodstream and is then carried to all parts of the body, multiplying rapidly and causing localized infection in any of the organs as well as a generalized blood infection.

This rapidly spreading infection can attack one organ system after another, resulting in severe destruction. If not recognized and aggressively treated (in a hospital), permanent damage to one or several organ systems—or even death—may result. Prompt evaluation and treatment of any infection—even the mildest, localized infection—is always vital because of the looming threat of this massive systemic infection.

Often, people are confused when they learn that there is an epidemic of a particular virus but then hear that one child has cold symptoms (fever, cough, and congestion), another child has pneumonia, another child has croup (infection of the area around the vocal cords), and yet another gets meningitis (infection of the coverings of the brain and spinal cord). How could this be?

The fact is, the same bacteria or virus can cause more severe and serious symptoms and illnesses in some children than in others. No one knows why this happens, but it appears to depend on each individual child's susceptibility at the time the microorganism invades the body and the extent of the contact, as well as his genetic strengths and weaknesses. There is nothing you can do to change this unfortunate natural phenomenon and ensure that your child would only get a cold if he was infected by the microorganism.

Therefore, infections have little to do with wet feet or cold drafts. They are caused by microorganisms and spread from one person (or animal or insect) to another person by some form of contact. If a child (or adult) is exposed to the microorganism, he or she is then at risk for a mild to severe illness (depending on the microorganism involved and the illnesses it can cause).

Let's put this into more concrete terms. When someone with a cold or flu coughs or sneezes (and doesn't cover his or her mouth and nose), the spray travels four to six feet—spreading droplets containing the microorganisms that caused the cold or flu. Obviously, anyone within that four- to six-foot path will be exposed. This is called "airborne" exposure and occurs when we inhale the microorganisms through our mouth or nose into the respiratory or digestive tract—even though we cannot see or feel them. Also, the droplets can invade our bodies through another opening (a cut, scrape, or scratch). In other words, there doesn't have to be "direct" contact with the person when it comes to some diseases.

Disease microorganisms that live in the respiratory tract (lungs, throat, nose, eyes, and mouth) are spread by coughing and sneezing, as well as by contact with saliva—for example, by drinking from someone's glass or cup or by using the same silverware, towel, washcloth, toothbrush, pillow, or sheets or by kissing. Be sure your child is properly immunized against the diseases that can be prevented, and use common sense in avoiding unnecessary exposure to children or adults who are sick. Common diseases spread through the respiratory tract (called "by droplet spread") include the following, to name a few:

- Many forms of so-called flu and viral infections
- Colds
- Measles
- Rubella (German measles)
- Strep infections
- Croup
- Infectious mononucleosis
- Some forms of meningitis
- Some types of pneumonia
- Chickenpox (also spread by skin contact)
- Pertussis (whooping cough)
- Diphtheria
- Polio (also spread by stool contact)

Other diseases are spread by skin contact—with an open lesion, sore, or parasite. Some of these diseases can also be spread by contact with clothing, towels, washcloths, and sheets. When one of these diseases is suspected, great care should be taken in handling contaminated clothing and the like. With young children, pay attention to toys, as well, particularly those that get or stay wet. Diseases that can be spread by contact with infected skin include the following:

- Chickenpox (this virus is spread by droplets, as well)
- Impetigo
- Scabies
- Herpes (cold sores)
- Head lice (which are spread by contact with infested hair, hats, and so on)

Still others are spread by contact with the stool (feces, bowel movement) of someone who has the disease or is a carrier of the disease. Careful hand-washing after using the toilet, changing diapers, changing clothing, and before handling food can help prevent these infections. Some infections spread by contact with stool include the following:

- Polio (which is spread by respiratory contact, as well)

- Pinworm

- Many intestinal parasites

- Most intestinal flus

- The common form of hepatitis

Some other diseases are transmitted by contaminated food or water. For example, food can be contaminated by sick food handlers or those who are ''carriers'' of the disease. Health departments screen food handlers for some of these diseases, and public eating places usually take great care to monitor their workers for these diseases. You can lower your risk of getting these diseases if you are careful to eat only in respectable eating establishments and be conscientious about handling food if you or your family members have one of these diseases. In addition, some of these diseases are spread by water that has been contaminated by sewage. Make sure to boil or chemically treat any water you suspect has been contaminated, and follow health regulations if you have your own sewer system or are doing your own work on plumbing. Still other diseases result from eating improperly prepared food, food left out of the refrigerator too long, or certain foods contaminated in the environment. Some infections that can be spread by contaminated food or water include the following:

- Strep infections (but these are more commonly spread by respiratory contact).

- Some diarrheas (especially bacterial diarrhea).

- Hepatitis (spread by food handlers, as well as contracted by eating seafood from contaminated waters).

- Tuberculosis.

- Intestinal parasites such as Giardia (spread by contaminated water), amoeba (water), and many others.

- Bacterial food poisoning (Salmonella infection).

- Toxic food poisoning (contracted by eating foods that have been improperly refrigerated or stored).

A few diseases are spread from animals, especially family pets, to children and/or their families. You can lower your child's risk of getting these infections if you dispose of animal waste promptly and safely, inspect your pets carefully for signs of any problems, get veterinary care for sick animals, keep animal immunizations up to date, and purchase pets from reputable sources. Some diseases that can be transmitted from pets or animals include the following:

- Scabies (from dogs with true mange).

- Toxoplasmosis (from cats).

- Salmonella, a form of gastroenteritis (from some pet turtles).

- Cat-scratch fever.

- Some forms of ringworm (from dogs).

- Repeated strep infections in some families (from the family dog).

- Rabies (from some wild animals and from domestic animals who are not properly immunized and have been infected).

- Psittacosis (a respiratory infection of birds).

Still other diseases are spread by certain insects or in certain contaminated environments. You can reduce your child's risk for getting some of these infections by: investigating the area you are going to ahead of time and taking precautions when camping or during other recreational activities; using effective insect repellents; avoiding known contaminated or risky areas; being alert to the signs of a problem; and taking care to control insects in your own area or on your own property. In addition, follow health department recommendations about immunizations and other precautions if you travel to areas of the world where certain diseases are prevalent. Some diseases that are carried by insects or result from contact with microorganisms in a contaminated environment include the following:

- Rocky Mountain spotted fever (ticks).

- Tick paralysis (ticks).

- Many forms of encephalitis (mosquitoes).

- Lyme disease (mosquitoes).

- Histoplasmosis (a fungus infection spread by contact with bird droppings).

- Coccidioidomycosis (so-called valley fever, a fungus infection prevalent in western desert areas).

- Tetanus (lockjaw, from contaminated soil or other objects in the environment).

- Malaria (mosquitoes).

- Many more unusual infections (fleas, mosquitoes, ticks).

While not all of the previously listed diseases have been discussed in this book, the lists serve to point out how easily diseases can be spread among people and from other sources in the environment.

Now that you know how some contagious diseases are transmitted, let's go back and take another look at the time you got wet in the rain and ended up with a cold, the friend who got pneumonia after being out in the snow without being dressed properly, and your child who didn't wear a hat and got an ear infection.

For one thing, all of these were coincidences, but they do have a few noteworthy factors in common. In the winter, in particular, or at other times of the year when there are days when it's cold, rainy, or snowing, people spend much more time inside (in enclosed areas). This allows for much closer contact with others who have colds or the flu or other infections. Infections are easily spread by those visiting your home or by you visiting theirs; by people at the shopping center, market, restaurant, school, ice hockey game, or basketball practice; or even by people traveling in a car or bus. Remember, one sneeze or cough could be the culprit.

Therefore, you may have gotten wet in the rain, but the cold you ended up with was the result of contact with someone who had a cold. The same is true of your friend who wasn't dressed properly for the snow and got pneumonia. The cold and snow had little to do with the pneumonia—but coming into contact with someone with the microorganism did. And your child with the ear infection probably got the microorganism from a little friend, so wearing the hat would have made no difference.

There are some things that can make a difference in some situations. In the last few years, it has become more and more evident that poor nutritional habits, poor sleep habits, lack of exercise, or too much stress make us more susceptible to disease. If a youngster has one of these problems, such as poor sleep habits (doesn't get adequate rest), that alone may make him more at risk for contracting an illness if he is exposed to it. His susceptibility increases with the number of problems he has.

For example, if he has poor sleep habits, poor nutritional habits, and is under stress, then his chances of contracting an illness he is exposed to are even greater. All of these are a matter of "lowered resistance." If a youngster is not getting enough rest, is not eating proper and adequate amounts of food, and is experiencing stress, then his defense system (immune system) just isn't at its peak and would be less able to fight off an invading microorganism.

Therefore, ensuring that your youngster gets proper rest, food, and exercise and has the means to lessen stress will at least keep up her resistance to infection. That doesn't mean she can avoid getting sick altogether, but it does mean her body and its defense system are as healthy as *you and she* can make them.

Natural Immunity: When It Begins and Ends

By and large, babies are born with "natural" immunity to most of the diseases their mothers had in their lifetimes. This special immunity usually lasts until between four and six months after birth, then begins to decrease, making them more and more susceptible to illnesses (even those their mothers had). This, however, is not a generalized immunity, as most people think. If the mother did not have that particular cold virus that's going around again, or that specific type of flu, then she cannot give the unborn baby immunity to those or any other diseases she has not had before.

Breast feeding does tend to give the baby a little more resistance for a longer period of time. Essentially, in nursing, the baby gets smaller "doses" of the same antibodies he received in the womb. Therefore, natural immunity (developed in the womb) combined with breast feeding can result in some resistance to diseases to which the mother has antibodies—until the baby is well into his second year of life. As noted, however, a baby will not be immune to the diseases his mother did *not* have at some time during her life. Because of this natural immunity, "immunizations" (for example, measles, mumps, and rubella [MMR] vaccine) are not given until the baby is fifteen months old—because this temporary natural immunity prevents the baby from developing his own antibodies to the diseases.

When to Expect Illness: To Everything There Is a Season!

Each of the viruses and bacteria, in particular, have a peak season of the year when they are more likely to appear in children. This does not mean diseases caused by them cannot appear at other seasons of the year, but it does mean that outbreaks of certain diseases can be more or less predicted.

For example, croup, bronchiolitis, and other respiratory illnesses are most common in the winter months and are even more common in cold climates, where people are indoors a great deal. Strep and other throat infections also occur most often during cooler months. On the other hand, skin infections like impetigo can be seen throughout the year but are especially common during the summer months.

Diarrheal illnesses are seen both in winter and in summer, but certain viruses called enteroviruses cause outbreaks of illness during the late summer and early fall months. Chickenpox appears in spring and early summer, while measles (which can be prevented through immunization) is a winter and spring disease. Meningitis caused by bacteria is most common during cooler months of the year, but viral meningitis is most common during warm months.

As you can see, certain times of the year bring certain diseases. Few people think of diseases as seasonal, but in fact, many are. Once a pediatrician or family practice physician sees a child or youngster with a certain contagious disease, the doctor can easily predict that he or she will be seeing many more young people with the same disease. Older children and teenagers are susceptible to the diseases they haven't had before and to those germs against which they haven't been immunized. For example, measles and rubella (German measles) are appearing in older children and teenagers who have "slipped through the system" and were not immunized during early childhood against these serious and potentially damaging diseases.

Getting Sick: Children Are Generous About Sharing Their Diseases

Most often, the first time a baby or child is exposed to other children (especially in a group setting), he or she is going to be more at risk for "catching" colds, flu, and other illnesses. It is at this time that parents become concerned because their baby or small child seems to get sick over and over again! Some children will have colds as often as once a month until they develop immunity to the viruses making their rounds.

Therefore, if a child is not exposed to other children—such as a group of friends or those in a day-care center, preschool, or group-care setting (defined as the care of children from two or more families)—until she is two years old, then the child will begin getting illnesses at that point. If the child is five years old before she is exposed to groups of other children, she will seem to get "everything" that comes along when she starts school.

Babies and small children who stay at home can get illnesses from older brothers and sisters who are exposed to these illnesses at preschool or elementary school. Adults are less likely to spread an illness to a baby or small child and even more likely to get one from the baby or small child. Children, in fact, are the most common sources of spreading contagious diseases. They are very generous about sharing their illnesses! Babies have contact with bottles and pacifiers, suck on their fingers, slobber on everything around them (including people), and put their hands into their diapers. All they need to do is transfer a virus, bacteria, or other microorganism through contact. Coming into contact with something that is wet from saliva is an excellent way to "catch" a respiratory disease.

Small children often cannot or do not cover their mouths when sneezing or coughing and can also spread "germs" through contact with their clothing, towels, blankets, and toys. Of course, kissing and hugging are also primary ways to spread illness and are almost impossible to avoid when you're talking about caring for a sick baby or small child who needs affection and the feeling of security when he or she is sick.

The point is, if your child experiences many illnesses at the time he or she is first exposed to a group or groups of other children—then this is usually normal. If, however, a child continues to get one illness after another for more than two years, then it's best to have the child evaluated by the doctor. It would be important to tell the doctor that the child seems to always be sick and appears to have a very low resistance to illness. The doctor can then examine the child and determine whether this is normal or not.

Special Considerations: Preschools, Day-Care Centers, and Other Group-Care Settings

Besides the bouts of the common cold, sore throats, the "flu," and other more minor illnesses, the diseases that tend to make their rounds in day-care centers, preschools, and other group-care settings (such as group baby-sitting and church nurseries) are quite predictable. Diarrhea—caused by standard viruses and bacteria, as well as by a parasite called Giardia—and a potentially more serious problem, hepatitis (viral infection of the liver), can be special problems in centers or group settings where young children are diapered.

The usual diarrheal diseases will more than likely take care of themselves with proper home care and attention to ensuring that the child does not become dehydrated (see Chapter 14 for more information about treating diarrhea). Giardia, on the other hand, requires that the child be given a special medication that destroys this parasite, which can cause persistent diarrhea, abdominal pain, and other symptoms. Any child with severe or persistent diarrhea should be under the care of a doctor, who can ensure that certain treatable bacteria or parasites are detected and treated.

Hepatitis (liver inflammation caused by viral infection) is particularly worth mentioning because it acts differently in small children than in adults. In small children, hepatitis is most often a mild disease that looks like stomach flu—with loss of appetite and vomiting. Very few children become seriously jaundiced (have yellow skin and eyes). They do, however, spread the virus to older children, teenagers, and adults—who get the infection by contact with the bowel movements, and sometimes urine or saliva, of infected children. Older youngsters and adults are likely to have a more serious infection and be jaundiced. In fact, caretakers or staff members at child-care centers who develop hepatitis are frequently the only clue that the outbreak of "stomach flu" in the center was actually hepatitis.

Outbreaks of hepatitis in group-care settings, while unusual, are generally seen when the children in the group are not toilet-trained and are diapered by their caretakers. Day-care workers, doctors, and health departments are alert to this problem and will want to investigate the cause of "stomach flu" outbreaks. If the cause is hepatitis, children and adults who have been exposed should be given an injection of gamma globulin, which can prevent the disease. Hepatitis outbreaks are a special problem in residential schools and hospitals for retarded and handicapped children, as well.

Another potentially serious bacterial infection risk seems to be emerging from day-care, preschool, and group-care settings. Called Hemophilus influenzae, this bacteria can cause serious infections such as meningitis (infection of the coverings of the brain), epiglottitis (infection of the epiglottis, which covers the windpipe), and cellulitis (inflammation of the tissues under the skin, usually around the eye or face). Until recently, it was believed that this bacteria and the disease it causes did not spread from one child to another in epidemic proportions. However, it has become apparent that young children in families or in group-care settings *are* at risk if another young child has an infection caused by the Hemophilus bacteria. Therefore, recommendations have been developed to treat exposed young children (those under six years old) with a medication (rifampin) to prevent this infection.

Usually, in the case of infants and young children with Hemophilus infections, all family members are treated with rifampin if there are other children in the household who are under six years old. In addition, young children in day-care, preschool, or group-care settings are also treated if one or more children in that group have this type of infection.

If you are informed that a child in your child's group has a Hemophilus infection, contact your doctor immediately for advice and proper treatment. (The treatment is most effective if started as close to the time of exposure as possible.) You should be aware that there is some controversy about preventive medication for this bacteria and that recommendations are changing frequently. Your doctor or local health department should be able to answer your questions about the current recommendations. (For further information about Hemophilus infections, see Chapter 3.)

Pinworm, lice, scabies, and impetigo also tend to make their rounds at preschools, day-care centers, and other group-care settings. It's important to remember that these diseases are not necessarily the result of a child's having poor personal hygiene. The cleanest, best-cared-for child can get pinworm, head lice, scabies, or impetigo if he or she happens to make contact with a youngster who has one of these problems. All of these problems spread rapidly if one child brings them to day care, group care, or preschool. Contact your doctor if your child brings home one of these unwanted visitors. He or she will recommend or prescribe effective treatment, which often must be given to your entire family.

Preventing Illness at Day-Care Centers, Preschools, and Other Group Settings

Often, parents ask if there is anything they can do to lessen the risk for their children's getting "everything that comes along" in a preschool, day-care center, or group-care setting. (We will discuss preventing or controlling the spread of infectious diseases overall later in this chapter.)

As you know, it is important to choose your child's preschool, day-care center, or group-care setting carefully, for a variety of reasons. Remember, this setting serves as an extension of your family and may care for your child for a great proportion of his or her week. You will want to know about the training and philosophy of the director and the staff, the overall program, whether there is a sense of structure or lack of it, and in general, whether your child and you will feel comfortable there. Be sure parents are welcome to visit unannounced—and then visit the school one or more times to see what really happens there.

One aspect of your decision about the appropriate place for your child's group care should involve health-care practices and ensuring the most healthful environment possible. Consider the following:

- Check to see if the facility is licensed, either locally or by your state. Check with the local or state licensing agency to see what requirements a facility must meet to be licensed.

- Find out what the health policies of the facility are. Be sure you are convinced that these policies are enforced by the director and staff. For example, there should be a general policy not to allow a child to be admitted if he has a contagious disease. There should also be a general policy that a child must be picked up if he becomes sick while at the facility.

- Try to choose a facility that meets all your requirements and cares for the smallest number of children possible (based on your budget constraints). Studies show that the more children there are from different families, the more illnesses children will experience, especially in their first few months in group care. Therefore, the fewer children there are from different families, the fewer illnesses you can expect in your child.

- If your child is toilet-trained, try to send him or her to a center or group where *all* the children are toilet-trained.

- If your child is still in diapers and must be cared for outside of your home, be sure to observe how the babies or children are diapered. Make sure great care is taken by the staff to wash their hands *before and after* diapering each baby or toddler, *before* tending to the needs of other children, and *before* handling food, bottles, and tableware. Check to see that caretakers help the children in washing their hands and faces frequently, as well, since the little ones have a tendency to get their hands into their diapers, then into their mouths; onto other children's hands, faces, and mouths; and onto toys, blankets, and so forth that other children play with or use.

- You will want to make sure that diapers are changed frequently and disposed of properly, to control or prevent the spread of potentially contagious diseases. Make sure you continue to provide an ample supply of disposable diapers to the staff, so that your baby or toddler can be changed frequently. You will need to know if you must bring a bag and dispose of used diapers or if the center staff disposes of them.

- For older children, is it the staff's policy to ensure that they are taken to or allowed to go to the toilet frequently, and encouraged and helped with hand-washing? Are there plenty of boxes of tissue available for nose-wiping?

- Check to see what kinds of toys are available for the children. Toys that are plastic and washable are better, as are those with few cracks and crevices to collect dirt and debris. Toys that stay wet and soggy may allow microorganisms (germs) to grow. Remember, when there are younger children, there is more mouth-to-toy contact, sharing of toys, and general "slobber" that goes onto everything and everyone, since the little ones touch everything and put everything into their mouths.

- If your child has a favorite blanket or soft toy (such as a stuffed animal) and is allowed to have it with him, be sure to launder it frequently.

- See if each baby or child has her own crib or sleeping/resting area.

- Check to see what kind of pets are kept at the facility. Are the pets well cared for, and are the children taught to respect them (and not abuse them)? Are the pets healthy, and are all shots up to date (when applicable)? How does the staff ensure the continued health of the animals? Are the babies, toddlers, and older children prevented from coming into contact with the urine and feces of the animals? Younger children, in particular, are curious and have no sense of clean and dirty. They pick up everything, eat anything, and get their hands into whatever is in their path. Be sure that animals that tend to bite are kept inside safe pens or cages and are handled only by adults.

It used to be that most children first caught everything that "made the rounds" when they were in kindergarten or when they had a brother or sister who started school. Kindergarten was the first large-group experience for children and became the breeding ground for sharing illnesses. Since the establishment and greater use of preschools, day-care centers, and other group-care arrangements, more children are exposed to large groups of other children at younger ages and are thereby exposed to more contagious diseases at an earlier age.

In addition to earlier exposure, other factors contribute to a higher incidence of infectious diseases when a young infant or child is exposed to groups at an early age. Small children must be diapered or helped with toileting, their noses must be wiped, they must be helped or reminded to wash their hands, and they must be fed or assisted with eating. They also share toys, have close physical contact when they play, and easily drool all over themselves and each other. At five or six years of age, children are more independent about nose-wiping, hand-washing, toilet use, and feeding themselves. In other words, there is less sharing and physical contact with other children, as well as with caretakers and teachers, who must also care for the needs of many other children.

You will notice that staff members at preschools, day-care centers, and other group-care settings tend to get sick more often than grade school teachers. That's because the risk for their contracting an infectious disease from the children they care for is quite high. In fact, you as a parent might find yourself in the same situation—you get everything your child brings home—because adults most often catch things from children and not the other way around! These teachers or caretakers generally experience more colds, more "flu" illnesses, and more of whatever the children are spreading. As with the children, they tend to be sick more often during their first few months or years in child care, then most of them develop immunity to more and more illnesses. However, a few aren't so fortunate and continue to get sick every time an illness is spread among the children.

Often, parents ask if it is detrimental for their children's overall health to be exposed to and catch contagious diseases at younger ages. Generally speaking, for healthy children, there is no serious risk, and these same children have fewer infectious diseases later. Basically, instead of getting things at five years of age, they get them at younger ages.

However, for some children, the risk of repeated infections is more of a problem in the younger years. For example, children who are prone to getting middle-ear infections with every cold can be expected to have repeated ear infections when they are faced with group care. A new ear infection may follow every cold—and that may happen as often as once a month. Since they do tend to "outgrow" the tendency to ear infections after the age of two or three, postponing group care for them can be a real health advantage. (For more information about middle-ear infection, see Chapter 14.) This same thing holds true for the infant or toddler who has asthma or a tendency to get pneumonia with colds.

The bottom line on preschool, day care, and group care is for you to assume that your child or children will experience more contagious diseases, at least for the first few months, because it is the first exposure to a large group of children. However, it is still vital that you evaluate the facility and its policies to make sure it is licensed and meets your requirements, as well. You should feel secure that all that can be done to prevent or control the spread of infectious diseases is being done.

Nonetheless, if you feel your child is sick too often or you are concerned about the situation, schedule an appointment with the child's pediatrician or family physician to make sure it's simply a matter of group exposure and not "low resistance," an immune-deficiency problem (a *rare* cause of repeated infections), or another chronic problem that would make the child unusually susceptible to contagious diseases.

While everyone would like to prevent contagious diseases at all ages, we must consider the practical needs of working parents and the need or desirability for some older preschoolers to have experience with groups of other children. In this context, you need to weigh the benefits and risks of group care for your child or children.

Preventing or Controlling the Spread of Infection: What You Can Do

Unfortunately, babies and children are often exposed to another child who is ill *before* the other child shows any signs or symptoms. Often, children (and adults) have been exposed and can spread the illness for twenty-four to forty-eight hours before they even begin to feel bad themselves. In this situation, there is really nothing you can do to prevent exposure, since you do not know the other youngster or adult is coming down with something.

Although there is little anyone can do when a child has no signs or symptoms of illness, there are some things that can be done when you *know* your child is sick. In fact, parents could really help each other out (and their children) if they did *not* send their sick children to school, parties, or out to play with other children.

Usually, a contagious illness can be spread for at least twenty-four hours before and twenty-four hours after the child shows signs and symptoms. If, however, the child has a fever or doesn't feel well after a twenty-four-hour period—she should continue to stay home until the fever is gone and she is feeling much better.

You'd be surprised how many children are sent to school, day-care centers, group activities, and out to play when they are sick *and* contagious. In some cases, the parent(s) work(s) and either cannot afford or has (have) not taken steps to find someone to care for the child or children when sick. It is important to make prior arrangements for your children so when they are sick or get sick while at school, there is someone to take care of them—if you cannot. Not allowing sick children to go to school or be around other children would markedly reduce the spread of infectious (contagious) disease to others.

Other steps you can take to prevent or control the spread of infectious diseases include the following:

- If possible, the sick child or youngster should be in a room separate from your other children or as far away from the others as possible—as long as he is contagious. (Assume the child is contagious for a twenty-four-hour period from the time he showed signs and symptoms; and assume the child is still contagious even after the twenty-four-hour period if he has a fever or still feels very bad.)

- Make sure the sick child or youngster uses separate towels, washcloths, clothing, sheets, pillowcases, blankets, tableware, and so forth.

- Be sure to wash all sheets, pillowcases, blankets, towels, washcloths, and clothing used by the sick child or youngster separately from those of other family members. These should be washed in hot water with soap.

- Teach older children to wash their hands after using the toilet, before eating, and after playing with or holding a baby or toddler who is sick (even if you aren't sure whether he or she is still contagious). The reason? These small ones slobber a great deal and, as you know, tend to get saliva all over themselves, as well as on everything and everyone around them. This is an easy way to spread a contagious disease. Likewise, avoid kissing sick children on the mouth and teach your older children to avoid this also. This prevents unnecessary exposure to saliva and respiratory secretions that might carry microorganisms.

- Since little children are often harder to "read" as to whether or not they are sick, don't send them to preschool, the day-care center, or group care if they show signs of pending illness. Each child is different, but since you know your child so well, it is often clear to you that he might be coming down with something, simply because of the way he is acting. If parents did this, it would surely lessen the exposure to other children when a child was most contagious (before showing overt signs and symptoms of an illness).

- Remember that anything that is wet is a breeding ground for microorganisms. Wet clothes, pillowcases, sheets, toys, washable books, and so on need to be laundered regularly and should not be shared with other children.

- Avoid unnecessary exposure of your children, especially young infants and toddlers, to groups of other children to reduce their risk of coming into contact with another sick child.

THE DON'TS

Don't forget that you can't prevent all exposure to contagious diseases. All children are eventually exposed to many contagious diseases and develop them during childhood.

Don't neglect to have your infant or child immunized against diseases that can be prevented by immunization. Be sure to have the immunizations given on the schedule recommended for good protection.

Don't ignore signs of infection in your child and allow him or her to expose other children unnecessarily. Use common sense about exposing your healthy child to other children who are sick.

Don't forget to weigh the risks and benefits of group care. Take all reasonable steps to choose a setting that will pose the least possible health risk to your child or children.

PLEASE NOTE: Now that you have a grasp of how to prevent or control the spread of infection, it would be extremely helpful for you to go back to the Quick Reference With the Steps in Detail and review it carefully. The more familiar you are with that material, the more useful it will be to you when you need it.

Understanding Common Tests and Procedures and Helping Your Child When Hospitalized

Just thinking about our children having to go through medical tests and procedures—even routine ones—isn't pleasant. We worry about how the youngster will handle the test or procedure and we worry about what the test or procedure might discover. These are legitimate concerns for any parent and, in fact, for anyone who knows and cares about children. Thinking about the possibility that our children may someday require hospitalization for an illness, injury or surgery is even more frightening.

When it comes to medical tests and procedures, as well as hospitalization, much has changed over the past forty years and even in the last five years. The good news is that these are two areas of medical care where *you can make an important, substantial, and lasting difference for your child!*

Over the years health care professionals have become keenly aware of the importance of meeting the emotional and educational needs, as well as physical needs, of children who require medical tests or procedures and/or hospitalization. Everyone has become more knowledgeable, more sensitive, and more aware.

Chapter 21 discusses some of the most common tests and procedures performed on children—as routine preventive medical care and when an illness or injury must be ruled out or identified. Emphasis is placed on what you and others can do to help your child if he or she ever requires a medical test or procedure.

Chapter 22 discusses the potential adverse effects that hospitalization can have on a child and what you and others can do to make hospitalization a more positive and less frightening experience.

Medical and hospital care have come a long way in the last several years. Along with advances in technology, new information about identifying and treating illness **679**

680

UNDERSTAND-
ING COMMON
TESTS AND
PROCEDURES
AND HELPING
YOUR CHILD
WHEN
HOSPITALIZED

and injury, and highly skilled health care professionals has come an awareness of treating the total child—not merely the illness or injury. There's no such thing as "the pneumonia" in room 307, "the hernia repair" in 208, or "the tantrum thrower" in 102. Children are no longer looked at as medical problems—but as human beings with special needs.

C H A P T E R 21

Some Common Tests
and Procedures

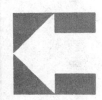

QUICK REFERENCE

With the Steps in Detail

Some Common Tests and Procedures

Be sure you get as much information as you can about any test(s) or procedure(s) the doctor recommends for your youngster.

▶ **ASK THE DOCTOR WHY HE OR SHE IS RECOMMENDING THE TEST OR PROCEDURE.**

- Is the test "routine" for a youngster this age?

- Does the doctor suspect some problem or illness? If so, what is he or she trying to pinpoint or rule out?

▶ **FIND OUT WHAT INFORMATION THE TEST OR PROCEDURE WILL PROVIDE AND HOW THE DOCTOR WILL USE THE RESULTS.**

681

682

UNDERSTAND-
ING COMMON
TESTS AND
PROCEDURES
AND HELPING
YOUR CHILD
WHEN
HOSPITALIZED

- Depending on the results of this test or procedure, will others be necessary?

- Will the doctor be able to determine treatment, if any, based on the results of this test or procedure?

▶ **ASK THE DOCTOR (OR HIS OR HER ASSISTANT) TO EXPLAIN HOW THE TEST OR PROCEDURE IS PERFORMED.**

- Will it be done in the office, or do you need to take the youngster to a laboratory, hospital, or other medical facility?

- How much discomfort will it cause the youngster?

- Are there any special preparations needed before the test or procedure is done?

- Will the youngster need any special care after the test or procedure?

- Are there any problems to look for after the test or procedure? If one or more of these occur, what action should you take?

- How soon will you be able to know what the test showed?

▶ **ASK THE DOCTOR (OR HIS OR HER ASSISTANT) WHAT THE RISKS OF THE TEST OR PROCEDURE ARE (IF ANY), AS WELL AS THE BENEFITS.**

- Discuss with the doctor (or assistant) whether the benefits of the test or procedure outweigh the risks.

▶ **IF THERE ARE RISKS INVOLVED IN THE TEST OR PROCEDURE, ASK IF THERE IS ANOTHER TEST OR PROCEDURE THAT COULD BE PERFORMED THAT HAS FEWER RISKS AND WOULD STILL PROVIDE THE SAME INFORMATION.**

If your youngster needs to have one or more tests or procedures, do your best to be supportive.

▶ **STAY WITH YOUR YOUNGSTER DURING AN UNPLEASANT, PAINFUL, OR FRIGHTENING MEDICAL TEST OR PROCEDURE—IF AT ALL POSSIBLE.**

- Be sure you understand what will be done, so you can explain what's happening to the child, and be as helpful as you can to both the youngster and the doctor or other health professional during the test or procedure.

- Help the youngster stay calm, and encourage her to cooperate during the test or procedure.

- Assist in holding the youngster still when this is important.

- Allow an older youngster or teenager to decide if she wants you to be with her or not.

▶ **BE HONEST WITH YOUR CHILD ABOUT THE TEST OR PROCEDURE.**

- Do not tell him it will not hurt if it will.

▶ **COMFORT YOUR YOUNGSTER AFTER THE TEST OR PROCEDURE IS COMPLETED, ESPECIALLY IF IT WAS PAINFUL.**

- A hug and praise for being brave (even if he screams, yells, or is uncooperative) are always appreciated! This praise and affection also send a message to the youngster—one he'll remember the next time he must have a test or procedure.

Common Tests and Procedures: What You Should Know

Most, if not all, youngsters undergo one or more medical tests or procedures during their infancy and childhood. While there are literally thousands of possible tests or procedures that could be recommended by your youngster's doctor, some are so common that it's helpful for you to be familiar with them. Others are very complex or not performed very often. Less common and more complex tests and procedures need to be explained (in detail) by your child's doctor.

Certain tests are recommended as a part of preventive medical care for infants, children, and older youngsters. These tests are usually designed to detect problems that are both relatively common and able to be successfully treated. The usual "requirements" for a test or procedure to be considered routine and therefore recommended frequently are as follows: 1) the condition the doctor is looking for is common; 2) the test is simple to perform and reliable in detecting a problem; 3) the test is safe for the youngster; and 4) the cost of the test is low enough to warrant its use in many youngsters

UNDERSTAND-
ING COMMON
TESTS AND
PROCEDURES
AND HELPING
YOUR CHILD
WHEN
HOSPITALIZED

(who may be perfectly normal), in hopes of finding the occasional one who has a problem.

Some tests (for example, newborn screening tests) detect uncommon but devastating problems that threaten an infant's overall health and well-being, as well as his mental development—if these problems are not discovered in their very early stages. As with many medical conditions, the conditions that these routine tests detect are best treated if they are discovered early, before a youngster has symptoms. Before your baby is born, it is wise to ask the pediatrician or family practice physician who will be caring for the baby what routine screening tests will be performed and what problems these tests will rule out or identify.

When a youngster is ill or injured, the doctor will first take a careful medical history (ask questions in detail about a youngster's symptoms and general health), then perform a careful physical examination. If these alone do not pinpoint the problem, the doctor may want to perform certain tests or procedures to correctly diagnose the youngster's condition. The doctor will choose a test or tests that will most accurately pinpoint a suspected illness (or rule it out), usually starting with the most simple and accurate test(s) possible. If the initial testing is not helpful and the problem is serious or potentially serious (or very bothersome), then further testing may be recommended. The doctor, like you, will not want to cause a youngster any more discomfort than necessary, nor expose him or her to unnecessary risks. This concept explains the step-by-step approach taken by most doctors when a child is ill or injured.

Many tests and procedures used to diagnose or treat illnesses and injuries are simple and cause little or no discomfort to the child. Others are uncomfortable and may carry risks. In these situations, the risks must be carefully weighed against the possible benefits of doing the test or procedure. Always ask the doctor about the risks of a test or procedure, and have the doctor explain to you why he or she feels the benefits outweigh the potential risks for your child.

So that you are well informed, it is important for you to understand some of the most common tests and procedures that are recommended for infants and toddlers, young children, older children, and teenagers. You also need to know when these tests or procedures might be indicated, what kinds of information the doctor can gain from them, their potential risks, and the usual benefits of doing them. We should point out that since each youngster is different, the reason(s) the doctor would recommend a particular test or procedure may vary from child to child. Therefore, be sure you ask your doctor about the specific reasons a test or procedure is being recommended for *your child* and what the risks and benefits of doing the test or procedure are for *your child*.

Hopefully, your youngster will need only those tests which are recommended as a part of excellent pediatric preventive care. However, if he or she is ill or injured and needs other tests or procedures, you will be better equipped to understand what is being recommended if you are familiar with some of the principles of certain medical tests and procedures.

Tests and Procedures: How You Can Help Your Youngster

Most medical tests and procedures—if not uncomfortable or downright painful—are still scary for youngsters (and adults). This is particularly true if the child doesn't know what will happen, when it will happen, if it will hurt, and how long it will hurt (if it will hurt). The most important thing we can do is *put ourselves in the child's place* and try to imagine the situation from his perspective. If you were an infant—how would you feel? If you were a toddler—how would you feel? If you were a young child—how would you feel? And, if you were an older child or teenager—how would you feel?

For example, if you were a baby and someone was going to give you a shot, there is no way you would understand what was going on! You would recognize the surroundings as unfamiliar, the people as unfamiliar, the smells as unfamiliar and maybe even a difference in your mother or father's "presence" or attitude. *But* (and this is the most important point), you would also recognize warmth, tenderness, compassion, caring, concern, emotional support, and love. These are recognizable to an infant by how he or she is talked to and touched. There are people who find it very strange or even funny to hear a mother, father, or health care professional talk to a baby as if he or she truly understands what is being said. Actually, there's nothing strange or funny about it! The infant *does understand* the tone of someone's voice—warm, sensitive, and loving, or terse, cold, and uncaring. The point is, what are you supposed to say? Making up gibberish is harder than gently and lovingly telling the infant or baby what is happening. "I know this will hurt for a second, but mommy (or daddy) is right here with you. I know that smells funny and is cold on your leg (the alcohol), but it will be over in a second. Here we go, we'll both hold on tight! Now, see it's over."

The baby can also *feel* as well as hear. Holding her tightly and securely and being loving and affectionate—as you talk—does make the experience tolerable and less frightening (even less painful for some children). Giving big hugs afterward and continuing to do so until the baby stops crying (if she cries) is very supportive and sends a special message that you care and know this wasn't such a great experience!

The same holds true for the toddler or nonverbal young child. Again put yourself in the child's position and respond from that point-of-view. Talk to him and hold him, if the test or procedure permits this. If you cannot hold him, then can you hold his hands, rub his head, or rub his feet? Sometimes you'll have to be innovative. When you talk to the child try very hard to say things in words that he may be able to understand or you know he can understand. Explain what is happening or will happen *in very simple terms—and always be honest*. If you're not sure the toddler or young child can understand, make sure your voice and your actions tell him that you are there, that you love him, and that this will be all right.

UNDERSTAND-
ING COMMON
TESTS AND
PROCEDURES
AND HELPING
YOUR CHILD
WHEN
HOSPITALIZED

The young verbal child and older child should be told in detail what will take place. She will understand what you say as long as you are careful to explain everything at the level she comprehends based on her age, ability, and experience. Ask the health care professional who will perform the test or procedure to please explain it to you and the child before it takes place. Also ask whether he or she will explain the procedure as it is being done—or if you should do it. The most important part of this is to let the child know when it will hurt and how long it will hurt (if pain is involved in the test or procedure). In this way the child has a few seconds to be prepared. Also, if you tell her the truth, she'll always have faith that she has nothing to worry about and can relax until you tell her, "OK, this part will hurt a little, too, so hold on."

Pain is a strange thing. Think about it. If you are told something will hurt, it often hurts *less* because you were prepared for it. On the other hand, if you are told something won't hurt and it does or the pain is unexpected and surprises you, it always seems to hurt *more*. Therefore, if a test or procedure will be uncomfortable, hurt a little, or really hurt—or is more scary than painful—be honest about it. If you don't know, tell the child you don't know, but you'll ask. Then make sure you ask and tell the child.

There's one other aspect of this to consider. If you tell a child that something won't hurt and it does, one or more of several repercussions can occur. Because you deceived the child, he may not believe you the next time you tell him something important or tell him something won't hurt. It may make the child feel that something is wrong with him, because you said it wouldn't hurt and it did (it wasn't suppose to, remember!). Or, it may make him feel that he wasn't brave because he cried or yelled over something you said wouldn't hurt.

If you take a moment to think back about your childhood, you may be able to remember one or more incidents in which you were lied to by your parents, a doctor, or nurse. They were well-meaning. The feeling then was, "Just get it over with and tell her it won't hurt!" The reason? Most people thought that children were better off not knowing. They feared children would be difficult or impossible if they knew something would hurt, or simply wouldn't understand. Research and clinical experience over the last several years have proved just the opposite.

The following is an example of how something *should not* be done. David goes to the pediatrician's office with his mother because he isn't feeling well. Once they get to the office, the doctor examines David, then tells his mother to take the eight-year-old over to the lab for a blood test and urine culture. Mind you, no one's talking to David, whose body it is that doesn't feel well and who has to go through the blood test and urine culture (whatever those big words mean). David probably understood the word "blood" so that may have already struck horror in him.

On the way over to the lab, David asks his mother where they are going and why. She answers his question, but in a way he, of course, cannot understand. "We're going to the laboratory for some tests." Very ambiguous. Now David is even more anxious. They get to the lab. David's mother goes to the desk and gives *David's name!* Now there's even more to worry about.

A lab technician comes out and calls *David's name*. His mother gets up and takes David by the hand. "Where are we going?" he asks. "Right in here," his mother says. David is told to sit in this funny-looking chair that has a place to put one arm—no place for the other arm. How odd! The technician gets all her things ready and then asks David to put his arm on the special place for it. Hold everything! David starts to panic. "No," he says, "I won't do it, no." He starts to whimper. The technician tells him this won't hurt and his mother agrees. David puts his arm out. The technician asks his mother to hold him (Why do I need to be held if it doesn't hurt? he wonders). The next thing you know, David sees the needle and the fight begins.

The test finally gets done but in the meantime it looks like a war was fought in the blood-drawing room. David is crying and screaming, his mother is embarrassed and upset, as well as feeling bad for David, and the technician is exasperated. The technician tells David that the urine culture is simple and doesn't hurt . . . and well . . . of course, he doesn't believe her, or his mother . . . and you can imagine the rest!

It would have been a lot easier if everyone had been honest with David. It would have been a lot easier to have David sit in his mother's lap (if he wanted to) or have her right next to him, holding his hand. It would have been easier for the technician to explain that a blood test hurts for just a minute. When it was going to hurt, she would tell him, so he could squeeze his mother's hand as hard as he could—but not move his other arm so the test would be over really fast!

When she was asked, David's mother could have told him that a lab or laboratory was a special place where they did all sorts of tests that helped the doctor find out why someone wasn't feeling well—and that David needed to have two tests done. One of the tests—called a urine culture—didn't hurt at all and she would help him. All he would have to do is go to the bathroom (or whatever language is used in the family for urinating) in a small container—like a jar. The other test—called a blood test—hurt a little for just a minute. The doctor needed to look at David's blood, so a tiny bit needed to be taken from his arm. She could have said that she has had a blood test many times (so has daddy and others she could think of) and that everyone said the same thing—it hurt for only a minute. David could have been reassured that if he was a little scared, it was all right—because everybody is a little scared when they go through something new to them.

Remember, the key is to be honest, talk warmly and gently to the child (whatever age), and be sure that your physical presence is somehow felt (either by holding the child, holding her hand or foot, or rubbing her head—whatever you can do within the limits of the test or procedure). If for some reason you can't be right there with her (as is the case in most X-ray studies and some other complicated procedures), then make sure she can hear you—and keep talking! Don't forget to comfort the child afterward. If a bandage or other visible sign of "bravery" is given after the test, be sure to talk about her special "bravery patch" or "badge of courage." This often makes the child feel better and the hurt disappear quickly. It also allows the youngster to feel proud of what she accomplished (again, even if the child screamed, cried, struggled, refused to do it at first, or was uncooperative).

688

UNDERSTAND-
ING COMMON
TESTS AND
PROCEDURES
AND HELPING
YOUR CHILD
WHEN
HOSPITALIZED

One important note: Don't be fooled by older children who *think* they have to be brave. Sometimes it helps if you say *you* need to hold his hand if that would be all right with him. A big hug afterward never hurt anyone! With teenagers, give them a choice. At that age some will want to go it alone, while others will want you with them. With all children—tell them the truth and be supportive, warm, and understanding. Again, whether you're two months old or eighteen years old, you can be frightened and want someone with you who really cares about you and really understands.

Routine Screening Tests

NEWBORN SCREENING TESTS

There has been a great deal of progress in routine newborn screening for hereditary diseases since the first tests to detect PKU (*phenylketonuria*) were developed approximately twenty years ago. It is now possible to screen an infant for more than twenty so-called inborn errors of metabolism on a single drop of blood taken from the baby's heel.

Currently, all fifty states require routine newborn screening for PKU and most include at least one or two others (most often congenital hypothyroidism and galactosemia) in their elaborate programs to detect potentially devastating hereditary or congenital (present at birth) diseases. Studies are currently in progress to determine the cost effectiveness of routine screening for many more similar but uncommon problems. The reason? The diseases for which testing is done lead to mental retardation and other serious abnormalities if they are not detected and treated soon after birth. With early detection and treatment, infants can lead normal or near-normal lives. This fact makes it worthwhile to screen all infants, with the hope that the few who have problems will be detected.

Phenylketonuria (PKU), the first disease for which accurate, cost-effective screening programs were developed, is a hereditary disease in which an infant is missing an enzyme needed to metabolize the amino acid phenylalanine, found in proteins. Abnormal buildup of phenylalanine and its by-products leads to mental retardation. If PKU is detected early and treated with a special diet that controls the amount of phenylalanine an infant gets, his or her development can be normal.

Congenital hypothyroidism is much more common than was previously thought when screening for its presence first began. Infants with this problem do not produce enough thyroid hormone, which is necessary for normal growth and development. Early detection and treatment with thyroid hormone can completely eliminate the effects of this devastating condition.

Galactosemia is another inborn error of metabolism which can be detected through newborn screening. Infants with this disorder cannot correctly metabolize galactose, a sugar which is formed from the lactose found in human and cow's milk. Galactose builds up in the blood, and can lead to listlessness, weight loss, liver damage, cataracts, brain damage, and even death. All these problems can be prevented simply by substituting a nonmilk formula which does not contain lactose.

TESTS FOR ANEMIA

Anemia refers either to a reduction below the normal level for a youngster's age in the number of red blood cells or to a reduction in the oxygen-carrying pigment (called hemoglobin) in the blood. Anemia can have many causes, but the two basic types of anemias are 1) those in which the bone marrow does not produce enough red blood cells or hemoglobin (for example, iron deficiency anemia), and 2) those in which the body destroys red blood cells too fast (for example, sickle cell anemia, in which red cells are destroyed because their abnormal hemoglobin changes their shape).

Anemia, especially the type caused by a deficiency of iron in a child's diet, is a common enough problem in infancy and childhood that periodic testing for its presence is recommended as a part of excellent health care. Testing is generally done at times when a youngster is most at risk for problems, especially with iron deficiency—at nine to twelve months of age, at the time of school entry, and during the early part of adolescence (especially for girls, who are or will be menstruating). Additional testing may be recommended for infants and children who are at risk for certain hereditary anemias (for example, black children from families in which sickle cell disease is a problem).

Testing for anemia is simple and quite inexpensive. An infant's heel or a child's finger can be pricked with a needlelike lancet, or a needle can be used to remove a small amount of blood from a vein. The blood is then analyzed in the laboratory. While there is always a slight amount of discomfort when blood is taken, this is the only risk involved with blood drawing.

The most reliable and complete test for anemia is the complete blood count (called a CBC), which gives the doctor the hemoglobin level, the hematocrit (the percent of the blood which is solid), the red blood cell count, the size of the red blood cells, and the concentration of hemoglobin in the red blood cells. In addition, it provides information about the numbers and types of white blood cells (the cells that fight infection) and the platelets (tiny particles important in blood clotting). In certain situations, screening for anemia involves measurements of the hemoglobin and/or hematocrit only, instead of doing a complete CBC.

ROUTINE URINE ANALYSIS

Urine analysis is recommended periodically during childhood in order to detect unsuspected problems with the kidneys and/or bladder. It is also recommended whenever the doctor suspects a problem about which a urine analysis will provide vital information

UNDERSTAND-
ING COMMON
TESTS AND
PROCEDURES
AND HELPING
YOUR CHILD
WHEN
HOSPITALIZED

(help rule out or identify a certain problem or problems). This simple test requires only a few drops of urine, but can provide important information about the way the kidneys are functioning. Urine testing is usually done at around one year of age, at the time of school entry, and every few years afterward.

A urine specimen is obtained from infants and toddlers who are not toilet trained by attaching a special plastic bag to the little one's genital area, then waiting until he or she urinates. Older children are asked to urinate into a container.

Urine is tested for its concentration (called specific gravity), and a special dipstick can be used to detect protein, sugar, acetone, blood, bilirubin, and acidity. Additional dipstick tests are now available to detect abnormal numbers of white blood cells and bacteria, and may become part of the routine urine analysis. In addition, a drop of urine is examined under the microscope to detect abnormal numbers of white and red blood cells, bacteria, and other abnormal elements.

TUBERCULOSIS TESTS

Periodic testing of infants and children for exposure to tuberculosis (TB) is an important part of routine health care. Tuberculosis is a serious respiratory disease that can be silent in young children. TB is easily treated if caught early—but can be a devastating problem if left undetected and untreated.

Tuberculosis skin testing is an easy, inexpensive, and quite reliable way of identifying TB in infants and children. The skin testing detects whether or not the youngster has made antibodies to TB. If the youngster has been exposed to TB, the test is "positive."

There are several types of TB skin tests. Two types of tests are most commonly used for "screening" children. One test (called a tine test) involves putting the testing material into the skin of the soft inner surface of the lower arm with tiny prongs, then looking for bumpy swelling two to three days later. A more reliable but more uncomfortable test (called a Mantoux test) involves injecting a "bubble" of liquid into the skin. The Mantoux test is performed if there is a serious risk of exposure to TB or if the prong-type test is positive.

TB skin testing is routinely recommended at one year of age or before the MMR vaccine is given, then every one to two years afterward. Exact recommendations depend on the risk for TB in your area. Check with your child's doctor or your local health department about specific recommendations for your area.

Tests and Procedures Recommended
When a Problem Is Suspected

BLOOD TESTS

In addition to the routine CBC discussed previously, there are literally thousands of tests that can be done on blood. Many of these tests can be performed on tiny amounts of blood in a very short period of time. Many are now automated, that is, done by a special, computerized machine which gives information in a matter of minutes. Some tests—called blood "panels"—are grouped together in order to give the doctor the most helpful, complete information about certain problems. This has both limited the amount of blood needed to do the tests and reduced the cost of testing.

Again, blood for many tests can be obtained from a simple finger or heel puncture, especially in infants and very young children. When larger amounts of blood are needed, a needle is used to withdraw blood from a vein in the youngster's arm or hand.

The following are among the most common blood tests performed on infants and children, along with some of the reasons they are recommended.

- The *complete blood count (CBC)*—in addition to information about whether or not a youngster has anemia, the test may tell whether or not there is infection or inflammation; or if a bleeding problem is caused by too few platelets.

- The *white blood count and differential* (part of the CBC)—can give clues about the presence and type of infection or inflammation. It may also detect abnormalities in the white blood cells themselves.

- Serum *electrolytes*—measure the amounts of sodium, potassium, chloride, and bicarbonate (body salts) in the liquid portion of the blood, and give information about dehydration, acid balance, and kidney function.

- *BUN (blood urea nitrogen) and creatinine*—measure the level of these waste products in the blood, giving information about whether the kidneys are functioning normally. (The levels are high if the kidneys are not working well.)

- Serum *bilirubin*—is measured if jaundice is present, especially in newborn infants. If the level of bilirubin, the chemical that causes jaundice, is too high, the baby may need treatment. In older infants and children, it is elevated in some liver diseases.

- *Blood culture*—detects bacteria in the bloodstream, if present, when overwhelming infection (sepsis) is suspected. Results of this test take one to three days. If there are bacteria in the blood, it takes this amount of time for them to grow in the laboratory so they can be identified.

692

UNDERSTAND-
ING COMMON
TESTS AND
PROCEDURES
AND HELPING
YOUR CHILD
WHEN
HOSPITALIZED

TESTS FOR URINARY TRACT INFECTION

When the doctor suspects a urinary tract infection (called a UTI), he or she will want to perform a urine analysis (as discussed previously), and will look for white blood cells and red blood cells, as well as bacteria. The doctor will want to confirm the suspicion that an infection is present by doing a *urine culture*. A urine culture involves adding a small amount of the youngster's urine to a special culture plate or plates, then placing the plate(s) in an incubator for one to three days. An infection is confirmed if bacteria grow in the laboratory, since urine is normally free of bacteria. The doctor can also request that the laboratory identify which antibiotic(s) will be effective in treating the infection.

A urine culture is reliable in diagnosing an infection only if the urine is collected correctly. Special care must be taken to ensure that the urine is not contaminated. A *"clean catch"* specimen is usually reliable in toilet-trained children and older young-sters. This involves carefully washing the external genitals, then urinating into a sterile container, hopefully after first urinating a small amount into the lavatory (this is called a mid-stream specimen). The urine must be processed in the laboratory immediately, or refrigerated until it can be processed. Even with excellent washing, clean catch specimens are sometimes contaminated, giving a false result that a urinary tract infection exists.

In a young infant or toddler who is not yet toilet-trained, a urine specimen can be collected by first washing the external genitals, then attaching a special plastic bag to the baby's genitals and waiting for the little one to urinate. This kind of specimen is often contaminated by bacteria on the skin, even when the baby or toddler is carefully washed. Therefore, the doctor might want to obtain a more reliable urine specimen so the culture results are more accurate.

When it is vital that urine culture results be accurate, urine is obtained by *bladder catheterization*. In this procedure, the external genitals are carefully washed by a nurse or physician's assistant. Then a tiny plastic catheter (tube) is inserted through the urethra (the tubelike structure that leads from the bladder to the outside of the body). Once the catheter is in the bladder, urine empties through the catheter and is collected in a sterile container. The catheter is then removed.

Bladder catheterization can range from a little uncomfortable to momentarily painful—depending on the youngster. For several hours afterward, there is usually a bit of burning or discomfort when the youngster urinates. This discomfort can be lessened if she drinks extra liquids (to make the urine less concentrated), or sits in a tub of water to urinate. There is a very slight risk of the catheterization causing a bladder infection when one did not exist before the procedure was performed.

As an alternative in infants under one year of age, a *suprapubic bladder aspiration* might be used to obtain a urine specimen for culture. This procedure, which involves inserting a needle through the lower part of the baby's abdomen directly into the bladder (after carefully washing the skin), then removing a small amount of urine with a syringe, is safer than catheterization for some young infants. It is about as uncomfortable as drawing blood, and carries a slight risk of causing a tiny amount of temporary bleeding in the bladder, and puncturing the intestine. However, it eliminates the risk of introducing infection into the bladder. This procedure is usually recommended when correct test results are vital—because a potentially serious infection is suspected and needs to be identified or ruled out.

TESTS FOR THROAT INFECTION

If the doctor suspects a throat infection caused by Group A beta hemolytic streptococcus (strep throat), he or she will usually take a *throat culture*. This procedure is simple (though momentarily uncomfortable), and involves wiping the throat and tonsils with a cotton swab. The secretions are then placed on a culture plate which is kept in an incubator for twenty-four to forty-eight hours to see if strep bacteria grow. If strep bacteria grow, the culture is "positive" and confirms the infection. If the culture is "negative" (no strep bacteria grow), the infection is caused by another type of bacteria or virus which usually does not need to be treated with antibiotics.

Currently there are several other tests for strep throat which take only a few minutes to a few hours for test results to be available. These rapid strep tests, which are performed on secretions collected from the throat with a cotton swab, appear to be quite reliable and are being used more and more. They allow the doctor to treat strep throat promptly and avoid using antibiotics to treat nonstrep infections. Results of these rapid strep tests are often confirmed by doing a throat culture, as well (with results available in one to two days).

TESTS ON STOOL (FROM A BOWEL MOVEMENT)

The most simple test performed on stool is a *test for blood*, which can be done in a minute or two. The doctor will do this test in the office on stool obtained during a rectal examination, or on a bowel movement that you have brought in. The test is helpful when a youngster is having problems with abdominal pain, constipation, or diarrhea, or when there is unexplained anemia.

A *stool culture* is a test used to look for certain bacteria (by growing them in the laboratory) that cause intestinal infection. The doctor will want to perform this test if a youngster has unusually severe or prolonged diarrhea, or if there is blood and/or mucus in the bowel movement. Results are available after two to three days. You might be asked to place your child's fresh bowel movement (stool) in a special container and take it to the laboratory, or the doctor may use a special cotton swab which is inserted a short distance into the rectum to obtain stool for the culture.

Tests for intestinal parasites are performed in the laboratory on very fresh stool. You will be given special instructions about collecting the bowel movement if these tests are recommended. It is important that you follow the instructions carefully so the tests are as accurate as possible.

UNDERSTAND-
ING COMMON
TESTS AND
PROCEDURES
AND HELPING
YOUR CHILD
WHEN
HOSPITALIZED

LUMBAR PUNCTURE (SPINAL TAP)

A lumbar puncture, also called an LP or a spinal tap, involves the removal of a small amount of spinal fluid so it can be examined in the laboratory. This procedure is recommended whenever the doctor suspects meningitis (infection of the coverings of the brain and spinal cord) or another serious infection or problem of the nervous system. It is also performed during the treatment of some children's cancers to inject medication into the spinal canal.

A lumbar puncture is performed with the youngster lying on her side (or sitting upright, if she is old enough) with her back rounded. Since it is vital that she hold very still during the procedure, an assistant will hold her securely in position so she doesn't move during the procedure. The doctor sits behind the youngster to perform the spinal tap.

After cleansing the skin of the lower part of the back (at the level of the hips) and placing sterile towels around the area, the doctor injects a small amount of local anesthetic into the skin and tissues to numb the area. This causes a stinging sensation for a moment or two. The doctor then carefully inserts a special needle into the back between two of the vertebrae and guides it into the spinal canal. The youngster will feel the pressure of the needle being inserted, and a popping sensation, as well as some pain, as the needle enters the spinal canal. The doctor may measure the pressure of the spinal fluid (in older youngsters who can cooperate), then collect a sample of spinal fluid, which drips slowly out of the needle into sterile tubes. If medication needs to be injected, it will be done through the same needle. The needle is withdrawn and a sterile dressing is placed over the puncture mark. The youngster may be asked to lie down to rest quietly for a short time after the procedure is finished.

A lumbar puncture is a procedure that really scares parents and others. The fact is, it is actually more frightening than painful. That's not to say it doesn't hurt. It does. But it is not as painful as it is so often dramatized in the movies—as excruciating, unbearable pain. It is the fear of the procedure—and fear about why it is being done— that really causes children (and adults) to panic. In addition, infants, children, and older youngsters object more strenuously to needing to be held for a spinal tap than to the actual insertion of the needle. Some cry and struggle before the procedure is started, and make no objection to the actual insertion of the needle!

Since lumbar puncture is recommended only when the condition(s) the doctor suspects are potentially very serious or life-threatening, the benefits of the procedure outweigh the risks. Spinal tap does not cause damage to the spinal cord or paralysis if done correctly (the needle inserted at the level of the waist or below). It does cause some pain at the time, and mild discomfort at the puncture site for a short time afterward. Interestingly, children do not often complain of so-called spinal headache, even if they do not rest after the procedure.

If your child needs a lumbar puncture, be sure to ask the doctor about his or her reasons for recommending the test, and review the risks and benefits of doing the procedure. Then ask if you can help your youngster by being with him to calm and reassure him. If you are asked to remain outside, be ready to comfort the youngster after the procedure is completed.

DIAGNOSTIC X RAYS

X rays are basically "pictures" that can be taken of any part of the internal structures of the body. Essentially, an X-ray beam is passed through a part of the body and onto a special photographic plate. An X ray looks very much like a black and white photograph negative. But, unlike the photograph negative, when you look at an X ray, you're looking at the actual "picture" (the positive, not the negative). X rays show the outlines of the different structures of the body because of differences in density of the various organs. Therefore, bone looks very white, and fat, air, and water are different shades of gray. If a contrast material is used (which will be discussed later in this chapter), then the internal structures and function of organs can also be visualized. (Contrast material makes organs look very bright or white).

X rays of the chest are the most common taken at any age, and can help the doctor detect or confirm pneumonia, other problems with the lungs, and some abnormalities of the heart. X rays of the bones can help the doctor diagnose the kind and exact location of fractures (broken bones), and a myriad of other bone problems. *X rays of the abdomen* can also be of assistance when there might be a bowel (intestinal) obstruction (blockage) or certain other abnormalities. X rays can be taken of the gallbladder, kidneys, bladder, pancreas, stomach, liver, heart, and all other internal organs. When an internal organ is involved, a contrast material is usually necessary.

The following (in addition to those studies noted previously) are the most common contrast X-ray studies performed to diagnose, confirm, or rule out problems in children:

- *Upper GI (Gastrointestinal) Series (also called a barium swallow)*—involves swallowing a special contrast material, barium, which tastes like a chalky malt. The barium moves through and coats the esophagus, stomach, and small intestine and/or bowel. Both "moving picture" (using a special camera called a fluoroscope) and conventional (still) X rays are taken so that the structure and function of these organs can be seen and evaluated. For the fluoroscope to be used the room must be darkened. The youngster should be told about this so it won't frighten him. If the bowel is to be included in the study, there will be a waiting period after the initial X rays have been taken (it takes time for the barium to reach the bowel). An upper GI series is not painful, but some youngsters complain of nausea or stomachache (due to the barium).

- *Lower GI (Gastrointestinal) Series (also called a barium enema)*—involves X-ray examination of the structure and function of the entire large intestine (colon). The youngster will be asked to lie on her left side so a tiny tube (attached to an enema bag filled with barium) can be carefully inserted into the rectum through the anus. The barium is released into the lower GI tract so that the X-ray series

696

UNDERSTAND-
ING COMMON
TESTS AND
PROCEDURES
AND HELPING
YOUR CHILD
WHEN
HOSPITALIZED

can be performed. This procedure is usually uncomfortable, but not painful. Most youngsters say they feel like they have to go to the bathroom. Again, moving and conventional X rays are taken, and the room is darkened so the fluoroscope can be used (as discussed previously).

- *IVP (Intravenous Pyelogram)*—allows the doctor to visualize and study the structures and function of the youngster's urinary tract, including the kidneys, ureters (the tubes that lead from the kidneys to the bladder), and the bladder. An IV (intravenous) solution is started and when the doctor is ready to begin the procedure, a special dye (contrast material) is injected into the vein via the IV tubing. The dye moves through the veins and passes through the kidneys (and is essentially processed like urine). X rays are taken as the dye passes through the urinary tract, allowing for sharp and clear pictures. When the IV is inserted (discussed later in this chapter), the youngster will experience the same type of discomfort or pain felt when getting a shot. Once the IV is in the vein, there is no discomfort. Also, when the dye/contrast material is first injected, the youngster may feel a warm flush for a few minutes and may say he has a strange taste in his mouth. This is normal and should only last for a few minutes.

- *Cystogram (also called a voiding cystourethrogram)*—allows the doctor to visualize and examine the structure and function of the bladder and urethra (the tubelike structure that leads from the bladder to the outside of the body). A catheter (see bladder catheterization, discussed previously) is placed into the bladder through the urethra so that contrast material can be put into the bladder. X rays are taken of the bladder, then the catheter is removed. The youngster is asked to urinate while more X rays are taken of the bladder and urethra (as they actually function). At times, the catheter must be reinserted and more dye instilled (if the initial X rays are not as clear and sharp as needed). As with bladder catheterization, the youngster will usually experience some discomfort or pain when the catheter is inserted, as well as some burning and discomfort when urinating after the procedure is over.

As is the case with all tests and procedures, you should discuss the risks versus the benefits of any X-ray procedure with your child's doctor. Radiation exposure (even in X-ray series) is minimal today because of advances in technology. However, reproductive organs are sensitive to repeated X-ray (radiation) exposure. Therefore, all children should be covered with a lead shield across the lower abdomen (if this does not interfere with the X-ray study being done). Since there is also concern about the possible effects of cumulative X-ray exposure over the years, you should be convinced that the child requires the recommended X-ray procedure (that the benefits outweigh the risks). It's also a good idea to list all X-ray studies (what kind of study and when it was performed) in your child's medical history. If the youngster (over the years) requires repeated or extensive X-ray studies, then this list should be shown to and discussed with the youngster's doctor. In this way, you and the doctor know how much

X-ray (radiation) exposure the youngster has experienced and can better determine if his future exposure should be limited, if at all possible.

Some youngsters (and adults) may be allergic to the contrast material used (particularly those which contain iodine). If you know your child is allergic or sensitive to iodine, be sure to tell his or her doctor if an X-ray procedure in which a contrast material is necessary is being recommended. Another contrast material might be used, or another diagnostic test recommended. If the youngster is not known to be allergic or sensitive to iodine or other materials, there is still some risk that an allergic reaction can occur. (If the child does have an allergic reaction to a contrast material, it usually takes place within a few minutes after the contrast material is given. Steps are then taken to treat the problem promptly.)

DIAGNOSTIC ULTRASOUND

Diagnostic ultrasound, which is also called ultrasonography, sonography, a sonogram, or simply ultrasound, is based on the principles of sonar. It is a painless procedure which can provide very useful information about the internal organs of the body. Ultrasound is frequently done before any other tests in order to guide the doctor in recommending further testing, and may eliminate the need for other more risky or uncomfortable tests. It is often recommended when the doctor suspects a problem in the child's abdomen, chest, head, or even heart, and is especially helpful during pregnancy, when it is used to detect problems with the developing fetus.

There is usually no special preparation for ultrasound, except that an older youngster might be asked to drink several glasses of water before the procedure and not urinate until afterward if the test involves the abdomen. Oil is rubbed on the skin over the area which will be examined, then the ultrasound transducer (which looks like a microphone) is moved firmly back and forth over the skin. This may cause some discomfort—particularly if the ultrasound transducer is moved across the skin above the bladder (it's like any other time when your bladder is full and someone pushes on it). The transducer sends out inaudible, high-frequency sound waves which hit the organs and internal structures of the body and bounce back at the transducer at different speeds. A sophisticated computer converts these waves into an image which appears on a monitor, and photographs can be made for further study. An even more sophisticated type of ultrasound (called real-time ultrasound) can provide very detailed moving pictures and allows the doctor to examine the function of an organ (for example, the heart).

So far, ultrasound appears to be a totally safe test (even for pregnant women). It is also an excellent diagnostic tool. Some harmful effects have been seen in the laboratory with very high sound waves and prolonged use. However, diagnostic (testing) levels used in the United States are far, far below those used in the laboratory on an experimental basis. Also, diagnostic ultrasound is a very short procedure—unlike the prolonged exposure experimentally tested in the laboratory. Therefore, experts agree that

698

UNDERSTAND-
ING COMMON
TESTS AND
PROCEDURES
AND HELPING
YOUR CHILD
WHEN
HOSPITALIZED

diagnostic ultrasound was a major medical breakthrough and continues to be one of the most useful, noninvasive, and painless diagnostic procedures available today.

CT (COMPUTERIZED TOMOGRAPHY) SCANNING

CT scanning involves the use of small amounts of X ray and a very sophisticated computer system to make very detailed images ("pictures") of deep-seated organs and structures in a matter of minutes. CT scanning is especially helpful in detecting bleeding, tumors, and other abnormalities inside the head, chest, and abdomen. It can be performed quickly in an emergency, giving valuable information so treatment can be started immediately.

Some CT scanning procedures involve the use of contrast materials ("dyes") to make the image more distinct. These must be injected through an intravenous (IV) needle. The IV is started before the procedure so the contrast material can be given at the time of the scan. CT scanning itself can be frightening to children, but is not painful. The youngster is placed inside the scanner's chamber and positioned. He is asked to hold perfectly still for a few minutes while the machine is turned on. (Infants and small children might need to be sedated beforehand so they will be still.) If contrast material is to be used, it will be injected through the IV and the scanner turned on again. The youngster is removed from the chamber and the procedure is finished.

Like diagnostic ultrasound, CT scanning was a major medical breakthrough and continues to be an excellent and potentially limitless diagnostic tool. (It also can be used to "guide" other procedures, such as certain types of surgeries.) The information the procedure gives is very precise. In fact, the CT scanner can visualize and record images of an organ, structure, or area of the body from many angles. It's amazingly close to actually "seeing" inside the body without making a surgical incision. This is possible because the computer actually makes images of the structure or organ in "slices." Once all the slices are put together by the computer, an extremely detailed image results.

CT scanning involves exposure to a very small amount of radiation. In addition, there is a slight risk of an allergic reaction if a contrast material/dye (usually iodine) is injected intravenously. Be sure to discuss these risks with your youngster's doctor. You will want to be sure that the benefits of the procedure outweigh the risks for your child.

MAGNETIC RESONANCE IMAGING

Magnetic resonance imaging (also called MRI, nuclear magnetic resonance imaging [NMRI], magnetic imaging, and other names) is the newest, state-of-the-art diagnostic tool available today. The procedure is totally noninvasive and produces very detailed images of body organs and structures. How this extraordinarily complex technology works is rather difficult to understand unless you have a very firm understanding of physics, chemistry, mathematics, computer science, and physiology. In very simple terms, the procedure uses magnetic fields coupled with highly sophisticated computers. This diagnostic landmark is still relatively new, but to date, it appears to have no risks associated with it. In many cases, it produces better or different information than is available with other tests.

The testing procedure is totally painless. However, the equipment (plus magnet) is massive, and a child may be frightened by it. It is therefore very important to explain that the procedure does not hurt and the big machine does not do anything but take a picture—even though it may look scary and make strange noises.

RADIOISOTOPE (RADIONUCLIDE) SCANNING

Radioisotope (or radionuclide) scanning can be performed on any organ or area of the body, and can provide the doctor with information about both the structure and function of various organs. This procedure is most often used to detect problems in the bone, liver, spleen, lungs, kidneys, and intestines.

Depending on what type of problem the doctor suspects, a small amount of one of several different kinds of radioactive substances—called radionuclides—is swallowed, inhaled, or injected. Then a special scanner is used to detect the location of the radioisotope. The scanner's sophisticated computer essentially "draws" a picture of the organ, structure, or area of the body being scanned. (There may be a waiting period of several minutes to several hours between the time the radionuclide is given and the time the substance "appears" in the organ, structure, or area of the body to be scanned, so the actual scan may not take place right after the radionuclide is given.)

Radioisotope scanning is painless, but the scanner is large and can be frightening to some children. It's important to explain that the procedure will not hurt them.

As with any procedure that involves the use of contrast material and radiation, the risks versus the benefits should be discussed with your child's doctor. It is possible for a youngster to have an allergic reaction to the radionuclide material. The amount of radiation exposure with radionuclide scanning is actually quite small and usually less than that of many complex X-ray series.

SWEAT CHLORIDE TEST

The sweat chloride test is a simple test that is recommended when the doctor suspects or wants to rule out cystic fibrosis. It involves collecting a sample of sweat from the skin, which is then analyzed in the laboratory for its salt content (chloride and sodium). In cystic fibrosis the chloride content of sweat is much, much higher than normal.

To collect the sweat, a small fiber patch is attached to the child's arm or leg. A tiny electrode which conducts electrical current is attached to the patch and the skin is stimulated for thirty to sixty minutes. A very minimal amount of electrical current is used to cause enough sweat to collect on the patch. The only risk from the procedure

700

UNDERSTAND-
ING COMMON
TESTS AND
PROCEDURES
AND HELPING
YOUR CHILD
WHEN
HOSPITALIZED

is that the infant or child may have some redness or mild blistering of the skin where the patch and electrode were placed.

ELECTROENCEPHALOGRAM (EEG)

An electroencephalogram (called an EEG or brain wave test) is helpful when a youngster has seizures (convulsions), or when the doctor suspects that a seizure problem might exist. The test records the patterns of the brain's electrical activity on paper so they can be analyzed.

Since the youngster needs to be quiet or even sleeping during the test, he may be given a sedative before the EEG is done. He is taken to a quiet room and small electrodes (wires) are attached to his scalp with paste. The electrodes are attached to a very complicated machine that detects the brain's electrical activity, which is recorded for fifteen to sixty minutes. (No electrical current is *given* during the test, so there is no chance of electrical shock, as many people fear, and there are no risks involved in the test.)

BONE MARROW ASPIRATION AND BIOPSY

Bone marrow examination is necessary whenever the doctor suspects a problem with how the blood cells are being formed, or if he or she suspects or wants to rule out leukemia and other types of children's cancers. Bone marrow (the tissue in the center of many of the bones of the body, which produces blood cells) is removed by bone marrow aspiration and/or biopsy and examined in the laboratory.

Most children are given a sedative in order to help them relax before a bone marrow sample is taken. The *aspiration procedure* consists of injecting a local anesthetic over the area where the special bone marrow needle will be inserted. Then the doctor inserts the bone marrow needle (it is hollow) very carefully. He or she attaches a syringe to the needle and pulls up on the plunger (usually several times) in order to remove (aspirate) a small amount of bone marrow. Pain is experienced momentarily when the local anesthetic is injected, and pressure and pain may be felt again as the special needle enters the bone. The youngster will usually feel some discomfort each time suction is applied.

A bone marrow *biopsy* procedure is performed similarly, except that the doctor inserts a small cutting needle through the center of the special bone marrow needle (once it is in place) and uses it to remove a small amount of bone marrow. When the bone marrow is being removed (in the biopsy procedure) the youngster will hear a grating sound and feel some discomfort.

When either of these procedures is completed, the special needle is removed, pressure is applied and a sterile dressing placed over the area of the needle puncture. There is usually some pain, discomfort, or soreness once the local anesthetic wears off. This discomfort can last for several days after the procedure.

Whenever bone marrow apiration or biopsy is recommended, it is important to discuss the procedure(s) in detail with your child's doctor. In general, the accurate, early diagnosis of potentially serious or life-threatening problems, such as cancers, bone infections, and other serious problems, allows for prompt treatment, and gives the youngster the best possible chance for effective treatment.

NEEDLE BIOPSY

Needle biopsy is the removal of tissue using a special needle, so the tissue sample can be examined in the laboratory in order to rule out or identify a potentially serious problem. If a surface lump or tissue is to be biopsied, then a local anesthetic is injected over the area. The biopsy needle is then inserted through the skin and into the lump or tissue. Some pressure or discomfort is usually experienced when the needle goes into the tissue to be biopsied. Tissue is withdrawn through the special (hollow) biopsy needle. The needle is then removed and a sterile dressing placed over the puncture mark.

When an internal organ is to be biopsied, the procedure is done in a hospital—often in the radiology department or using ultrasound if the doctor needs assistance in locating the exact area to be biopsied. Sometimes a sedative is given to relax the youngster before a needle biopsy of the internal organ is performed. The same procedure is performed as with the surface lump or tissue, except that the youngster will feel some pain or discomfort when the biopsy needle is inserted beyond the skin (which is anesthetized). The tissue sample from a needle biopsy of an organ is taken to the laboratory and tests performed to rule out or identify potentially serious or life-threatening problems.

The risks and benefits of needle biopsy depend upon both the organ or tissue involved, and the exact problem the doctor suspects. It is vital for you to discuss in detail the exact procedure being recommended for your child with his or her doctor.

PNEUMOGRAM

A pneumogram is a test which helps the doctor determine if a baby's breathing pattern is normal. A pneumogram is usually recommended if there is a suspicion that an infant has an abnormal breathing pattern, is at risk for infant apnea (stopping breathing suddenly and unexpectedly), or at risk for sudden, unexpected death—called SIDS (Sudden Infant Death Syndrome, also known as crib death).

A simple pneumogram records breathing pattern and heart rate only, and can be completed at home or in a hospital or sleep center. In some situations, air flow through the nose, blood oxygen, brain waves, and blood carbon dioxide, as well as breathing pattern and heart rate, are recorded, in order to give even more information about the baby's potential problem. This more extensive testing must be performed in a hospital or sleep center.

UNDERSTAND-
ING COMMON
TESTS AND
PROCEDURES
AND HELPING
YOUR CHILD
WHEN
HOSPITALIZED

For this test the infant is attached to a special monitor which records his breathing pattern during sleep for eight to twelve hours. Special electrodes (sensors) are taped onto his chest or held in place with a belt. Special sensors may also be attached to the scalp, nose, and fingertip or toe if more detailed information is needed. The monitor is simply turned on and the baby goes to sleep as usual. The baby's activities are recorded by a nurse or technician (for example, sleeping, crying, awake, or playing). When the test is completed the monitor is turned off and the information evaluated by the doctor.

There is no risk or pain associated with the test. However, in a few infants it may give a false-positive result (that is, it indicates that the baby has a breathing problem or is at risk for apnea or SIDS when he is not). Conversely, it may also give a false-negative result (thereby missing an infant or baby who later experiences a breathing problem, apnea episode, or SIDS). It is therefore important to discuss the test and its results in detail with your baby's doctor.

pH PROBE MONITORING

When the doctor suspects serious gastroesophageal reflux (regurgitation of stomach contents into the espohagus), he or she may recommend pH probe monitoring in order to both detect the reflux problem and determine how extensive the problem is. This test is done in a hospital and takes from eight to twenty-four hours.

A special probe (sensor) which detects acidity is passed through the youngster's nose and into the lower portion of the esophagus. Part of the probe is taped onto the child's nose so it stays in place. The other end of the probe is then attached to a machine which records the acidity as a graph on paper. A nurse or assistant records the youngster's position, feedings, and activity as the test proceeds.

The most difficult part of this test is that the probe causes discomfort, and the youngster's movement and activity are limited because of the machine. Infants and toddlers usually need to be restrained so they do not pull out the probe.

Common Treatment Procedures

INTRAVENOUS (IV) INFUSION

Usually simply called an IV, an intravenous infusion involves placing a small needle or catheter (tube) into a vein through the skin to allow liquids to be administered. IVs are inserted so that liquids and body salts can be administered directly into the vein when liquids and/or solid foods cannot be taken by mouth, to prevent or treat dehydration and to keep in balance or rebalance body chemicals. They can also be used to administer medications, eliminating the need for repeated, painful injections. In addition, they are needed when contrast materials must be used for certain X-ray and other diagnostic procedures, as previously discussed. As always, ask the doctor why the IV is recommended and discuss any risks with him or her.

In children, IVs can be inserted into veins in the top of the foot, the ankle, the hand, or the arm. In infants, veins in the scalp can be used, as well. When the hand, arm, ankle, or foot is used, a thin board (much like a splint) may be taped down to keep the child from bending and disturbing the IV once it is in place.

Before the IV is started, the nurse or doctor wraps a thin rubber tourniquet around the arm or leg above the area where the IV will be inserted (or places a rubber band around a baby's head at the hairline, if a scalp vein will be used) so the veins stand out. This makes them easy to see or feel. The area over the vein is cleaned with an antiseptic solution. Then the special IV needle is inserted through the skin into the vein, and the tubing from the bottle (of IV solution) is attached. The needle and part of the tubing are securely taped down. The youngster usually experiences some pain when the needle is inserted (much like any shot/injection), but once the needle is in the vein, there is little or no discomfort.

If a plastic catheter is used, local anesthetic may be injected right over the vein before the catheter is inserted. A special needle guides the catheter into the vein. Once the catheter is in place, the needle is removed, and the IV tubing is attached to the end of the catheter. The catheter and part of the IV are securely taped in place, but a board-type splint may not be needed. The child may experience a stinging pain if local anesthetic is given over the vein and some discomfort when the catheter is inserted into the vein.

Even with the best of care, IVs are precarious in infants and children, and may need to be replaced often because the needle or catheter comes out of the vein or punctures the side of the vein. Be sure you follow the suggestions given to you by the nurse about handling your child, and don't be tempted to remove the restraints without asking—even when the youngster asks you to do so or cries because of the restraints. You can usually find a way to comfort your child without disrupting the IV.

PHOTOTHERAPY

Phototherapy involves the use of fluorescent lights to treat jaundice (a temporary condition that causes yellow skin) in newborn infants. Certain wavelengths of light are capable of changing bilirubin (the yellow chemical which causes jaundice) in the skin into a form which can be eliminated from the infant's body. Phototherapy is recommended when an infant's bilirubin level is rising rapidly or approaching a dangerous level. It treats the jaundice, but not the cause of the jaundice. While phototherapy is usually performed in the hospital, it can be used safely at home in a few special circumstances.

During phototherapy, the infant is undressed (except for his diaper) and his eyes

704

UNDERSTAND-
ING COMMON
TESTS AND
PROCEDURES
AND HELPING
YOUR CHILD
WHEN
HOSPITALIZED

are carefully covered with eye patches to completely protect them from the light. He is usually placed in an incubator (isolette) or in an area that is warm to keep his body temperature at its proper level. The phototherapy lights are switched on and the baby is turned periodically so all areas of his body are exposed to the lights. The lights are on continuously during treatment—except during feedings.

The infant's blood bilirubin is checked regularly throughout phototherapy treatment in order to determine the effectiveness of the treatment. Once the bilirubin has dropped to a safe level, the phototherapy treatments are stopped. The bilirubin level in the baby's blood may be checked one or more times after phototherapy treatment is stopped to ensure that safe levels are maintained.

Babies who are treated with phototherapy must be watched carefully to be sure their temperatures stay normal. They also require more fluid than usual to prevent dehydration. Careful eye patching is vital since damage to the retina of the eye can occur due to exposure to phototherapy lights.

NEWBORN CIRCUMCISION

Newborn circumcision is the most common surgical procedure performed in the United States. It is the surgical removal (cutting off) of the part of the foreskin which normally covers the end of the penis. The decision about whether circumcision will be done is made by parents. It is important that you make the decision (if you have not already done so) based on facts and not emotion and custom.

There is no medical reason for routine circumcision of newborn boys to be recommended, and in fact, most pediatricians recommend that it not be done. Why then are so many boys circumcised? If we eliminate the boys who are circumcised for religious reasons, we are left with social concerns and custom in the vast majority of families. "He will be different." This is the easiest argument to counter—the uncircumcised boy is exactly the way he was made!

In the past, doctors argued that circumcision prevented cancer of the cervix in one's sexual partners. This belief has been shown to be false. While it is true that circumcision does reduce the risk of cancer of the penis, this is one of the most rare of cancers, and is easily detected in its earliest stages if a young man is taught to examine his penis regularly for its signs.

Cleanliness is also an issue—one that can be easily dealt with by teaching a boy to practice good hygiene as soon as he is able. Cleanliness almost always prevents infections that can lead to the need for later circumcision in older boys or adults. (There is no quarreling with the fact that later circumcision is very painful.)

Newborn circumcision is usually performed in the first day or two of life, but may be delayed in premature or sick infants. The baby is strapped to a special board so he cannot move. Most often, anesthetic is not used. After cleaning the penis, the doctor makes a cut in the top of the foreskin, then removes the rest of the foreskin. He or she may use a metal clamp which actually cuts off the skin, or use a plastic ring with string tied around it. If the plastic ring (called a Plastibel) is used, the ring falls off five to ten days later.

Circumcision is intensely painful for babies, although they probably don't remember the pain. They do, however, show signs of irritability for twelve to twenty-four hours after the operation. Some of the pain could be lessened if a local anesthetic were given.

The major risks of circumcision are bleeding, which may vary from mild to serious, and infection. In addition, later complications ranging from tightness of the cut foreskin to more serious damage or deformity of the penis are possible. Circumcised boys are also prone to irritation and ulceration of the end of the penis during the time they wear diapers. This can lead to scarring and narrowing of the opening of the urethra.

THE DON'TS

Don't hesitate to ask the doctor to explain the risks versus the benefits of any test or procedure recommended for your child. It's important for you to be an active partner in your child's health care.

Don't forget to ask the doctor what the test or procedure involves. One of the best ways to help your youngster is to understand the test or procedure, so any questions he has can be answered.

Don't hesitate to ask why the test or procedure is being recommended and what information the doctor hopes to glean from it. This is important because you should not only know why a test or procedure is being recommended, but what the doctor is looking for or trying to rule out. This makes you a well-informed partner in your child's health care.

Don't forget to do all you can to explain (in simple terms) the test or procedure to the youngster. It's important that the child not be lied to and be told if and when something will hurt.

Don't hesitate to offer assistance in helping your child through a test or procedure. Remember the youngster trusts and loves you and needs your physical and emotional support.

Don't let anyone make you feel that your questions or concerns are silly or unnecessary. It's often the questions that you think are silly, stupid, or unnecessary that are precisely the important ones that need answers.

Don't forget to comfort and praise the youngster after the test or procedure is over. Affection and understanding go a long way.

PLEASE NOTE: Now that you have a grasp of how and why some common medical tests and procedures are performed, as well as how to help your youngster if he or she ever requires a medical test or procedure, it would be extremely helpful for you to go back to the Quick Reference With the Steps in Detail and review it carefully. The more familiar you are with that material, the more useful it will be to you when you need it.

C H A P T E R 22

When Your Child Needs Hospitalization

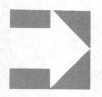

QUICK REFERENCE

With the Steps in Detail

When Your Child Needs Hospitalization

▶ **ALWAYS BE HONEST WITH THE CHILD—NO MATTER WHAT AGE HE OR SHE MAY BE.**

- Never tell him a lie or he will never trust what you say again.

- If something will hurt, then tell her it will hurt and for how long it will hurt.

- If you tell your child that you will be gone for a few minutes, then make sure you are back in a few minutes. It's a terrible thing to be deceived. With the best of intentions, parents have told their children they will be right back (because it's time for bed), then return in the morning. Frequently children wait all night for their parents to return and become frightened when they do not.

▶ **TAKE GREAT CARE IN EXPLAINING WHY THE CHILD MUST GO TO THE HOSPITAL AND EXACTLY WHAT WILL HAPPEN TO THE YOUNGSTER WHILE IN THE HOSPITAL.**

- Be sure to talk to the child in terms he can understand. Base this on age and understanding level. Often talking to your child's doctor about what to say or having the doctor explain it to the youngster with you is very helpful.

- Remember that even a small child should be told—in very simple terms—the whys and whats of her hospitalization. Also, take "time" into consideration when you talk to a child. Remember that children under five years old have no concept of time. Everything is now! So, it's important to tell the smaller ones about what will happen right before it does. (For example, going to the hospital might be explained one or two days before he has to go. Explaining a test or procedure should be done right before and during the test or procedure.)

- If the hospital offers a Pre-Admission Tour, make sure you take the child on the tour. This will help make the hospital and the people working there more familiar to her and therefore less frightening. If there is no Pre-Admission Tour, then take the child on one yourself or ask your child's doctor if there is someone at the hospital who can take you and the child for a tour.

▶ **INVOLVE THE CHILD IN HIS TREATMENT AND CARE AS MUCH AS YOU OR THE HEALTH CARE PROFESSIONALS CAN.**

- Be creative. The little child can help hold the tape if an IV must be inserted. She can help put on a bandage or help you wash her face.

- The older child or teenager can be even more helpful and should be encouraged to take as active a role in his treatment and care as he wants to.

▶ **MAKE SURE YOU, AS PARENTS, BECOME INVOLVED IN THE CHILD'S CARE AND TREATMENT. ENCOURAGE OTHER FAMILY MEMBERS TO DO THIS AS WELL.**

- Becoming involved is not only helpful for the child and makes her feel more comfortable and secure, but it's important for you, as well. When a child is hospitalized most parents feel helpless. It's as if their role as parents—caretakers—has been suddenly snatched away. This causes anxiety and frustration. Besides providing all the warmth, security, and love the child craves even more than usual because she is in the

708

UNDERSTAND-
ING COMMON
TESTS AND
PROCEDURES
AND HELPING
YOUR CHILD
WHEN
HOSPITALIZED

hospital—become involved in her care and treatment whenever possible.

- Change your baby's diapers, feed him, and help with tests and procedures. Be creative!

- Help feed your small child if she needs help (instead of letting the nurse do it), help her get in and out of bed, go to the bathroom with her, and help with tests and procedures. Be creative!

- Give your older child or teenager choices about whether or not you should help. Some older children and teenagers will want to do things for themselves, while others will enjoy the attention and want you to "baby" them a little.

▶ **TRY TO ALLOW THE CHILD TO MAKE CHOICES WHENEVER POSSIBLE.**

- In children's hospitals and most hospitals with children's units, nurses and other health-care professionals are specially trained to work with children. Often it's easy to follow their lead. You may notice that a nurse will say something like, "Cathy, your doctor wants you to drink a lot of liquids. So, what will it be? Do you want apple juice, 7-Up, or cold water?"

- Remember, it's the little things that add up and help make a child feel like he has some control over what is happening to him. For example, "Do you want to brush your teeth first or help me give you a bath—right here in your bed!" Or, "It's important for you to have this shot. It will hurt for just a second. Do you want the nurse to give you the shot while you lie in your bed or would you like to lie across my lap? Which do you want to do?"

▶ **STAY OVERNIGHT WITH THE CHILD, IF THE HOSPITAL ALLOWS THIS.**

- This is very important to a baby, toddler, or small child—really a must, if at all possible.

- Give older children and teenagers a choice, but be sure to ask them in private. Watch for signs that "no" really means "yes." On one hand, you certainly don't want to embarrass the youngster who wants to be his own person and test his "growing up." On the other hand, you don't want to leave a youngster who is scared but unable to admit it. Sometimes it's helpful for you to say, "Jane, I would really like to spend the night here with you. The hospital allows that and provides a cot (or bed). It would make me feel better to be here with you. Is that all right with you, or do you want to be alone? If you do, I'll understand and respect your decision."

- If the child (of any age) is really sick or badly injured—don't ask the child—just stay. If the youngster is in an intensive care unit, the hospital often provides a room or area for the parents or family so they can be near the young person and go in to see him or her as often as they want.

▶ **ENCOURAGE BROTHERS AND SISTERS, OTHER RELATIVES AND FRIENDS TO VISIT THE CHILD (NO MATTER WHAT AGE), IF THE HOSPITAL ALLOWS THIS.**

- If the child is not restricted to bed, many hospitals have special play rooms, teen lounges, and other areas where children can meet, talk, and play records or games.

- If the youngster must stay in bed, then be creative and have the brother, sister, other relative, or friend bring something they can do together (such as play a game, crossword puzzle, and so on). If the child isn't able or isn't up to socializing, then still have visitors come (that's a very important part of getting better and feeling better), but restrict the visits to five or ten minutes—enough time for some talk, but most of all for the youngster to see others and know they care.

▶ **IF THE HOSPITALIZATION IS SUDDEN AND UNEXPECTED, IT IS STILL IMPORTANT TO TALK TO THE CHILD, TELL HIM WHAT HAPPENED, WHAT IS NOW HAPPENING, AND WHAT WILL HAPPEN NEXT.**

- All of the previous information still holds true even in an emergency or sudden, unexpected hospitalization. The difference to keep in mind is that neither the child nor you have had any time to prepare for this. Therefore, more support, more talking, more physical contact (if possible) is vitally important.

- Even if the child is sedated, unconscious, or in a coma—it is important to tell him or her what happened, what is now happening, and what will happen next. Often a child who has survived serious, sudden illness or injury later talks about: hearing his parents, brother or sister, grandparents, or other relative speaking to him; knowing he was not alone—that someone was with him and helping him; smelling his mother's perfume or father's aftershave; knowing that someone was holding his hand, and so on.

710

UNDERSTAND-
ING COMMON
TESTS AND
PROCEDURES
AND HELPING
YOUR CHILD
WHEN
HOSPITALIZED

➤ **IF A NEWBORN IS IN AN INFANT SPECIAL CARE UNIT (SOMETIMES CALLED NEWBORN OR INFANT INTENSIVE CARE) OR A BABY, TODDLER, YOUNG CHILD, OLDER CHILD, OR TEENAGER IS IN A PEDIATRIC INTENSIVE CARE UNIT (SOMETIMES CALLED CHILDREN'S INTENSIVE OR SPECIAL CARE), IT IS VITALLY IMPORTANT TO VISIT THE CHILD, TALK TO HIM, TOUCH HIM AND HOLD HIM (IF POSSIBLE).**

- Even very tiny babies—although weak and sick—are very sensitive to sound and touch.

- It has become very clear that children of all ages respond to their parents' voices and touch. Older babies, children, and teenagers also respond to sight. So don't think your child wouldn't know you are there or that your presence or lack of presence won't make a difference. It does!

- Again, it's vital to talk to the child, explain what is happening and what will happen. Emphasize that you are there and that the people in the hospital are doing everything they can to help her feel better and get better.

Hospitalization: What You Should Know

For a child, hospitalization can often be a nightmare. It's a strangely bizarre place where people wear funny clothes, wear masks, and seem to always say things he or she can't understand. It's a place that smells strange and has weird, frightening equipment. All in all, it can be a frightening and impersonal place for any child.

Put yourself in the child's place. For a moment you're three years old, six years old, or thirteen years old. Suddenly, your entire world is interrupted—shattered, torn apart, turned upside-down—all because of illness, injury, or a need for surgery. Although you may not feel well—or even hurt—you don't understand this thing they call "a hospital," this big place where you feel all alone and helpless.

You've probably already been to the doctor where you were pushed, probed, squeezed, and poked—while having no clothes to protect you! Strange, mostly cold instruments were put on you . . . a light was shined in your eyes . . . and maybe even a needle was put into your arm and blood withdrawn. When all this was over, things were written down and the doctor talked to your parents. (Who was it anyway who was just probed and poked?) Then everyone looked worried. You noticed that . . . just like you noticed everything else that was going on.

Next thing you knew, you were told you were going to the hospital—and now here you are—helpless, forced to cope with something you don't understand. All you know is fear . . . overwhelming fear!

In some situations, that's about how things happen. They never should! The emotional strain of hospitalization can literally tear a child apart. She is vulnerable. She wants to fight the assaults upon her. She protests these insults upon her body and her person. She may scream, holler, and cry. She may be uncooperative, struggle, and resist. All children have fighting spirits and built-in self-protective mechanisms. Why not? As far as she knows, she is fighting for her life—or at least trying to hold on tight to her own identity.

And parents? Obviously, they are anxious and afraid. Their role is suddenly taken from them. People they don't even know are caring for their child . . . trying to meet the youngster's needs. In a real way, the hospital staff is taking *their* place . . . giving the orders . . . making the decisions. Parents feel almost as helpless and fearful as the child . . . and inadequate.

This is not the way it should be—although it once was the rule and not the exception.

When a child is hospitalized all the things he thrives on are threatened—love, comfort, security, consistency, and a continuation of his normal activities (seeing his friends, being with his brother or sister and parents). When in the hospital these needs are MAGNIFIED. Remember that any change of environment is difficult for a child. Things are foreign to him—even the language he hears—and he must somehow cope with this, in addition to being sick or injured or needing surgery (which he doesn't understand). Things that we accept, as adults, seem ridiculous or frightening to him.

Hospitalization: From the Child's Point of View

The following are a few true stories that have occurred in hospitals. They are important because they allow us to see things—in the hospital—from the child's perspective. It's vital that we keep this perspective in mind if our children ever require hospitalization. In this way, we can be more in tune to the youngster's needs and more in touch with the value of explaining everything in as much detail as he or she requires. If we keep this in mind, there is a better chance that the youngster will not misinterpret or misunderstand what is being said, what will happen and what the hospital will be like.

Eight-year-old Bobby sat in his hospital bed almost as if he was frozen in one position. No one could quite figure out what was wrong. When his mother came into the room, she realized immediately that something was terribly wrong—or at least Bobby thought so.

"What's wrong, Bobby," his mother asked? "You'd better go home, Mom," he replied. "Why? Can you tell me why I need to go home?" she asked. Bobby became very silent and looked around.

712

UNDERSTAND-
ING COMMON
TESTS AND
PROCEDURES
AND HELPING
YOUR CHILD
WHEN
HOSPITALIZED

"I don't think I'm supposed to tell you, 'cause you won't like it a bit, 'cause I don't like it a bit."

His mother was perplexed. Bobby's mother buzzed the nursing station and the nurse soon appeared. She asked what Bobby needed. "I need," Bobby said, "for my mother to go home before it's too late!" Now the nurse and his mother were perplexed.

Bobby was getting panic-stricken. "Please, Mom, go home, now!"

Reason wasn't going to work, so Bobby's mother became demanding. "Robert James, I'm not going anywhere until you tell me what is wrong, and I mean right now!"

Bobby grimaced and then exhaled. "I'm going to explode any minute now, so you have to get out of my room!"

After much discussion it was discovered that Bobby thought since the IV (intravenous) fluid was going into his arm—and not his stomach—that it had no way of getting out of his body. He logically concluded that he was simply going to blow up like a balloon . . . and pop!

Obviously, no one had explained anything to Bobby about IV feeding, so he arrived at his own conclusion. If you think about it, his deduction was not only creative, but reasonable!

Another true story.

Midnight. Empty halls except for nurses checking patients and charts. An occasional "mommy" or "daddy" is whispered in the darkness—a nurse responds. Bedtime is early here—the patients are young.

A resident (a doctor in training to be a pediatrician) stands at the nurse's station going through a chart, a nurse checks the rooms through her control board. All is quiet except for the sounds of sleepy breathing.

One at a time she checks each room. She stops, flips back to the last one. The resident turns toward the board and looks at the nurse—they both listen. Someone's out of bed—playing, moving around the room.

"Katie," the nurse says gently over the intercom, "get back into bed now. I want you to go to sleep." Rustle of clothing, the quick patter of pajama'd feet hurrying across the room, the squeak of the bed, the whoosh of covers being pulled up quickly . . . rapid breathing, a hard gulp.

Softly the child says, "Is that *You*, God?"

It's a cute story, but for Katie, it was a very scary moment. There she was in a dark, unfamiliar room—knowing she was very much alone (and obviously doing something she wasn't supposed to be doing)—when suddenly out of the darkness came this ominous, authoritative voice that echoed in the room. The nurse went and got Katie, brought her back to the nurse's station and showed her the intercom. After explaining what an intercom was, she took Katie back to her room and showed her that she, too, had an intercom in her room and could talk to someone at the nursing station anytime she needed something.

Then there was the twelve-year-old boy who told his mother that he didn't want to have his operation because he was afraid he couldn't love her, his father, sisters, or brothers anymore! The surgery involved fixing a minor heart defect. For him—based on what he had heard and seen about hearts, Valentine's Day, and love—love came directly from your heart. He took this literally. The youngster, therefore, thought that if the doctors did something to his heart—*changed his heart*—that it would also change how he felt; change his love or ability to love. Slogans like "have a heart," "from your heart," "love comes from the heart," and so on, needed to be explained in great detail. His mother did an excellent job of explaining—while at the same time not making her son feel foolish, stupid, or silly.

Little Jennifer's parents had their own story to tell. It is not about a child's misunderstanding or drawing her own conclusions about a medical test or procedure, nor about any aspect of hospitalization. The story, nonetheless, is abstractly related to what can happen in terms of medical tests or procedures or when a child is hospitalized. As Jennifer's parents said, this event constantly reminds them about the importance of *listening to the child and asking questions* until you learn specifically "what" the child's concerns are or what she "wants to know!"

Here's what happened. Jennifer's parents came to visit their bright-eyed five-year-old who had been in the hospital for a major surgical procedure. She had done very well and was now in the final stages of her recovery period and would be going home in a day or two. As they passed the nursing station, Jennifer's parents were told that she had a new roommate—just admitted today. When they reached Jennifer's room, she was bubbly and energetic—obviously feeling well and excited about her new friend.

After talking about her day and her new friend for a while, Jennifer paused as if deep in thought. Her mother asked if anything was wrong. The little girl looked at her parents very seriously then asked, "Mommy and Daddy, where do I come from? Valerie and me were talking about it and . . . well . . . she knows where she came from . . . but I told her I didn't know where I came from . . . but I'd ask you because you would know that."

Well, they thought, here we go. Both parents sat down and explained and explained. Jennifer looked rather perplexed the entire time. She tried to interrupt a few times, but her mother and father just kept explaining. Finally, Jennifer's mother stopped, looked at her husband and said she didn't think Jennifer was ready for this . . . that they should try to discuss it later.

The room was very silent for several minutes. Jennifer continued to look perplexed. Suddenly and unexpectedly Jennifer exhaled loudly. "Well," she said quite innocently, "I don't know what to tell Valerie. Where I come from is different than where Valerie comes from. You know . . . Valerie comes from Chicago! It sounds like a really neat place!"

Both parents almost fell over! All Jennifer wanted to know is what city she came from, but when she asked, "Where do I come from," her parents automatically thought they *knew* what she was asking. As her father put it, "We just assumed she meant how was I made and how was I born! All we had to do is ask her one question— 'Jennifer, what do you mean?'—and she probably would have told us that Valerie

714

UNDERSTAND-
ING COMMON
TESTS AND
PROCEDURES
AND HELPING
YOUR CHILD
WHEN
HOSPITALIZED

came from Chicago. Then we would have *known* what she was really asking, not assumed that we knew.''

Jennifer's mother said that after that experience, they realized how important it was to ask questions until they were sure what concerned Jennifer or what information she really wanted from them. ''We tried to be much more attentive to the details of Jennifer's questions, more perceptive and sensitive about what she was asking—and we realized how important it was to really listen.

''This was especially helpful,'' her mother emphasized, ''when Jennifer started asking about why she had to stay in the hospital longer for more tests, why she couldn't go back to school right away, why she still had to see her doctor at his office a few more times, why her incision looked the way it did. We found out that by talking to her, asking her questions and listening that what she really wanted to know was often hidden under her original question. For example,'' her mother explained, ''she really didn't want to know why her incision looked the way it did—which was her original question—but if it would always look like it did and would her friends make fun of it. Jennifer taught both of us a good lesson—never assume anything when it comes to questions from your children, always ask questions and listen, listen, listen until you know exactly what they want to know and what's bothering them.''

It's important to remember, too, that children ''pick up'' on how a parent feels. If you appear panic-stricken or frightened, the child will feel this and respond accordingly. If you are calm and confident, the child will feel this, too. That is not to say that parents and others should be dishonest. Just the opposite! However, there are times that we are really frightened because our child must have surgery. We don't want him to have to go through this, we don't want him hurt, we don't want him to be sick or injured, and we are so afraid that something will go wrong and our child will die. These are legitimate concerns, because we love our child. But, often our anxieties and fears are transferred to the child who is doing well and is not frightened. In this situation, we do not want to transfer our parental anxieties and fears to the child.

One mother handled this very well—after she realized what had happened! Her husband had died in Vietnam and she had to raise three children on her own. Because of the death of her husband, she always feared losing someone else she loved—in particular, one of her children. Therefore, when thirteen-year-old Melinda needed her appendix out suddenly—she was immediately panic-stricken. Melinda, who was in a great deal of pain, but doing well before the surgery, got very quiet and started to cry every time her mother entered her room. Finally she asked the question she feared most. ''Mom, I'm going to die, aren't I? I can tell, you look so scared and you're shaking. I wish someone would tell me the truth!''

Melinda's mother suddenly realized what was happening. Her daughter had been doing fine. The doctors and nurses had explained why she hurt so much, what had to be done, how the surgery would be performed, how she'd feel afterward. They had said that it was all right for her to be a little scared, because all of us are *always* a little scared when we hurt and go through something we've never experienced before.

But, that she would be just fine. Melinda understood and believed them. The problem? Her mother was sending totally opposite signals.

Being sensitive and perceptive, Melinda's mother immediately realized what had happened and sat down to hug her daughter. "The doctors and nurses did tell you the truth," she said. "I'm sorry if I've frightened you, Melinda, and made you feel that you were not told the truth. I love you and sometimes when you love someone very much, you just overreact, you panic . . . often when there's no reason to be scared. We'll talk more about this later when you're feeling well, okay?" Melinda nodded. "But, for now, let's concentrate on your getting well. You'll be going into surgery in about twenty minutes—and when you come out of surgery, I'll be right here waiting for you! I do love you!" Finally, Melinda believed her and smiled—even though she hurt. Everything was going to be all right.

One last, true story.

Benjamin had just turned six and was still celebrating his birthday when he was told he would have to go to the hospital to have the lump in his lower left side fixed. His parents were very supportive, open, honest, and prepared Benjamin well for his pending hospitalization. It was an excellent children's hospital and all the members of the staff were specially trained to work with children . . . talk to children about what was to be done, when, where, and how.

Benjamin was doing just fine. His brother visited that afternoon and his mother was going to stay overnight in his room. The routine, minor hernia repair was scheduled for the next morning and things couldn't have been going more smoothly.

The anesthesiologist dropped by Benjamin's room to explain his role in the surgery. After he left, there was a notable difference in the (up-to-now) cheerful boy. "What's wrong, Ben?" his mother asked. Benjamin said nothing. "Ben, can you tell me what's wrong, I'd like to know." Still Benjamin sat quietly, saying nothing for a long time.

Finally the silence was shattered. Benjamin jumped from his bed—over the rail—holding his side and limping toward the door. "I'm going home. Take me home, Mama."

His mother reached him as he rounded the corner . . . out of the door. She hugged him, but he just wiggled and squirmed to get loose. "Benjamin, it's okay to be scared," she said gently. "Everyone gets scared, but then it goes away." Then to everyone's surprise and shock—Benjamin threw a temper tantrum—the first one in his entire life. He screamed, cried, hollered, bellowed, rolled on the floor, beat on the walls, and generally disrupted the place to the point that other children started crying, too.

Benjamin's mother was half mortified and half frightened. What was happening to Benjamin?

With the help of the nurses, his mother was able to calm him down enough to get him back into bed. Couldn't he tell her what was wrong? she asked him. "I'm not gonna have that operation. I'm gonna go home. You can't make me have it . . . I'm going home." When Benjamin's father arrived, he asked everyone to leave the room. He wanted to talk to Ben alone. Fifteen minutes later his father came out of Ben's

716

UNDERSTAND-
ING COMMON
TESTS AND
PROCEDURES
AND HELPING
YOUR CHILD
WHEN
HOSPITALIZED

room with an embarrassed smile on his face. Waiting outside was Benjamin's doctor, the nurse, his mother, and his older brother.

"Todd." Ben's father looked at his older son. "When Trixie died, did you tell Ben she was 'put to sleep'?" Todd wasn't sure what to say. When the family dog died everyone was crushed—particularly Ben—and he didn't want his little brother too upset about it. "Yes," Todd said, reluctantly, "I did because it was the truth."

"Well, Todd, it's not exactly the truth. The truth for Ben—what he could understand—was that Trixie was very old, very sick, and because of that, she died. I know you really meant well, but how she died was too complex for him. The problem right now is that the anesthesiologist just explained to Benjamin that tomorrow morning, he would simply be *put to sleep* and then they would do the operation. The reason Ben is so hysterical is that he believes that he is going to be put to sleep—like Trixie— never to return—to die. Because you told him that, he's not going to believe anyone but you! Todd, you're going to have to go talk to your brother and explain. He loves you, looks up to you and will believe you."

Benjamin did believe Todd and had his surgery the next morning. He did just fine. Again, whenever a child is hospitalized, what he has heard and how he interprets information may be very different from how we mean it. Therefore, it is very important that we are sensitive to his needs and how he perceives the information given him.

There are countless stories that could be told, but the most important thing to remember is that children perceive things differently than adults—and differently based on their age, ability to understand what is being said to them, and their experiences. What we have to do is be keenly aware and sensitive to their needs and wants. To answer all questions honestly and in terms the child can understand. To never assume. If we are not sure what is being asked—what the child's real concern or question is— to keep asking questions until we know. And to constantly tell ourselves—over and over again—to look at this from the child's point of view, and respond and act based on that perspective.

Hospitalization: Then and Now

In the 1940s, parents were allowed to visit their child in the hospital twice a week for one hour. Exceptions were made if the youngster was seriously ill or injured—then parents could visit daily. It was thought that children did better when their parents and others were not there. Children were not told the truth about what was wrong with them—especially if it was serious or life-threatening. No one explained tests, procedures, or surgeries. Little was known about the psychosocial needs of children when hospitalized—and therefore little was done about these needs. All in all, children were seen as little adults. It was better, everyone thought, for children to know very little. Therefore, the job of doctors, nurses, and others was to care for the child's physical needs, period! If this was done, then obviously everything would be fine.

Instead, hospitalized children (of all ages) experienced terrible emotional trauma. Changes came about slowly but consistently over the years. As more was known about how hospitalization affected children, how children responded to clear and simple information that was also true, and what psychosocial needs they had when in the hospital, more and more changes took place. In fact, the hospital today—in particular, children's hospitals and major medical centers with special children's units—are quite different than they were forty years ago or even five years ago. Progress continues yearly!

Today, parents, siblings, other relatives, and friends are not only welcomed to visit a child when he or she is in the hospital, but encouraged to do so. The staff at children's hospitals across the country also emphasize the importance of having one parent stay overnight with a baby, toddler, young child, and even older child (and teenager, if he or she wishes the parent to stay). Health care professionals have become more aware that even the very little, apparently insignificant things that are said to a child can have a profound effect on him. It has become clear, too, that it is vitally important to be totally honest with a child (of any age) and to involve him in his own health care. Children, it has been discovered, understand more than we often give them credit for and want to be involved in their care—to have some control.

It has also become clear that children respond differently to the same thing—depending on their age, ability to understand, and experiences. In other words, a two-year-old will not react to having a shot (injection) the same way a four-year-old or five-year-old will, or the same as a youngster of eight or nine or twelve or thirteen or sixteen or seventeen. Because of this, health professionals who work with children often have (and should have) special additional training in working with hospitalized children of different ages. Today, the emotional support of children—from parents and all members of the hospital staff—is of paramount importance when children are hospitalized.

Special child-life programs (found in almost all children's hospitals across the country) have highly trained professionals who encourage children to express their feelings, anxieties, and hostilities in art work, music, using puppets and dolls, and by talking openly. There are also dolls with casts on, IVs to "put" into dolls, and cardiac catheterization models, to name a few. All these aspects of play therapy are very helpful for the child when hospitalized. Most of these activities take place in a special play room (for younger children). Some children's hospitals also have a teen lounge where teenagers can gather, talk, play video games, table games, read, or play music.

Emphasis is placed on youngsters becoming better acquainted with their illnesses or injuries and how to manage their chronic problems (such as insulin-dependent diabetes or asthma). Therefore, while youngsters are being emotionally prepared and equipped to deal with being in the hospital, they learn a great deal about their bodies and their problems. The point is to try to meet the emotional, physical, and educational needs of all children who require hospitalization and to continue the support for youngsters with a chronic, serious, or long-term illness or injury.

Parents now play a vital and active role in their child's care. Health care professionals

UNDERSTAND-
ING COMMON
TESTS AND
PROCEDURES
AND HELPING
YOUR CHILD
WHEN
HOSPITALIZED

realize that children do better (not worse) when parents are there, supportive and involved. Parents are encouraged to help feed their child, change a diaper or pajamas, help with baths, and be with the child and help them through any tests or procedures that are required.

If your child requires hospitalization (especially in a children's hospital), you should feel free to seek the help of the child life staff if you are unsure about how your child is doing emotionally or are concerned about your child's emotional well-being. These specially trained professionals are there to assist you in helping your child deal with being in the hospital, going through tests, procedures, surgeries, and being ill or injured. The point is to make the hospital experience a more positive and less frightening one.

It's also important to be aware of the fact that youngsters often respond in ways we often don't understand. Some children act very confident, happy-go-lucky, are quite outgoing and act very brave about everything—but are confused and frightened inside. Other children are downright obnoxious and always difficult—it's their way of having control, of rebelling against what is happening to them—in the only way they know how. Still other children are withdrawn, submissive, and uncommunicative. Others are supportive of other children in the hospital—kind, gentle, and acting as if they are handling all of this stress, discomfort, and even fear very well. The child-life program staff is trained to get children involved, to talk and express how they really feel, how they are really doing, and help them to deal with their true feelings and fears—no matter what they show on the outside.

You will also notice that children's hospitals or special units for the care of children in major medical centers are bright, colorful, and full of pictures, photographs, toys, stuffed animals, and other items that help the child feel more "at home." Emphasis is placed on making the hospital setting cheerful and hopeful. In fact, if you've been to visit a youngster in a children's hospital (or other hospitals) lately, you may have been surprised because nurses and doctors didn't look like the traditional white coat/ white dress/white cap stereotype that everyone has of them. You would have also noticed that it was pretty noisy—music, chatter, and little red wagons flying down the halls and shrieks of laughter. Great strides have been made. Nurses, pediatricians, psychiatrists and other physicians, psychologists, child-life specialists, social workers, and many others have made a substantial impact on how children do when in the hospital and when long-term medical care is necessary. So have parents.

Actually, hospitalized children do very well when their emotional, social, and physical needs are met—and when they are encouraged to express their feelings openly and honestly. No one likes being ill or injured (even adults). Let's face it—it's not a wonderful experience and one we'd all prefer to avoid, if possible.

We can, however, make a child's hospitalization a positive experience, a learning experience, and a less frightening experience. We must respect each youngster as an individual. We must also learn to listen and to hear—and, when necessary, to read between the lines (if you will). We must, in essence, *be there* for the child—both physically and emotionally. And we must do all we can to be open, honest, supportive, understanding, affectionate, and loving.

Repeated Hospitalizations: What You Can Do

In essence, all the information previously discussed holds true for the child who must have repeated hospitalizations due to chronic or serious illness or injury. The difference is that everything is intensified. Because of this, the child needs to really understand—as much as is possible for his age—what the problem is, what caused the problem (if known), what treatment is necessary to follow at home, why he must go to the hospital periodically (and/or to the doctor's office), and what will happen when he goes to the hospital (or doctor's office).

A child with a chronic, serious, or life-threatening illness or injury also needs as much emotional support as possible. It's important to utilize all the hospital's resources, if necessary, to help the child deal with what is happening to her. Most children's hospitals and major medical centers with children's units already have a network set up to help meet the child's psychosocial needs. This network often consists of social workers, child psychiatrists, child psychologists, child-life professionals, fully credentialed schoolteachers, and other professionals who work with the child, her parents, doctors, and nurses.

Many times, the child feels isolated, different, and rightfully angry that he has something wrong with him that he cannot control. Children often ask, ''Why me?'' With everyone's support, encouragement, and understanding, many of the youngster's questions can be answered. ''Why me?'' is often one of those questions that cannot be answered. With help, however, the child can better understand that he did nothing to deserve this—and that sometimes not so good things happen to very good people.

Intensive Care: How You Can Help Your Child

Intensive care medicine is so misunderstood that just hearing that a child is in an intensive care unit (ICU) frightens people. Therefore, before we discuss how you can help your child—if he is ever in an intensive care unit—we thought it best to explain why children are placed in intensive care units. It is true that children who are seriously ill or injured and those with life-threatening problems are cared for in intensive care units, but it is also true that children may be placed in an intensive care unit as a precaution. In this case, being in such a unit is the best preventive medicine. For example, a youngster may require special monitoring and/or around-the-clock intensive nursing supervision to ensure that a serious or life-threatening problem doesn't occur. And if a problem does occur, the child is in a unit where intensive medical intervention can take place immediately to treat the problem.

Therefore, a premature infant may be placed in an intensive care nursery (also called infant special care, infant intensive care, newborn intensive care, and so on) because he is sick or has a problem requiring intensive treatment, or so he can be watched and

720

UNDERSTAND-
ING COMMON
TESTS AND
PROCEDURES
AND HELPING
YOUR CHILD
WHEN
HOSPITALIZED

monitored in order to detect a problem immediately if it occurs. A baby, toddler, young child, older child, or teenager may be placed in a pediatric intensive care unit (also called pediatric special care or children's intensive care) because he has a serious or life-threatening illness or injury. Or the child may be placed in the pediatric intensive care unit (or an intermediate care unit) because he requires sophisticated monitoring and twenty-four-hour intensive nursing supervision (due to a surgery, for example) to ensure that if a problem occurs immediate treatment can be initiated. Therefore, an intensive care unit is often the best place an infant, child, or teenager can be—when the situation warrants this level of medical supervision and/or medical care.

When an infant, child, or teenager is in an intensive care unit, it's even more important that parents and other family members (if allowed) visit the child and let their presence be "felt." Years ago, children who required intensive medical care were essentially isolated from family and friends. Today, it is well recognized that children (of all ages) *need more, not less emotional support* when seriously ill or injured or when needing more intensive medical supervision. Therefore, it is vitally important to apply all of the same principles previously discussed in this chapter— whenever an infant, child, or teenager is in an intensive care unit.

For example, very tiny and even very sick infants who are in an infant special care unit are quite sensitive to touch and sound. It has become rather evident over the years that these babies need their parents and others to touch them, hold them (if possible), and to talk to them. They do respond—especially to their parents. Health care professionals know that infants do better when parents are as actively involved as possible in their infant's care (with consideration to the limits imposed by being in a special care unit).

Some parents feel that such young or sick infants are too fragile to hold (if this is possible) or to even touch. They are fearful of hurting the infant. They are also frightened by all of the "things" attached to the infant. It is true that some of the medical equipment is noisy and rather ominous, but most parents don't even hear it and get used to its presence very quickly. Tubes, oxygen hoods, special lights, monitors, IV setups, and other vital medical paraphernalia that some infants require tend to make parents intimidated and feel out of place. Since the infant must be in an isolette (a special type of incubator), parents feel that they cannot get close to the infant. Although parents (as well as doctors, nurses, and other health care professionals) are required to scrub and wear gowns each time they enter the special care nursery to see their baby (to prevent the spread of illness to the infant and other infants), parents are still fearful they may "give" the infant something. It's important to remember that all infant special care units have very strict rules to protect the infants in the unit, and if these are followed carefully, parents cannot endanger the well-being of their baby. Also, specially trained and skilled nurses and doctors are always glad to help show parents how to hold and touch their baby so they won't hurt him or disrupt any medical equipment that is monitoring or assisting the baby.

The fact is, parents need to feel a special part of the "team" that is caring for their baby. If ever in this situation, you need to know what you can do to help your baby and what limitations there are. (These often change as the baby improves.) You also need to understand what is wrong with the baby or why he or she requires special monitoring and care, what is being done for the baby, and why this treatment or monitoring is recommended, as well as how the baby is doing each step of the way. You should feel free (and be encouraged) to spend as much time as you can with the infant. Again, even very sick and weak infants recognize and need warmth, affection, and love. Your presence does make a difference—because the infant does respond to your voice, your touch, and your love.

The same holds true for the older baby, toddler, young child, older child, or teenager when in an intensive care unit. Whether the child is in the unit because he is seriously ill or injured or because he requires specialized monitoring and nursing supervision—he needs his parents to be there as often as possible. Parents (and others allowed to visit the child) should talk to the child, hold him (or hold his hand if the medical equipment limits your ability to hold the child). It's still important to tell the child what is happening to him (in terms he can understand) and to be open and honest with him. It's also vital that the youngster understand what all the medical equipment is, what it does, and why it makes noise (if it does), so it doesn't frighten him.

Even if the youngster is sedated or unconscious, it is still vital to tell her what is happening and what will happen before or as it does. She needs to be encouraged, talked to often, and held or touched. (It's amazing how reassuring a hand on a shoulder can be.) It is remarkable that some children who were sedated, unconscious, or in a coma have later said that they knew that their mother and/or father talked to them, held their hand, kissed them, told them they loved them or that everything was going to be all right. Others have said that they knew their parents were in the room because they could smell their mother's perfume or father's cologne or aftershave. Therefore, no matter what the situation is, talk to the youngster and touch her—because she may, indeed, be able to feel your presence in some way.

If your child ever requires intensive medical care, be sure to ask the doctor what is wrong with the youngster or why he needs special monitoring and care, and what is being done (or going to be done) for the child, as well as what this treatment and/or monitoring will hopefully do to help the youngster. Be sure to let the nurses know you want to be kept up-to-date about the child's condition. Ask, too, what limitations there are (for example, you may not be able to hold a small child because of all the medical equipment and support he requires). You need to know what you can do to help your child and not disturb the medical equipment. Most of all, never underestimate your importance to your child!

Emergency Hospitalization: Making a Difference

Again, all of the previously discussed principles about helping a child when hospitalized apply when a youngster experiences an emergency hospitalization. The difference is

722

UNDERSTAND-
ING COMMON
TESTS AND
PROCEDURES
AND HELPING
YOUR CHILD
WHEN
HOSPITALIZED

that *everything is greatly intensified*. Since there is no warning and therefore no time to prepare the child (or yourself)—events seem to occur quickly and often decisions must be made in rapid succession. This is an enormously frightening situation for parents and the youngster (who is suddenly and unexpectedly ill or injured and thrust into a medical setting he or she doesn't understand).

Therefore, everyone involved—parents and all members of the health care team— must do even more to help the child deal with this experience. At times, a child is quite aware, alert, and frightened—and needs to be talked through his fear and pain. At other times, the youngster isn't really aware of what has happened, what is happening, and what will happen (although it is still important to talk to him about it and to be there for him). In these situations, once the child is conscious or more able to understand, it's vital to repeat all that you have told him and be as comforting, reassuring, and loving as possible. As always, the child needs to feel secure and safe, as well as loved. With everyone's help, the youngster will be able to deal with this sudden, unexpected, stressful, frightening, and often painful situation.

Don't Forget Your Needs, Too!

Keep in mind that you, too, need support, warmth, affection, and love when your child requires hospitalization (whether the child is in the general pediatric unit, an infant special care unit, pediatric intensive care unit, has a chronic or serious problem that requires repeated hospitalizations, or is admitted to the hospital on an emergency basis). Allow family and friends to be supportive, to help you with other children at home (although you need to spend some time with your other children, as well), to visit the child (if possible), or just be there for you off and on, and to listen and talk when you need to do so. Don't hesitate to seek help from the health care professionals who are there to work with parents, other family members, and the child.

The fact of the matter is—you cannot help your child (and other children at home) if you do not have the support and help *you need during this often very stressful time*. Whenever a child requires hospitalization, it affects the entire family—not just the child. It's important to keep this in mind and deal with any problems that may occur. Sometimes just talking to the doctor, your child's nurse, the social worker, or child-life professional can make a big difference. If you don't understand *what* is going on, what to expect, what you can do for your child who is hospitalized and for your other children (if you have other children), who may be very frightened—and *what* to do for *yourself* in order to deal with fear, anxiety, frustration, and even anger—then you can't possibly expect to get through this in one piece. The situation is bound to be destructive to members of your family, yourself, and the child.

Therefore, it is not selfish to need some time to yourself. It is not selfish to want to go home and take a shower. It is not selfish to seek affection from your husband or wife. It is not selfish to want to spend time with your other children. You are not being weak if you seek the assistance of professionals to help you and your family—and your child—get through this ordeal. When it comes to hospitalization of a child who is seriously ill or injured or has a chronic problem, you have every right to take advantage and should indeed take advantage of the network of professionals there to help.

Most children who require hospitalization do very well because of great advances in medicine over the years. Most also do quite well emotionally—if they are treated with respect, given support, affection, and love, and feel secure. Most parents do quite well, too. If the situation is serious, however, then it's always best to take advantage of all the hospital has to offer in terms of helping your child, your family, and you!

THE DON'TS

Don't forget how important honesty is to the child. No matter what age the child is, it's important to be open and honest, and to answer all questions in terms the child can understand.

Don't underestimate a child's ability to understand what you say and how you really feel. Even very young children are quite perceptive and insightful. We often make the mistake of not giving them enough respect for their intelligence.

Don't forget to try to see things from the child's perspective—based on his or her age, ability to understand, and experiences. It's easy for us, as adults, to forget what it is like to be afraid of a shot (injection), people we don't know, unfamiliar surroundings, and the unknown.

Don't hesitate to ask for help from the health care professionals who are specially trained and skilled to work with children, parents, and other family members—if your child requires hospitalization. Never feel apprehensive or foolish about seeking help—if you feel help is needed or may be needed.

Don't underestimate the power of affection, warmth, love—and just being there for the child. The youngster needs to feel secure and confident and to be able to trust those who are taking care of him or her. You can make a significant difference in how the child responds to the situation—by your presence, support, and expressions of affection and love.

PLEASE NOTE: Now that you have a grasp of what your youngster's needs might be if he or she is hospitalized and how you can help, it would be extremely helpful for you to go back to the Quick Reference With the Steps in Detail and review it carefully. The more familiar you are with that material, the more useful it will be to you when you need it.

YOUR SPECIAL ROLE:

The Bottom Line

Over the years it has become more and more clear that each of us has a very special and vital role in our children's health care. Long gone are the days when parents (and others) were simply left in the dark when it came to their children's health and well-being. Long gone are the days when doctors and other health-care professionals essentially worked alone—making decisions that affected children and their families without involving them in the decision-making process.

The fact is, there has been a slow but continual revolution in this country that has resulted in a changed attitude—from "whatever the doctor says" to "let's talk about the risks and benefits in detail and make a cooperative decision." This change came about, in part, because parents and others wanted to know more, do more, and be more involved. Also, some very sensitive doctors and other health-care professionals recognized the value and importance of such a change and encouraged it (supporting the development of some of the original health-education programs both for patients and the public at large, brochures for distribution, and magazine articles and books written specifically for the public).

The bottom line? Parents (and others who care for children) have a special role as vital members of their child's (or children's) health-care team. In a real way, *we can* make a significant difference in our children's overall health care and well-being. What we know, how prepared we are for life-threatening medical emergencies (for example, taking a CPR certification course, learning water safety and rescue techniques, knowing how to control serious bleeding, relieving airway obstruction, and so on), the decisions we make when our children are ill or injured, and the steps we take to prevent illness and injury and to better ensure a safe environment—all are part of our special role. **725**

So is teaching our children (as they grow older) about prevention, safety, good health habits, what actions to take in a medical emergency, and how and when to properly utilize medical care.

Remember how important it is to establish and maintain an excellent relationship with your child's doctor. He or she is a vital resource and the person to turn to when you have questions and concerns about your child's health or well-being, and when the youngster requires medical evaluation and/or treatment.

Ultimately, however, *you* are the bottom line in your child's overall health care. How seriously you take your special role can make an enormous difference in your youngster's health, safety, and well-being.

The proper performance of "your special role" involves recognizing and accepting the scope and depth of that role, as well as making a strong and lasting commitment to learn all you can and to be prepared. It also includes never being afraid or embarrassed or feeling foolish or stupid about asking questions (when you have them), and being insistent (when necessary) that your questions be answered—and answered in language you can understand. By taking these steps, you will feel confident about the decisions you make and the actions you take.

Remember, too, that your role is made easier if a similar responsibility and commitment are properly assumed by "significant others" who care for your child. Therefore, whether that person is a grandparent, other relative, friend, teacher, baby-sitter, or someone who cares for or works with children in some other capacity, the role he or she plays in the health and well-being of your child should not be underestimated! If *you are* a "significant other" who has read *Should I Call the Doctor?* and will now use it as a continual resource, you should be applauded! As noted previously in the book, taking the time to be well-informed, prepared, and more involved means that you care deeply, recognize the importance of your role, and take that responsibility quite seriously.

Whether you are a parent or a "significant other," we hope that *Should I Call the Doctor?* has been (and will continue to be) instrumental in making your special role easier and well defined—and the problems and decisions you may face clear and understandable. If it has, then we couldn't be more pleased!

A reminder: If you have just finished reading *Should I Call the Doctor?* in its entirety, you may find it helpful to review the broad-based Emergency Quick Reference guides in Chapter 1 (as well as any other Emergency Quick Reference or Quick Reference guides, Assessment Checklists, the Injury Assessment, and any other areas of the book you wish to review). In this way you will be as confident as possible in your ability to evaluate problems and take action, and you'll be totally comfortable and familiar with the quick reference information and able to find it when you want it promptly or need it urgently.

BIBLIOGRAPHY

American Academy of Pediatrics Committee on Accident and Poison Prevention. *Protect Your Baby* factsheets (from birth through the teenage years). Evanston: American Academy of Pediatrics, 1978.

American Heart Association Working Group on Cardiopulmonary Resuscitation (CPR) and Emergency Cardiac Care (ECC) in Infants and Children. "Part III: Basic Life Support in Infants and Children." *Emergency Medicine* (August 1980):95–165.

Baker, Susan P., M.P.H. "Motor Vehicle Occupants Deaths in Young Children." *Pediatrics*. Volume 64, No. 6 (December 1979):860–861.

Bennett, William I., M.D., ed. "Are Accidents Accidental?" *The Harvard Medical School Health Letter*. Volume VII, No. 10 (August 1982):5.

Bennett, William I., M.D., ed. "The Trouble with Immunization." *The Harvard Medical School Health Letter*. Volume X, No. 11 (September 1985):3–5.

Berger, Lawrence R., M.D. "Childhood Injuries: Recognition and Prevention." *Current Problems in Pediatrics*. Volume XII, No. 1 (November 1981).

Bergman, Abraham B., M.D. *Preventing Childhood Injuries*. Report of the Twelfth Ross Roundtable Report on Critical Approaches to Common Pediatric Problems. Columbus: Ross Laboratories (in collaboration with the Ambulatory Pediatric Association), 1982.

Branch, David. "Panel Says Heimlich Maneuver In, Back Blows Out." *Pediatric News*. Volume 19, No. 10 (October 1985):3–57.

Carey, Anne, R.N. *The Children's Pharmacy*. New York: Warner Books, 1985.

Centers for Disease Control. "Aquatic Deaths and Injuries—United States." *Morbidity and Mortality Weekly Report*. Volume 31, No. 31 (August 1982):417–419.

Centers for Disease Control. "State Action to Prevent Motor Vehicle Deaths and Injuries among Children and Adolescents." *Morbidity and Mortality Weekly Report*. Volume 31, No. 35 (September 1982):488–490.

Centers for Disease Control. ''Unintentional and Intentional Injuries—United States.'' *Morbidity and Mortality Weekly Report*. Volume 31, No. 18 (May 1982):244–248.

Feldman, Kenneth W., M.D. ''Prevention of Childhood Accidents: Recent Progress.'' *Pediatrics in Review*. Volume 2, No. 3 (September 1980):75–82.

Fleisher, Gary, M.D., and Stephen Ludwig, M.D., eds. *Textbook of Pediatric Emergency Medicine*. Baltimore: Williams & Wilkins, 1983.

Freeman, Roger K., M.D., and Susan C. Pescar. *Safe Delivery: Protecting Your Baby During High Risk Pregnancy*. New York: Facts on File, 1982.

Gellis, Sydney S., M.D., ed. ''Ingestion of Small Flat Disc Batteries.'' *Pediatric Notes*. Volume 7, No. 9 (March 1983):36.

Heimlich, Henry J., M.D., and Milton H. Uhley, M.D. ''The Heimlich Maneuver.'' *Clinical Symposia*. Volume 31, No. 3 (1979):3–32.

Jackson, Douglas W., M.D., and Susan C. Pescar. *The Young Athlete's Health Handbook*. New York: Everest House, 1981.

Johnson, Susan Ann [Susan C. Pescar]. *First Aid for Kids*. New York: Quick Fox/Putnam, 1981.

Los Angeles County Department of Health Services. ''Haemophilus Influenza Type b Vaccine.'' *Public Health Letter*. Volume 7, No. 8 (August 1985):29–30.

Los Angeles County Department of Health Services. ''Hazards of Hot Tubs.'' *Public Health Letter*. Volume 4, No. 7 (July 1982):1–2.

McCann, Michael, *Artists Beware*. New York: Watson-Guptill Publishers, Inc., 1979.

McIntire, Matilda S., M.D., ed. *Handbook on Accident Prevention*. Hagerstown: Harper & Row, 1980.

Montgomery, William H., M.D., and Thomas J. Herrin, M.D., eds. *Student Manual for Basic Life Support: Cardiopulmonary Resuscitation*. Dallas: American Heart Association, 1981.

National Center for Health Statistics/U.S. Department of Health and Human Services. ''Advance Report of Final Mortality Statistics, 1980.'' *Monthly Vital Statistics Report*. Volume 32, No. 4 (August 1983).

National Center for Health Statistics/U.S. Department of Health and Human Services. ''Changing Mortality Patterns, Health Services Utilization, and Health Care Expenditures: United States, 1978–2003.'' *Vital & Health Statistics*. Series 3, No. 23 (September 1983).

National Electronic Injury Surveillance System/National Injury Information Clearinghouse. *Product Summary Report: All Products*. Washington, D.C.: U.S. Consumer Product Safety Commission, 1983.

National Health Survey/National Center for Health Statistics/U.S. Department of Health, Education, and Welfare. ''Current Estimates from the Health Interview Survey: United States–1978.'' *Vital and Health Statistics*. Series 10, No. 130 (November 1979).

Nelson, Christine A., M.D. ''Chapter 25 Pediatric Illness and Emergencies.'' *Emergency Care: Principles and Practices for the EMT-Paramedic* (2nd edition). Alan B. Gazzaniga, M.D., ed. Reston: Reston Publishing Co., 1982.

O'Shea, John S., M.D., Edward W. Collins, M.D., and Christine B. Bulter, R.N., P.N.P. ''Pediatric Accident Prevention.'' *Clinical Pediatrics*. Volume 21, No. 5 (May 1982):290–297.

Pescar, Susan C., and Christine A. Nelson, M.D. *Where Does It Hurt: A Guide to Symptoms and Illnesses*. New York: Facts on File, 1983.

Rivera, Frederick, P., M.D., M.P.H. ''Epidemiology of Childhood Injuries.'' *American Journal of the Diseases of Children*. Volume 136 (May 1982):399–405.

Rushford, Patricia, R.N. *The Care & Feeding of Sick Kids*. Palm Springs: Ronald N. Haynes Publishers, Inc., 1983.

Saxena, Kusum, M.D. "The Basic Principles in the Treatment of the Poisoned Patient." *Resident & Staff Physician* (March 1983):47–57.

Temple, Anthony R., M.D., and Frederick H. Lovejoy, M.D., eds. *Cleaning Products and Their Accidental Ingestion* (fifth edition). New York: The Soap and Detergent Association, 1980.

U.S. Consumer Product Safety Commission. "High Chairs." *Product Safety Fact Sheet*. Number 70 (revised August 1981):1–3.

Wegman, Myron, E., M.D. "Annual Summary of Vital Statistics—1981." *Pediatrics*. Volume 70, No. 6 (December 1982):835–842.

White, Roger Dean, M.D., F.A.C.C. "CPR: Basic Life Support." *Clinical Symposia*. Volume 34, No. 6 (1982):3–31.

Yates, Alayne, M.D. "Stress Management in Childhood." *Clinical Pediatrics*. Volume 22, No. 2 (February 1983):131–135.